BHASKER RAO and ROY CHOWDHURY'S

# Clinical Gynecology

Fifth Edition

Editor **S Rathnakumar**

Universities Press

Bhasker Rao and Roy Chowdhury's CLINICAL GYNECOLOGY (FIFTH EDITION)

UNIVERSITIES PRESS (INDIA) PRIVATE LIMITED

*Registered Office*
3-6-747/1/A & 3-6-754/1, Himayatnagar, Hyderabad 500 029, Telangana, India
info@universitiespress.com, www.universitiespress.com

*Distributed by*
Orient Blackswan Private Limited

*Registered Office*
3-6-752 Himayatnagar, Hyderabad 500 029, Telangana, India

*Other Offices*
Bengaluru, Bhopal, Chennai, Guwahati, Hyderabad, Jaipur, Kolkata
Lucknow, Mumbai, New Delhi, Noida, Patna, Vishakapatnam



First published 1984
Reprinted 1984
Second edition 1988
Reprinted 1989
Third edition 1992
Reprinted 1994 (Twice)
Fourth edition 1999
Fifth edition 2019

501586

*Cover image source:* # 98083311, 123RF

ISBN 978 93 86235 23 7



*Typeset in* Life 10.5/13.3

*Printed in India by*
Rasi Graphics Private Limited
Chennai 600 014

*Published by*
Universities Press (India) Private Limited
3-6-747/1/A & 3-6-754/1, Himayatnagar, Hyderabad 500 029, Telangana, India

# Preface to the Fifth Edition

Gynecology has undergone a sea change over the past decades, necessitating an updation of the existing book. The fifth edition of Clinical Gynecology has been written by well experienced faculty members from different medical colleges. It has incorporated the recent evidence-based investigations, interventions and management of various gynecological conditions. Though recent concepts have been incorporated, the time-tested earlier concepts are retained wherever necessary. This gives a comprehensive idea as to the evolution of various techniques over a period of time.

I am thankful to all the contributors for their contributions and suggestions. My thanks to Dr Anita, Asst. Prof. of Obstetrics and Gynecology, Govt. K G Hospital, for the diagram on fibroid. I also express my thanks to Dr Umarani Ramesh from Institute of Obstetrics and Gynecology for helping me with the clinical cases. My thanks to Mr Gangadharan for his secretarial assistance. My sincere thanks to Dr Sudha Ganesan and Ms Parvath Radha of Universities Press for their help and assistance throughout the preparation of the book.

I sincerely hope this book would be of immense use to the readers.

**S Rathnakumar**

# Preface to the First Edition

In this volume, the editors have aimed at providing concisely and clearly the basic facts necessary in the study of clinical gynaecology. Appropriate attention has been given to fundamentals in the anatomy (including embryology), physiology and pathology of the female reproductive tract for the proper understanding of the causation, diagnosis and management of gynaecological disorders. Some of the important operative procedures are discussed in detail separately at the end of the book.

The order of presentation has been the same as adopted in most medical schools. Though planned as a textbook for undergraduate students, it is sufficiently comprehensive to be useful to practising physicians and residents working in gynaecological wards.

The recent advances in the field of gynaecological endocrinology, genetics, contraceptive technology, applied ultrasonography and endoscopy have been considered in writing this volume. The editors are grateful to some of the senior teachers in gynaecology from different parts of India for their valuable contributions. Thanks are also due to Dr S Suresh of Mediscan Systems, Madras, for the microphotographs and ultrasonographs.

We are indebted to Professor M K Krishna Menon, doyen among gynaecologists in India, for writing a foreword to this textbook.

We are obliged to Orient Longman for all their cooperation and assistance in the preparation of this book.

**K Bhasker Rao**
**N N Roy Chowdhury**

# Contributors

**S Rathnakumar** BSc, MD, DGO
Formerly Professor of Obstetrics and Gynecology
Madras Medical College and Institute of Social Obstetrics and Govt. K G Hospital, Chennai

**Ramani Rajendran** MD, DGO
Formerly Professor of Obstetrics and Gynecology
Madras Medical College and Institute of Social Obstetrics and Govt. K G Hospital, Chennai

**V Madhini** MD, DGO, MNAMS
Formerly Director
Institute of Obstetrics and Gynecology and Madras Medical College, Chennai

**Radha Bai Prabhu** MD, DGO, MNAMS, FRCOG, FRCS, PhD
Formerly Director
Institute of Obstetrics and Gynecology and Madras Medical College, Chennai; Presently, Professor of Obstetrics and Gynecology, Meenakshi Medical College, Enathur, Kancheepuram

**A Kalaiselvi** MD, DGO, Dip. NB
Formerly Professor of Obstetrics and Gynecology
Govt. Kilpauk Medical College and Hospital, Chennai

**K Kalaiselvi** MD, DM
Professor and Head, Dept. of Medical Oncology, Madras Medical College and Rajiv Gandhi Govt. General Hospital, Chennai

**Revathy Janakiraman** MD, DGO, MNAMS FICOG, FICMCH
Professor Emeritus, The Dr MGR Medical University, Tamil Nadu, Retd. Director, Institute of Obstetrics and Gynecology and Madras Medical College, Chennai

**Poonam Verma Shivkumar** MBBS, MD, Advance Course in SHRS
Professor and Head, Dept. of Obstetrics and Gynecology, Mahatma Gandhi Institute of Medical Sciences, Sevagram, Wardha

**Shila Shelke** MBBS, DGO, DNB
Assistant Professor, Mahatma Gandhi institute of Medical Sciences, Sevagram, Wardha

**S Chhabra** MD, DGO
Director Professor, Obstetrics and Gynecology, CEO, Aakanksha Shishu Kalyan Kendra, OSD, Melghat Project, MGIMS, Sevagram, Wardha

**N Sanjeeva Reddy** MD, DGO
Professor and Head of Department of Reproductive Medicine, Sri Ramachandra Medical College and Research Institute, Sri Ramachandra University, Chennai

**Srinivas Krishna Jois** MS, DGO, DNB, MNAMS, PGDMLE, FICOG, MA
Assitant Professor of Obstetrics and Gynecology, Bangalore Medical College and Research Institute and Vanivilas Hospital, Bangalore

**K Lavanya** MD (OG), DCH
Registrar and Assitant Professor of Obstetrics and Gynecology, Madras Medical College and Institute of Social Obstetrics and Govt. K G Hospital, Chennai

**J Sarala** MD, DGO
Formerly Professor of Obstetrics and Gynecology, Madras Medical College and Institute of Obstetrics and Gynecology, Chennai

**Thomas Samuel Ram** MD
Professor, Radiation Oncology, Christian Medical College, Vellore

**V Radha** MBBS, DGO, DNB, PhD
Associate Professor, Department of Reproductive Medicine, Sri Ramachandra Medical College and Research Institute, Sri Ramachandra University, Chennai

**Amardeep Tembhere** MBBS, MS (Obstetrics and Gynecology)
Associate Professor, Department of Obstetrics and Gynecology, Mahatma Gandhi Institute of Medical Sciences, Sevagram, Wardha

# Contents


**PART I: Approach to Gynecological Evaluation**

1. Gynecological History and Physical Examination — 1
   — *S Rathnakumar*
2. Clinical Evaluation and Symptomatic Approach in Gynecology — 11
   — *S Rathnakumar*

**PART II: Basic Science in Gynecology**

3. Anatomy of the Female Reproductive System — 16
   — *S Rathnakumar*
4. Physiology of Menstruation and Ovulation — 34
   — *K Lavanya*

**PART III: Paediatric and Adolescent Gynecology**

5. Congenital Anomalies of the Genital Tract — 43
   — *S Rathnakumar*
6. Adolescent Gynecological Problems — 54
   — *S Chhabra*

**PART IV: Benign Gynecological Disorders**

7. Abnormal Uterine Bleeding — 64
   — *V Madhini*
8. Benign Diseases of the Vulva and Vagina — 77
   — *S Rathnakumar*
9. Benign and Premalignant Lesions of the Cervix — 91
   — *Ramani Rajendran*
10. Benign Diseases of the Uterus — 106
   — *J Sarala*
11. Benign Tumours of the Ovary and Fallopian Tube — 121
   — *S Rathnakumar*
12. Pelvic Inflammatory Disease — 131
   — *Radha Bai Prabhu*

**PART V: Infertility, Menopause and Hormones in Gynecology**

13. Infertility — 140
   — *A Kalaiselvi*
14. Polycystic Ovarian Syndrome — 158
   — *A Kalaiselvi*
15. Endometriosis — 165
   — *Radha Bai Prabhu*
16. Amenorrhea — 176
   — *S Rathnakumar*
17. Menopause — 191
   — *Revathy Janakiraman*

18. Hormones in Gynecology 200
— *Srinivas Krishna Jois*

**PART VI: Premalignant and Malignant Diseases**

19. Malignant Diseases of the Vulva, Vagina and Fallopian Tube 215
— *S Rathnakumar*

20. Malignant Lesions of the Cervix 223
— *Ramani Rajendran*

21. Malignant Neoplasm of the Uterus 233
— *Poonam Verma Shivkumar and Shila Shelke*

22. Malignant Ovarian Tumours 245
— *Srinivas Krishna Jois*

23. Gestational Trophoblastic Disease 257
— *Revathy Janakiraman*

24. Chemotherapy in Gynecology 263
— *K Kalaiselvi*

25. Radiotherapy in Gynecological Cancer 274
— *Thomas Samuel Ram*

**PART VII: Pelvic Organ Prolapse and Urogynecology**

26. Uterovaginal Prolapse 283
— *Poonam Verma Shivkumar and Amardeep Tembhere*

27. Disorders of the Urinary System 301
— *S Rathnakumar*

28. Genitourinary Fistula 314
— *S Rathnakumar*

**PART VIII: Imaging in Gynecology**

29. Radiological Investigations in Gynecology 327
— *S Rathnakumar*

30. Endoscopy in Gynecology 335
— *N Sanjeeva Reddy*

**PART IX: Miscellaneous Topics**

31. Operative Gynecology 343
— *S Rathnakumar*

32. Pain in Gynecology 361
— *S Rathnakumar*

33. Contraception 365
— *S Rathnakumar*

*Appendix* 381

*Key to MCQs* 393

*Index* 394

# Gynecological History and Physical Examination

## At a Glance

Gynecological History
- Menstrual History
- Marital History
- Obstetric History
- Previous History
- History of Medications
- Other Complaints
- Pain
- Urinary Symptoms
- Rectal Symptoms

Physical Examination
- General
- Chest Examination
- Breast Examination
- Abdominal Examination
- Pelvic Examination
- Rectal Examination
- Rectovaginal Examination

## INTRODUCTION

History taking is an important aspect of medical practice and in gynecological practice too, it is important to obtain a detailed history before a gynecological examination. A hurried enquiry or an incomplete history (often given by someone other than the patient) may lead to wrong diagnosis. The actual history should be elicited tactfully from reticent patients who may not tell the physician about certain sexual problems such as dyspareunia. In such instances the physician's sympathetic attitude encourages the patient to narrate the salient points in her history. Some statements may be irrelevant but frequent interruptions and enquiring only about the so-called relevant details may lead to a wrong diagnosis if vital facts relating to the case do not emerge. Depending on the main complaint of the patient, the physician is of course always free to ask for additional details. It is always necessary to avoid technical terms and also to ensure that the patient enjoys some degree of privacy during the interview.

**Social and environmental factors** have an influence on gynecological complaints especially dysmenorrhea, premenstrual tension, infertility, vaginal discharge or PID.

A **family history** of tuberculosis, diabetes or pelvic malignancy should alert the gynecologist to any early evidence of these conditions in the patient during the check-up.

The main complaints should be noted down briefly in the words used by the patient, along with the duration (in its sequence), type of onset and the present status of each complaint.

## GYNECOLOGICAL HISTORY

### Menstrual History

The following factors are of particular importance:

1. Age at menarche, regularity, duration and length of cycle.
2. Date of last normal menstrual period.
3. Premenstrual symptoms, for example, mastalgia, tension, headache, weight gain.
4. Whether menstruation is associated with pain, and facts relating to it; for example, the site of pain, time of onset and subsidence, accompanying nausea or vomiting.
5. Amount of flow, judged by the number of pads or tampons used per day. If the person is menopausal, the age at menopause and associated menopausal symptoms, if any, should be ascertained.

#### Pictorial Blood Assessment Chart (PBAC) scoring

The PBAC scoring chart is shown in Fig. 1.1.

### Marital History

This would include facts relating to

1. Age at marriage, duration of the marriage

| PBAC SCORING | | | | | | | | |
|---|---|---|---|---|---|---|---|---|
| Name of Patient | Days | | | | | | | Score |
| Sanitary pads | 1 | 2 | 3 | 4 | 5 | 6 | 7 | |
| | | | | | | | | |
| | | | | | | | | |
| | | | | | | | | |
| Tampons | | | | | | | | |
| | | | | | | | | |
| | | | | | | | | |
| | | | | | | | | |
| Clots/Flooding | | | | | | | | |
| 1 Point | For each small clot | | | | | | | |
| 5 Point | For each large clot | | | | | | | |
| 5 Point | For each episode of flooding | | | | | | | |

**For sanitary pads**
1 = Lightly stained
5 = Moderately stained
20 = Completely stained

**For tampoons**
1 = Lightly stained
5 = Moderately stained
10 = Completely stained

**For clots/flooding**
Each small clot = 1 point
Each large clot = 5 points
Each episode of flooding = 5 points

**Fig. 1.1** PBAC scoring chart

2. Frequency of coitus and whether or not it is associated with dyspareunia
3. Type of contraceptive used
4. Duration of use of contraceptive and side-effects if any

## Obstetric History

The obstetric history should include information about the following:

1. The number of pregnancies—normal or associated complications like preeclampsia, anaemia, etc.
2. Deliveries—preterm or full term.
3. Nature of delivery—spontaneous, instrumental, cesarean section.
4. The condition of the babies at birth—live birth, fetal or neonatal death.
5. Weight of the babies at birth.
6. Postpartum complications like PPH, eclampsia, puerperal sepsis, puerperal psychosis, wound sepsis (episiotomy, or Cesarean section wound)
7. Duration of breast feeding.
8. Resumption of menses after the delivery.
9. The number of abortions, if any, the period of gestation at each termination, whether abortion was spontaneous or induced (with method of induction) and postabortal complications, if any.
10. The date of the last pregnancy and delivery or abortion.

In cases of genital fistulae or prolapse following delivery, more details are necessary, for example, the duration of labour especially in the second stage, the method of delivery and how long after the delivery the complaint arose.

## Previous History

Information about any major previous illness such as tuberculosis, appendicitis or surgery involving the abdominal or pelvic viscera should be recorded with details. The indication, findings at surgery, details of the procedure and the pathology report on the tissue/organ resected would be useful. Efforts should be made to obtain the relevant notes from the physician or institution concerned if they are not readily available with the patient. This is helpful in the management of infertility, chronic pelvic pain or in dealing with recurrent pelvic masses.

## History of Medications

It is important to find out whether the patient has been taking any drugs such as cortisone, antihypertensives, anti-tuberculous agents or sex steroids recently. The information is important if surgery is contemplated.

## Other Complaints

Information about abnormal bleeding, vaginal discharge and pain (abdominal or pelvic) and urinary or bowel symptoms should also be carefully noted down.

### Abnormal bleeding

In cases of abnormal bleeding, its relation to the periods (intermenstrual, premenstrual or postmenopausal) or to coital experience (postcoital) must be established.

- Frequency and duration of bleeding
- Information about periods of amenorrhea, if any
- The type of contraceptive used (whether hormonal or an intrauterine device)

- The quantum of flow
- Whether it is associated with clots and pain
- Whether the periods are profuse or prolonged *(menorrhagia)*
- Whether frequent *(polymenorrhea)*
- Whether irregular with bleeding between the periods *(metrorrhagia)*

### Abnormal vaginal discharge

The following points are to be noted whenever there is abnormal vaginal discharge.

- The quantum (profuse or scanty)
- Colour (white, yellowish, bloodstained, brownish or mucoid)
- Nature (curdy or frothy) (as in *Trichomonas vaginalis*) (Fig. 1.2)
- Odour (offensive, urinary or ammoniacal)
- Relation to the menstrual cycle (intermenstrual or premenstrual)

Associated symptoms such as pruritus and burning micturition should be ascertained.

An ulcerated lesion in the genital tract (cancer, polyp) will result in an irregular bloodstained discharge.

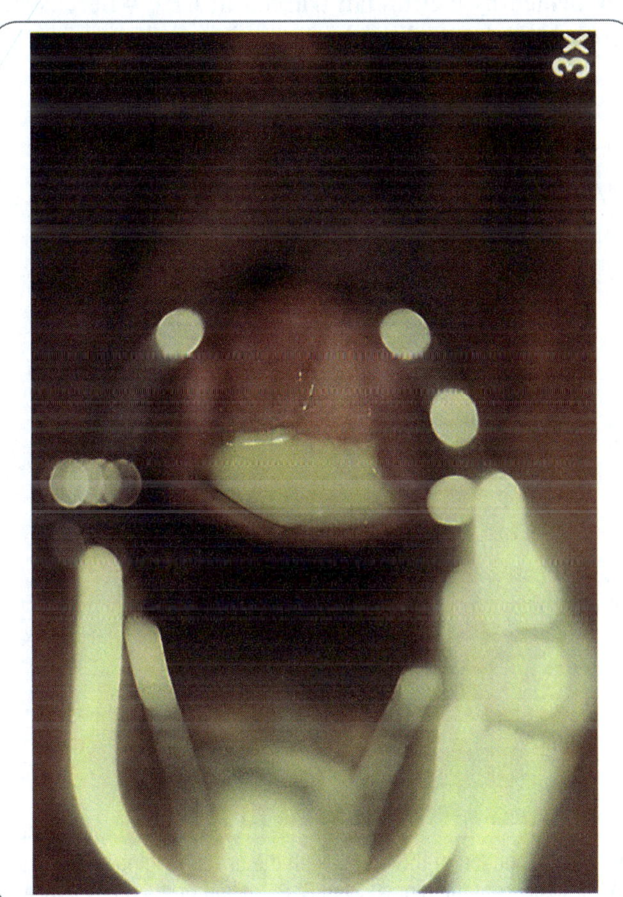


**Fig. 1.2** Trichmonas infection (*Source:* PHIL)

If the growth is infected and covered over with slough, the discharge is likely to be offensive. In a rectovaginal fistula, the discharge may be fecal.

## Pain

Menstrual pain may be spasmodic (colicky during periods) or congestive (dull pain with the approach of periods). In some cases, it may be present a few days preceding the periods, during and two to three days following the periods as in endometriosis.

If there is abnormal abdominal or pelvic pain, the following are to be recorded.

- Type—sharp, stabbing, dull, bearing-down or colicky
- Nature—acute, chronic or intermittent
- Onset—gradual or sudden
- Location or distribution
- Relation to the periods and to food, posture and urination.

The nature of pain under various diseased conditions is listed in Table 1.1.

Backache of gynecological origin is generally secondary to PID, endometriosis and malignancy of the cervix. But in most women, backache may be ascribed to orthopedic causes, or is musculoskeletal in origin. This is discussed in Chapter 32.

### Dyspareunia

Pain during sexual intercourse may be due to functional or organic factors. It may be felt at the introitus (inflammatory lesions, urethral caruncle, Bartholinitis) or may be deep-seated (PID, endometriosis, prolapsed ovary). It is of a functional nature if intercourse takes place in a situation of fear or anxiety.

In cases of infertility, a detailed history relating to frequency and timing of coitus and where indicated, a history of STD, tuberculosis, previous curettage or induced abortion should be elicited.

**Table 1.1** Nature of pain under various disease conditions

| Condition | Nature of pain |
|---|---|
| Tubal rupture | Acute at onset and associated with fainting or collapse |
| PID | Acute or chronic depending on the stage of the disease, but may be associated with fever, vaginal discharge and other symptoms |
| Submucous myoma | Colicky |
| Twisted ovarian cyst | Abdominal pain sudden and severe with the tumour appearing tense on palpation |
| Genital prolapse | Pain in the lower back, which is dull and prolonged |

## Urinary Symptoms

Typical complaints are a burning sensation during micturition, frequency of or difficulty in micturition, and retention of urine. Frequency of micturition is often due to cystitis; difficulty may be associated with genital prolapse or marked cystocele, pelvic hematocele, soon after a vaginal surgery or even after an episiotomy is sutured.

Urinary incontinence may be false (as in stress or urge incontinence) or true (as in urinary fistulae). A vesicovaginal fistula is often preceded by either prolonged, neglected labour or by pelvic surgery. An ureterovaginal fistula usually follows a hysterectomy.

## Rectal Symptoms

The patient may complain of constipation, diarrhea or dysentery. In some cases of complete perineal tear or rectovaginal fistula, there is fecal incontinence.

# PHYSICAL EXAMINATION

## General

This should include assessment of height, weight, nutritional status including degree of anemia and examination of the neck to rule out any goitre, prominent veins or supraclavicular nodes. Blood pressure and pulse rates must be recorded.

## Chest Examination

This should include the heart, lungs and the breasts.

## Breast Examination

Though many patients are shy at first, they may agree to having their breasts examined after assurance and explanation. Next to cancer of the cervix uteri, cancer of the breast is the most common cancer in Indian women.

> **Clinical Importance**
>
> Any suspicious areas or gross pathology found in clinical breast examination warrants immediate referral to surgeon for confirmation and further treatment.

**Clinical Breast Examination (CBE) differs from breast self-examination (BSE) in that the former is performed by a clinician trained in CBE whereas the latter is performed by the woman herself.**

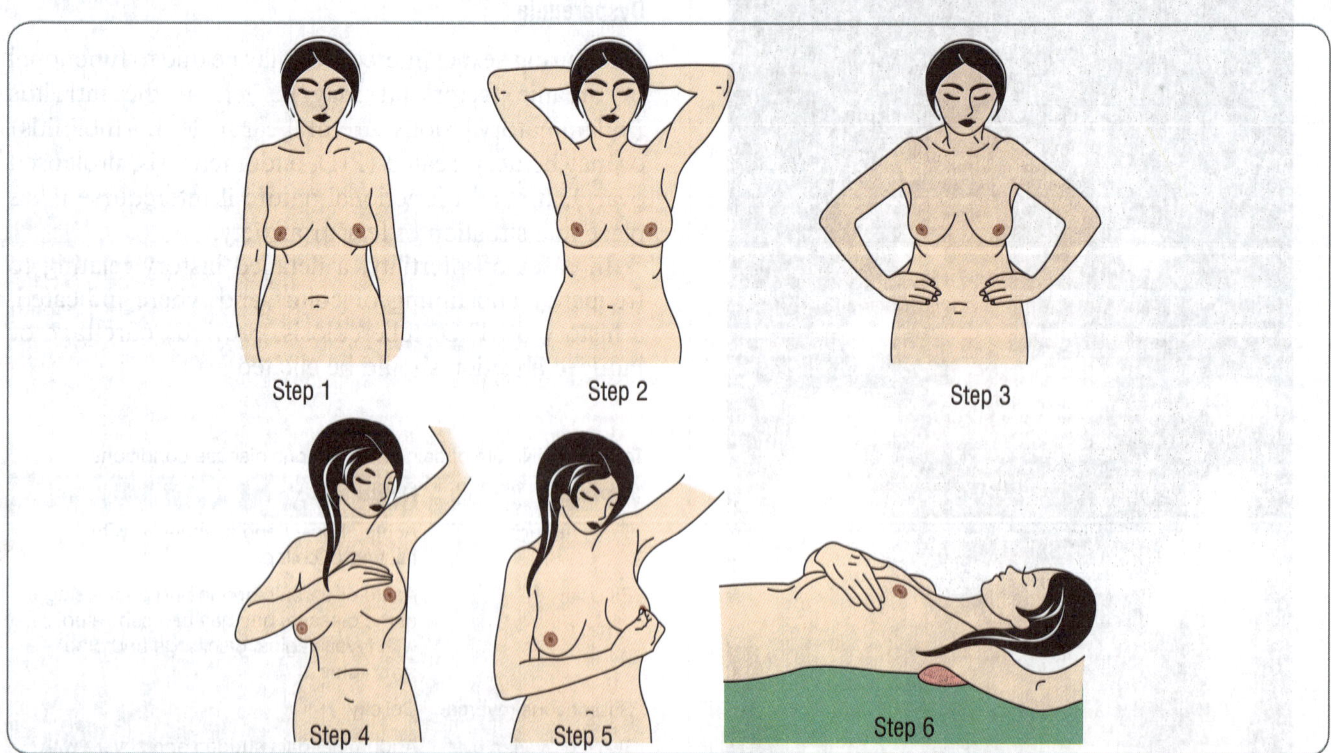


**Fig. 1.3** A pictorial example of breast self-examination in six steps. Steps 1–3: Inspection of the breast with the arms hanging next to the body, behind the head and in the side; Step 4: Palpation of the breast; Step 5: Palpation of the nipple; Step 6: Palpation of the breast while lying down.

### Breast self-examination (BSE)

Breast self-examination is the method by which the woman herself examines her breast for any lumps, swelling or discharge (Fig. 1.3). Though it was once very actively promoted as a screening method for early detection of breast cancer, large randomised controlled trials have found it not effective in either detecting or preventing deaths due to cancer breast. Moreover, it increased the number of biopsies, surgery and anxiety. It is not routinely recommended as a routine screening method. However, It may be appropriate in women who have a high risk of developing breast cancer. In spite of its ineffectiveness, it is still being promoted in low-resource settings.

### Clinical breast examination (CBE)

CBE (Fig. 1.4) involves a systematic search pattern that ensures that all breast tissue is examined. During the examination the patient should be in supine position and her hands should be above her head. An inspection of the size, shape of the breast, skin over the breast tissue, looking specifically for any puckering, any ulcer over the skin, nipple discharge and any visual mass is performed. The area of CBE extends from the clavicle, medially to the midsternum, laterally to the midaxillary line, and to the inferior portion of the breast. **In addition, the examination should include the axillary tail of Spence and the axilla to search for palpable lymphadenopathy.**

CBE is carried out using the pads of the 2nd, 3rd, and 4th fingers. The three search patterns commonly described are the following.

i. **Concentric circle method** The breast is examined in larger or smaller concentric circles (Fig. 1.4a).
ii. The **radial spoke method** This is the method in which the breast tissue is examined beginning at the periphery toward the nipple in a radial pattern (Fig. 1.4b).
iii. **The vertical strip pattern** In this method, the breast tissue is examined in overlapping vertical strips across the chest wall (Fig. 1.4c).
iv. **Redness/Pain** This is suggestive of inflammation and/or infection (Fig. 1.4d).

## Abdominal Examination

This is done with the patient in a dorsal recumbent position with her knees slightly flexed as it promotes

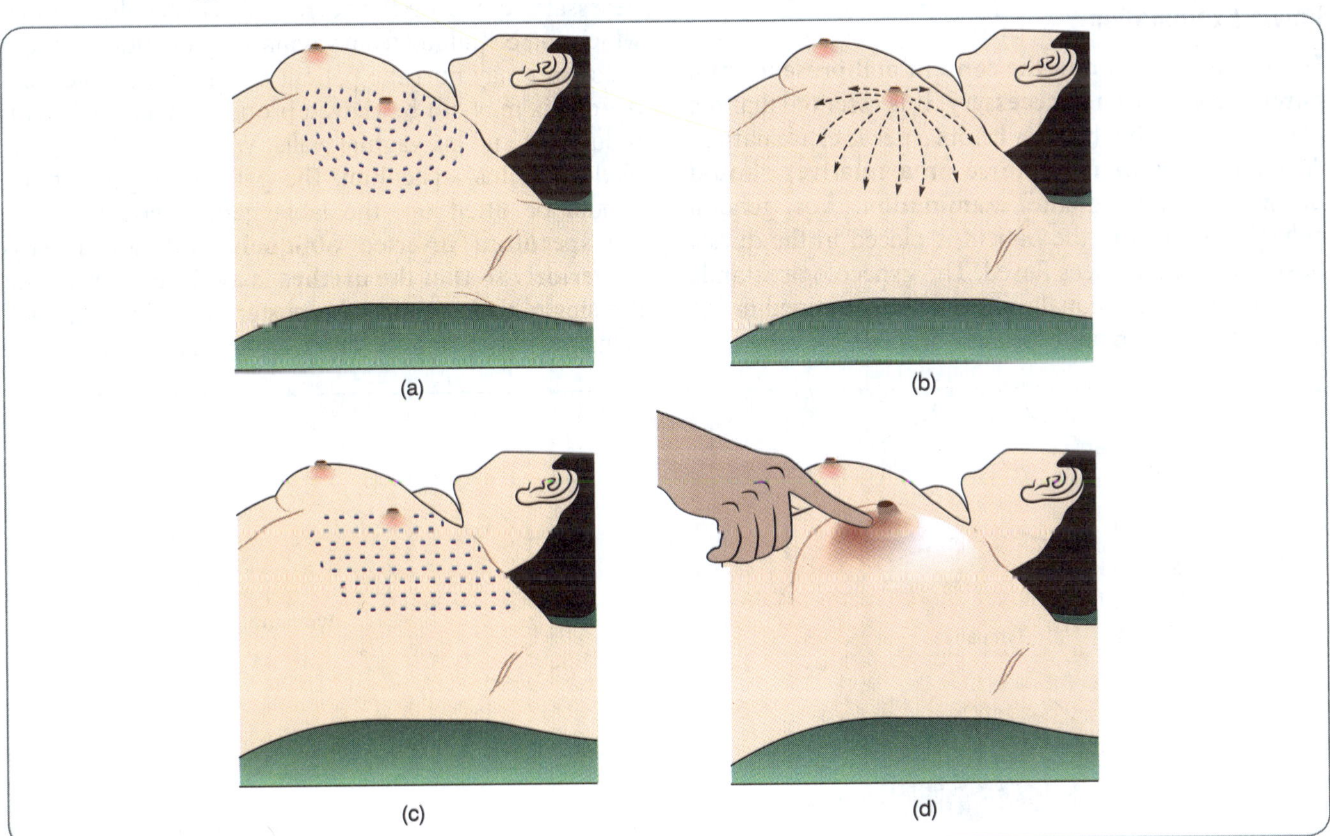


**Fig. 1.4** Clinical breast examination: (a) Concentric circle method; (b) Radial spoke method; (c) Vertical strip pattern; and (d) Redness/Pain: Suggestive of inflammation and/or infection.

abdominal relaxation. The inspection reveals whether the abdomen moves freely on respiration; it also indicates enlargement or prominence, scars from previous surgery and skin changes which have, for instance, followed earlier pregnancies, or radiation.

While palpating, the gynecologist should also look for enlarged liver or spleen, any tenderness or muscle-guarding, mass over the abdomen including the groin and hernial orifices.

Tenderness in the costovertebral angle may suggest pyelonephritis.

If any mass is felt, it should be described in detail with reference to its location, size, consistency (hard, firm or cystic), contour (smooth, lobulated or nodular), sensitivity (tender or not), mobility (freely mobile and in what direction, restricted mobility or fixed), and dullness (Fig. 1.5a and b) or resonance on percussion. Free fluid or shifting dullness have to be looked out for in association with abdominal or pelvic tumours.

Tenderness in the right iliac fossa may be due to adnexitis, ectopic gestation, appendicitis or amebiasis. Other relevant points in the history and findings may be useful in reaching a probable diagnosis.

## Pelvic Examination

**In the case of a minor, the consent and presence of a parent or guardian is necessary**. It is essential that the patient empties her bladder before a pelvic examination. **A female attendant (a nurse or a relative) should be present during the examination**. For general pelvic examination, the patient is placed in the dorsal position with the knees flexed. The gynecologist stands on her right. Occasionally she may be examined in the lithotomy position appropriately draped.

### Inspection of the external genitalia

The first step is to establish whether the vulva is healthy, inflamed, ulcerated or leukoplakic, to determine the size of the clitoris, and to look for perineal relaxation or tears. Discharge of any kind from the urethral meatus (redness and purulent discharge), the vaginal or hymenal orifices and the opening of Bartholin's ducts must be noted. The patient is asked to strain or cough to see whether there is a cystocele or prolapse of the uterus. If the main complaint is stress incontinence she must not urinate prior to the examination and must be asked to cough to check if any urine escapes in the process through the urethra. If the hymen is intact or if the patient is a virgin, the vaginal examination usually does not proceed further. If necessary, a rectal examination or examination under anaesthesia is carried out.

### Speculum examination

This is carried out mainly to view the cervix and the vagina and to determine whether they are healthy or not. This is also necessary for obtaining smears for cytology and for biopsy of the cervix. **Sim's and Cusco's speculum** (Figs. 1.6 and 1.7) are commonly used. It is necessary to choose the correct-sized speculum, a fact which can be judged from vaginal examination. A larger speculum may hurt the patient and with a smaller one the cervix may not be viewed properly in a person with redundant and lax vaginal walls. When introducing the blade of Sims' speculum, the patient's right buttock should be lifted up, the labia gently separated and the **speculum inserted obliquely and not antero-posteriorly so that the urethra is avoided**. Depressing the single blade against the posterior vaginal wall will bring the cervix and the anterior vaginal wall into view.

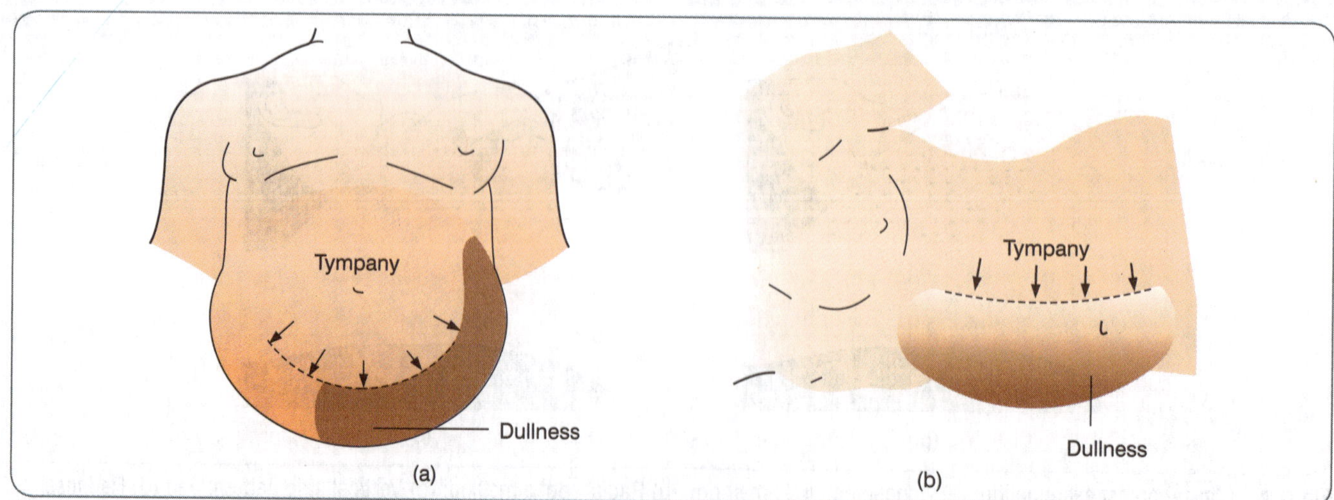


**Fig. 1.5** (a) Flank dullness and (b) Shifting dullness

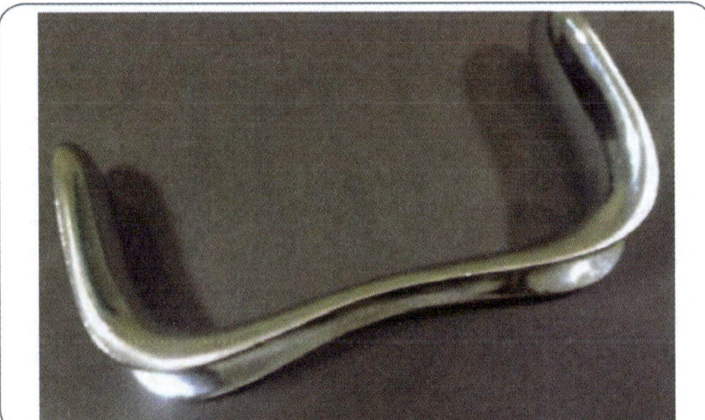

Fig. 1.6 Sim's speculum (*Source:* Wikimedia)

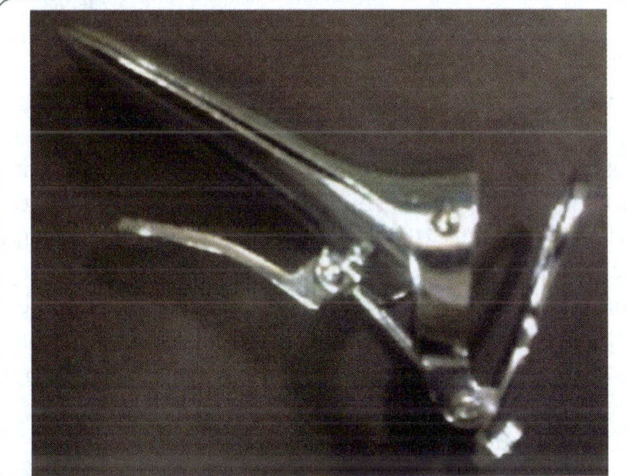

Fig. 1.7 Cusco's speculum (*Source:* Wikimedia)

Cusco's speculum is inserted with the blades closed, and after the blades have met the cervix or vaginal vault, they are opened to retract the anterior and posterior vaginal walls, thus exposing the cervix fully. The blades can be fixed in position by tightening a screw. Since it is a self-retaining speculum, the physician is then free to do any tests: collect cytologic smears with Ayre's spatula, obtain material for culture with a platinum loop, do a biopsy of the cervix, twist off a mucus polyp protruding through the external os or attend to the posthysterectomy granulation tissue seen sometimes at the vaginal vault.

A good torchlight or a focusing lamp is essential for viewing the cervix clearly. Some specula have a light-source attached to the device.

The cervix is usually pink in colour or there may be a red area around the external os which is known as ectropion (Fig. 1.8).

Presence of ulcer, growth, tumour or cyst should be looked for. Any secretion should be collected for further examination.

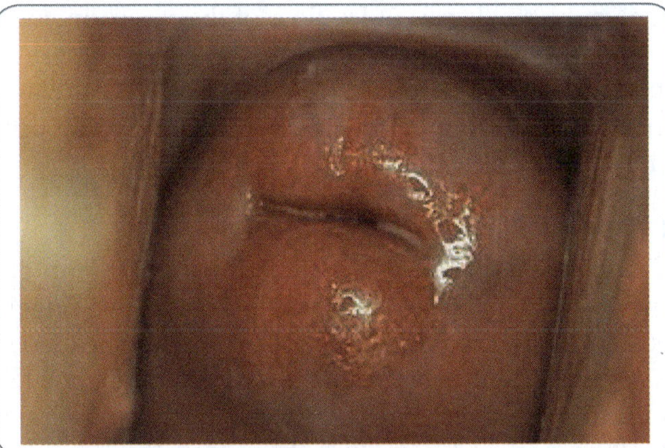

Fig. 1.8 Ectropion (*Source:* Wikimedia)

As the speculum is being withdrawn gradually, the vaginal walls are examined carefully. Instead of the pink thick rugose mucosa, one may find it bluish in pregnancy, congested or covered with discharge in vaginitis, or ulcerated due to pathological lesions. During its withdrawal, one can also make out the cystocele anteriorly or the pouch of Douglas hernia posteriorly.

#### Internal or digital examination

The labia are gently separated and two lubricated fingers (index and middle finger) of the gloved right hand are carefully introduced into the vagina. If there is any difficulty, the fourchette is gently depressed and the fingers passed into the vagina avoiding the more sensitive clitoris and the urethra anteriorly.

##### *Cervix*

The cervix is felt as the fingers are passed into the vaginal vault. If the uterus is anteverted, the anterior lip is the first to be felt, and if it is retroverted, the external os or the posterior lip will be palpated first.

In nulliparous women, the cervix is conical and firm and the external os is circular. But in multipara, it may be enlarged or hypertrophied and the external os is often slit transversely. Rarely, it may show evidence of cervical laceration as a result of the trauma in a previous delivery.

The cervix is now lightly outlined with the fingers to identify the size, position, consistency, texture and dilation of the os. It is normally smooth and firm. In pregnant women the cervix is soft. Its surface around the external os may feel velvety in cases of erosion. In carcinoma, it is ulcerated, friable and bleeds easily. Occasionally, there may be a polyp protruding through the os. By digitally moving the cervix, the gynecologist can gauge the degree of freedom of the cervix. In cases of pelvic inflammation and tubal gestation, there is tenderness when the cervix is moved. The patient is then asked to strain to see whether there is any descent or prolapse of the uterus.

### *The perineal body and the levators*

These are examined next. By keeping the thumb externally over the perineum and flexing the two fingers posteriorly in the vagina, the tone of the perineal body is assessed. Similarly the tone of the levator can be felt with the thumb externally over the labium majus and two fingers flexed laterally in the vagina. If there is any abnormality such as ulceration, scarring, a septum or cyst in the vagina, the location and extent are noted.

### *Bimanual examination*

**Technique** In bimanual examination (examination with both hands), one hand is placed over the patient's lower abdomen and two fingers of the other hand are inserted into the vagina. The cervix, uterus are palpated between the fingers in the vagina and the hand over the abdomen. The patient is requested to breathe through the mouth to avoid making the abdominal wall tense. The two internal fingers which are placed in the anterior vaginal fornix against the anterior lip of the cervix (and the lower part of the corpus) press the uterus upwards while the external hand placed over the lower abdomen pushes it downwards. The uterine outline between the two hands can now be clearly noted (Fig. 1.9). If the uterus is retroverted, the internal fingers are inserted in the posterior fornix to push up the uterus and thus felt more easily. In obese or tense patients, it is difficult to palpate the pelvic organs easily. It is only with experience that the physician can identify the pelvic organs clearly by this method of examination.

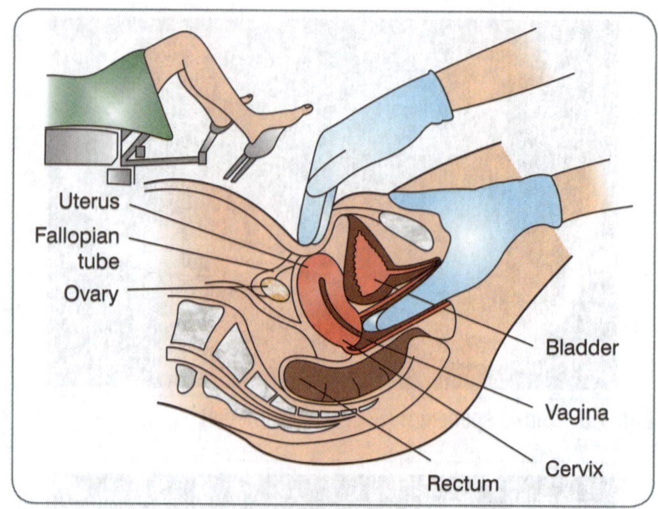


**Fig. 1.9** Bimanual palpation of the uterus

When the uterus is felt, one has to determine its position, size, consistency, contour and mobility. Normally it is in the midline in the upper half of the pelvis with the external os in the same plane as the ischial spine. The uterine fundus is directed forwards and is said to be anteverted. It is normally pear-shaped, firm and smooth. Normal or abnormal size can be made out only with some experience as in the relationship of the size of the cervix to that of the corpus (Fig. 1.10).

If the uterus is firm, nodular and enlarged, it suggests myoma of the uterus. In adenomyosis, it may be enlarged.

The uterus has some degree of mobility in all directions. The mobility is restricted in PID (due to peritoneal adhesions or parametrial fixation), endometriosis, impacted fibromyoma and advanced carcinoma of the cervix.

**Adnexa** For palpation of the adnexa, the fingers in the vagina are placed in the lateral fornix and the

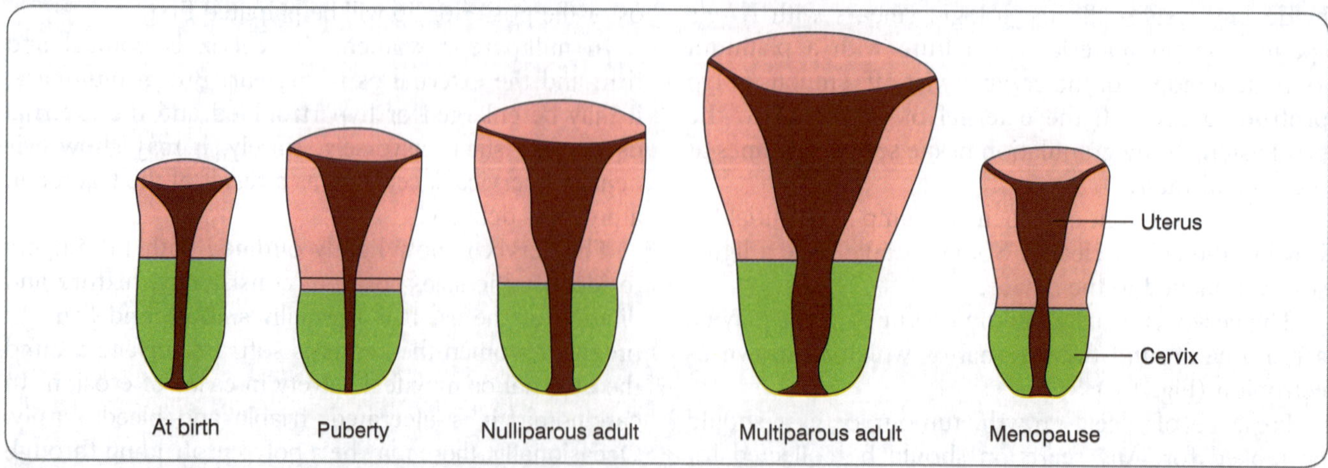


**Fig. 1.10** Ratio of the length of the uterus and the cervix from birth to menopausal age

external hand is pressed down over the vaginal fingers in an attempt to outline the uterine adnexa (Fig. 1.11). Normally, the healthy tubes are not palpable but the ovaries may be felt when prolapsed, cystic or enlarged.

In acute PID, the fornices may be tender and in chronic cases a thickened tube or a fixed, tender, retort-shaped pyosalpinx may be felt on one or both sides of the uterus.

In tubal gestation, the tube may be tender and pulsatile or it may be felt as a tender boggy mass when there are blood clots around it.

In pelvic cellulitis, there is tenderness and induration on one or both sides of the uterus extending up to the pelvic wall, giving an impression of a frozen pelvis.

In pelvic endometriosis, of which the ovary is the most common site, it may be felt as an enlarged tender swelling on one or both sides surrounded by nodular endometriotic deposits in the posterior fornix.

The pouch of Douglas can be felt through the posterior fornix. In this pouch, one may find the body of the uterus when it is retroverted, an adnexal inflammatory swelling, endometriosis, pelvic hematocele, pelvic abscess, the lower pole of an ovarian tumour, a myoma arising from the posterior uterine wall or secondary malignant deposits.

In postmenopausal women with an adnexal mass the possibility of an ovarian malignancy should be ruled out. If the rectum is loaded, one may feel the fecal masses and lack of experience may lead to a wrong diagnosis. The rectal examination supplementing the vaginal examination always gives useful information concerning the contents of the pouch of Douglas.

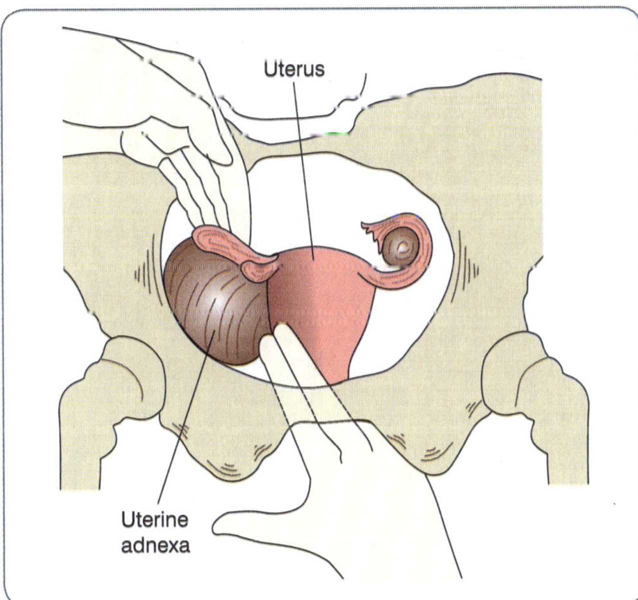


**Fig. 1.11** Bimanual palpation of the uterine adnexa

In some pelvic tumours palpable through the abdomen, it is difficult to determine whether they arise from the uterus or from the adnexa.

> **Clinical Importance**
>
> If the uterus is not felt separately from the pelvic swelling and if on moving the swelling with the external hand, the cervix also moves in the same direction as the swelling, it is likely to be a uterine tumour.

An adnexal swelling is diagnosed only when it is clearly distinguished from the uterus. Apart from the differentiating feature mentioned above, another possible clinically distinguishable feature is the **presence of a groove between the uterus and the adnexal tumour** palpable better with a rectal examination. In rare cases, a pedunculated myoma may be mistaken for an adnexal tumour, or an adnexal mass adherent to the uterus may be diagnosed as a uterine tumour.

## Rectal Examination

### Indications

Rectal examination is an important part of gynecological examination and is particularly indicated in children and in virgins. It is indicated in the following:

- Cases of congenital or acquired vaginal atresia
- Tumours in the pouch of Douglas
- Pelvic endometriosis
- Carcinoma of the cervix
- Rectocele
- In patients with rectal symptoms or low backache

Besides digital palpation, the rectal examination gives a fund of useful information often supplementing the vaginal examination.

During rectal examination, the upper part of the vagina, the cervix, the pouch of Douglas and its contents, and the posterior wall of the uterus can be felt. The parametrium on either side of the uterus and the uterosacral ligaments posteriorly can also be felt. The anterior rectal wall can be easily palpated. Whenever there is a pathology or suspicion, proctoscopy should be performed.

## Rectovaginal Examination

This examination (Fig. 1.12) performed as a bidigital examination with the middle finger in the rectum and the index finger in the vagina can reveal whether the tumour arises from the ovary or the rectum.

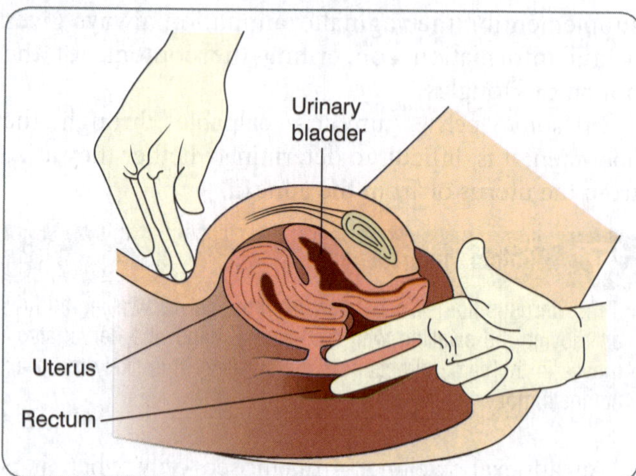


**Fig. 1.12** Bidigital (rectovaginal) examination

### Indications

- Doubtful pelvic tumour
- Evaluation of the rectovaginal septum
- Evaluation of the levator ani muscle
- Diagnosis of rectovaginal fistula

As a final step, the patient may be examined standing. She can be asked to cough or strain and the hernial orifices checked for a suspected inguinal or femoral hernia. This may also be necessary in some cases of stress incontinence.

After the examination is over, the gynecologist should review the salient points in the history and the physical findings with the patient and indicate the most probable diagnosis. She should also be informed about the investigations needed to confirm the diagnosis or to carry out the treatment. A brief discussion with the patient about the form of therapy indicated is an essential part of the consultation and helps not only in making her aware of her problems but also in planning further therapy. It may be useful to invite her husband or a close member of her family (with her consent) when this final discussion is held.

# Chapter 2

# Clinical Evaluation and Symptomatic Approach in Gynecology

**At a Glance**

Common Gynecological Symptoms
- Vaginal Discharge
- Absent or Delayed Menarche
- Pain During Menstruation
- Menstrual Disorders
- Lower Abdominal Mass
- Mass Descending Per Vaginum
- Acute/Chronic Abdominal and/or Pelvic Pain
- Urinary Symptoms
- Bowel Symptoms

The female anatomy is unique, so also are the problems of women; also, the same problem may present with an entirely different set of signs and symptoms during different periods of life. Moreover when women have confidence in and develop a good rapport with their gynecologists, they tend to approach the gynecologist first for non-gynecological problems as well. Hence it is imperative to be familiar with the common gynecological problems, their mode of presentation and their diagnosis and management.

## COMMON GYNECOLOGICAL SYMPTOMS

The most common gynecological symptoms are:
- Vaginal discharge
- Absent or delayed menarche
- Pain during menstruation
- Menstrual disorders—absent, scanty, profuse, frequent, infrequent or delayed flow, intermenstrual bleeding, postcoital bleeding and postmenopausal bleeding
- Lower abdominal mass
- Mass descending per vaginum
- Acute/chronic abdominal and/or pelvic pain
- Urinary symptoms
- Bowel symptoms

### Vaginal Discharge

Vaginal discharge could be **physiological** or **pathological**.

**Physiological** vaginal discharge could occur:
- Due to transfer of maternal estrogen in utero; the newborn could have vaginal discharge or even vaginal bleeding for few days after birth
- Prior to ovulation
- Prior to menarche and during pregnancy; there could be vaginal discharge due to increased estrogen production

Physiological discharge is usually a diagnosis of exclusion. The discharge is clear and non-purulent. The discharge varies with the phase of the menstrual cycle.

Once the diagnosis is made, the management is mainly reassurance.

**Pathological** causes of infective vaginal discharge are:
- Bacterial vaginosis
- Candida infection
- *Trichomonas vaginalis*
- *Chlamydia trachomatis*
- *Neisseria gonorrhoeae*

The **non-infective causes** of vaginal discharge are:
- Cervical ectropion
- Foreign bodies like tampon, condom
- Chemical irritants like spermicidal creams, jelly

Vaginal discharge is also specific for the age group. They can also be classified according to their common occurrence in a particular age group:

#### In children

- Poor perineal hygiene
- Foreign bodies—small pebbles, eraser and small sticks have often been identified and removed in children
- Infections—particularly *Enterobius vermicularis* (pinworm), candida, streptococcal and staphylococcal infections

- Chemical irritants like soap, soap nut, etc.
- Sexual abuse

#### In women of reproductive age

- Trichomonal infection
- Candidal infection
- Bacterial vaginosis
- Pelvic inflammatory disease
- Foreign bodies (forgotten tampon, condom)

#### In women of postmenopausal age

- Atrophic vaginitis
- Chemical vulvitis due to irritation from urine or faeces
- Malignancies like cervical or endometrial cancer

The initial investigation for vaginal discharge is usually a **vaginal smear**. Based on the result of the smear study, further investigation and treatment are decided. The diagnosis and management of these conditions are dealt with in detail in the corresponding chapters.

### Absent or Delayed Menarche

The parents of the girl are more anxious about this condition. Though there is no definitive age limit for attaining menarche, different societal groups fix their own upper limit for attaining menarche and seek medical advice when this is not happening. **However, a girl who has not attained menarche by the age of 13 years with absent or poorly developed secondary sexual characters needs investigation.**

**Primary amenorrhea** (when the girl has not attained menarche at all) could be due to:

- Developmental defects of genital tract like complete absence of vagina, transverse septum, partial absence of upper part of vagina and imperforate hymen
- Chromosomal anomalies
- Hypothalamic, pituitary and ovarian causes
- Thyroid and adrenal dysfunction
- Unresponsive or absent endometrium

Primary amenorrhea is also differentiated based on the hormonal pattern as:

- Hypergonadotropic hypogonadism,
- Hypogonadotropic hypogonadism and
- Eugonadism (pubertal delay with normal gonadotropins)

A thorough physical examination will give lot of clue as to the underlying pathology. For example, history of regular, periodic lower abdominal pain would point towards an imperforate hymen as the possible etiology for absence of menstruation. Similarly, examination of secondary sexual characters is also important. The details of examination, diagnosis and management are dealt with in Chapter 16.

### Pain During Menstruation

Though almost all women experience some amount of pain during menstruation, it becomes a distressing symptom when the pain is unbearable and lasts for a long time. This pain during menstruation is known as **dysmenorrhea**. It is customary to classify dysmenorrhea as

1. Spasmodic or primary dysmenorrhea
2. Congestive or secondary dysmenorrhea

#### Spasmodic dysmenorrhea

This is the more common of the two varieties and is seen very often in the adolescent age group. It is not associated with any identifiable gynecological abnormality. This **colicky pain** is felt in the suprapubic region and lasts for 12–24 hours. The pain usually disappears on the second day of the period. It may be associated with nausea or vomiting. The treatment consists of psychological support and reassurance. Any cause of emotional stress should be corrected. Analgesic drugs may be helpful.

#### Congestive dysmenorrhea

In this type of dysmenorrhea, there is a **dull, dragging type** of premenstrual lower abdominal pain, which is relieved with the onset of periods. This is due to increased vascularity of the pelvic organs before menstrual periods. There is some pelvic pathology such as myoma, adenomyosis or pelvic endometriosis. Management consists of treating the underlying pathology.

#### Pelvic congestion syndrome

In this condition, the patient has congestive dysmenorrhea without any gross pelvic pathology. The pain in this condition is attributed to disorder of the autonomic nervous system producing gross vascular congestion with pelvic varicosities. There is pain on movement of the pelvic organs and supporting structures. It is a functional disorder and treatment may not yield satisfactory results.

#### Mittelschmerz

This German term means middle pain or mid-cycle pain which is caused by ovulation. It is temporary, usually felt mid-cycle, often in the right or left iliac fossa. The pain or discomfort is related to ovulation and is due to follicular distension or intraperitoneal leakage of fluid from the Graafian follicle after ovulation. Apart from slight tenderness in the iliac fossa there is no other sign. The pain is relieved by analgesics.

## Menstrual Disorders

This is another common symptom for which patients approach the gynecologists. The menstrual disorders range from absent menstruation to irregular bleeding patterns.

### Absent menstruation

**In all patients in whom menstruation has ceased after being regular, pregnancy should be ruled out.** The other causes of secondary amenorrhea could be weight loss/anorexia, polycystic ovarian syndrome, hypothyroidism, pituitary tumour, Sheehan syndrome, premature ovarian insufficiency (POI) (formerly known as premature ovarian failure), Asherman syndrome, ovarian tumour.

### Alteration in menstrual flow

Average menstrual cycle has a frequency of 28 ± 7 days with flow for 5 ± 3 days with a volume of 50 ± 30 ml. Gross deviation from these limits leads to abnormal uterine bleeding which may be oligomenorrhea, polymenorrhea, menorrhagia, etc. The conditions are dealt with in detail in Chapter 7.

### Intermenstrual bleeding

This could be due to pregnancy-related causes like ectopic pregnancy or gestational trophoblastic disease. The non-pregnancy-related causes are combined oral contraceptive pills, recent vaginal investigative procedures like pap smear, endocervical/cervical polyp, ectropion, cervical erosion, intrauterine contraceptive device and cervicitis. Malignancy should always be ruled out. Clinical examination including a speculum and bimanual pelvic examination will most often reveal the pathology. Additional investigations like pap smear, ultrasound, hysteroscopy, colposcopy, cervical biopsy may be required.

### Postcoital bleeding

Causes associated with intermenstrual bleeding can also be responsible for postcoital bleeding. Cervical erosion, ectropion, polyps, coital trauma and malignancy, particularly cancer cervix, can be associated with postcoital bleeding.

### Postmenopausal bleeding

This could be due atrophic endometrium, polyp, endometrial hyperplasia, endometrial cancer, cervical cancer and other malignancies. Hormone replacement therapy and infections also can cause postmenopausal bleeding. This condition is described in detail in Chapter 17.

## Lower Abdominal Mass

Lower abdominal mass can present at any age. Sometimes even a large mass may be asymptomatic and may be detected accidentally. The lower abdominal swelling could be genital or extra genital in origin. Similarly some masses are more common in a particular age group. Though malignant tumours are usually associated with older age group women, some tumours might occur in young women and children also.

### In adolescents

It is not uncommon to see lower abdominal mass in adolescents. Hematometra produced by imperforate hymen or other Mullerian anomalies often present as lower abdominal mass in this age group. This would also hold true for hematocolpos and rarely hematosalpinx. The benign mass seen in this age group are:

- Functional cyst
- Paraovarian cysts
- Benign cystic teratoma
- Tubo-ovarian abscess
- Germ cell tumours.
- Malignant teratoma, dysgerminoma and embryonal cell carcinoma.

> **Clinical Importance**
>
> Sometimes an appedicular abscess/mass may be mistaken for gynecological tumour and operated upon.

### In women of reproductive age

Pregnancy should always be ruled out in a woman of reproductive age. All genital organs can have a pathology contributing to lower abdominal mass.

#### *Myomas*

The most common lower abdominal mass is myoma uterus. Though myoma is usually associated with menstrual disturbances, some might be completely asymptomatic also. Pain in a myoma usually indicates the fibroid is undergoing degeneration and should be investigated and managed more effectively. Adenomyosis can also present as lower abdominal mass though the size is usually small. The symptoms may be similar to myoma. Both these conditions could be diagnosed during investigation for infertility also. However, the tendency to blame all myoma as the cause for infertility should be resisted. A cervical fibroid can cause distressing urinary symptoms like hesitancy, dribbling or urinary retention.

#### *Tubo-ovarian masses*

These are also common in this age group though they are much smaller in size compared to myoma or other tumours. Endometrioma can also present as a lower abdominal mass.

#### *Benign epithelial tumours of the ovary*

Some of these tumours like serous or mucinous cystadenoma can be large. Other ovarian tumours like follicular cyst, corpus luteum cyst, Brenner tumour can all present as lower abdominal mass. Large theca lutein cysts also present as lower abdominal mass. Malignant tumours of the ovary like serous and mucinous cystadenocarcinoma, malignant teratoma can all present as lower abdominal mass. Metastasis either from a primary in the genital organs or from extragenital primaries can present as abdominal mass.

### In women of postmenopausal age

Most of these masses tend to be malignant but benign tumours can also occur in the postmenopausal women. Uterine myoma can still occur and so also benign ovarian epithelial tumours like cystadenoma. The more common are malignant tumours of the uterus and ovaries, such as the following:

- Sarcoma of the uterus
- Malignant epithelial tumours of the ovary like cystadenocarcinoma
- Germ cell tumours
- Secondaries from genital and extra genital primaries

The benign tumours usually present with menstrual irregularities as in the case of myoma. The malignant tumours, particularly the ovarian malignancies produce symptoms only much later and it varies from pain and pressure effects to jaundice (liver secondaries), hemoptysis (lung secondaries).

The diagnosis is usually by clinical examination and imaging modalities like ultrasound and CT/MRI. Tumour markers are useful more as a prognostic aid.

The treatment is discussed in the relevant chapters.

## Mass Descending Per Vaginum

Though the mass descending per vaginum is usually associated with pelvic organ prolapse, other conditions should also be considered before arriving at a final diagnosis. They are:

- Vaginal cysts
- Cerival polyp
- Infravaginal elongation of cervix—diagnosed most often during investigation for dyspareunia, infertility
- Pelvic organ prolapse
- Cystocele
- Rectocele
- Procidentia
- Chronic inversion of uterus

### Diagnosis

These conditions are diagnosed based on the clinical findings. Vaginal cysts, though classified here, do not protrude out of the introitus. But a cervical polyp can be seen coming out of the introitus and its origin is easily traced by speculum examination. The deep fornices differentiate an infravaginal elongation of the cervix from a prolapsed uterus in which the fornices are shallow. Whereas cystocele is an anterior projection, the rectocele is seen more posteriorly. Procidentia is a condition in which the whole uterus is seen coming out of the uterus and it is diagnosed by palpating the fundus of the uterus outside the introitus. In chronic inversion, the cervix will not be visible as the uterus has come out through the cervix.

The management of these conditions is discussed in Chapter 26.

## Acute/Chronic Abdominal and/or Pelvic Pain

Pain is an important gynecological problem because of its frequency and the diversity of its causes. In about 40 per cent of cases it may be of gynecological origin but in the rest it is due to orthopedic, urologic, neurologic and other factors.

**Clinical Importance**

The most important cause of sudden **acute pain** in a woman of reproductive age is ectopic pregnancy. This should always be ruled out as missing the diagnosis could be fatal.

The other causes of acute pain are:

- Abortion
- Degenerating fibroid
- Adenomyosis
- Endometriosis

- Pelvic inflammatory disease
- Tubo-ovarian abscess
- Rupture of ovarian cyst
- Mittelschmerz

### Chronic pain

The American College of Obstetrics and Gynecology (ACOG) defines chronic pelvic pain (CPP) as continuous or non-cyclical pelvic pain of longer than 6 months duration that localises to the anatomic pelvis, abdominal wall at or below the umbilicus, lumbosacral back, or the buttocks and is of sufficient severity to cause functional disability or lead to medical care.

#### *Causes*

1. *Menstrual disorders* These have been dealt with earlier.
2. *Iatrogenic cause* Intrauterine contraceptive devices
3. *Dyspareunia* This may be functional or due to organic causes. Dyspareunia may be superficial, at the introitus (caruncle, bartholinitis) or deep-seated as in cervicitis, endometriosis or prolapsed ovaries.
4. *Inflammatory conditions* Chronic PID, adnexitis, pelvic cellulitis, pelvic abscess.
5. *Neoplasms*
   Benign—adenomyosis, endometriosis, myoma and ovarian tumours
   Malignant pelvic neoplasms where pain is late due to infiltration into neighbouring organs and nerves.
6. *Thrombophlebitis* Following surgery, delivery or abortion, thrombophlebitis of the pelvic veins may occur, which may give rise to low-grade fever and pain in the lower abdomen and legs. There is a risk of thromboembolism in some of these patients.
7. *Residual ovary syndrome* This is caused by the ovary(ies) left behind during hysterectomy. It can cause chronic lower abdominal pain and dyspareunia.
8. *Remnant ovarian syndrome* In this condition a part of the ovary left behind during early surgery causes constant or cyclic lower abdominal pain.
9. *Non-gynecological causes* Appendicitis, intestinal obstruction, diverticulitis, hernia or postoperative adhesions.
10. *Urologic* Urethral caruncle, urethritis, cystitis, perivesical abscess, pyelonephritis or ureteral colic.
11. *Low backache* This is a symptom very common in women. It may be postural, fibromuscular or bony in origin. Fibromyositis, spondylitis, spondylolisthesis, disc lesions and sacralisation of the fifth lumbar vertebra are important causes.
12. *Functional cause* The pain may be functional in origin, when no obvious lesion is found, but organic causes must always be ruled out before this diagnosis is arrived at.

The various conditions producing pain and their diagnosis and management are dealt with in detail in Chapter 32.

## Urinary Symptoms

The most common urinary symptom in women is dysuria. This is due to urinary tract infection. The short length of the urethra, the proximity of the rectum to the moist vulva and sexual intercourse results in urinary tract infections.

Incontinence of urine could be a true incontinence as in the case of a urinary fistula or due to stress or urge incontinence. These have been dealt with in detail in Chapters 27 and 28.

## Bowel Symptoms

Irritable Bowel Syndrome (IBS) is a bowel condition very frequently seen in gynecological practice. A higher incidence of dysmenorrhea and premenstrual syndrome has been noted in women with IBS. Abdominal pain, bloating, constipation are some of the common symptoms in women, with or without IBS, during menstruation.

Fecal and flatus incontinence can occur in women with rectovaginal fistula.

It is imperative that a detailed history is taken and the patients are encouraged to explain the symptoms in their own way. Analysing the symptoms will lead the clinician in the right direction. This would ultimately lead to correct diagnosis and proper treatment and alleviation of patient's symptoms.

## RECAP

- The last few decades have seen enormous advancement in diagnostic aids and many are of undeniable value to the clinician. But there is no substitute for a thorough clinical examination and to arrive at a tentative diagnosis. The confirmation could be done with these investigative and diagnostic modalities. Similarly the symptoms with which the patient comes gives a lot of clue to the clinician for arriving at a correct diagnosis. There is no substitute for clinical evaluation.

# Anatomy of the Female Reproductive System

## At a Glance

External Genitalia
- The Vulva
- The Vagina

Internal Genitalia
- The Uterus
- The Uterine Appendages
- The Fallopian Tubes
- The Ovary

Urinary System—Parts Associated With the Female Reproductive System
- The Female Urethra
- The Urinary Bladder
- The Ureter

Posterior Gastrointestinal Parts Associated With the Female Reproductive System
- The Rectum
- The Anal Canal

Pelvic Musculature

Pelvic Cellular Tissue

Pelvic Blood Vessels

The Pelvic Lymphatics

Nerve Supply
- To the Vulva and the Perineum
- To the Pelvic Viscera

A thorough knowledge of the anatomy of the female genital organs is essential for understanding the various anomalies and the diseases associated with them.

The organs of the female reproductive system may be divided into the **external** and **internal genitalia**. The external genitalia are the vulva and vagina. The internal genitalia are the uterus with the cervix, Fallopian tubes, ovaries and other supporting structures. These internal organs can be visualised only with instruments such as the speculum for the cervix and the laparoscope for the uterus, tubes, ovaries and other organs.

## EXTERNAL GENITALIA

### The Vulva

The vulva comprises the following (Fig. 3.1):
- the mons pubis
- the labia majora
- the labia minora
- the clitoris
- the vestibule
- the external urinary meatus
- Bartholin's (vulvovaginal) glands
- the hymen
- the navicular fossa
- the fourchette

1. **The mons pubis (veneris)** is a mound of fat overlying the symphysis pubis and the lower part of the anterior abdominal wall. It is covered with coarse dark hair at puberty.

> **Clinical Importance**
>
> The normal female escutcheon is triangular in shape with the base facing upwards unlike in the male where the base of the triangle is downwards and the apex is towards the umbilicus.

2. **The labia majora** correspond to the scrotum in the male and consist of two rounded, longitudinal folds of skin extending from the mons veneris to enclose the pudendal cleft. They merge into the **perineum** about 3 cm anterior

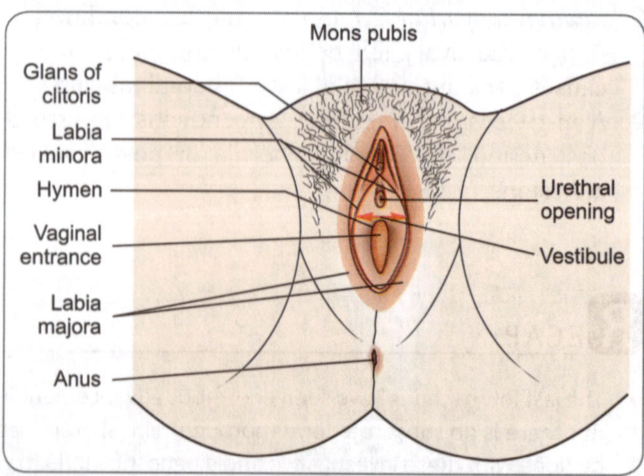


**Fig. 3.1** The female external genitalia

to the anus. At puberty, they are more prominent, pigmented and covered with coarse hair, especially over the outer surface. The labia majora contain

- areolar tissue
- sebaceous glands
- sweat glands (and their special variety, the apocrine glands)
- hair follicles
- the terminal portion of the round ligament anteriorly

**Clinical Importance**

In view of these structures the labia majora may become the seat of folliculitis, sebaceous cysts, rarely, a hydradenoma (a tumour arising from the apocrine glands) and endometriosis of the terminal part of the round ligament. Because of the loose areolar tissue, edema is marked in these labiae as in the eyelids.

3. **The labia minora** are smaller, smooth, thin folds located medial to the labia majora. They are lined by stratified squamous epithelium and do not contain hair follicles, sweat or sebaceous glands. Anteriorly, the labium minus splits to enclose the **clitoris** forming its hood or prepuce in front and the frenulum of the clitoris behind. The labia extend posteriorly and join to form the **fourchette** in the midline. This transverse fold is often torn at child birth.

**Extent of Labium Minus**

| | |
|---|---|
| Anteriorly | Labium minus splits to enclose the **clitoris** forming its hood or prepuce in front and the frenulum of the clitoris behind. |
| Posteriorly | The labia extend posteriorly and join to form the **fourchette** in the midline. |

4. **The vestibule** is located between the labia minora. The **external urinary meatus** opens into it. The boat-shaped **navicular fossa** is situated in front of the fourchette and is bounded in front by the hymen.
5. **The hymen** is a thin membrane covered by squamous epithelium on each side and surrounds the vaginal orifice. It partially covers the vagina enabling only the tip of the finger to pass through the introitus. However, the hymenal membrane is torn or ruptured in coitus, and further lacerations occur during childbirth resulting in small tags of skin known as **carunculae myrtiformis**.

   Presence of an intact hymen was once considered as an indication of virginity. Though tearing of hymen during first intercourse happens frequently, intercourse is not the only condition where the hymen could be torn. Conditions like injury, medical examination, masturbation, use of tamponade or physical exercise can also cause hymenal tear. For these reasons, the state of the hymen is not a reliable indicator of virginity. According to the WHO, "The hymen is a poor marker of penetrative sexual activity or virginity in postpubertal girls." (WHO -Strengthening medico-legal response to sexual violence, 2015). Similarly, according to the Independent Forensic Expert Group's Statement on virginity testing (2015) "Virginity testing (virginity examination) is a gynecological examination that is intended to correlate the status and appearance of the hymen with previous sexual contact. ... The IFEG concludes that virginity examinations are medically unreliable and have no clinical or scientific value." Hence too much significance should not be given to the state of hymen as far as virginity is considered.

**Clinical Importance**

Though the hymenal membrane is generally annular, it is sometimes cribriform or sieve-like with holes in it. Occasionally it may completely close the vaginal orifice. In such cases the vagina may become distended with the menstrual discharge after menarche to give rise to **cryptomenorrhea** and **hematocolpos.**

6. **The external urinary meatus** lies between the clitoris in front and the vagina behind. It appears like a circular or slit-like opening with raised margins. It is lined with transitional epithelium, with the vascular mucosa often protruding through it. Immediately within the urethra on its posterolateral aspects are two small orifices leading to shallow tubular ducts known as **Skene's glands** which are homologous to the prostate in the male.

**Clinical Importance**

The Skene's glands are susceptible to gonococcal infection.

7. **Bartholin's (vulvovaginal) glands** are situated posterolaterally around the vaginal orifice, deep to the bulbospongiosus muscle and superficial to the outer layer of the triangular ligament. The gland is about 10 mm in diameter and **lies at the junction of the middle and posterior third of the labium majus.** Its duct, about 2 cm long, passes forward and inwards to open external to the hymen on the inner side of the labium minus. These glands are of a compound, racemose type and the acini are lined by low columnar epithelium.

Though the surface epithelium lines the orifice of these ducts, deeper down it is lined by transitional epithelium. Bartholin's glands are **'coital lubricators'** as they secrete clear mucus during sexual excitement.

**Clinical Importance**

Though normally these glands are not palpable, they can be felt when enlarged or inflamed mostly due to gonococcal infection, to form Bartholin's abscess or cyst. Rarely, they are the seat of adenocarcinoma of the vulva.

## The Vagina

The vagina is a tubular, muscular canal extending from the hymenal orifice below to the cervix uteri above. As it is attached to the cervix slightly higher up posteriorly, the posterior vaginal wall is longer (10–11 cm) and the posterior fornix deepest compared to the anterior vaginal wall which is about 8 cm. Its anterior and posterior walls are ordinarily close together except in its upper part where it is most distensible. The direction of the vaginal canal is slightly curved and directed upwards and backwards. The vaginal walls are thrown into transverse folds or **rugae** in nulliparous women but in the multiparae they are usually stretched out.

In the anterior vaginal wall, **three transverse sulci** establish themselves as important landmarks: **below the external urinary meatus, at the vesico-urethral junction, and near the vagino-cervical junction where the bladder is attached to the anterior vaginal wall.**

### Anatomical relations of the vagina

The anterior vaginal wall is in close contact with the urethra in its lower half and with the base of the bladder in its upper half, and is separated from it by a **vesicovaginal space**. Posteriorly, the vagina is related to the anal canal in its lower third (separated from it by the perineal body), to the rectum in its middle third and to the pouch of Douglas in its upper third. Laterally, from below upwards, the vestibular bulb, the superficial perineal muscles, the levator ani (separating the vagina from the ischiorectal fossa), the pelvic cellular tissue or paracolpos and Mackenrodt's ligaments (with the ureter) are related to the vaginal canal.

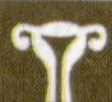

**Clinical Importance**

Due to the intimate relationship of the vaginal wall with the base of the bladder and with the urethra, a cystocele and sometimes a urethrocele form when the anterior vaginal wall prolapses.

**Relationship of the Vagina**

| | |
|---|---|
| Anterior vaginal wall | Is in close contact with the urethra in its lower half and base of the bladder in its upper half |
| Posteriorly | Anal canal in its lower third separated from it by the perineal body to the rectum in its middle third, pouch of Douglas in its upper third |
| Laterally, from below upwards | the vestibular bulb<br>the superficial perineal muscles<br>the levator ani<br>the pelvic cellular tissue or paracolpos<br>Mackenrodt's ligaments |

### Structure of the vaginal wall

The vaginal wall consists of

- mucosa
- a sub-mucosal layer composed mainly of areolar tissue
- blood vessels
- lymphatic follicles but no nodes
- a muscular layer (outer longitudinal and inner circular) surrounded by paravaginal fascia beyond it

The mucosa varies in its thickness and structure depending on the age and phase of the menstrual cycle. It consists of stratified squamous epithelium which is thin before puberty and after menopause. During reproductive life, it becomes thicker and multilayered with basal cuboid cells, a middle layer of prickle cells and superficial layers of cornified epithelium in response to the sex hormones. The top layers are rich in glycogen (estrogen-dependent) and some of these squames are shed and acted on by the gram-positive Doderlein bacilli present in the vagina, converting this glycogen into lactic acid. This action is responsible for maintaining the pH of the vagina at about 4.5 and preventing the growth of pathogens.

**Clinical Importance**

However, with menopause (and also prior to puberty) the vaginal mucosa is thin and devoid of glycogen due to the absence of estrogenic stimulus, and hence the pH of the vagina is alkaline. Therefore the vagina is vulnerable to gonococcal or other bacterial infections which lead to conditions such as gonococcal vaginitis and senile vaginitis.

The vaginal pool contains desquamated epithelial cells from the cervix, uterus and vagina. These cells are aspirated and the smears are Papanicolaou-stained for the early detection of genital cancer, especially of the cervix.

## INTERNAL GENITALIA

### The Uterus

The uterus is an inverted pear-shaped organ 8 cm × 5 cm × 3 cm located at right angles to the vagina, and with the bladder below and in front of it (Fig. 3.2).

The uterus is divided into two parts at the level of the internal os

- the corpus or body
- the cervix

**Clinical Importance**

The internal os is an important landmark as the peritoneum is reflected from the superior surface of the bladder to the anterior surface of the uterus. It is also at this level that the uterine artery reaches the uterus after traversing the base of the broad ligament and courses upward along its side wall.

The junctional tissue between the uterus and the cervix is called the **isthmus** (Fig. 3.3) and it lies between the endometrium of the corpus and the endocervix. The isthmus is hardly 6 mm wide in the non-pregnant condition.

**Relationship of the Isthmus**

| | |
|---|---|
| Above | The anatomical internal os |
| Below | The histological internal os |

During pregnancy it grows to form the lower uterine segment and is about 10 cm wide at term.

#### The cervix uteri

The cervix is about 2.5 cm in length and in diameter and is divided equally into the vaginal and supra-vaginal portions.

The **vaginal portion** protrudes into the vaginal vault to form the anterior, lateral and posterior fornices. It is a firm, fibro-muscular structure through which the spindle-shaped cervical canal traverses and opens below into the vagina at the external os.

In the **supra-vaginal portion,** the canal communicates above with the uterine cavity through the internal os. The mucous membrane of the vaginal portion is continuous with that of the vagina. The endocervical lining is columnar and in some areas, it forms folds or crypts extending into the muscular tissue to form mucus-producing 'glands'. It is now known that these are infoldings of the mucus-secreting membrane. **The clear mucus secretion from the cervix is thinnest and most abundant at the time of ovulation, thus facilitating sperm migration.** It also gives rise to **ferning** in the follicular phase.

**Clinical Importance**

In these crypts, gonococci may be harboured and can give rise to gonococcal cervicitis.

The **external os** is circular in nullipara but during parturition, the circular muscle fibres at the external os tear to produce a slit-like appearance and give rise to the anterior and posterior lips of the cervix.

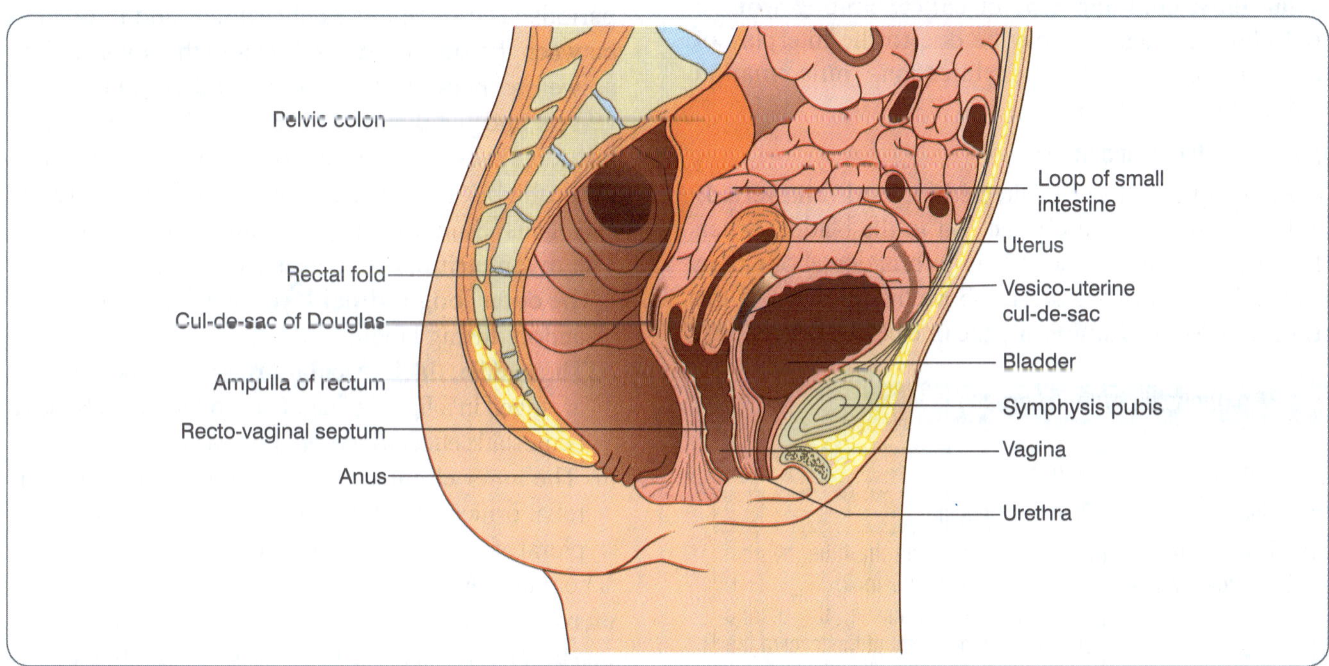


**Fig. 3.2** Median section through the female pelvis showing the pelvic viscera (*Source:* etc.usf.edu)

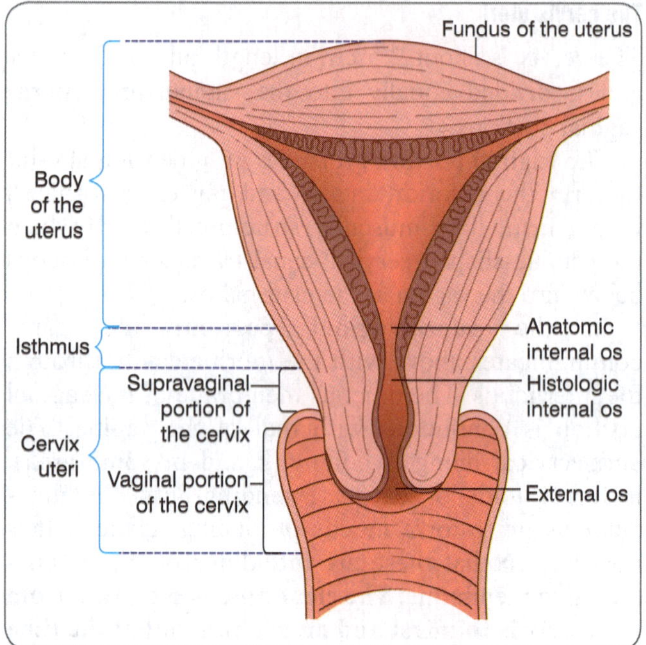


**Fig. 3.3** Coronal section of the uterus and the cervix

The external os is the site of the junction between the columnar and the squamous epithelium. The vaginal part of the cervix around the os, in certain conditions, shows evidence of erosion or replacement of the thick squamous epithelium with the thin columnar epithelium of the endocervix. Similarly the chances of severe dysplasia, carcinoma-in-situ and invasive squamous cell carcinoma are relatively high at this site. **Squamous cell carcinoma arising in this area is the most common type of cancer among women in India**. Perhaps this may be due to the interplay of different forces—hormones, infections, inflammation and trauma—at this site.

### Normal position of the uterus

The body of the uterus is directed forward (**anteverted**) and bent on itself (**anteflexed**) on to the bladder when the latter is empty. The uterus is broader above than below. The part of the uterus above the insertion of the tubes is called the **fundus** and the one below, the **corpus.**

**Relationship of the Uterus**

| | |
|---|---|
| In front | Bladder |
| Behind | Pouch of Douglas |
| Laterally from above downwards | Broad ligament (with the tube, ovarian and round ligaments in it) (Fig. 3.4), the pelvic cellular tissue, the uterine vessels and the ureter at the level of the cervix and to Mackenrodt's ligaments |

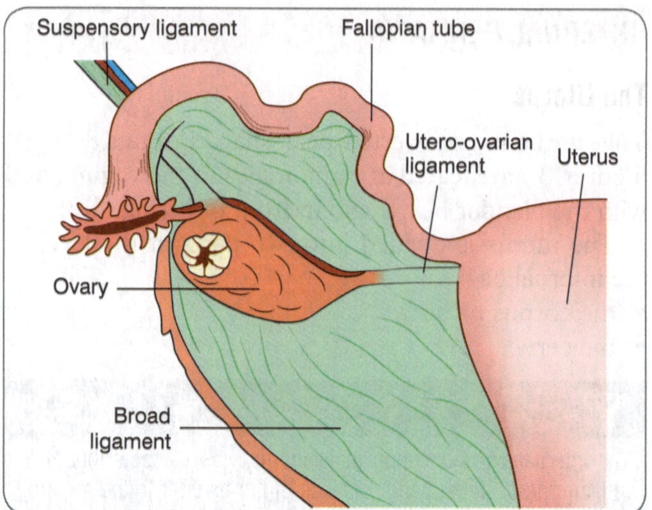


**Fig. 3.4** The structures in the broad ligament

### Structure of the uterus

The uterus consists of three layers:

- the inner mucosa or the endometrium
- the middle muscular layer or the myometrium
- the outer serosal layer, the perimetrium or peritoneum

1. The **endometrium** varies in thickness (3–7 mm) during the menstrual cycle and forms the decidua during pregnancy in response to the hormones.

   The **surface epithelium** is cuboidal or low columnar and ciliated. The endometrial glands are simple tubular in the postmenstrual phase and become tall and tortuous with the approach of the periods. The stroma is richly cellular and intervenes between the surface epithelium and the myometrium as well as between the glands, and contains blood vessels and lymphatics. Except for its deeper basal portion, most of the endometrium is discarded cyclically but regenerates rapidly in response to the estrogens. Similarly, it regenerates after delivery.
2. The **myometrium** also consists of three layers:
   i. The **outer longitudinal layer** which has a detrusor action during labour.
   ii. The **middle, thick vascular layer** which, because it is arranged in a figure of eight around the vessels, has a hemostatic effect to prevent postpartum hemorrhage.
   iii. The **inner circular layer** which is seen around the tubal orifices, the internal and external ora (ora = plural of 'os'), and probably has a sphincteric action.
3. The **peritoneum** covering the bladder forms the uterovesical pouch as it passes on to the front of the uterus and is later densely attached to the uterus anteriorly over the fundus and posteriorly covering

the uterus fully. It also extends downwards to clothe the posterior surface of the supra-vaginal cervix and the upper third of the vagina before it passes over the rectum to form the **pouch of Douglas**.

The non-pregnant uterus weighs about 80 g and has an endometrial cavity which can hold 5–7 mL of fluid. But with pregnancy, the uterus grows to about 1000 g at term and has a capacity of 4000 ml.

The pouch of Douglas is the deepest part of the peritoneal cavity and any fluid, exudate, blood or pus in the peritoneum is collected in this pouch. In endometriosis or malignancy of, say, the ovary, the cells or tissue deposit here to form nodular deposits. This pouch can easily be reached in pelvic examination (rectal rather than vaginal) and the pathology in this area can easily be identified by rectal examination.

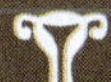
**Clinical Importance**

By culdocentesis, the pus or blood collected in the Douglas pouch can be readily aspirated in suspected cases of pelvic abscess or in ruptured tubal pregnancy.

## The Uterine Appendages

### The broad ligaments

These are thin folds of the peritoneum extending from each side of the uterus to the pelvic side wall. They enclose the **Fallopian tube** at the upper border, the round ligament and ovarian ligament, the **Wolffian duct** and its vestiges, the areolar tissue and the ureter at the base. The portion of the broad ligament between the tube and the ovary is called the **mesosalpinx** (Fig. 3.5). The outer border of the broad ligament forms the **infundibulopelvic ligament** which is prominent when the ovary is lifted. This ligament which connects the infundibular portion of the tube to the pelvic side wall contains ovarian vessels.

### The round ligament

This ligament arises from the uterine cornu. It passes laterally and forwards in the anterior layer of the broad ligament and enters the internal inguinal ring to traverse the inguinal canal and terminates in the substance of the labium majus. It is homologous to the gubernaculum testis and is continuous with the ovarian ligament. It consists of connective tissue and plain muscle. These ligaments are usually lax except during labour when they anchor the uterus.

The round ligaments are supplied by a branch of the ovarian artery derived from its anastomosis with the uterine artery.

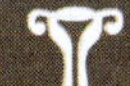
**Clinical Importance**

The lymphatics from the fundus of the uterus drain along the round ligament into the superficial inguinal group. This has to be kept in mind while managing an endometrial carcinoma.

### The ovarian ligaments

These ligaments lie in the posterior peritoneal fold of the broad ligament and connect the inner pole of the ovary to the posterior part of the uterine cornua just below the tubal insertion. They are about 2–5 cm long and are morphologically and structurally similar to the round ligament.

## The Fallopian Tubes

Each tube is about 10 cm long and extends from the uterine cornua outwards and backwards in the broad ligament to connect the uterine cavity to the outside, near the ovary, for picking up and transporting the ovum. It consists of four parts.

1. The **interstitial or intramural part** is enclosed within the cornual myometrium. This is the shortest and narrowest part (the lumen is 1 mm in diameter) of the tube.
2. The **isthmial part** is about 2.5 cm long and the tubal lumen is about 2 mm in diameter.
3. The **ampullary part** is the longest (7 cm) and widest portion.
4. The **infundibular** or funnel-shaped part opens as fimbriae or finger-like processes. One of the fimbriae, the **ovarian fimbria**, is longer and connects to the ovary.

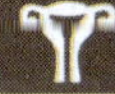
**Clinical Importance**

Just before ovulation, the tube becomes turgid and expands medially over the ovary to 'catch the egg'.

### *Structure*

The tubal wall consists of

- the serosa or peritoneum which covers most of it except the cornual portion and the inferior border
- the muscular layer, consisting of the outer longitudinal and inner circular fibres
- the mucosa which has two or three folds near the isthmial region but is thrown into innumerable folds or plicae when traced laterally

These tubal plicae consist of cellular stroma lined by tubal epithelium (which is mostly ciliated columnar or low cuboidal) to help propel the tubal contents towards the uterus. Besides the ciliated epithelium, there are

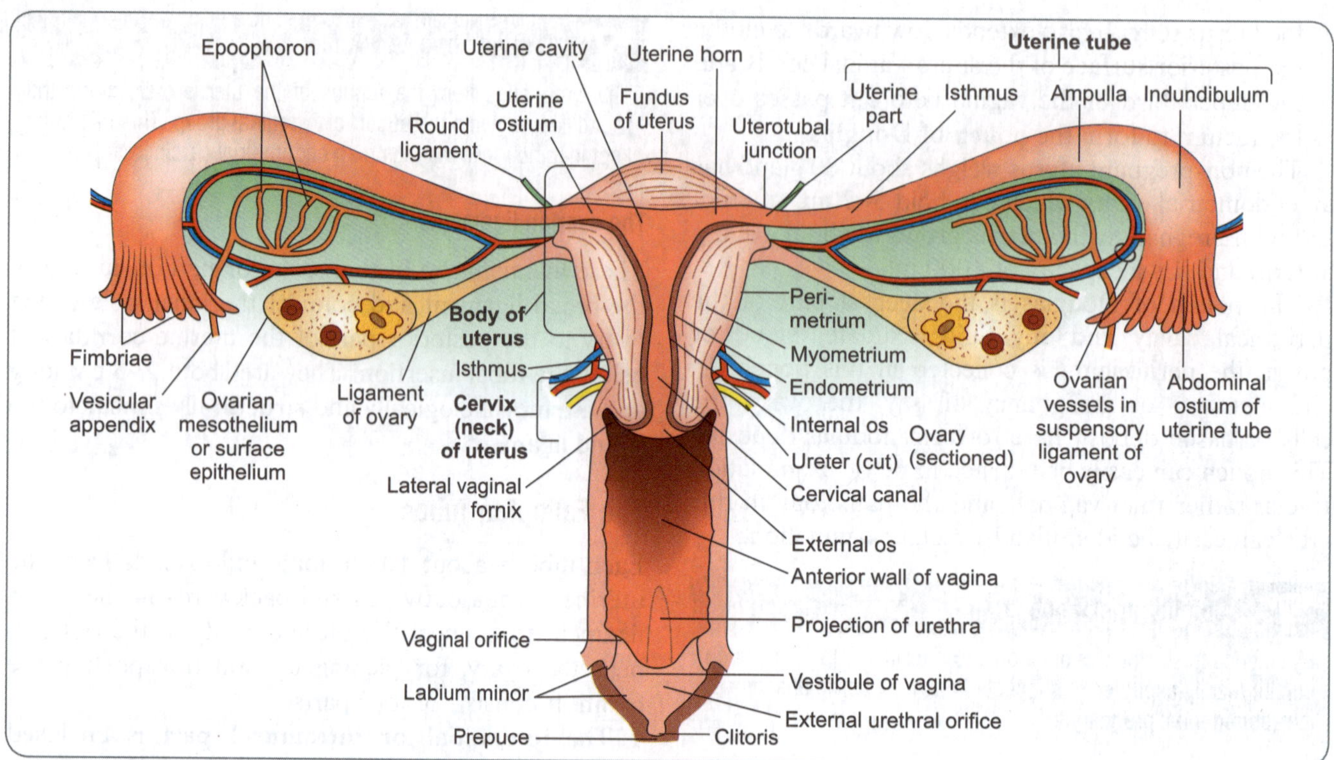

**Fig. 3.5** Posterior surface of the broad ligament and other adnexa

goblet-shaped non-ciliated cells and intercalary, rod-shaped or peg cells. **The tubal mucosa also responds cyclically to the hormones during the menstrual cycle.**

### *Tubal functions*

**The Fallopian tube is derived from the cranial end of the Müllerian duct** and its lumen is therefore continuous with the uterine cavity and the cervical canal. Sperms can thus easily travel upwards through the cervix and uterus into the tubal lumen to fertilise the ovum. Dye injected through the cervix should pass into the peritoneal cavity to confirm tubal patency.

### *Blood supply*

The Fallopian tube has a **dual blood supply**—the medial half is supplied from the tubal branch of the uterine artery and the lateral half from the tubal branch of the ovarian artery.

The **tubal lymphatics** communicate with those of the uterine fundus and of the ovary to drain along the infundibulopelvic ligament to the aortic group.

## The Ovary

The ovaries form the gonads in the female. Each ovary is an ovoid structure about 3.5 cm × 2.0 cm × 1.5 cm. They are a dull white and are attached to the superior aspect of the broad ligament by a short peritoneal fold called the **mesovarium.**

**Surface of the Ovary**

| | |
|---|---|
| In children | Ovary is smooth |
| In young adults | Follicles or corpus luteal cysts may be seen |
| In postmenopausal women | Ovary is atrophied with its surface grooved or pitted |

### *Anatomical relationship*

The ovary often lies in the ovarian fossa below the bifurcation of the common iliac artery with the internal iliac artery.

**Anatomical Relationship of the Ovary**

| | |
|---|---|
| Posteromedially | internal iliac artery ureter |
| Anterior and above | Fallopian tube |
| Anterior | attached to the broad ligament at the hilum |
| Medially | the ovarian ligament connects it to the uterine cornu |
| laterally | the ovarian fimbria to the tube |

### *Structure*

On section, the ovary can be divided into two areas:

- the cortex which is dense and compact
- the medulla which is soft and vascular

**The cortex** consists of a specialised ovarian stroma with numerous follicles in different phases of development and atrophy.

It is covered by the thick tunica albuginea which lies just below the so-called germinal epithelium (germ cells are not derived from this layer) which in turn is continuous with the peritoneum.

In the hilar area, occasionally there may be a few large polyhedral cells.

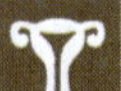

**Clinical Importance**

The ovary is not static in its location but moves with the uterus and the broad ligament, especially during pregnancy and after delivery. The tubes and ovaries, often collectively called the **uterine adnexa**, are so intimately related to each other that when the tube is inflamed, the ovary is also affected resulting in salpingo-oophoritis.

The ovary is the most common site of endometriosis and, rarely, becomes the seat of extrauterine gestation.

**The epoophoron** consists of several vestigial tubules in the mesosalpinx (between the tube and the ovary) and can be easily recognised on stretching the mesosalpinx. The **paroophoron** consists of a few vertical tubules in the mesosalpinx above the ovary and medial to the epoophoron. Both these structures are derived from the Wolffian body.

The **Wolffian duct** or **Gartner's duct** runs parallel to the Fallopian tube in the mesosalpinx just below the tube. Later, it descends by the side of the uterus to the level of the internal os merging into the substance of the cervix. It finally runs forward on the anterolateral aspect of the anterior vaginal wall to the level of the hymen.

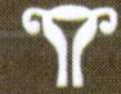

**Clinical Importance**

Though it is imperfectly developed, the Gartner's duct may lead to cysts in the anterior part of the vagina known as **Gartner's cyst.**

## URINARY SYSTEM—PARTS ASSOCIATED WITH THE FEMALE REPRODUCTIVE SYSTEM

### The Female Urethra

The urethra is about 4–5 cm long and 6 mm wide (though dilatable). It extends from the neck of the bladder through the pelvic cavity along the anterior vaginal wall to end at the external meatus. Most of its lining consists of stratified squamous epithelium though further up it is transitional. Deeper to the mucosal layer are veins, connective tissue and smooth muscle. As it pierces the triangular ligament, the voluntary compressor urethrae surround it.

### The Urinary Bladder

The urinary bladder is located between the uterus and the symphysis pubis. It is pyramidal in shape when empty, with its apex directed upwards as the urachus which is continuous with the median umbilical ligament extraperitoneally.

- The bladder has a triangular base or fundus related to the cervix and the upper part of the anterior vaginal wall.
- Its superior surface is covered by peritoneum and its two inferolateral surfaces are related to the retropubic pad of fat.
- The trigone of the bladder is a smooth triangular area formed by the two ureteric orifices above and the internal urinary meatus below (Fig. 3.2).

#### *Structure*

The bladder wall consists of three layers:

- the mucosa which is lined by transitional epithelium and underlying loose connective tissue (favouring its distension)
- the muscle, mainly the detrusor, which helps in emptying the bladder
- the peritoneum

At the vesico-urethral junction, there is a complicated set of smooth muscle slings around the bladder neck and upper urethra, which form a smooth muscle sphincter or internal sphincter. Some of these involuntary muscle fibres pass down to the urethra. The voluntary muscles such as the anterior fibres of the puborectalis which surround the urethra also possess some sphincteric action. The compressor urethrae located between the layers of the triangular ligament also act as an external sphincter preventing the escape of urine. It helps in emptying the urethra at the end of micturition.

#### *The bladder and the urethra during micturition*

The anatomy of the vesico-urethral junction is important in understanding the physiopathology of micturition. Normally the bladder is at rest and the urethra forms a well-marked angle of 100° posteriorly.

During micturition, this posterior urethro-vesical angle (PUV angle) is abolished as it straightens out to 180°. In most women with urinary stress incontinence this angle is obliterated completely both at rest and during coughing or straining.

**Clinical Importance**

A line drawn from the upper urethra to the perpendicular forms an angle of 35°. This angle is disturbed in cases of urinary stress incontinence.

The normal capacity of the bladder is about 500 ml. When it reaches about 250 ml, there is a desire to micturate but this can be ignored and the bladder muscle can accommodate more with the intravesical pressure still remaining at 10 cm of water. When the volume exceeds 500 ml, there is an urgent desire to empty the bladder. If the time and place are convenient, signals are sent through the higher centre, the hypothalamus and S2, 3 and 4, to the detrusor to contract, raise the intra-abdominal pressure by contraction of the abdominal muscles and obliterate the PUV angle. The intravesical pressure rises to 50–100 cm of water, the internal sphincter opens from above downwards, the compressor urethrae relax and the urine is voided. At the end of micturition, the urethra closes from below upwards and the compressor urethrae return the residual urine to the bladder.

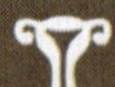

**Clinical Importance**

The closeness of the bladder to the anterior vaginal wall explains why the bladder descends as a cystocele whenever there is descent of the vagina. It also explains the risk of injury, direct or indirect, to the bladder resulting in vesicovaginal fistula during surgical repair of the anterior vaginal wall (as in genital prolapse) or due to prolonged compression by the fetal head in cases of neglected labour.

### *Blood supply to the bladder*

The bladder neck is supplied by the **vesical artery—a branch of the internal iliac artery**—and by anastomotic vessels from the vagina and cervix. Venous drainage is to the hypogastric vein.

The urethra is supplied by the terminal branches of the **internal pudendal artery.**

### *Lymphatic drainage*

The urethral lymphatics drain to the superficial inguinal group of nodes and the vesical into the hypogastric group of nodes.

## The Ureter

### *Anatomy*

The ureter is 25 cm long and half of it lies in the pelvis (Fig. 3.6).

- It crosses the pelvic brim at the bifurcation of the common iliac artery.

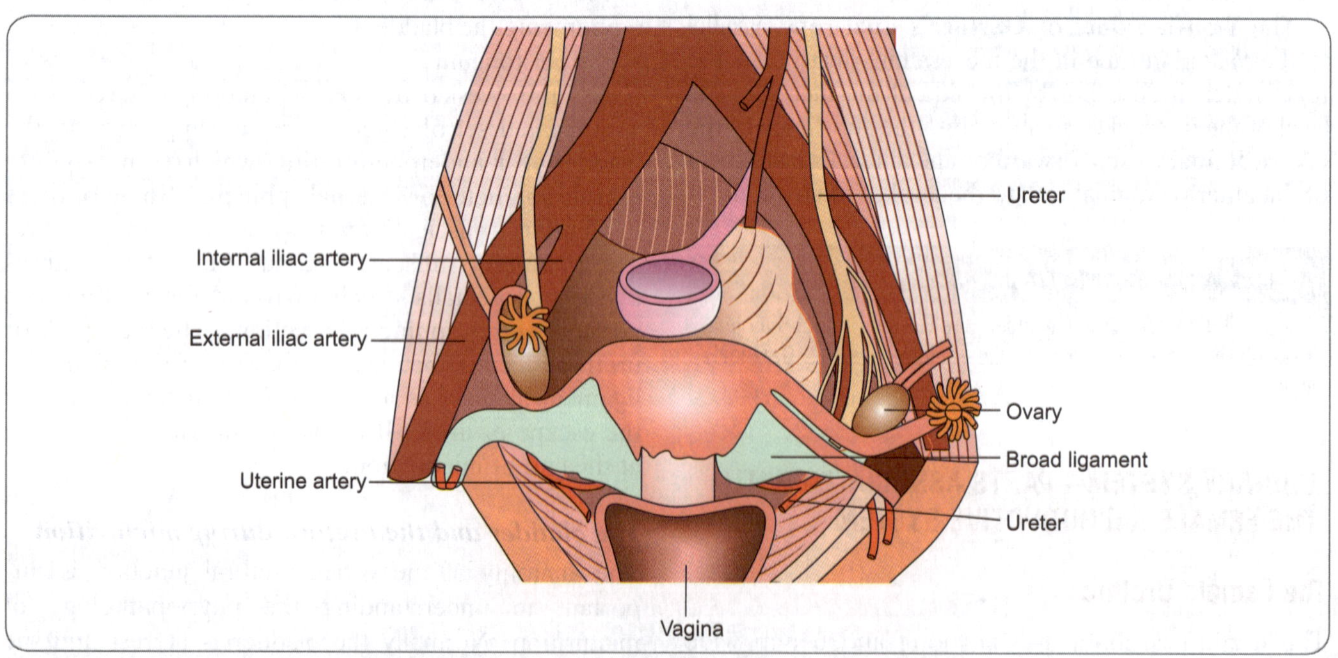


**Fig. 3.6** Anatomy of the pelvic part of the ureter

- It runs over the front of the internal iliac artery sub-peritoneally in the side wall of the pelvis posteroinferior to the ovary.
- At the level of the ischial spines, it curves forwards and medially at the base of the broad ligament piercing Mackenrodt's ligament to enter the ureteric canal.
- It passes below the uterine artery and veins at the level of the internal os.
- After leaving this canal, it passes forwards and medially to reach the bladder, piercing its posterosuperior angle.

The ureter can easily be recognised during surgery by its peristaltic movements and also by the way it feels (like a cord). Rarely, the ureter may be duplicated.

**Clinical Importance**

- When the ureter is stripped during radical surgery, there is a risk of ureteric fistula due to avascular necrosis.
- In advanced cervical carcinoma, the ureter may become obstructed leading to hydroureter, hydronephrosis and uremia. It may be displaced by tumours (especially broad ligament tumours or cervical myomas) or may be densely involved in pathological lesions such as adnexitis (pelvic inflammatory disease) or endometriosis. It is important for the gynecologist to know its course and its displacements so as to preserve it during gynecological surgery.
- The ureter is most likely to be injured during hysterectomy when the uterine vessels are clamped near the internal os. The ureter is very close by, passing under the uterine artery at this level (Fig. 3.7).

### *Blood supply to the pelvic ureter*

The ureter receives blood supply from the common iliac, internal iliac, uterine and inferior vesical arteries which form a rich anastomotic network over its wall (Fig. 3.8).

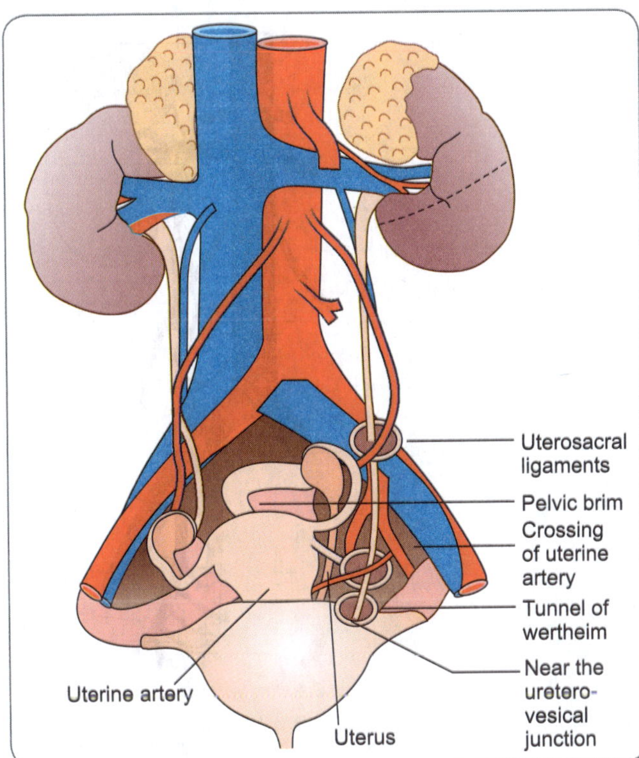


**Fig. 3.7** Sites of ureteric injury

## POSTERIOR GASTROINTESTINAL PARTS ASSOCIATED WITH THE FEMALE REPRODUCTIVE SYSTEM

### The Rectum

#### *Anatomy of the rectum*

The sigmoid colon continues to form the rectum at the level of the third sacral vertebra.

- It is about 12 cm long and follows the curve of the sacrum and coccyx in the sagittal plane and an S-shaped curve in the coronal plane before it ends as the anal canal.
- It is surrounded by the rectal fascia.
- The rectal wall consists of a thick outer longitudinal smooth muscle and inner circular muscle fibres.
- The larger part of the rectum is more distended and is called the ampulla.
- The peritoneum covers it anteriorly and on the sides in the upper third, and in the front in the mid-third; it does not cover it in its lower third.
- The upper part of the rectum is related to the pouch of Douglas and the ampulla to the vagina.
- Laterally, the uterosacral ligaments, and at its lower end the puborectalis muscle fibres, are attached to it; the ischiorectal fossa is lateral to the rectum and the anal canal.
- Posteriorly it lies over the sacrum and coccyx with nerve trunks, the middle sacral artery and loose areolar tissue.
- It is surrounded by the rectal fascia.

The rectal wall consists of a thick outer longitudinal smooth muscle and inner circular muscle fibres. The submucosa is loose and contains venous plexuses which when distended cause hemorrhoids or piles. The mucosa is thick with simple tubular glands.

#### *Blood supply to the rectum*

The rectum receives its blood supply from the superior hemorrhoidal branch of the inferior mesenteric artery, the middle rectal branch from the anterior division of the internal iliac artery, and the inferior hemorrhoidal

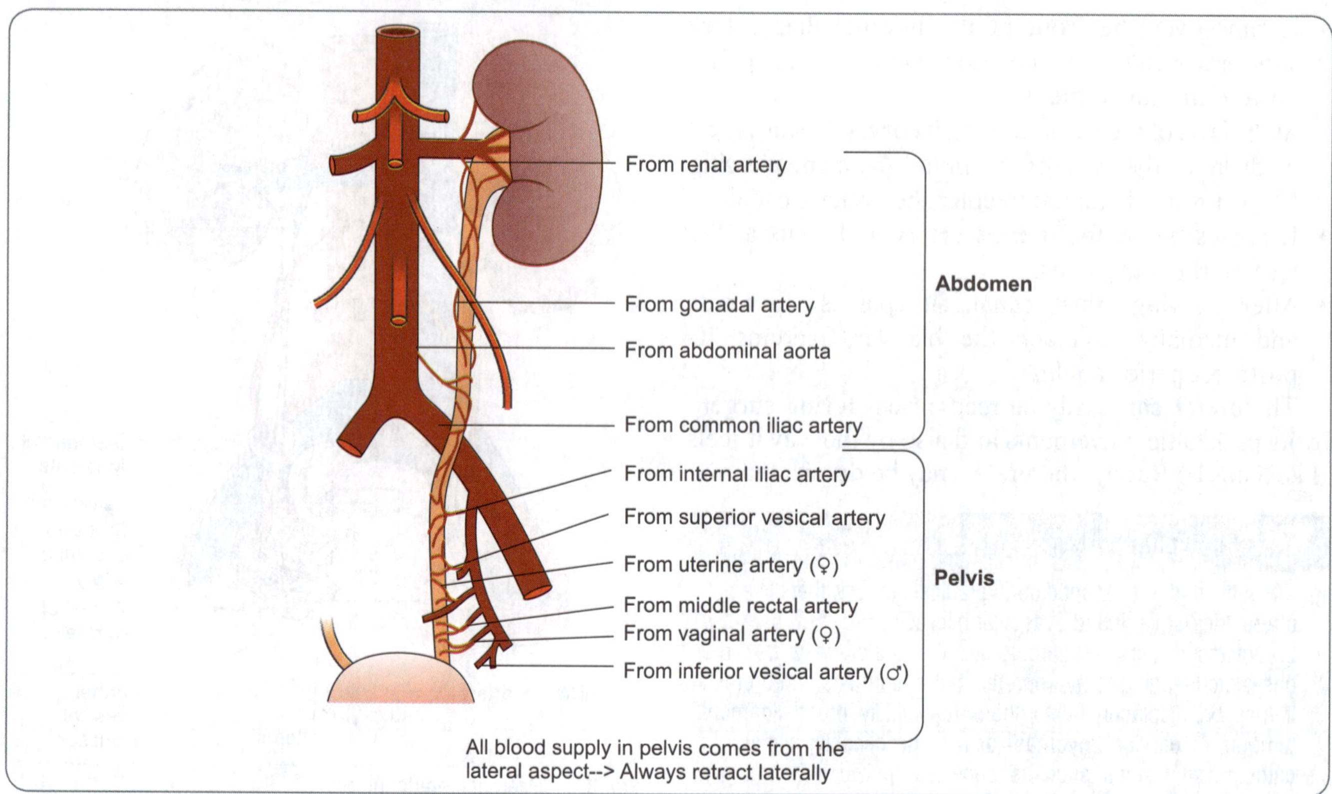


**Fig. 3.8** Blood supply to ureter

branch of the internal pudendal artery. The veins drain into the portal-systemic anastomosis.

## The Anal Canal

The terminal part of the large bowel or the anal canal is about 4 cm long. The lower third of the anal canal is lined by stratified squamous epithelium. It descends posteroinferiorly between the levator ani muscles to end at the anus. The internal sphincter is formed by the thickening of the circular smooth muscle of the upper two-thirds of the anal canal. The external sphincter surrounds the lower two-thirds of this canal. The puborectalis muscle surrounding the sides and posterior aspect of the anorectal junction acts as a voluntary sphincter. The mucosa of the canal in its upper two-thirds forms longitudinal ridges (**anal columns**) which are united below at a mucocutaneous junction by the horizontal semilunar folds (**anal valves**). These may be torn or infected to cause **'fissure in ano'**. The lower third of the anal canal is lined by stratified squamous epithelium.

The lymphatics from the lower part of the anal canal and perineum drain to the superficial inguinal group; those from the upper part drain to the internal iliac artery; other rectal lymphatics pass to the sacral, the common iliac and lumbar nodes.

### Perianal abscess

An anal abscess is a painful condition in which pus collects near the anus. Perianal abscess is the most common type of anal abscess. Perianal abscess is a painful condition with all signs of symptoms of inflammation.

#### *Causes of anal abscesses*

- Anal fissure
- Sexually transmitted infections
- Blocked anal glands
- Colitis
- Inflammatory bowel disease such as Crohn's disease or ulcerative colitis
- Diabetes
- Diverticulitis
- Pelvic inflammatory disease

The most common symptoms are constant, throbbing, acute anal pain. This is usually associated with localised swelling, erythema and flatulence. This can be differentiated from other causes of acute anal pain such as anal fissure and thrombosed external hemorrhoid by history and gentle visual inspection. Usually a rectal examination would be sufficient to diagnose the condition, but sometimes an examination under anesthesia may be required.

The treatment of perianal abscess is incision and drainage. The drainage should be as close to the anus as possible to reduce the length of any subsequent fistulous tract.

## PELVIC MUSCULATURE

There are three groups of pelvic muscles:
- the levator ani and the coccygeus which together form the pelvic diaphragm
- the deep transverse perineal muscle in the urogenital diaphragm
- the superficial muscles of the pelvic floor

These three layers of muscles, from the fascia covering the levator ani above to the perineal skin below, constitute the pelvic floor.

1. The **levator ani** is a wide, fan-shaped, curved sheet of muscle.

**Origin and Insertion of the Levator Ani Muscle**

| | |
|---|---|
| Originates from | posterior aspect of the pubic bone, the ischial spine, and from the white line of the obturator fascia between these two points |
| Inserted into | anococcygeal raphe and the coccyx |

Together, the two levator ani muscles, one on either side, form a V-shaped gutter or the pelvic diaphragm allowing the urethra, vagina and rectum to pass through the space between them (Fig. 3.9).

Each levator ani is subdivided into three parts depending on its origin and location:
- the pubococcygeus (the medial-most)
- the iliococcygeus
- the ischiococcygeus

The inner fibres of the **pubococcygeus** which pass lateral and posterior to the rectum (designated puborectalis by some) form a sling to prevent the passage of faeces from the rectum to the anal canal.

Some of the **puborectalis** fibres are said to cross between the vagina and the rectum and these decussating fibres may tear during childbirth contributing to laxity of the pelvic floor and eventually leading to genital prolapse.

These muscles are covered by pelvic fascia and separate the pelvic cavity from the ischiorectal fossa.

The **pelvic diaphragm** made of the two levators supports the pelvic viscera. These levators act together to raise the pelvic diaphragm, and help in increasing intra-abdominal pressure during vomiting and defecation. These muscles also act as a sphincter to the rectum and the vagina. During labour, the mechanism of internal rotation is facilitated by the contraction of these muscles as they have a fixed origin anteriorly and a mobile insertion below and behind, so that the presenting part of the fetus which touches the pelvic floor first gets rotated forwards and inwards.

2. The **deep transverse perineal muscle** is situated between the two fascial layers of the urogenital diaphragm which extend from the pubic arch anteriorly to the central point of the perineum. This

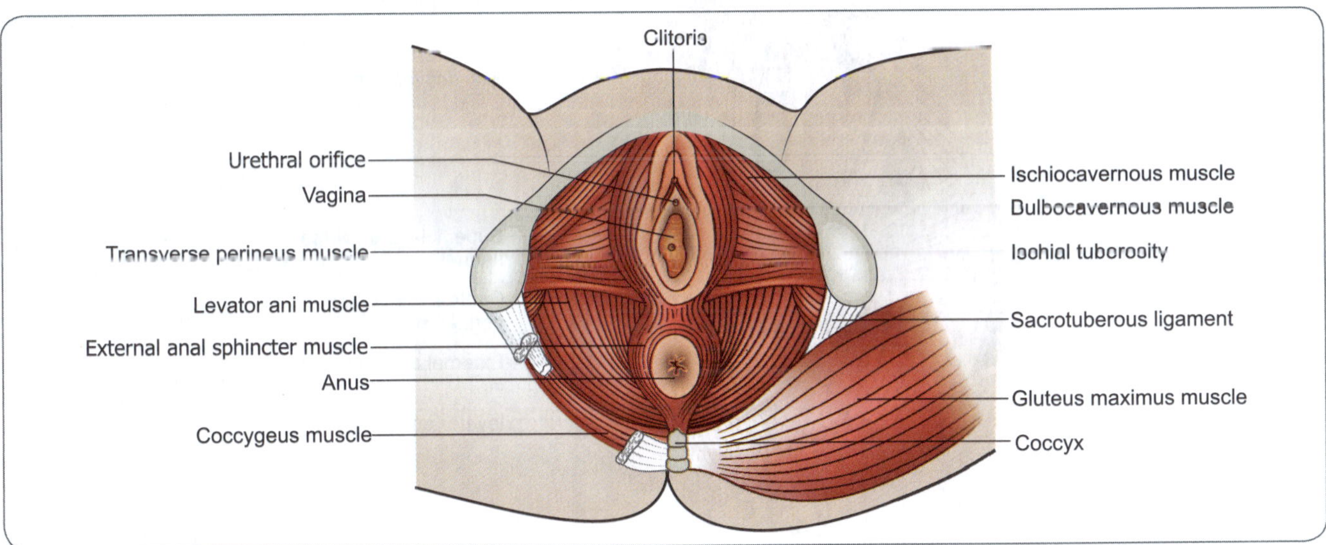


**Fig. 3.9** The levator ani muscles

muscle is poorly developed. The striated voluntary sphincter urethra also lies between the two layers of the triangular ligament.

3. The **superficial perineal muscles** consist of
   - the external sphincter ani which surrounds the anus and is attached to the central point of the perineum (Fig. 3.10).
   - the bulbospongiosus or the sphincter vagina which stretches on either side of the vagina from the central point of the perineum to the symphysis pubis anteriorly
   - the ischiocavernosus extending on either side from the ischial tuberosity to the crus of the clitoris
   - the superficial transverse perineal muscle extending laterally from the centre of the perineum to the pubic ramus on either side

   **The perineal body** comprises a pyramidal fibromuscular structure located between the lower third of the posterior vaginal wall and the anterior wall of the anal canal. The base is formed by the perineum and the apex is at the junction of the middle and lower third of the posterior vaginal wall.

   From below upwards, it consists of
   - superficial perineal muscles (the external sphincter ani, bulbospongiosus and superficial transvers perinei)
   - the deep transverse perinei enclosed in the triangular ligament
   - the medial fibres of the levator ani muscles

The tone of the perineal muscles can be gauged by palpating with two fingers in the vagina, and with the thumb applied externally.

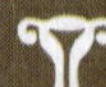 **Clinical Importance**

The perineal body may be lacerated leading to a patulous vagina and later to genital prolapse. In cases of complete perineal tear the patient will complain of fecal incontinence.

## PELVIC CELLULAR TISSUE

### *Anatomy*

The pelvic floor muscles support the pelvic organs only indirectly. The uterus is held in its position of anteversion and anteflexion slightly below the pelvic brim with the external os at about the level of the ischial spines. The levators are well below this level. Therefore the uterus is supported here mainly by ligaments and the connective tissue fills the space between the peritoneum above and the pelvic fascia covering the levator ani below. Laterally it extends to the fascia covering the obturator internus, and medially to the lateral wall of the uterus and the upper half of the vagina. It is continuous with the loose areolar tissue of the subperitoneal and perinephric spaces.

That part of the pelvic cellular tissue which surrounds the uterus is called the **parametrium** and which surrounds the vagina is called the **paracolpos,** which also covers the bladder, the supra-vaginal cervix and

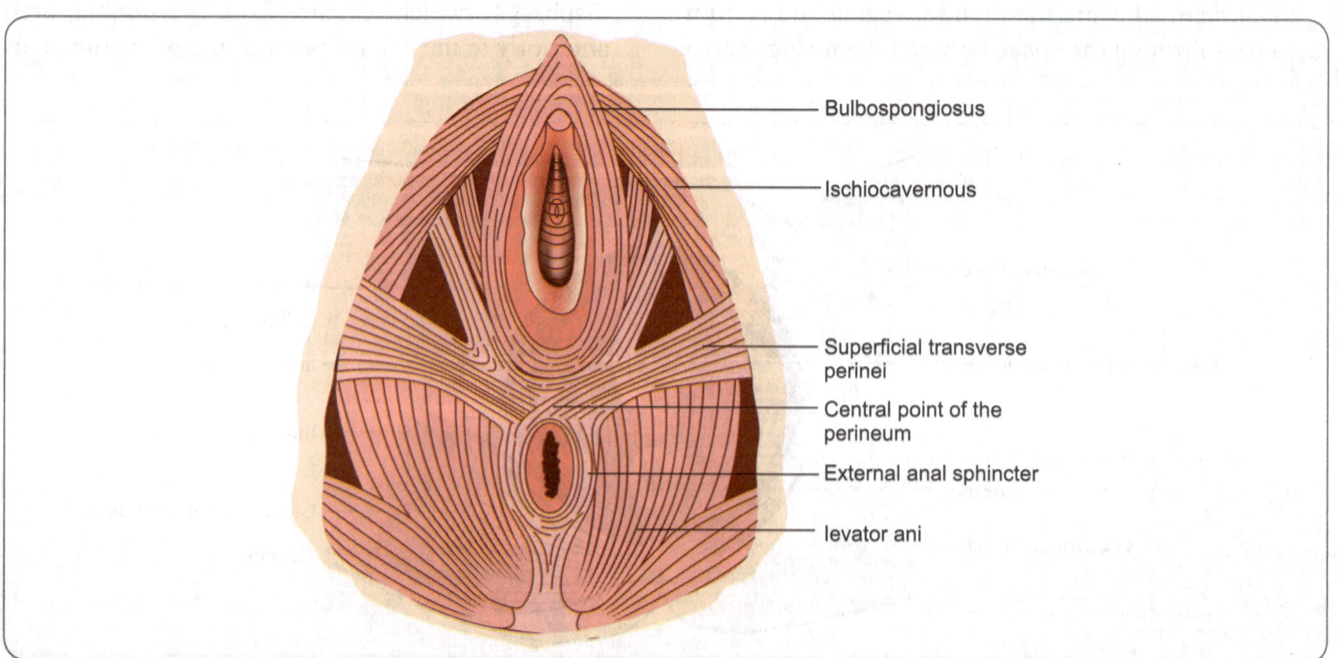


**Fig. 3.10** The superficial perineal muscles

rectum, forming fascial coverings to these organs. In the pelvic cellular tissue, there are uterine arteries, veins, lymphatics, sympathetic nerve ganglia and nerves, besides the ureters.

### *Ligaments supporting the uterus*

The pelvic cellular tissue is condensed to form ligaments supporting the uterus and other pelvic structures and fixing them to the side of the pelvis (Fig. 3.11).

- The **uterosacral ligaments** pass from the supravaginal portion of the cervix and the vagina backwards lateral to the rectum to be inserted into the second and third sacral vertebrae.
- The **transverse cervical ligaments, Mackenrodt's ligaments** (also called cardinal ligaments), extend from the cervix and from the upper part of the vagina, or to the side wall of the pelvis.
- Anteriorly, the **pubo-vesico-cervical ligament** plays an important role in supporting the cervix and the bladder.

While the uterosacral ligaments keep the uterus anteverted by pulling the cervix behind, the transverse cervical ligaments help prevent the descent of the uterus whenever there is increased intra-abdominal pressure.

**Clinical Importance**

When these three ligaments weaken, stretch due to repeated childbirths or atrophy with menopause, the uterus and the bladder descend leading to genital prolapse.

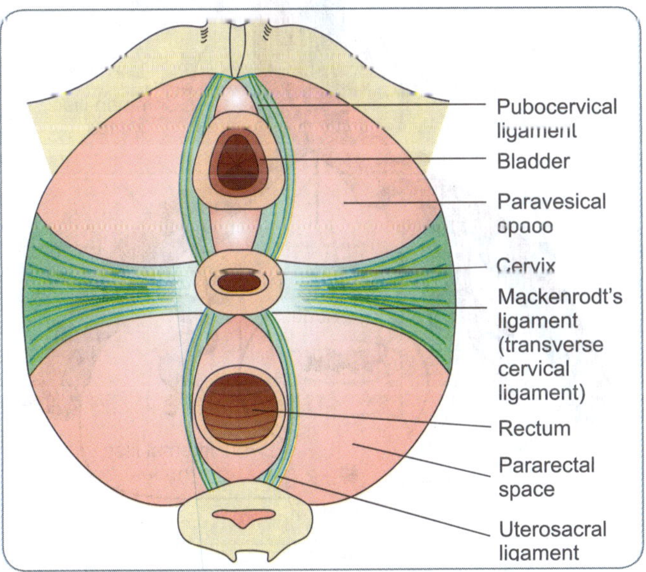


**Fig. 3.11** The pelvic cellular tissue and the ligaments of the cervix

**Clinical Importance**

In pelvic cellular tissue inflammation (pelvic cellulitis or parametritis), the lesion easily spreads from one side of the uterus and vagina to the side wall of the pelvis on either side because of its continuity. In rare cases, it may extend above the inguinal ligament or even up to the perinephric space.

In cases of pelvic inflammatory disease (PID) or malignancy of the cervix, a rectal examination reveals the extent of involvement of the pelvic cellular tissue by the pathological process.

## PELVIC BLOOD VESSELS

### The ovarian artery

- It arises from the aorta just below the renal artery.
- It runs downwards over the psoas muscle to the pelvic brim.
- At that level, it crosses the ureter and the external iliac artery before entering the infundibulopelvic fold of the peritoneum.
- Its branches supply the ovary and the outer part of the Fallopian tube, and anastomose with the terminal branches of the uterine artery.

### The uterine artery

- It is a branch of the anterior division of the internal iliac artery (Fig. 3.12).
- It passes along the base of the broad ligament.
- It then crosses medially above the ureter about 1.5–2 cm from the internal os to run tortuously along the lateral margin of the uterus.

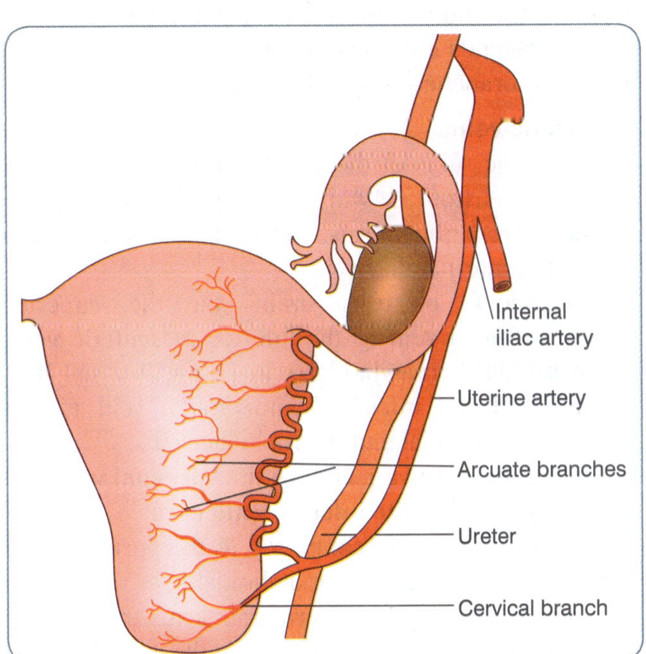


**Fig. 3.12** Blood supply to the uterus

- Finally, it anastomoses with the ovarian artery.
- During its course, it supplies a branch to the ureter, cervix and the upper part of the vagina, and sends several arcuate branches to the substance of the uterus.

### The vaginal arteries

- These arise from the anterior branch of the internal iliac artery and supply the lower part of the vagina.
- The upper part of the vagina is supplied by the vaginal branches of the uterine artery.

### The internal pudendal artery

- It mainly supplies the perineum and the external genitalia.
- It originates from the internal iliac artery.
- It then passes forwards over the sacral plexus.
- It leaves the pelvis through the inferior part of the greater sciatic foramen.
- Then it winds round the ischial spine to enter the ischiorectal fossa.
- At this point it gives off two branches: the inferior hemorrhoidal artery to the rectum and the transverse perineal artery supplying the perineum and the external sphincter.
- The main pudendal artery pierces the genital diaphragm and branches again to supply the posterior part of the labia and the erectile tissues around the vaginal orifice.
- It terminates as the dorsal artery of the clitoris.

### The superior hemorrhoidal artery

- It is the continuation of the inferior mesenteric artery and descends into the base of the pelvic mesocolon.
- Its two branches supply the rectum.

### The pelvic veins

- The pelvic veins of the bladder, uterus, vagina and rectum anastomose with each other freely.
- Those from the uterus, vagina and bladder drain into the internal iliac vein.
- The rectal plexuses drain via the superior hemorrhoidal vein to the inferior mesenteric vein, the middle hemorrhoidal vein to the internal iliac vein, and the inferior hemorrhoidal vein to the internal pudendal and internal iliac veins.
- **The left ovarian vein ends in the left renal vein and the right one in the inferior vena cava.**
- The pelvic veins are connected to the portal system through the superior hemorrhoidal vein which also communicates with the vertebral plexus through the middle and lateral sacral veins and the lateral lumbar veins.
- This explains occasional intracranial metastases from a primary pelvic cancer without any evidence of pulmonary involvement.

## THE PELVIC LYMPHATICS

Knowledge of the lymphatic drainage of the pelvic organs is essential for the management of pelvic malignancies. The lymphatics are one-way drainage channels from the organs; the nodes, on the other hand, act as filter points so that macrophages may destroy malignant cells before the lymph drains into the bloodstream through the thoracic duct.

The lymphatics from the genital organs drain into the following six groups of lymph nodes (Fig. 3.13):

**The hypogastric group** Most of these are located below the bifurcation of the common iliac artery. A few of the glands in this group are in the obturator fossa, below and behind the obturator nerve, and are often called the obturator group.

**The gland of the parametrium** This is an inconstant node situated at the point where the uterine artery crosses the ureter.

**The sacral group** This consists of a group lateral to the rectum and a medial group in front of the sacrum.

**The inguinal group** This consists of horizontal and vertical groups. The former lie superficially along the

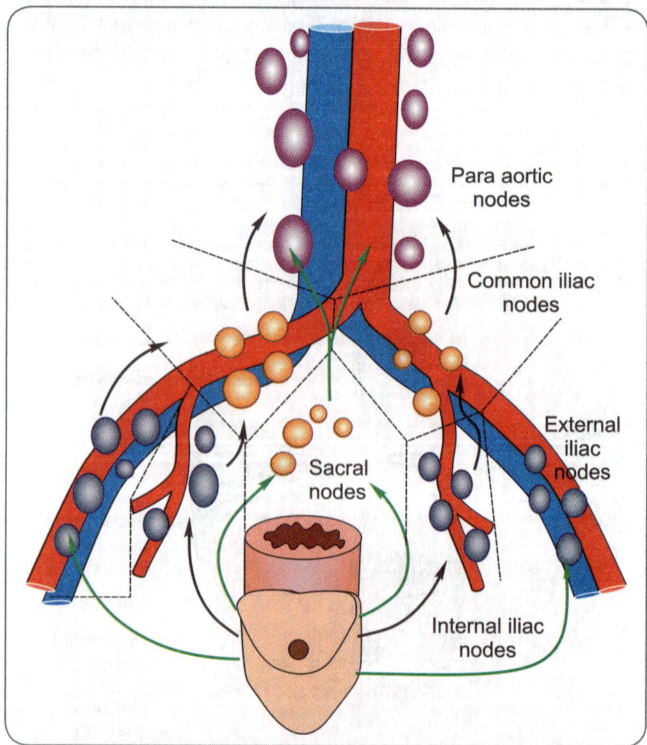


Fig. 3.13 Lymphatic drainage of the pelvic organs

inguinal ligament but the latter follow the course of the saphenous and femoral veins and are called the deep femoral glands. The uppermost of this femoral group is often called the **gland of Cloquet** and lies beneath the inguinal ligament in the femoral canal.

**The external iliac group** These glands are situated along the external iliac artery and vein. They drain the hypogastric group into the common iliac artery which in turn drains into the lumbar group.

**The lumbar or para-aortic group** This consists of two groups: the superior group near the origin of the ovarian artery and the inferior group below the origin of the inferior mesenteric artery.

These nodes receive most of the lymph from the other pelvic groups. They drain into the lumbar lymphatic trunk and the cisterna chyli at the level of the second lumbar vertebra. The lymph from the pelvis is finally carried by the thoracic duct through the thorax to be emptied into the junction of the left subclavian vein and the internal jugular veins.

The lymphatic vessels from different parts of the genital tract drain into the various lymph nodes as follows:

**The cervix** The cervical vessels drain laterally into the hypogastric and obturator groups besides the gland of the parametrium. Those along the uterosacral ligaments are received by the lateral sacral group.

**Lymphatic Drainage of Pelvic Organs**

| Organ | Node of lymphatic drainage |
|---|---|
| Cervix | Laterally to hypogastric and obturator groups |
| Body of the uterus | From lower part of the corpus into the hypogastric group.<br>From the fundus into the superior lumbar along with the ovarian lymphatics; some drain into the superficial inguinal group along the round ligaments. |
| Tubes and ovaries | Pass upwards along the infundibulopelvic ligament close to the superior lumbar group.<br>Free communication present between the ovarian lymphatics of each side across the fundus of the uterus |
| Vagina | Lower third of the vagina drain into the superficial inguinal group.<br>Upper two-thirds pass upwards to join the cervical lymphatics draining into the hypogastric group. |
| Tubes and ovaries | Pass upwards along the infundibulopelvic ligament close to the superior lumbar group.<br>Free communication present between the ovarian lymphatics of each side across the fundus of the uterus |
| Vagina | Lower third of the vagina drain into the superficial inguinal group.<br>Upper two-thirds pass upwards to join the cervical lymphatics draining into the hypogastric group. |
| Vulva | Vessels from the labia pass to the superficial inguinal glands.<br>From the clitoris, the lymphatics pass to the inguinal group and to the gland of Cloquet.<br>Those from Bartholin's glands into the deep femoral group through the gland of Cloquet to the external iliac group. |
| Bladder and urethra | Drain into the hypogastric group and those from the lower urethra to the vulval group. |
| Rectum and anal canal | Those from rectum drain into the hypogastric and inferior lumbar group.<br>Those from the anal canal flow into the superficial inguinal nodes. |

**The body of the uterus** The vessels from the lower part of the corpus drain into the hypogastric group and those from the fundus into the superior lumbar along with the ovarian lymphatics; some drain into the superficial inguinal group along the round ligaments.

**Tubes and ovaries** These pass upwards along the infundibulopelvic ligament close to the superior lumbar group. There is free communication between the ovarian lymphatics of each side across the fundus of the uterus.

**The vagina** The lymphatic vessels of the lower third of the vagina drain into the superficial inguinal group and those from the upper two-thirds pass upwards to join the cervical lymphatics draining into the hypogastric group.

**The vulva** The vessels from the labia pass to the superficial inguinal glands. From the clitoris, the lymphatics pass to the inguinal group and to the gland of Cloquet. Those from Bartholin's glands drain into the deep femoral group through the gland of Cloquet to the external iliac group.

**The bladder and urethra** These drain into the hypogastric group and those from the lower urethra to the vulval group.

**The rectum and anal canal** The vessels from the rectum drain into the hypogastric and inferior lumbar group whereas those from the anal canal flow into the superficial inguinal nodes.

## NERVE SUPPLY

### To the Vulva and the Perineum

**The pudendal nerve** This is derived from the S2, S3, S4 segments and issues out of the pelvis through the greater sciatic notch, crosses behind the ischial spine and passes through the lesser sciatic foramen into Alcock's canal on the lateral wall of the ischiorectal fossa. Here it gives off the inferior hemorrhoidal nerve and divides into two terminal branches: the larger, perineal branch supplying the posterior part of the labia and the muscles of the perineum, and the smaller, dorsal nerve of the clitoris.

#### Clinical Importance

1. The pudendal nerve is important as it plays a role in the mechanism of copulation (erection and ejaculation in the male), parturition, micturition and defecation. The levator ani muscles are supplied directly from $S_3$ and $S_4$.
2. In a pudendal block, the pudendal nerve is infiltrated around the ischial spines. It provides effective vulval and perineal anesthesia enabling one to perform obstetric procedures such as forceps delivery.

**The ilio-inguinal nerve (L1)** This issues out of the superficial inguinal ring and supplies the sensory fibres to the skin of the mons and the upper part of the labium majus.

**The genitofemoral nerve** Through the genital branch (LI and L2), this nerve carries the sensory impulses from the inner aspect of the thigh and the outer aspect of the labium majus.

### To the Pelvic Viscera

The nerve fibres from the pre-aortic plexus of the sympathetic nervous system continue with those of the **superior hypogastric plexus** lying in front of the last lumbar vertebra. It is often incorrectly referred to as the presacral nerve. This plexus is triangular and is 5–6 cm long with its apex at the bifurcation of the aorta. It also receives fibres from the sympathetic trunk. The superior hypogastric plexus then divides into two hypogastric nerves and terminates in the **inferior hypogastric plexus**. This plexus, also called the **uterovaginal plexus** or the **plexus of Frankenhauser**, is located in the loose areolar tissue posterolateral to the cervix, below the uterosacral folds of the peritoneum. Parasympathetic fibres from the S2, S3 and S4 nerves join the uterovaginal plexus. From here, the nerve fibres pass to the ureter, bladder, rectum, uterus and vagina.

**The ovarian plexus** is derived from the celiac and renal ganglia. These fibres accompany the ovarian vessels to reach the ovary, tube and the fundus of the uterus.

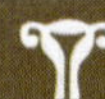

#### Clinical Importance

In presacral neurectomy, the presacral nerve is excised to relieve intractable dysmenorrhea, but the procedure is more of historical significance as a treatment for endometriosis. In hysterectomy for benign lesions, the uterovaginal plexus is not disturbed but in extended radical hysterectomy (Wertheim's operation) atony of the bladder is seen due to the division of the sacral connections to the uterovaginal plexus. The uterus has the intrinsic power of contractility even when denervated. The myometrium has alpha and beta adrenergic receptors as well as cholinergic receptors. In the non-pregnant state, their role is uncertain; but in pregnancy the beta receptors can be stimulated with beta mimetic drugs such as isoxuprine to inhibit uterine activity.

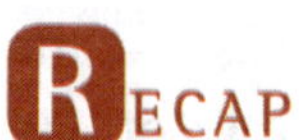

## ECAP

- The organs of the female reproductive system may be divided into the external and internal genitalia.
- The external genital organs consist of the vulva and the vagina.
- The internal genitalia are composed of the uterus with the cervix, Fallopian tubes, ovaries and other supporting structures.
- The vulva comprises the mons pubis, the labia majora, the labia minora, the clitoris, the vestibule, the external urinary meatus, Bartholin's (vulvovaginal) glands, the hymen surrounding the vaginal orifice, the navicular fossa, and the fourchette.
- The vagina is a tubular, muscular canal extending from the hymenal orifice below to the cervix uteri above. As it is attached to the cervix slightly higher up posteriorly, the posterior vaginal wall is longer (10–11 cm) and the posterior fornix is the deepest compared to the anterior vaginal wall which is about 8 cm.
- The uterus is an inverted pear-shaped organ 8 cm × 5 cm × 3 cm located at right angles to the vagina and with the bladder below and in front of it. It is divided into two parts, the corpus or body and the cervix, at the level of the internal os.

- The internal os is an important landmark as the peritoneum is reflected from the superior surface of the bladder to the anterior surface of the uterus. It is also at this level that the uterine artery reaches the uterus after traversing the base of the broad ligament and courses upward along its side wall.
- The cervix is about 2.5 cm in length and in diameter and is divided equally into the vaginal and supra-vaginal portions.
- There are three groups of pelvic muscles: the levator ani and the coccygeus which together form the pelvic diaphragm, the deep transverse perineal muscle in the urogenital diaphragm, and the superficial muscles of the pelvic floor. These three layers of muscles, from the fascia covering the levator ani above to the perineal skin below, constitute the pelvic floor.
- The ovarian artery arises from the aorta just below the renal artery and runs downwards over the psoas muscle to the pelvic brim where it crosses the ureter and the external iliac artery before entering the infundibulopelvic fold of the peritoneum.
- The uterine artery is a branch of the anterior division of the internal iliac artery. It passes along the base of the broad ligament, crosses medially above the ureter about 1.5–2 cm from the internal os to run tortuously along the lateral margin of the uterus and finally anastomoses with the ovarian artery.
- The vaginal arteries arise from the anterior branch of the internal iliac artery and supply the lower part of the vagina.
- The internal pudendal artery mainly supplies the perineum and the external genitalia.
- The pelvic veins of the bladder, uterus, vagina and rectum anastomose with each other freely. Those from the uterus, the vagina and the bladder drain into the internal iliac vein.
- The left ovarian vein ends in the left renal vein and the right one in the inferior vena cava.

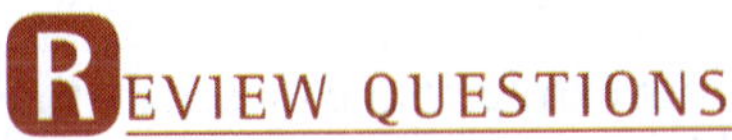

## REVIEW QUESTIONS

### Long-Answer Question

1. Discuss the course of ureter in the pelvis and the points at which it is liable for injury.

### Short-Answer Questions

1. Discuss the lymphatic drainage of the pelvic organs.
2. Write short notes on the perineal body and its clinical importance.

### MCQs

**1. The infundibulopelvic ligament is formed by the**
a) inner border of the broad ligament
b) outer border of the broad ligament
c) outer border of the round ligament
d) outer border of the ovarian ligament

**2. The round ligaments are supplied by**
a) a branch of the ovarian artery derived from its anastomosis with the uterine artery
b) the uterine artery
c) the ovarian artery
d) a branch of the internal iliac artery

**3. The longest part of the Fallopian tube is**
a) the isthmial part
b) the ampullary part
c) the interstitial part
d) the fimbriae

**4. The ovarian artery arises from**
a) the aorta just below the renal artery
b) the uterine artery
c) the internal iliac artery
d) the inferior hemorrhoidal artery

# CHAPTER 4

# Physiology of Menstruation and Ovulation

## AT A GLANCE


Theories of Menstruation
Organic Structures Involved in the Menstrual Cycle
- Ovaries
- Uterus

Phases of the Menstrual Cycle
1. Menstrual Phase
2. Proliferative Phase
3. Secretory Phase
- Changes in Pregnancy

Neuro-endocrinal Control of the Menstrual Cycle
- Hypothalamic-Pituitary-Ovarian (HPO) Axis

Ovulation
- Methods of Detecting Ovulation
- Hormones in Ovulation
- Fine-Tuning


Menstruation is the normal cyclical uterine bleeding seen in female primates. It starts with menarche and ends with menopause. Age of menarche in humans is approximately 14 years. With better and improved nutrition standards, the age of onset of menarche has gradually come down to 12.6 years in Indian girls, which is comparable to that in the developed world; menarche varies with genetic composition, climate and nutrition status.

## THEORIES OF MENSTRUATION

The various theories that were postulated to explain menstruation include:

**1. Galen's plethora theory** This theory explains menstruation as the periodic letting of blood to get rid of excess blood.

**2. Lunar theory** This theory relates causation of menses to the lunar cycle.

Even after the discovery of the ovary by von Baer in 1827, many years elapsed before Pflueger in 1863 formulated a well-defined theory which explained that menstruation was due to the presence of ovaries.

## ORGANIC STRUCTURES INVOLVED IN THE MENSTRUAL CYCLE

1. Anterior pituitary
2. Ovaries
3. Uterus (endometrium)

### Ovaries

The ovaries are derived from extracelomic mesenchyma of the genital ridge. At birth, each ovary in its stroma has 80,000 to 1,00,000 primordial ova, each measuring 35–45 micron (μ) in diameter. At puberty, there are about 30,000 ova in each ovary and only about 500 of these reach maturity during the reproductive period of a woman's. The majority never develop beyond the primitive stage but regress and remain as white spots—**Atretic follicles**. At term, the fetal ovary is 10–15 mm long.

#### Structure

The ovary consists of the surface epithelium, connective tissue, parenchymal zone (cortex) and vascular zone (medulla) (Fig. 4.1). The cortex contains a collection of egg cells and primordial follicles in different stages of development.

The **primordial follicle** measures about 0.25 mm in diameter and consists of a single, eccentrically placed, large, well developed, sex cell (primordial ovum) surrounded by an epithelial layer of small flattened dark-staining granulosa cells. The primitive ovum is about 20 μ in diameter and its nucleus is about 10 μ and consists of a small nucleolus.

#### Graafian follicles

The Graafian follicle is ovoid or spheroidal in shape and consists of two layers—**theca interna** and the **granulosa cells** (Fig. 4.2). The theca interna lies close to the stroma where the cells appear large

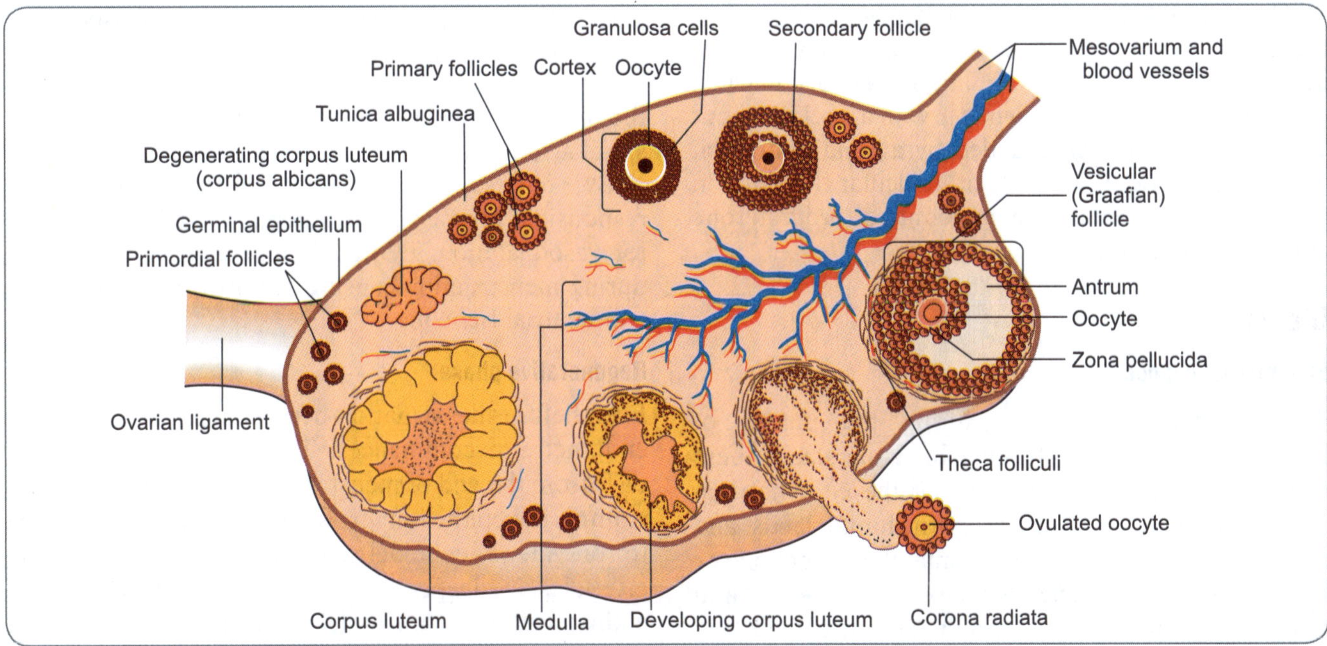


**Fig. 4.1** Structure of ovary showing sequential development of follicles

and polyhedral in the mature follicle. Multilayered granulosa cells are derived from the original epithelial cells surrounding the ovum; they have deeply staining nuclei with very little cytoplasm. The granulosa cells have no blood vessels of their own and derive their nutrition from the theca interna. Between the two layers is the basement membrane on which granulosa cells are arranged.

The ovum is enclosed in a well-defined projection of cells called **cumulus oophorus**. Scattered among the granulosa cells are vacuoles or globules known as the **Call–Exner bodies** characteristic of the granulosa cells.

**Clinical Importance**

Call–Exner bodies are also seen in granulosa cell tumours of the ovary.

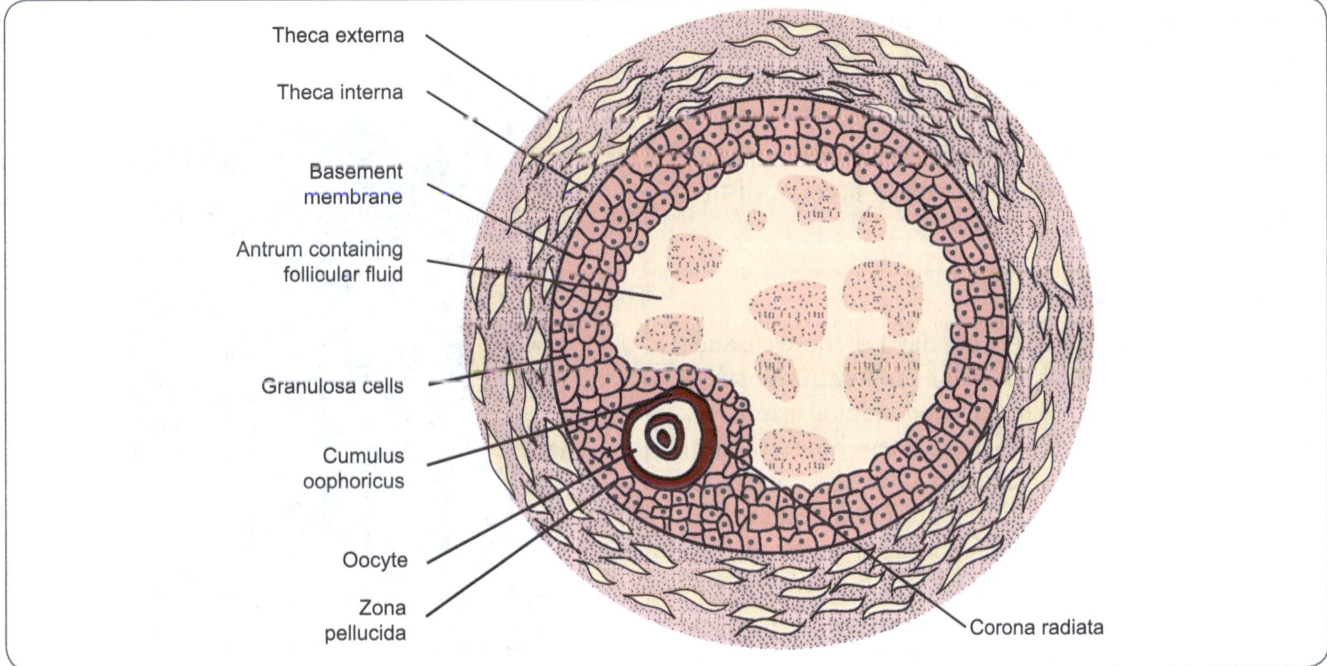


**Fig. 4.2** Graafian follicle

The granulosa cells immediately surrounding the ovum form the **corona radiata,** which remains attached to it even after ovulation. The ovum when mature is about 130 μ in diameter with a nucleus about 20 μ in size and is surrounded by a **zona pellucida**. The **liquor folliculi** is the viscid follicular fluid rich in estradiol 17 β besides small amounts of progesterone and androstenedione.

## Uterus

### Endometrial changes

The endometrial changes during the phases of menstruation are significant. To understand these changes, it should be realised that the endometrium consists of cuboidal surface epithelium, glands and specialised connective tissue stroma; the upper zone or upper 2/3 form the functional layer. The deeper basal layer is closer to the myometrium. Similarly, the blood supply to the endometrium is also arranged in such a way that vasoconstriction of the coiled arteries supplying the functional layer occurs during menstruation and subsequent improvement in blood supply occurs by the short and straight arteries supplying the basal layer.

## PHASES OF THE MENSTRUAL CYCLE

The menstrual cycle has always been considered as consisting of the proliferative and secretory phases. Though these two phases are more significant, the menstrual cycle actually consists of three phases, viz.,

1. Menstrual phase
2. Proliferation phase/follicular phase
3. Secretory/luteal phase

Here, there will be a brief description of the menstrual phase followed by a detailed account of the proliferative and secretory phases.

## 1. Menstrual Phase

The menstrual cycle extends from day 1 of the cycle and lasts for 4–6 days. The thickened endometrium is shed as menstrual bleeding. Markedly coiled spiral arterioles undergo intense vasoconstriction a few hours before the onset of menstruation causing severe hemorrhagic necrosis of the superficial layer of endometrium and extravasation of blood. The superficial layers along with the epithelial lining glands and stroma disintegrate and are thrown into the uterine cavity. The proteolytic enzymes help in digesting the endometrium rather than allow its prolonged sloughing. During the menstrual phase, the straight arterioles undergo vasospasm to reduce the blood loss.

By day 2, most of the functional layers are shed and the bleeding is reduced as the clotting factors plug the spiral arterioles.

By day 3, regeneration occurs. PGF2α is responsible for vasoconstriction. PGE2 is responsible for vasodilatation. PGF2α is higher in concentration during menstruation causing arteriolar vasospasm and endometrial ischemia.

### Regenerative phase

Even before menstruation ceases, regeneration of the endometrium commences. This is completed in two days from the end of menstruation. From the glandular stumps, the epithelium grows over the denuded stroma to provide a cuboidal epithelial lining. The spiral arterioles in deeper parts show very few coils. The endometrium is 2 mm thick. The stromal cells have a thin rim of cytoplasm around the nucleus.

## 2. Proliferative Phase

The proliferative phase extends from day 6/7 to day 14 of the cycle. The glands are initially simple tubular but as the endometrium proliferates, they become longer and columnar. The stroma becomes edematous and arterioles become more coiled. The endometrium is now 5–6 mm in thickness including 1 mm of the basal layer (Fig. 4.3). Intense vascularity towards the end of

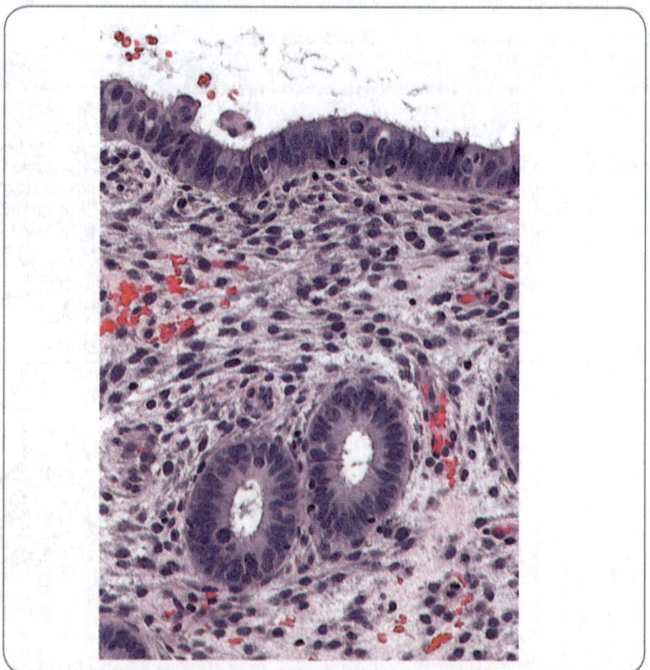

**Fig. 4.3** Proliferative endometrium (*Source:* Wikimedia)

this phase may lead to slight oozing of blood into the uterine cavity causing intermenstrual spotting.

Histologically, proliferating glands have multiple mitotic cells and their organisation changes from a low columnar pattern in the early proliferative period to a pseudo-stratified pattern before ovulation (Fig. 4.3).

### 3. Secretory Phase

In the typical 28-day cycle, ovulation occurs on day 14 of the cycle. Within 48–72 hours following ovulation, the proliferative endometrium is converted to secretory endometrium (Fig. 4.4) by the action of progesterone. This is marked by presence of eosinophilic protein-rich secretory products in the glandular lumen. The earliest evidence of secretion is the appearance of subnuclear vacuolation in the glands and is due to the progesterone from the corpus luteum.

During the secretory phase, endometrial glands form characteristic **glycogen-containing vacuoles that stain positive for periodic acid–Schiff (PAS) stain** (Fig. 4.4). Vacuoles initially appear subnuclearly and progress towards the glandular lumen. The nuclei can be seen in the mid-portion of cells and ultimately undergo apocrine secretion into the glandular lumen often by day 19 or 20 of the cycle. On postovulatory day 6 or 7, secretory activity of the glands are generally maximal and the endometrium is optimally prepared for implantation of the blastocyst.

Stroma shows progressive increase in edema. Spiral arteries progressively lengthen and coil during the remainder of the secretory phase. On day 24, eosinophilic staining pattern known as **cuffing** is visible in the perivascular stroma. This staining pattern of edematous stroma is termed **pseudodecidual** because of its similarity with the pattern that occurs during pregnancy. Approximately 2 days before, there is dramatic increase in the number of polymorphonuclear lymphocytes that migrate from the vascular system, and

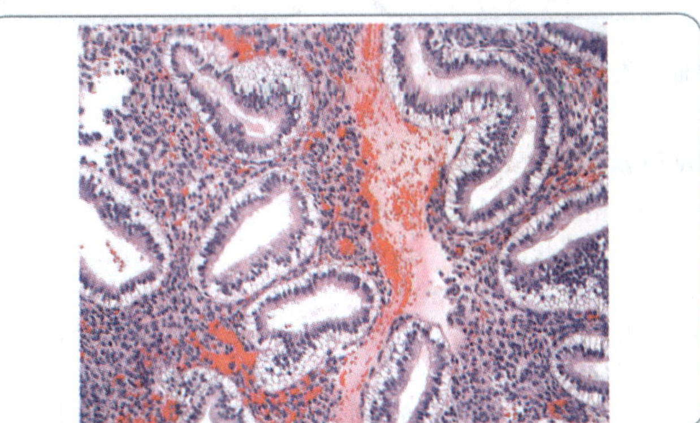

**Fig. 4.4** Secretory endometrium (*Source:* Wikimedia)

this heralds the collapse of the endometrial stroma and the onset of menses.

### Changes in Pregnancy

In pregnancy superficial compact and spongy layers are well marked. The glandular lining appears saw-toothed or crenated with secretion in its lumen. The stromal cells are large and markedly edematous. The stellar or polygonal cells with a zone of cytoplasm are rich in glycogen and are arranged in mosaic or tile-like pattern. The basal layer is devoid of lymphoid tissue.

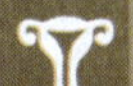

**Clinical Importance**

Similar but pseudodecidual reaction is likely to be produced in the endometrium by oral contraceptive pills and progestational drugs but there will be no chorionic villi in such endometrium.

## NEURO-ENDOCRINAL CONTROL OF THE MENSTRUAL CYCLE

### Hypothalamic-Pituitary-Ovarian (HPO) Axis

The cyclical changes in the ovary and the endometrium during the menstrual cycle are coordinated and controlled by the neuro-endocrinal mechanism (Fig. 4.5). The normal functioning of the hypothalamic-pituitary-ovarian axis is dependent on synchronisation of the time of release and the quantity of hormones involved (Fig. 4.6).

#### Two Cell – Two Gonadotropin hypothesis

Granulosa and theca cells have specific hormone receptors. FSH acts on the granulosa cells to produce estrogens and also progesterone if luteinised.

LH acts on theca cells and produces androgens which are aromatised and converted to estrogen (Fig. 4.7).

#### Gonadotropin-releasing hormone (GnRH)

GnRH is a decapeptide synthesised by specific neuronal nerve endings in the anterior medial basal hypothalamus and it is secreted into the portal vessel running a short course to the anterior pituitary. GnRH is released in a pulsatile fashion as its half-life is only 2–4 minutes. This dictates the pattern of release of two gonadotropins LH and FSH. Pulsatile release of GnRH and fluctuations in the pattern of this pulsatility are thus integral features in the normal functioning of the ovulatory cycle.

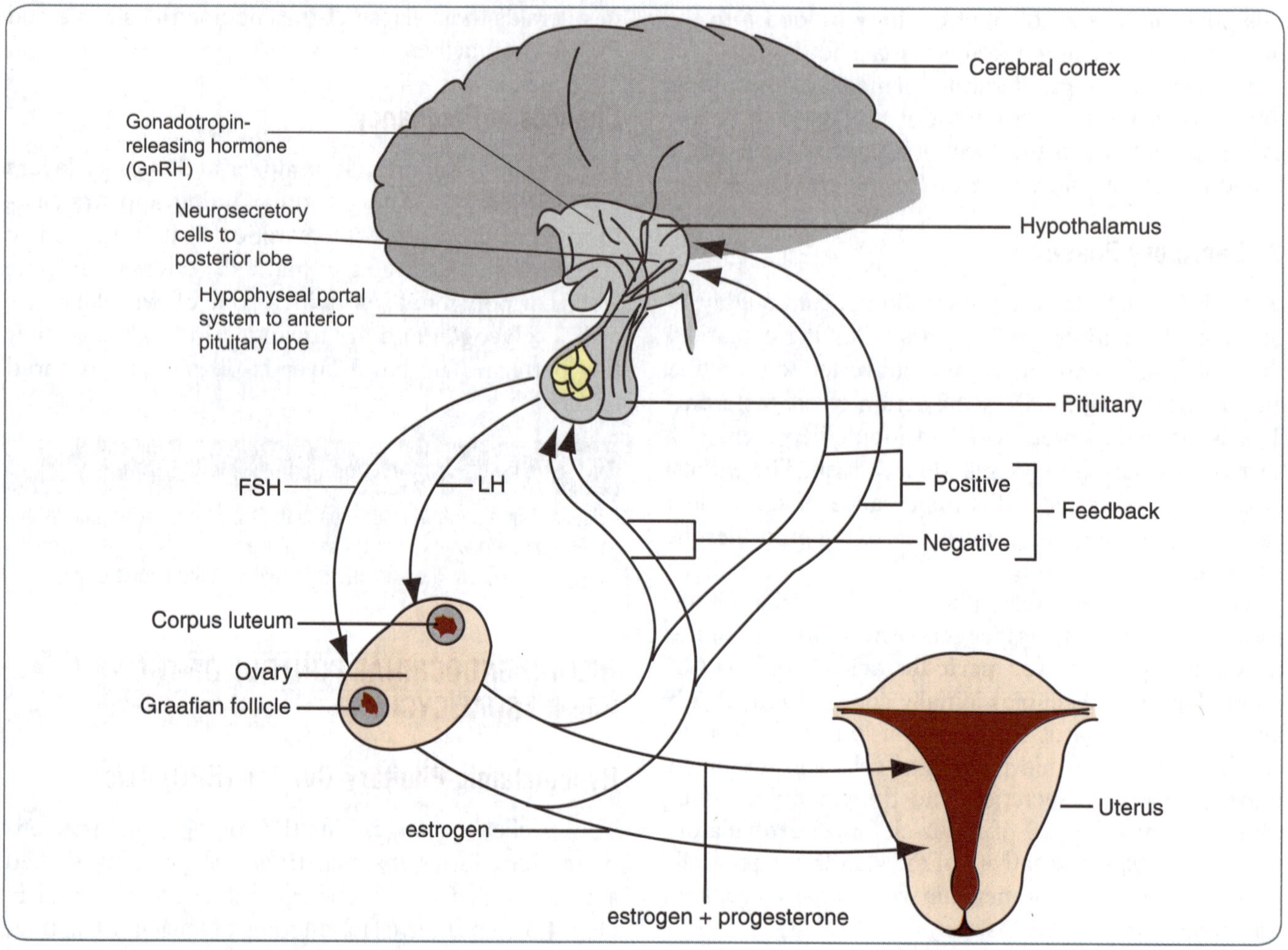

**Fig. 4.5** Neurohormonal control of ovarian function

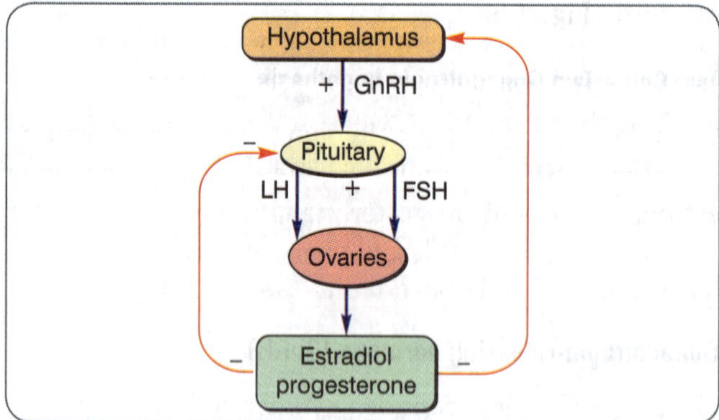


**Fig. 4.6** Origin, target organs and feedback mechanisms of the principal hormones involved in the hypothalamic-pituitary-ovarian axis.

### Follicle-stimulating hormone (FSH)

The amount and timing of FSH release from the anterior pituitary changes throughout the ovulatory cycle. The rise in FSH concentration stimulates the growth of a group of follicles, granulosa cell proliferation and differentiation.

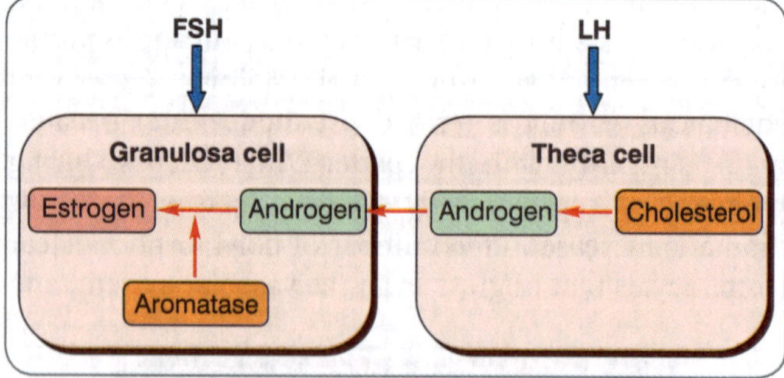


**Fig. 4.7** The two cell – two gonadotropin hypothesis

#### *Role of FSH*

1. Granulosa cell proliferation
2. Antral follicle development
3. Estrogen production
4. Induction of LH receptors on the dominant follicle
5. Inhibin synthesis

FSH activates aromatase which converts androgen into estrogen. Rise in estrogen level results in negative feedback mechanism on FSH secretion. Decrease in FSH with increasing estrogen level plays a role in selection of the dominant follicle and prevents development of multiple follicles.

### Luteinising hormone (LH)

During the early and mid-follicular phases, secretion of LH is relatively quiet with pulse every 60–90 mins. LH surge occurs in the late follicular phase, 36 hours prior to ovulation.

Pre-ovulatory LH surge has a number of key functions:

1. Triggering of ovulation and follicular rupture about 36 hours after the surge
2. Disruption of cumulus–oocyte complex
3. Stimulation of oocyte meiotic maturation
4. Luteinisation of granulosa cells

## OVULATION

Ovulation (*see* Fig. 4.1) refers to release of viable ovum from the ovary. Ovulation occurs when the ovum surrounded by the corona radiata escapes out of the Graafian follicle. It is quickly picked up by the tubal fimbriae, which hugs the ovary at ovulation. Ovulation requires a peak level of 75 ng/mL of LH (Fig. 4.8).

The rupture of the Graafian follicle occurs because of contraction of micromuscle present over the theca externa. The contractions are brought about by prostaglandin secreted under the influence of LH. The process of maturation and ovulation can be minutely studied by serial ultrasonography. The Graafian follicle grows at the rate of 1–2 mm daily and attains the size of 20 mm or more at ovulation. Knowledge of the timing of ovulation is needed in in vitro fertilisation, in artificial insemination and in the control of fertility.

**Signs of Ovulation**

- Sudden shrinkage in the size of the follicle
- Appearance of free fluid in the pouch of Douglas
- Regrowth of the collapsed cyst

**Features Responsible for Follicular Rupture**

1. Increased intrafollicular pressure
2. Proteolytic enzyme activity on follicular wall
3. Morphological changes in the stigma
4. Perifollicular ovarian smooth muscle contractions
5. Vascular alterations in the perifollicular vessel

Ovulation is estimated to occur 14 days before the first day of the succeeding cycle, and this interval is more or less fixed.

In case of irregular cycles, it is the follicular phase which varies, but the luteal phase remains more or less constant at 14 days. However, we do encounter cases of infertility with a short luteal phase, when menstruation begins in less than 14 days after ovulation.

**Clinical Importance**

Normally, one single ovum is discharged from the Graafian follicle. However, multiple ovulations can occur and result in a multiple dizygotic pregnancy. Multiple ovulations can also be therapeutically induced with hormones during in vitro fertilisation.

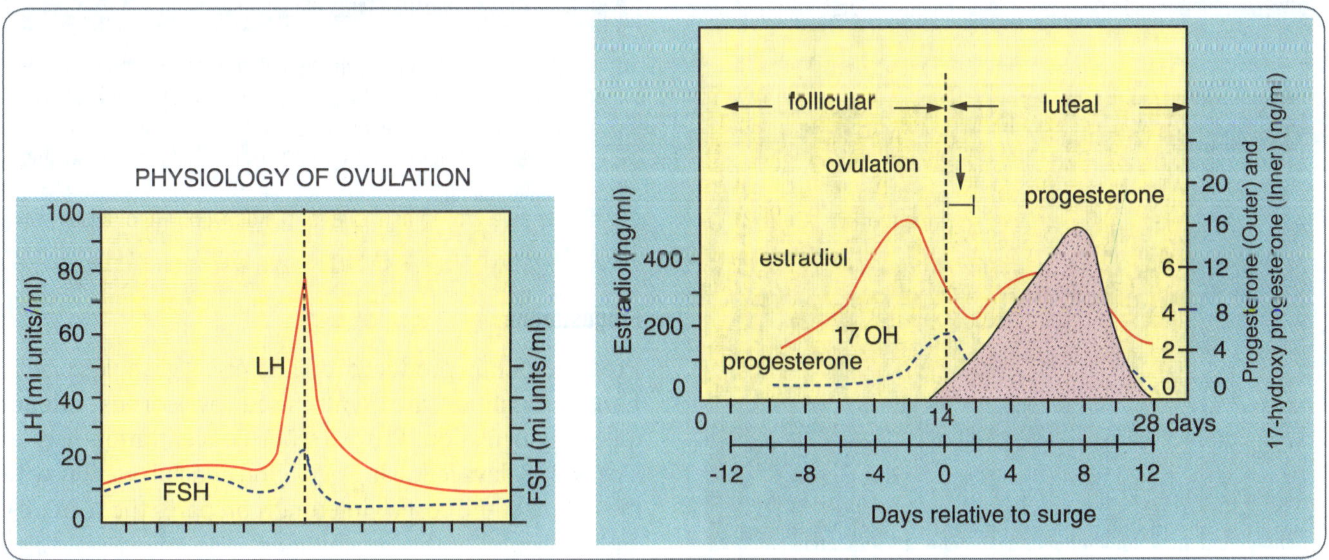


**Fig. 4.8** Levels of FSH and LH in the plasma during the ovarian cycle. Note that the cycle is divided into the follicular and luteal phases on both histological and endocrine criteria.

The aperture through which an egg escapes from the ovary is called the **stigma**, which on laparoscopy appears as a red spot that heals in 3–4 days' time.

## Methods of Detecting Ovulation

The indirect methods of detecting ovulation are based on serial vaginal cytology, serial cervical mucus study, premenstrual endometrial biopsy, observing daily basal body temperature (BBT) and estimation of blood progesterone levels (or urinary pregnanediol levels) in the postovulatory or immediate premenstrual phase. However, with the routine use of ultrasound (Fig. 4.9), these tests are not routinely used anymore; instead, follicular growth and rupture are visualised by serial ultrasonography.

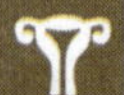

### Clinical Importance

Rarely, rupture of the Graafian follicle fails and the follicle grows into a corpus luteum. This is termed **luteinised unruptured follicle**, which may cause infertility.

Ovulation occurs once a month between the time of menarche and menopause. Oocyte release is preceded by estrogen-induced distinctive changes that prepare the reproductive tract.

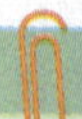

### Changes that Occur Towards Ovulation

1. pH of vagina becomes less acidic.
2. Cervical mucus becomes more copious and less viscous.
3. Cervical os becomes more patulous.

All these changes favour the progress of the motile sperm towards the released oocyte.

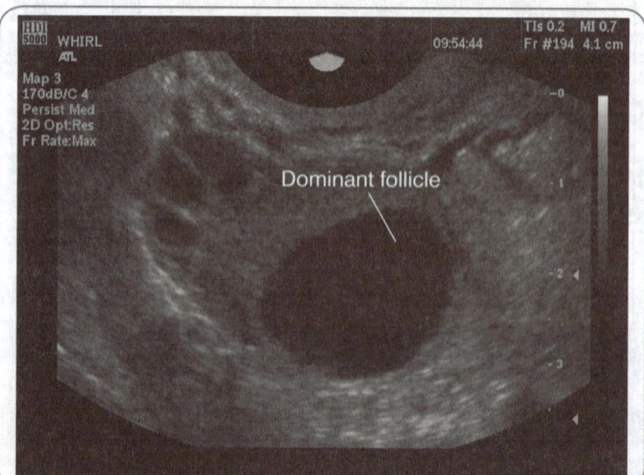


**Fig. 4.9** Transvaginal sonography showing a dominant follicle (*Source:* ©Chizen, D, Pierson, R, Glob. libr. women's med.)

Estrogen serves as a growth factor for the endometrium and prepares it for transition from the proliferation to the secretory phase. The secretion of estrogen and progesterone from the corpus luteum prepares the uterus for possible nidation of fertilised egg.

Corpus luteum is formed from
- Collapsed ovarian follicle
- In-growth of capillaries and fibroblasts from theca cell layer
- Luteinisation of the granulosa cells.

**LH mid-cycle surge** activates a cascade of inflammatory response in the dominant follicle leading to the breakdown of follicular boundary wall and escape of oocyte with its cumulus oophorus.

## Hormones in Ovulation

The ovary is the most dynamically changing organ in the female body during its reproductive lifespan. The hormones involved in ovulation are
1. Estrogen
2. Progesterone

### Estrogen

Estrogens are the basic female hormones. The three types of estrogens are **esterone**, **estradiol** and **estriol.** Of these, estradiol is the most important in the ovulatory cycle. FSH stimulates the enzyme aromatase, CYP19, to convert the substrate of basic androgens, androstenedione and testosterone to estradiol in granulosa cells.

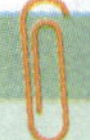

### Key Features of Estradiol

1. By negative feedback mechanism it suppresses the secretion of FSH aiding in the selection of the dominant follicle and preventing multifollicular development.
2. It triggers LH surge in mid-cycle by initiating a positive feedback.
3. It acts as a growth hormone for the development of endometrium.

### Progesterone

Progesterone is produced by luteinised granulosa cells. Large quantities are synthesised by corpus luteum following ovulation. Progesterone concentration rises to a peak 7–8 days following ovulation and falls rapidly with the failure of the corpus luteum. It prepares the secretory endometrium for the implantation of an embryo and also maintains the endometrium throughout the early weeks of pregnancy until trophoblastic/placental hormones take over this role. Under the influence of progesterone, endometrial glandular stroma increase greatly in number and become more tortuous.

## Fine-Tuning

Factors involved in fine-tuning of ovulation are
1. Inhibin
2. Activin and follistatin
3. Growth factors

### Inhibin

Inhibin is secreted by granulosa cells. Inhibin A reaches its peak in the mid-luteal phase, but Inhibin B peaks in the early to mid-follicular phase and again at ovulation. Estrogen and inhibin B are both inhibitory factors for the secretion of FSH.

### Activin and follistatin

Activin increases FSH secretion, inhibits androgen production and also promotes ovarian follicular development. Follistatin is also known as activing-binding protein. It binds with and neutralises the action of activin.

### Growth factors

Many growth factors form a network of interactions within the ovary and its compartments. The most well known are the **Insulin like growth factors (IGF) 1 and 2** which are very active.

The **transforming growth factor (TGF)** and **epithelial growth factor (EGF)** also play a passive role in the regulation of gonadotropin activity within the follicles.

### *Anti-Müllerian hormone (AMH)*

AMH, a dimeric glycoprotein and member of the transforming growth factor β family, is produced by ovarian follicular granulosa cells in the late preantral and small antral follicles. It regulates folliculogenesis by
1. restricting the progression of development of primordial follicles
2. inhibiting the sensitivity of antral follicle to FSH and inhibition of aromatase activity during an ovulatory cycle.

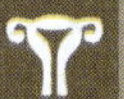

**Clinical Importance**

AMH concentration reflects ovarian reserve, i.e., the number of small antral follicles.

## RECAP

- GnRH is produced in the arcuate nucleus of the hypothalamus and secreted in a pulsatile fashion into portal circulation, where it travels to the anterior pituitary.
- Ovarian follicular development moves from a period of gonadotropin-independence to a phase of FSH dependence.
- As the corpus luteum of the previous cycle fades, luteal production of progesterone and inhibin-A decreases, allowing FSH levels to rise.
- In response to FSH stimulus, the follicles grow, differentiate and secrete increasing amount of estrogen and inhibin-B.
- Estrogen stimulates growth and differentiation of the functional layer of the endometrium, which prepares for implantation. Estrogen works with FSH in stimulating follicular development.
- The two cell – two gonadotropin theory dictates that with LH stimulation, the ovarian theca cells will produce androgens that are converted by the granulosa cells into estrogens under the stimulus of FSH.
- Rising estrogen and Inhibin levels negatively feedback on the pituitary gland and hypothalamus and decrease the secretion of FSH.
- The one follicle destined to ovulate each cycle is called the dominant follicle.It has relatively more FSH receptors and produces a larger concentration of estrogen than the follicles that will undergo atresia.It is able to continue to grow despite falling FSH levels.
- Sustained high estrogen levels cause a surge in pituitary LH secretion, which triggers ovulation, progesterone production, and a shift to the secretory or luteal phase.
- Luteal function is dependent on the presence of LH. The corpus Luteum secretes estrogen, progesterone and inhibin-A, which serve to maintain gonadotropin suppression.without continued LH secretion. Corpus luteum will regress after 12 to 16 days.The resulting loss of progesterone secretion results in menstruation.

- If pregnancy occurs, the embryo secretes hCG, which mimics the action of LH by sustaining the corpus luteum.
- The corpus luteum continues to secrete progesterone and supports the secretory endometrium, allowing the pregnancy to develop further.

## REVIEW QUESTIONS

### Long-answer Question

1. Discuss the phases of menstrual cycle in detail.

### Short-answer Questions

1. Briefly describe the role of estrogen and progesterone in ovulation.
2. Describe the changes in the endometrium during the secretory phase of the menstrual cycle.

### MCQs

**1. How many hours after LH surge does ovulation occur?**
a) 24 hours
b) 12 hours
c) 36 hours
d) 48 hours

**2. Among the following, which is the most potent estrogen?**
a) Estrone
b) Estriol
c) Estradiol
d) Estronate

**3. Androgen is converted to estrogen in the granulosa cell by**
a) 5-alpha reductase
b) 21-alpha hydroxylase
c) 17-beta estradiol
d) Aromatase

**4. According to the Two Cell – Two Gonadotropin hypothesis,**
a) FSH acts on the granulosa cells to produce estrogens and also progesterone if luteinised.
b) LH acts on the granulosa cells to produce estrogens and also progesterone if luteinised.
c) Both FSH and LH act on the granulosa cells to produce estrogens and also progesterone if luteinised.
d) TSH acts on the granulosa cells to produce estrogens and also progesterone if luteinised.

### Further Reading

Berek JS, editor. Berek & Novak's Gynecology, 15th ed. Philadelphia: Wolters Kluwer Health/Williams and Wlkins; 2012.

Farage MA, Sallie Neill S, MacLean AB. Physiological changes associated with the menstrual cycle: a review. Obstet Gynecol Surv. 2009 Jan;64(1):58–72.

Homburg R. The Mechanism of Ovulation. Glob. Libr. Women's Med. 2014. http://www.glown.com. Accessed 29 Feb, 2016.

Ross JW. The Endocrinology and Physiology of Menstruation. Journal of the National Medical Association. 1951 May;43(3): 184–7.

# CHAPTER 5

# Congenital Anomalies of the Genital Tract

**AT A GLANCE**


Development of the Gonad
Development of the Internal Genital Organs
The Müllerian Ducts
Development of the External Genital Organs
Chromosomal Sex and Sexual Differentiation
Genital Tract Anomalies
Aplasia and Hypoplasia
Atresia
Congenital Absence of the Vagina
Fusion and Septal Defects


Congenital anomalies of the genital tract though present at birth are often identified only later. They are recognised mostly when menarche is delayed, when women complain of sterility, reproductive wastage or recurrent fetal malpresentations in pregnancy. On the other hand developmental errors in the external genitals or in the gonads are often genetic in origin and pose problems during infancy or childhood. These are discussed in Chapter 6.

For a proper understanding of the congenital anomalies of the female reproductive tract, it is essential to appreciate the different stages in the normal development of the gonads, the Müllerian and mesonephric ducts and the factors that regulate their development along normal lines. **All the organs of the female urogenital tract except the vulva, bladder and urethra develop from the intermediate cell mass or the urogenital ridge which is first noticed at about the 21st day after fertilisation.**

## DEVELOPMENT OF THE GONAD

Medial thickenings in the urogenital ridge are the earliest evidence of undifferentiated gonads. These are seen at about the fifth week of intrauterine life. At this stage the gonads are bisexual and bipotential with a primitive cortex and a medulla. **The presence or absence of the Y chromosome determines whether the undifferentiated gonad becomes an ovary or a testis.** In the short arm of the Y chromosome is present the testicular determining factor (TDF), which acts via a cell-surface antigen, H-Y antigen, to bring about this differentiation. Therefore, in the presence of the all-important Y chromosome, the gonad develops into a testis with maturation of the medulla to form the interstitial and Sertoli cells and seminiferous tubules.

In the absence of the Y chromosome, the gonad develops into an ovary by week 10. If there are two normal X chromosomes, there is proper development of the gonadal cortex. In Turner's syndrome (45 XO), there is **cortical dysgenesis** and in Klinefelter's syndrome (47 XXY), there is **medullary dysgenesis**. In the rare case of a true hermaphrodite, there is a formation of both the male and female gonadal tissues. The gonad from its fairly cephalad position in the genital ridge later descends to its normal site before birth. The ovary descends into the pelvis and the testis into the scrotal sac though it may sometimes get arrested en route.

## DEVELOPMENT OF THE INTERNAL GENITAL ORGANS

### The Müllerian Ducts

The Müllerian or paramesonephric ducts appear in the intermediate cell mass close to and lateral to the gonads about the seventh week of intrauterine life. They are formed by the invagination of the celomic epithelium. As they grow caudally, these ducts approach each other in the mid-line and cross the mesonephric or Wolffian ducts. There is partial fusion between the two Müllerian ducts growing towards the common cloaca where the mesonephric and Müllerian ducts terminate. The upper ends of the Müllerian ducts form the Fallopian tubes, and the fused portion gives rise to the uterus, cervix and the upper three-fourths of the vagina (Fig. 5.1). The caudal ends of the Müllerian ducts end as the Müllerian tubercle in the urogenital sinus. From

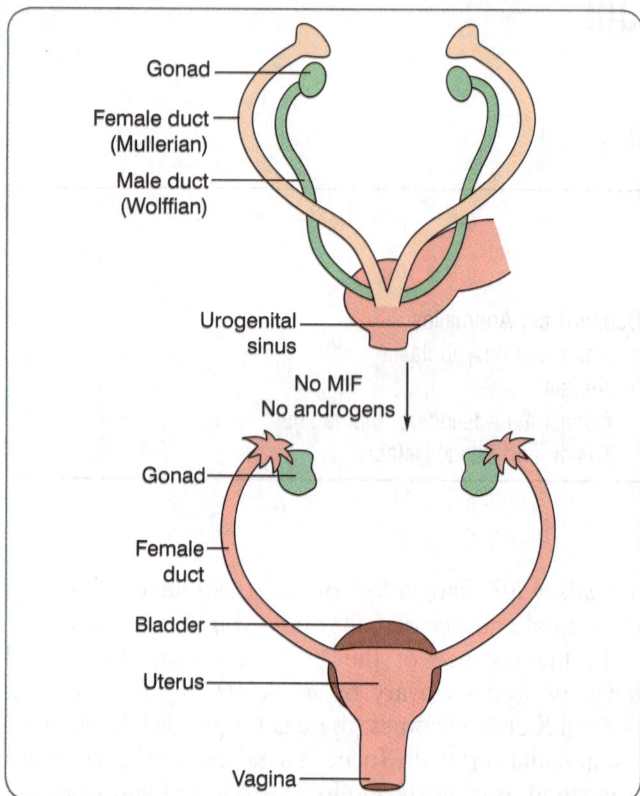


**Fig. 5.1** Development of the internal genital organs

the urogenital sinus, the sinovaginal bulbs growing upwards meet the terminal ends of the Müllerian ducts and later canalise to form the lower part of the vagina.

The growth of the Müllerian system in the male embryo is arrested by the androgens as well as the Müllerian inhibitory factor (MIF), which is a polypeptide, causing regression of the Müllerian ducts. The MIF is also responsible for the stimulation of the Wolffian duct in forming the collecting system and the vas deferens. If the androgens and the MIF are not present, as in the normal female or as in Turner's syndrome, the Müllerian system continues to develop naturally into the female type of the Fallopian tubes, uterus, cervix and vagina. The Wolffian system in these individuals may remain vestigial as an epoophoron, paroophoron and mesonephric (Gartner's) duct.

The MIF seems to have only a local inhibitory effect; so in the case of a true hermaphrodite, there is a testis on one side with inhibition of Müllerian development, and an ovary on the other with a well-developed uterus from the opposite Müllerian system.

At week 16, the mesoderm around the fused portion of the Müllerian ducts forms the muscle wall of the uterus and the cervix. The ducts get canalised, and the septum formed by the fusion is absorbed.

## DEVELOPMENT OF THE EXTERNAL GENITAL ORGANS

In week 6 of embryonic life, the cloaca is seen divided by a septum into a rectal and a urogenital portion. A genital tubercle now appears as a cervical prominence in the genito-urinary portion of the cloaca leading to the development of indifferent or bisexual external genitals. On either side of the genital tubercle, genital ridges (folds) are seen, and external to these, labioscrotal swellings are noticed (Fig. 5.2).

In the absence of androgenic influence, the external genitalia develop into the female type: the genital tubercle becomes the clitoris, the genital folds form the labia minora and the swellings become the labia majora.

In the male, due to the androgenic hormone from the testis, the "indifferent" external genitalia will develop into the male type: the genital tubercle becomes the penis, the genital folds fuse to form the penile urethra and the labioscrotal swellings join to form the scrotum into which the testes will descend later, before birth. At this critical stage of development (before week 12), if the androgens are produced in the female fetus by the fetal adrenal gland (as in adrenal cortical hyperplasia) or are transferred to the fetus across the placenta from the mother (either due to an ovarian neoplasm or from exogenous sources such as oral androgens or progestogens), the external genitalia will exhibit varying degrees of masculinisation even though the gonads and Müllerian ducts are properly developed. Similarly, in the male, 5α-reductase deficiency and failure of conversion of testosterone into dihydrotestosterone by the local cells or non-response to androgens by the end organs can lead to the female type of external genitalia as in the testicular feminising syndrome.

The bladder and the urethra develop from the urogenital sinus. The development of the kidney and ureter are closely associated with the development of the Müllerian system and so whenever there are anomalies in the development of the uterus, defects in the development of the kidney and ureters should also be looked for. If there is a unicornuate uterus (or development of only one Müllerian duct), there may be a single ectopic kidney. Therefore, all cases of uterine anomaly should also be investigated for urological anomaly before any surgery is planned.

The abnormalities in the development of external genitals and sex chromosomal anomalies are discussed in the following sections.

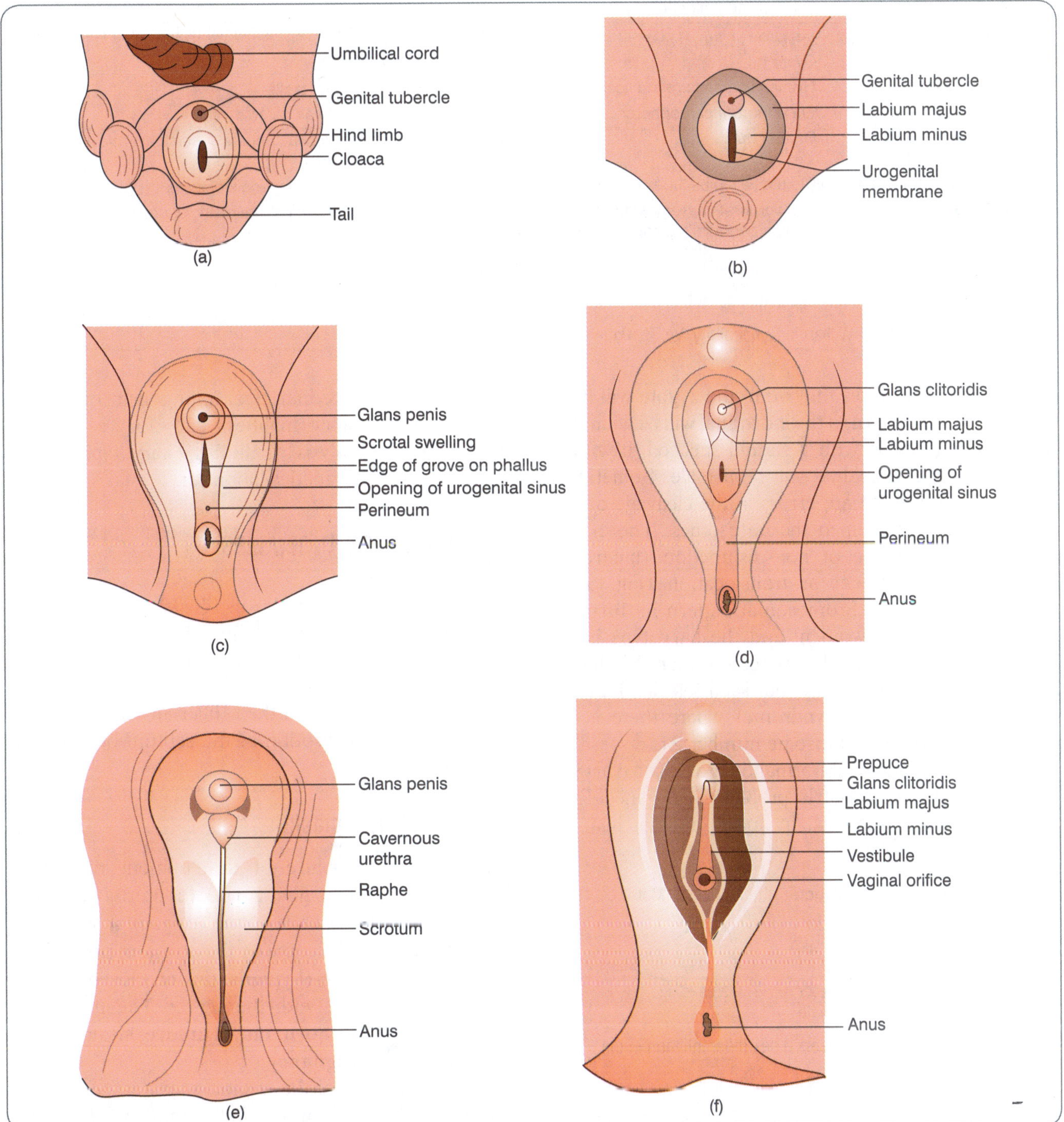


**Fig. 5.2** Development of the external genital organs in both sexes. (a) Common development; (c), (e) Male development; (b), (d), (f) Female development.

## CHROMOSOMAL SEX AND SEXUAL DIFFERENTIATION

Each cell in the human body consists of 46 chromosomes, that is, 22 pairs of autosomes and one pair of sex chromosomes—XX in the female and XY in the male.

The ovum after ovulation undergoes a reduction division (meiosis). The spermatozoon also displays a similar reduction in the number of chromosomes before fertilisation so that the resultant zygote could have the species-specific number of 46 chromosomes as shown in Fig. 5.3. If by chance the X-carrying

**Table 5.1** Embryological structures and their derivatives

| Embryological structure | Female | Male |
|---|---|---|
| Gonad | Ovary | Testis |
| Gubernaculum | Ovarian ligament; round ligament | Gubernaculum testis |
| Mesonephric tubules | Epoophoron; paroophoron | Efferent ductules paradidymis |
| Mesonephric ducts | Gartner duct | Epididymis; ductus deferens; seminal vesicle; ejaculatory duct |
| Paramesonephric ducts | Uterus; Fallopian tubes; upper vagina | Prostatic utricle; appendix of testis |
| Urogenital sinus | Bladder; urethra; vagina; urethral and paraurethral glands; bartholin's glands and vestibular glands | Bladder; urethra; prostatic utricle; prostate glands; bulbourethral glands |
| Genital tubercle | Clitoris | Glans penis |
| Urogenital folds | Labia minora | Floor of penile urethra |
| Labioscrotal swellings | Labia majora | Scrotum |

(*Source:* Modified from William's Gynecology, Vol 2, Page 484)

spermatozoon fertilises the ovum, the zygote will have 46 XX chromosomes and the individual will be a female. If the spermatozoon with Y should succeed, it will be 46 XY and the individual will be a male. Sometimes during meiosis, there are errors in the cleavage of sex chromosomes or even in the autosomes. The errors for example, may be of non-disjunction (failure to separate), displacement or translocation (Fig. 5.4). Thus 45 XO is the chromosomal pattern in Turner's syndrome found in women; and the karyotype is 47 XXY in Klinefelter's syndrome seen in men. Similarly, autosomal anomalies may be seen as in Down's syndrome (trisomy 21 syndrome) where there is an extra chromosome in autosome number 21.

These chromosomal abnormalities give rise to varying gynecological and pediatric problems. In gynecology they present as intersex, primary amenorrhea or

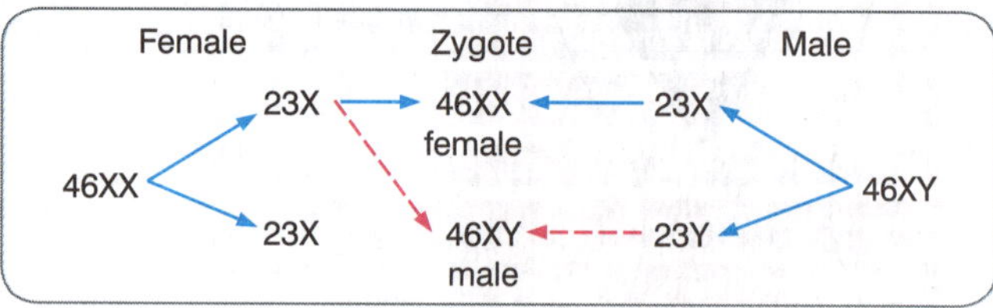


**Fig. 5.3** Meiosis and chromosomal sex differentiation in the zygotes

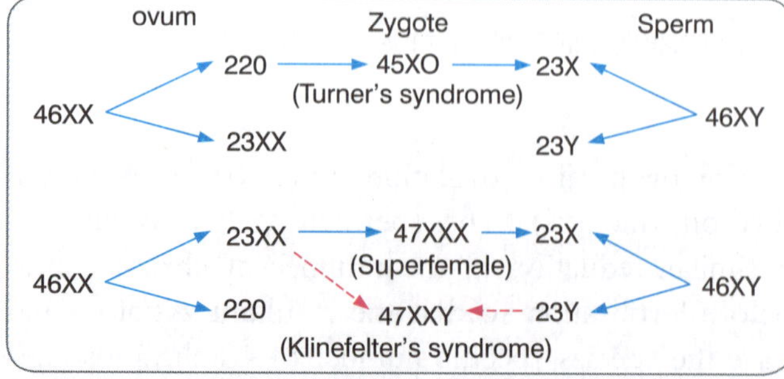


**Fig. 5.4** Chromosomal anomalies resulting in anomalous fetus

infertility, and in pediatrics as mongolism or stunted growth. Such abnormalities call for a detailed chromosomal analysis including karyotyping with assistance from a genetics laboratory.

## GENITAL TRACT ANOMALIES

Genital tract anomalies may be due to
- aplasia or failure of development
- hypoplasia (rudimentary or poor development)
- atresia or non-canalisation
- failure in the fusion of the Müllerian ducts
- failure in the resorption of the septum between the ducts

### Aplasia and Hypoplasia

Rarely, there is failure of development of one of the Müllerian ducts giving rise to uterus unicornis (Fig. 5.5) or the absence of the urogenital system on the opposite side. In some of these, the opposite horn may be rudimentary (**hypoplastic**) or closed, that is, non-communicating with the cervix. **The pregnancy in a rudimentary horn may rupture simulating a ruptured tubal pregnancy.**

In some patients, the vagina may fail to develop either partially or along its whole length. If the uterus is well-developed in such cases, an artificial vagina has to be constructed.

### Atresia

Vaginal atresia and agenesis are congenital anomalies of the female genital tract. The American Society for Reproductive Medicine (ASRM) classifies vaginal atresia as a Type I anomaly. These are also known as complete and partial vaginal agenesis. The most common

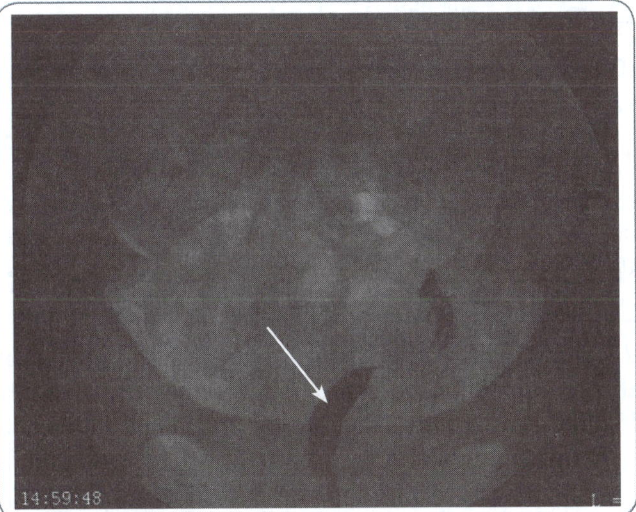


**Fig. 5.5** Hysterosalpingogram picture of unicornuate uterus (*Source:* Wikimedia)

complete vaginal atresia is Mayer–Rokitansky–Küster–Hauser (MRKH) syndrome (MRKH syndrome) in which vaginal agenesis is associated with Müllerian agenesis. This is dealt with in detail in Chapter 16.

Partial vaginal agenesis which is also known as a variant of vaginal atresia is actually a variant of a transverse vaginal septum.

The most common form of atresia is an **imperforate hymen** (Fig. 5.6).

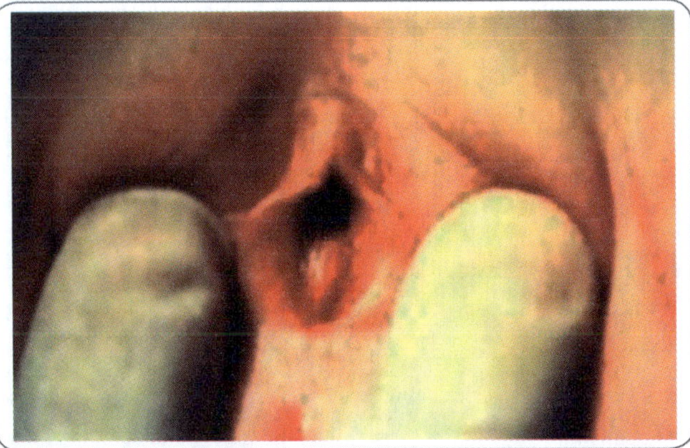

**Fig. 5.6** Imperforate hymen (*Source:* © Syed-Ansari, T, Murray, P, et al, Glob. libr. women's med).

### Signs and symptoms of imperforate hymen

This usually escapes attention until puberty when there is no menstruation but she has periodic attacks of lower abdominal pain. With recurrent menstrual cycles, the menstrual blood collects in the vagina behind the hymenal membrane, becomes thicker due to absorption of the serum and gradually distends the vagina to form a **hematocolpos** (Figs. 5.7 and 5.8). After several months there is over-distension of the vagina because of this cryptomenorrhea or hidden menstruation, difficulty in micturition and a painful lower abdominal swelling. In a few progressive cases, besides the hematocolpos, the uterus **(hematometra)** or even the tubes **(hematosalpinx)** may be involved.

**Examination** reveals a lower abdominal midline swelling due to hematocolpos and uterus will be found lifted on top of it. On inspection of the vulva, the bluish hymenal membrane is seen bulging with the menstrual blood.

### Treatment

The treatment recommended is a **hymenectomy.** A cruciform incision is made initially to drain off all the blood collected in the vagina. The four bits of the septum are excised and the cut edges are approximated with a few hemostatic sutures.

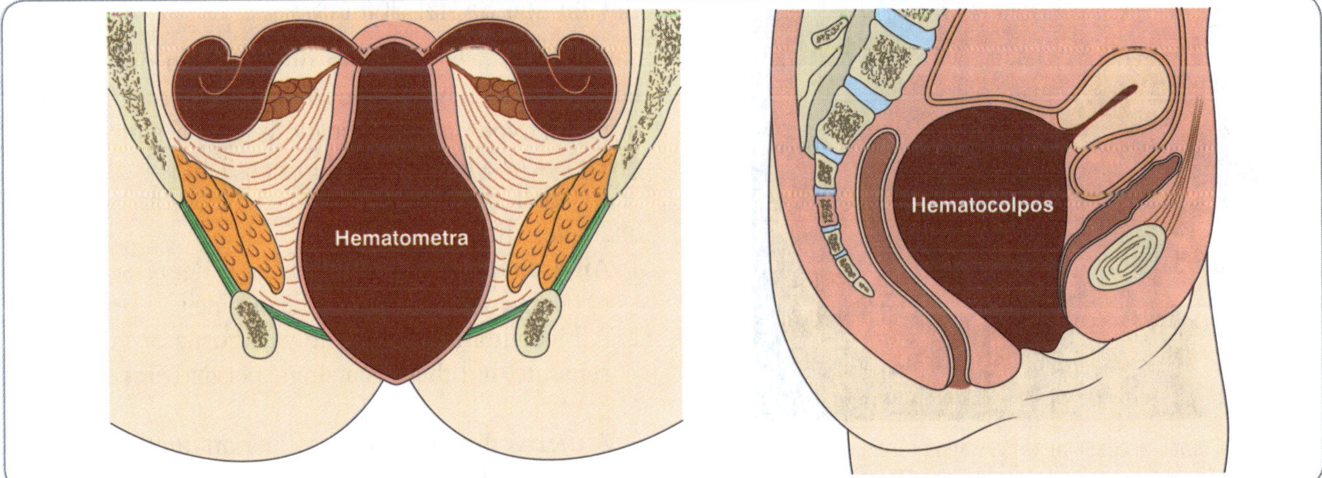


**Fig. 5.7** Imperforate hymen causing hematocolpos and hematometra

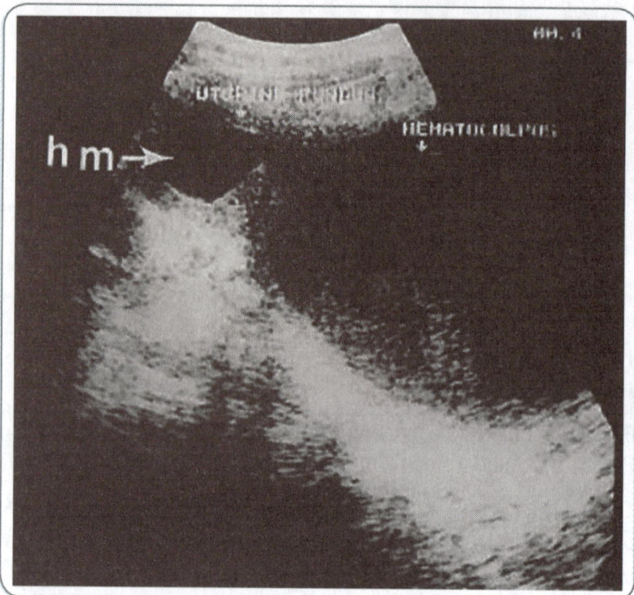

**Fig. 5.8** Ultrasonographic image of hematocolpos and hematometra (*Source:* ©Wade, R, Bliss. Glob. libr. women's med.)

In rare cases of imperforate hymen in children, the vagina may get distended by mucus accumulation resulting in **mucocolpos** which requires excision and drainage.

## Congenital Absence of the Vagina

This may be due to either absence of development or vaginal atresia. It typically involves the upper two-thirds or the whole of the vagina with an absent or rudimentary non-functional uterus and tubes (Fig. 5.9). In these cases, however, the ovaries are present and function normally. In rare cases, a normal uterus may coexist with the rudimentary vagina and give rise to a hematometra.

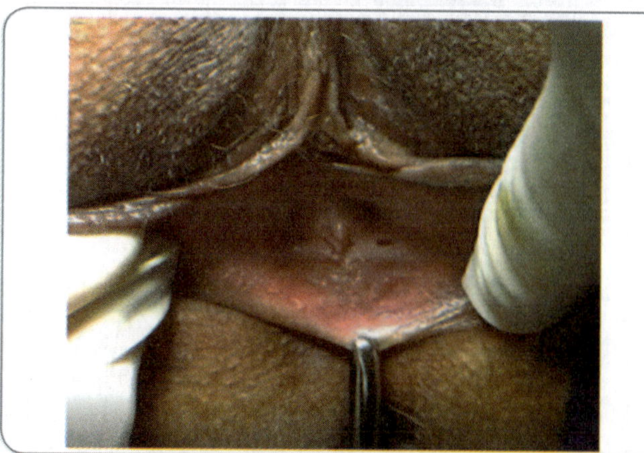
**Fig. 5.9** Complete absence of the vagina (*Source:* Dr. Girija Wagh, Professor, Obstetrics & Gynecology, Bharati Vidyapeeth University Medical College)

### Treatment

If a functioning uterus is diagnosed early, reconstructive vaginal surgery carries a good prognosis.

In all other cases of congenital vaginal atresia, surgery for artificial vagina should be delayed till sexual activity is likely or imminent. If surgery is performed earlier, the vagina may narrow or close down with functional disuse. In these cases there is no chance of menstruation or reproduction. Various surgical procedures are advocated for this condition:

1. ***McIndoe's operation*** The space between the rectum and the bladder is opened up carefully avoiding injury to these organs and a plastic mould of a suitable size covered with a full-thickness of skin graft is placed in this space for two weeks. The skin graft 'takes', in most cases, and lines the artificial vagina (Fig. 5.10).
2. ***William's operation*** Here the artificial vagina is lined by the labia minora with no attempt made to open the space between the urethra and the rectum. The results are satisfactory as the tunnel between the labia minora forms a good 'vagina'.
3. Instead of a skin graft, an isolated loop of ileum or large bowel with its mesentery and blood supply may be used to line the space between the rectum and the bladder. The upper end of this bowel segment is closed and its lower end is sutured to the perineal skin.
4. ***Frank's method*** In this non-surgical method, an artificial vagina is created by the application of gradually progressive pressure at the appropriate site over the perineum using rounded pyrex tubes everyday for several months. The results are often not satisfactory.

## Fusion and Septal Defects

These form a large group of Müllerian duct anomalies and are seen in about 1 in 700 births. There are different types of classifications and a simple one is given below and illustrated in Fig. 5.11.

In fusion defects (Fig. 5.12), the following characteristics are seen:

1. **An arcuate uterus** The fundus is depressed instead of being convex. The uterine outline is heart-shaped.
2. **A bicornuate uterus** The two horns or cornua are separate, but there is a single cervix (Figs. 5.13 and 5.14).
3. **A uterus didelphys** The Müllerian ducts have failed to unite along their whole length. Each develops into a separate uterus, cervix and vagina. In septal

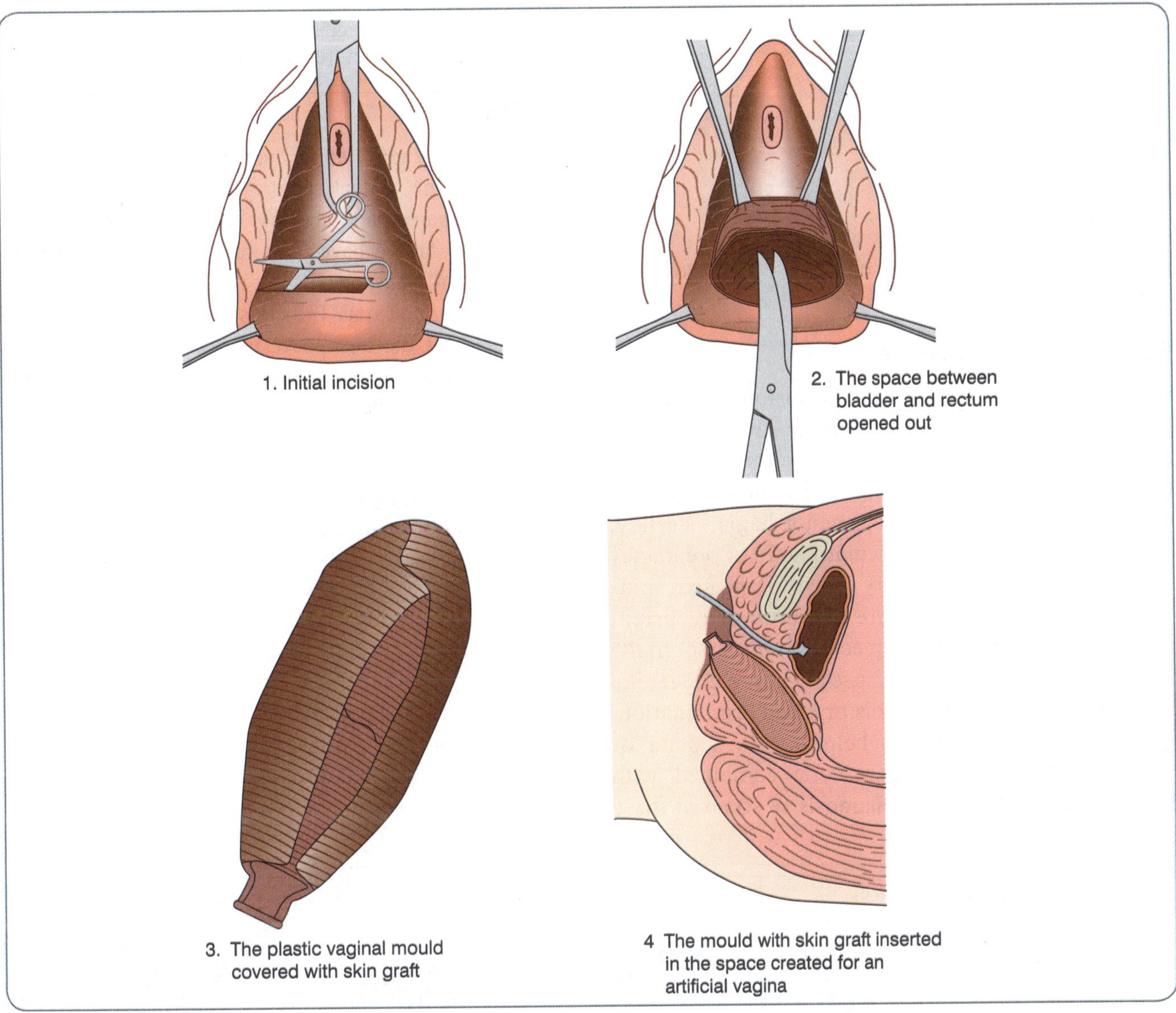


**Fig. 5.10** McIndoe's operation for complete absence of the vagina. Note the main steps of the operation.

defects the uterine outline appears normal but there is a septum of variable length in the uterine cavity or vagina. The following are characteristic.

a) *A uterus subseptus* The ducts have fused but a septum extends from the fundus into the uterine cavity.

b) *A uterus septus* The septum extends from the fundus down to the cervix and sometimes even to the vagina (Fig. 5.15).

c) *A septate vagina* This may be associated with a septate uterus, or the septum may be limited to the vagina only.

The other classification is ASRM (now known as American Fertility Society (AFS)) classification which is as follows:

**Classification of Müllerian Anomalies**

I. Segmental Müllerian hypoplasia or agenesis
   a. Vaginal
   b. Cervical
   c. Uterine
   d. Tubal
   e. Combined
II. Unicornuate uterus
   a. Rudimentary horn with cavity, communicating to unicornuate uterus
   b. Rudimentary horn with cavity, not communicating to unicornuate uterus
   c. Rudimentary horn with no cavity
   d. Unicornuate uterus without a rudimentary horn

III. Uterine didelphys
IV. Bicornuate uterus
  a. Complete bifurcation (bicollis)
  b. Partial bifurcation (unicollis)
V. Septate uterus
  a. Complete septation
  b. Partial septation
VI. Arcuate uterus
VII. Diethylstilbestrol-related anomalies

(*Source:* William's Gynecology, Eds. Barbara L. Hoffman, John O. Schorge, Joseph I. Schaffer, et al., page 496 Edition 2, 2012.)

### Signs, symptoms and diagnosis

In most cases of duplication or fusion defects, no symptoms are present and the diagnosis may be accidental. Most of these women are fertile and have normal term deliveries. Some patients, however, complain of dysmenorrhea, menorrhagia, sterility, dyspareunia or report with hematometra or pregnancy in a rudimentary accessory horn. Repeated mid-trimester abortion, premature deliveries or recurrent malpresentations (such as breech or transverse) in the absence of a demonstrable cause suggest a congenital uterine anomaly. Besides history and examination, a hysterosalpingography is helpful in a septate or a bicornuate uterus. Laparoscopy combined with hysteroscopy helps in the diagnosis of some of these anomalies. A urological evaluation is required to determine the associated urinary tract defects.

### Treatment

Very few cases of uterine duplications call for surgical corrections. The vaginal septum can be removed easily in cases of dyspareunia or sterility. Where all other causes of reproductive failure have been ruled out and the woman has recurrent abortions or premature deliveries uterine unification is indicated. The classical Strassman operation is reserved for the bicornuate uterus. The separate horns are united after resection of the central septum, in the fundus and/or in the cervix. In Strassman's series of 128 cases, prior to surgery, only 4 per cent had term deliveries, 70 per cent had recurrent abortions and 15 per cent delivered prematurely. Following surgical unification, 85 per cent delivered at term and most of them vaginally. With septate uterus, the septum could be resected through operative hysteroscopy. The results are better and, as there is no scar in the uterus, the chances of subsequent vaginal delivery are good in these cases.

If there is a symptomatic rudimentary horn (accessory or not), it requires excision. The larger horn is capable of normal function including carrying a pregnancy to term.

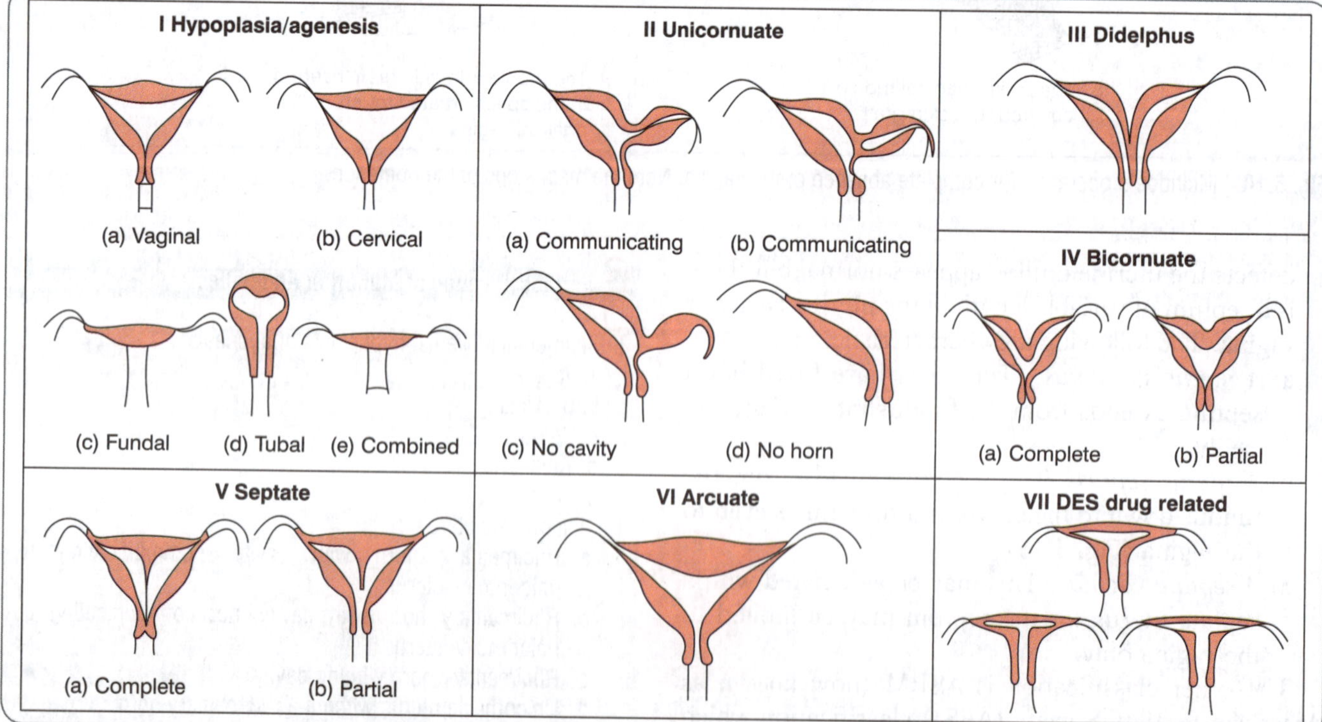


**Fig. 5.11** Classification system of Müllerian duct anomalies used by the American Fertility Society

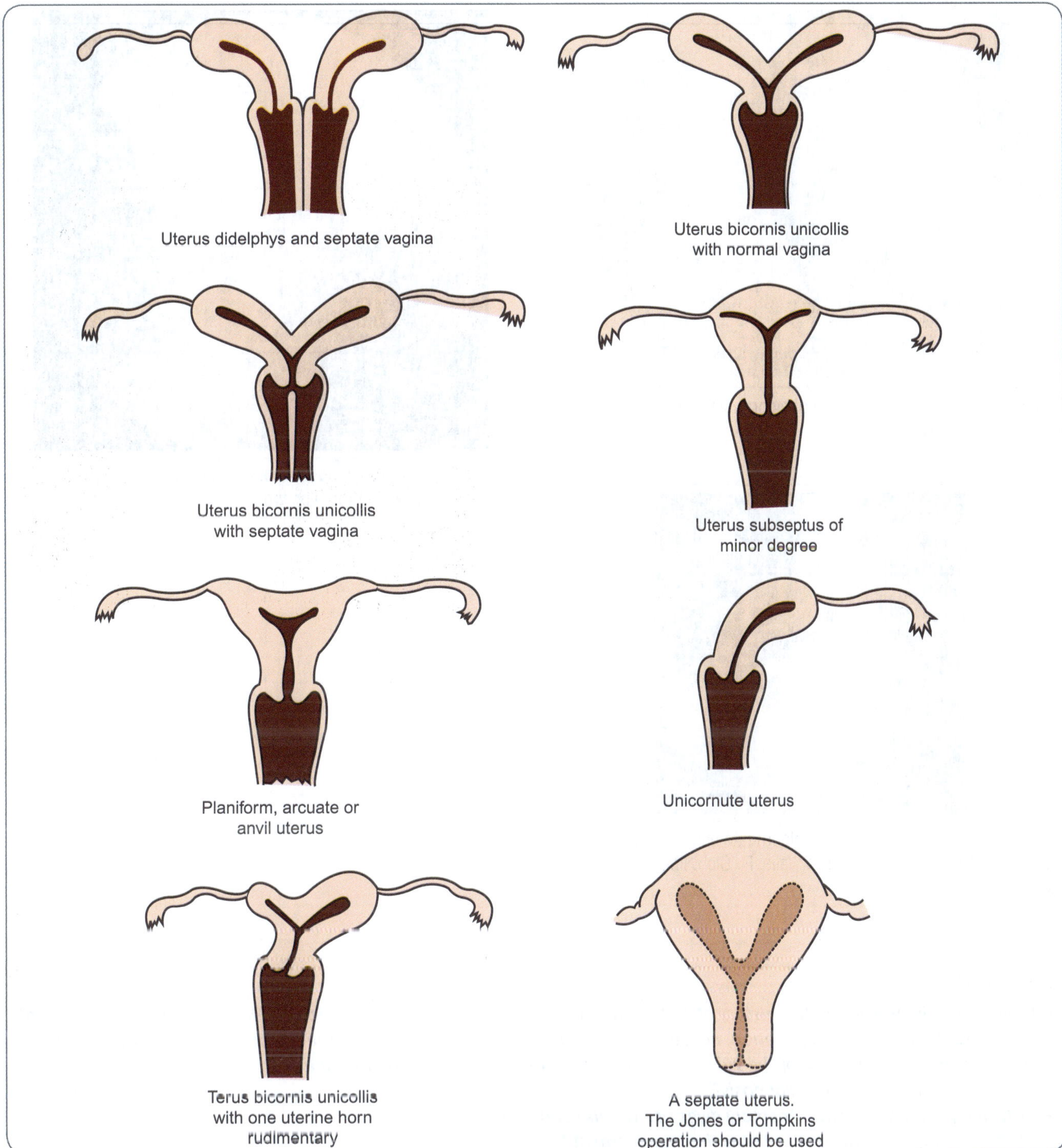


**Fig. 5.12** Fusion and septal defects

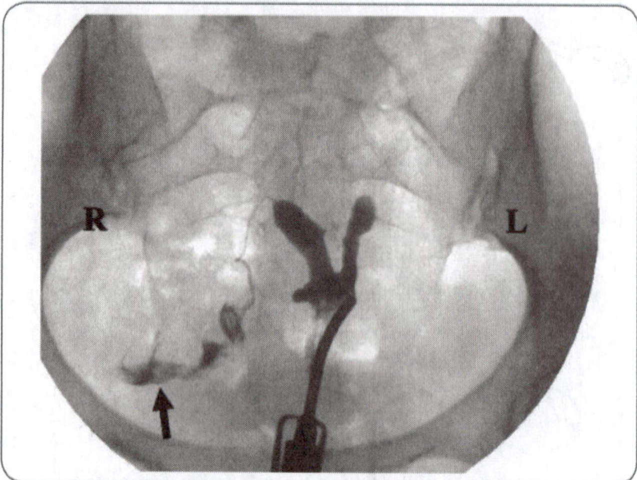


**Fig. 5.13** Hysterosalpingogram of bicornuate uterus (*Source:* Radiopedia ©Aditya Shetty)

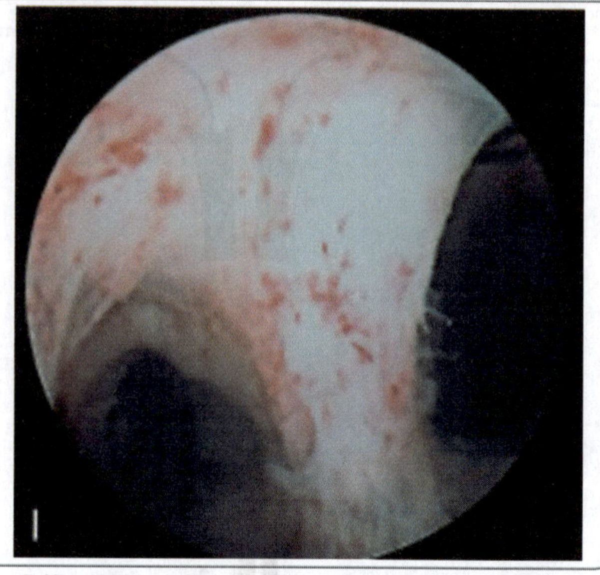

**Fig. 5.15** Hysteroscopic view of complete uterine septum (*Source:* ©Valle, R, Glob. libr. women's med.)

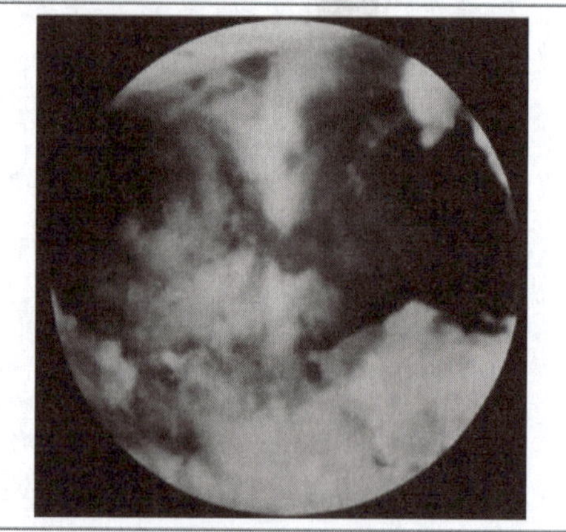

**Fig. 5.14** Hysteroscopic view of bicornuate uterus (with pregnancy in one horn) (*Source:* ©Valle, R, Glob. libr. women's med.)

***Case study***

*A 16-year-old girl presents with a history of cyclic abdominal pain of eight months duration and lower abdominal swelling of three weeks duration. On examination, her secondary sexual characters are normal. There was a tender, cystic suprapubic mass of 20 cm size. Inspection of the vulva revealed a bluish bulging hymenal membrane.*

- *What is the most probable diagnosis?*
- *Which type of genital tract anomaly gives rise to this condition?*
- *If the diagnosis is confirmed, what is the management?*

## REVIEW QUESTIONS

### Long-answer Question

1. What are fusion and septal defects? Describe the signs, symptoms and diagnoses of fusion and septal defects?

### Short-answer Questions

1. Discuss briefly the diagnosis and management of imperforate hymen in a 16-year-old girl.

2. Briefly discuss the development of external genital organs with particular reference to female sex.

## MCQs

1. **The earliest evidence of undifferentiated gonads is**
   a) Urogenital ridge
   b) Medial thickenings in the urogenital ridge
   c) Presence of TDF
   d) Presence of H-Y antigen
2. **Müllerian ducts appear by about**
   a) Fourth week of intrauterine life
   b) Twelfth week of intrauterine life
   c) Seventh week of intrauterine life
   d) Tenth week of intrauterine life
3. **Hematocolpos is due to**
   a) Distension of vagina with blood
   b) Distension of cervix with blood
   c) Distension of tubes with blood
   d) All of them
4. **Which of these is not a surgery for creating artificial vagina?**
   a) Strassman operation
   b) McIndoe's operation
   c) William's operation
   d) None of them

### Further Reading

Edmunds DK Malformations of genital tract. In: Dewhursts Practical Paediatrics and Adolescent Gynaecology. London: Butterworth; 1989. 27 p.

Hoffman BL, Schorge JO, Schaffer JI et al., editors. William's Gynecology. 2nd ed. New York: McGraw-Hill; 2012.

Jones HW Jr., Rock JA. Surgical treatment of female infertility. WHO symposium on advances in fertility regulation (Moscow, 1976). Geneva: WHO; 1977. 181 p.

Jones LD. Fundamentals of obstetrics and gynecology, 3rd ed. London: Faber and Faber; 1982. 3 vol. 33 p.

Williams EA. Progress in Gynaecology. M.L.Taymor ML, Green TH, editors. New York: Grune and Stratton; 1989. 6 vol. 671 p.

# Chapter 6

# Adolescent Gynecological Problems

**At a Glance**

Physical and Endocrinal Changes
Tanner Staging
Causes of Premature Pubertal Development
Precocious Puberty
Central Precocious Puberty (True Precocious Puberty)
Peripheral Precocious Puberty
Heterosexual Precocious Puberty
Variations in Normal Puberty
Conditions Associated With Pubertal Delay
Common Gynecological Complaints and Disorders in the Adolescents
Menstrual Disorders
Abdominal Pain
Congenital Genital Anomalies
Rupture of Functional Ovarian Cyst
Sexually Transmitted Diseases
Tubo-ovarian Torsion
Endometriosis
Neoplasms
Polycystic Ovarian Syndrome
Genital Prolapse
Genetic Problems
Miscellaneous

Adolescence is the period of life beginning with the appearance of secondary sex characteristics and terminating with the cessation of somatic growth.

It is a period of many social and physical changes, a time of transition. Adolescence is the period of life during which the carefree child transforms into a responsible grown up.

The various changes that take place during adolescence are as follows:

- Biological—sexual development, reproductive maturity
- Psychological—cognitive development, emotional patterns of adulthood
- Social—relative economic and social independence from parents

Thus, marked morphological changes occur in all the organs and systems. All these changes during adolescence are reflected as:

i) Physical and Endocrinal
ii) Psychological

## PHYSICAL AND ENDOCRINAL CHANGES

- **Gonadarche** is the maturation of the hypothalamic-pituitary-gonadal axis,and sexual maturity.
- **Menarche** is the onset of menstruation which is dependent on normal hypothalamus–pituitary–ovarian–uterine axis. The development of the female reproductive tract is a complex process that involves cellular differentiation, migration, fusion, and canalisation with probable apoptosis.
- **Adrenarche** is increase in secretions of the adrenal androgens and is independent of the process of sexual maturity (gonadarche) and is responsible for **pubarche** which is the development of the pubic and axillary hair.The growth of pubic and axillary hair is due to an increased production of adrenal androgens at puberty. Considerable evidence supports a dissociation of the control mechanisms that initiate adrenarche. Premature adrenarche is a condition in which pubic and axillary hair appear before 8 years of age (precocious appearance of pubic and axillary hair). However this is not associated with a parallel abnormal advancement of gonadarche.
- In true precocious puberty (before 6 years of age), gonadarche precedes adrenarche.
- In hypergonadotropic hypogonadism (gonadal dysgenesis) or in hypogonadotropic states such as Kallmann's syndrome, adrenarche occurs despite the absence of gonadarche.
- When adrenarche is absent, as in children with cortisol-treated Addison's disease (hypoadrenalism), gonadarche still occurs.
- **Thelarche** is breast budding.

## Tanner Staging

Tanner Staging has been used as a scale for assessing the physical development in children, adolescents and adults (Fig. 6.1). It is more often employed in conditions like altered sexual development and growth. The two aspects that are commonly assessed using this scale are the development of breast and pubic hair.

Tanner's staging of breast and pubic hair development are given in Tables 6.1 and 6.2.

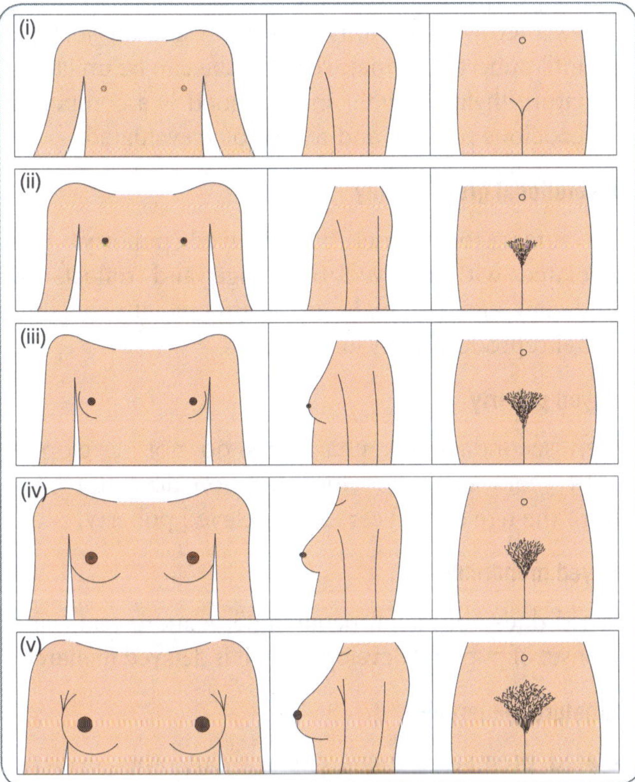


**Fig. 6.1** Tanner's staging of breast and pubic hair development

**Table 6.1** Tanner's staging of breast

| | |
|---|---|
| **Tanner I** | No glandular tissue: areola follows the skin contours of the chest (prepubertal) (typically age 10 years and younger) |
| **Tanner II** | Breast bud forms, with small area of surrounding glandular tissue; areola begins to widen(10–11.5 years) |
| **Tanner III** | Breast begins to become more elevated, and extends beyond the borders of the areola, which continues to widen but remains in contour with surrounding breast (11.5–13 years). |
| **Tanner IV** | Increased breast size and elevation; areola and papilla form a secondary mound projecting from the contour of the surrounding breast (13–15 years) |
| **Tanner V** | Breast reaches final adult size; areola returns to contour of the surrounding breast, with a projecting central papilla. (15+ years) |

**Table 6.2** Tanner's staging of pubic hair development

| | |
|---|---|
| **Tanner I** | No pubic hair at all (prepubertal) (typically age 10 years and younger) |
| **Tanner II** | Small amount of long, downy hair with slight pigmentation at the base of the penis and scrotum (males) or on the labia majora (females) (10–11.5 years) |
| **Tanner III** | Hair becomes more coarse and curly, and begins to extend laterally (11.5–13 years) |
| **Tanner IV** | Adult-like hair quality, extending across pubis but sparing medial thighs (13–15 years) |
| **Tanner V** | Hair extends to medial surface of the thighs (15+ years) |

## CAUSES OF PREMATURE PUBERTAL DEVELOPMENT

Premature pubertal development may be due to:
- Central precocious puberty
- Peripheral precocious puberty
- Heterosexual precocious puberty and
- Variation of normal puberty

### Precocious Puberty

This is defined as the onset of menstruation accompanied by other evidence of puberty such as the development of breasts and pubic hair before the age of 8 years, or before 10 years (if ±2 years is considered) (Fig. 6.2).

### Central Precocious Puberty (True Precocious Puberty)

**Etiology** This condition is rare. It could be due to CNS tumours like astrocytomas, adenomas, gliomas or germinomas. Congenital anomalies like hamartomas, hydrocephalus and empty sella syndrome can also lead to this condition.

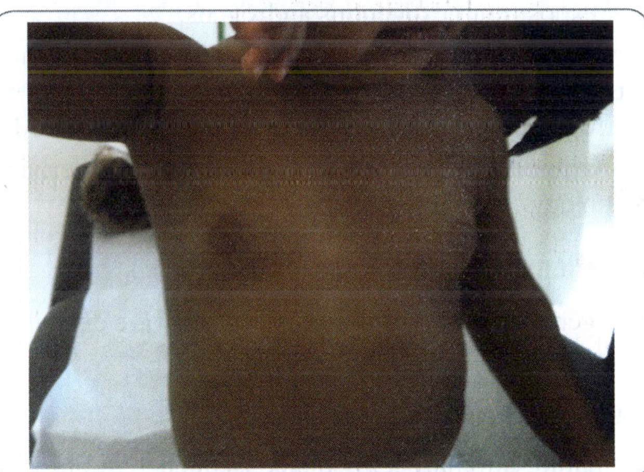

**Fig. 6.2** Precocious puberty (*Source:* Wikimedia)

In central precocious puberty, the hypothalamo-pituitary-ovarian axis is activated early leading to increased GnRH secretion resulting in increased gonadotropin formation.

**Signs and symptoms** These are like that of precocious puberty. However bone age assessment and evaluation of serum FSH, LH and estradiol levels will help in differentiating this condition from precocious puberty. In central precocious puberty, bone age would be more than that expected for the age and the FSH, LH and estradiol levels also would be in the pubertal range.

**Management** Using GnRH agonists like leuprorelin, buserelin or goserelin.

## Peripheral Precocious Puberty

**Causes, signs and symptoms** Less commonly, ovarian cysts could be the cause of elevated estrogen levels, and this is known as peripheral precocious puberty. This is characterised by absence of GnRH pulsatile release, low levels of pituitary gonadotropins but increased serum estrogen levels.

**Etiology** The most common ovarian tumour causing this condition is granulosa cell tumour. Other causes could be adrenal disorders, iatrogenic disorders, and primary hypothyroidism.

**Management** Discontinuation of estrogen source which may be hormonal pills or creams. An estrogen-secreting ovarian or adrenal tumour should be surgically removed. Hypothyroidism is treated with thyroid hormone replacement.

## Heterosexual Precocious Puberty

**Causes** This condition is most commonly caused by androgen-secreting ovarian or adrenal tumours, congenital adrenal hyperplasia, Cushing's syndrome, and exposure to exogenous androgens.

**Signs and symptoms** The clinical signs and symptoms are related to androgen excess. However, androgen excess with virilisation is rare in childhood.

**Management** Depends on addressing the underlying pathology.

## Variations in Normal Puberty

The general variations in normal puberty are described in detail below:

### Premature adrenarche

Premature adrenarche, is the consequence of an early modest increase in the adrenal androgens. Treatment is not necessary because the transient acceleration in growth and bone maturation has no major influence on puberty or final height. Surveillance of these patients should be continued because, although not certain, it has been suggested that they have an increased incidence of anovulation, hirsutism, and hyperinsulinemia.

### Premature thelarche

This refers to breast budding without pubertal growth, which might occur in the first few years of life and is usually self-limiting, requiring no therapy. Follow-up has revealed that most of these children experience normal growth and development. The breast growth may regress after a few months, wax and wane for years, or last until puberty. Premature thelarche can be unilateral. Premature thelarche later in childhood is a component of precocious puberty and needs to be evaluated.

### Constitutional growth delay

This refers to normal but delayed puberty. It is associated with delayed bone age and reflects the adolescent's genetic make-up. Ultimately it results in a normal reproductive system.

### Delayed puberty

When secondary sex characters do not develop by 13/14 years and when menstruation does not begin before the age of 16 years, it is delayed puberty.

### Delayed menarche

If a girl does not attain menarche 5 or more years since the onset of pubertal development, it is delayed menarche.

### Premature menarche

Isolated premature menarche without other evidence of maturation is an exceedingly rare presentation of precocity. Infection, foreign body, abuse and trauma, or local neoplasms should be considered. Normal growth, development, and fertility are not affected.

# CONDITIONS ASSOCIATED WITH PUBERTAL DELAY

The ability to diagnose and manage disorders of female pubescence requires a thorough understanding of the physical and hormonal events that mark the evolution of the child into a sexually mature adult capable of reproduction.

The normal pubertal development and subsequent normal menstrual cycles are a reflection in part of the general health of a girl. The maturation of the hypothalamic pituitary ovarian axis requires a given body mass with a certain percentage of distribution of fat also. When the transition is confounded with the addition of any medical illness or disability, it becomes a challenging situation. Nearly one-third of adolescents with Crohn's disease present with pubertal delay, weight loss, or amenorrhea without gastrointestinal symptoms. Any disease that causes malabsorption, such as cystic fibrosis or coeliac disease, can result in growth and/or menstrual disturbances. Sickle cell disease, thalassemia major, HIV, and renal disease are commonly associated with delayed puberty and menstrual irregularities. Undertreated endocrinopathies, particularly thyroid disease and diabetes mellitus, are known to affect the general growth and menstrual function. Primary or secondary amenorrhea often are the signs of anorexia nervosa.

## COMMON GYNECOLOGICAL COMPLAINTS AND DISORDERS IN THE ADOLESCENTS

Sometimes female neonates' mothers or family members complain that the baby has vaginal discharge or slight bleeding. This is due to withdrawal of maternal hormones. What is needed is assurance to the mother and the family that this is normal. The best way to reassure them is to let them know that such a complaint in a neonate is only proof that the child has a functioning genital system. Some of the gynaecological problems that affect adolescents can also affect children, even infants, and need to be tackled with sensitivity.

> Gynecological disorders in the adolescents could be structural and functional dysfunction of genital tract due to various reasons including uterine abnormalities either of obstructive variety or absent uterus which manifest during adolescence.

**Incidence** Out of the gamut of problems, menstrual disorders are the most common. Since menstrual problems are subtle, the problems often get unreported. Of the girls who report to a gynecologist as outpatients, the percentage of various menstrual complications are listed in Table 6.3.

**Table 6.3** Incidence of various menstrual complications in adolescents

| Complication | Percentage of occurrence |
|---|---|
| Menstrual disorders | > 50% |
| Vaginal white discharge (leucorrhea) with or without bad odour, with or without itching | 25% |
| Genital infections | 7% |
| Menorrhagia (cyclical heavy bleeding) or frequent or infrequent menstrual cycles with less or more bleeding | 35–50% |
| Oligomenorrhea/Hypomenorrhea (infrequent menstruation or less bleeding during menstruation) | 10–12% |
| Primary amenorrhea | 10% |
| Secondary amenorrhea | 5–6% |

**Symptoms** Dysmenorrhea, i.e., painful menstruation, is the most common complaint.

- Dysmenorrhea occurs in 70–80% of girls. Some report to hospitals, others live with the problem. Some do not go to school/college/work. Others take action as per tradition of the family.
- Other common complaints are abdominal pain, lump in pelvis or lump in abdomen.
- With obstructive uterine abnormalities and amenorrhea, there is cyclic pelvic pain, mass in lower abdomen due to haematocolpos, haematometra and haematosalphinx and pressure symptoms like retention of urine.
- Other gynaecological complaints with which girls present are genital tract injuries (1–2%). Ovarian tumours constitute about 1% and of them 40% are malignant, mainly germ cell tumours.

### Menstrual Disorders

#### Dysmenorrhea

**Primary dysmenorrhea** is a cramping pain in the lower abdomen. It is the most common menstrual disorder in young girls and is reported to occur in 70–80% of girls, though the real numbers are not known because some report while others do not. Also the pain is difficult to measure partly because it depends on the individual, and is affected by the mental make-up of the person experiencing pain, and also because it is accompanied by other unpleasant symptoms and many other visible/invisible issues. **It is so common that many women fail to report it even in medical interviews, even when the pain poses restrictions on their daily activities.** During the last decade, substantial progress has been made towards understanding the nature and potential management of dysmenorrhea, however it still manages to confound clinicians. Although it is only temporarily disabling, its regularity, frequency and effects make it worthy of renewed appraisal. Some girls just take rest. Others take help of quacks. Some go to health professionals, nurse, doctor who prescribe antispasmodics, analgesics.

**Prevention** Simple measures are taken for prevention and therapy of dysmenorrhea.

- **Drugs** The most common approach is to prescribe one of the non-steroidal anti-inflammatory drugs (NSAID). Most girls have relief with antiprostaglandin drugs started at the onset of the menses and continuing for the first 1–2 days. However if NSAID drugs are contraindicated or produce undesirable side effects, an alternative is tramadol hydrochloride tablets. Tramadol is a centrally acting analgesic.
- **Dietary changes** during menstruation are believed to be beneficial in decreasing blood loss and pain. Some girls avoid only spicy food, others nonvegetarian food. Some take more of vegetables and fruits. But more research is needed in this field, which will not only help in prevention and treatment of dysmenorrhea but can also lead to information about other related disorders. There is need to work on reverse pharmacology.

### Premenstrual syndrome (PMS)

PMS is also common. Sometimes it becomes severe enough to interfere with interpersonal relationships. PMS is a psychoneuroendocrine disorder of unknown etiology, often noticed just prior to menstruation. There is cyclic appearance of a large number of symptoms during the last 7–10 days of the menstrual cycle. The exact cause is not known.

#### Treatment

Symptomatic therapy is advocated. Lifestyle modification and cognitive behaviour therapy are important steps. Non-pharmacological therapy includes assurance, yoga, stress management and diet manipulation. Avoidance of salt, caffeine and alcohol especially in the second half of the cycle improves the symptoms.Vitamin D therapy is believed to be a safe, effective and convenient method for improving the quality of life in young women with severe hypovitaminosis D and concomitant mood disorders associated with PMS.

### Puberty menorrhagia—excessive menstrual bleeding

A common menstrual problem in adolescent girls is cyclical excessive menstrual loss, in amount and/or duration.

Normal menstrual loss is up to 80 mL per cycle and normal duration of menstruation is 3–5 days, but 2–7 days is normal.

Anything beyond normal amount of loss or duration of menstruation is abnormal. Sometimes bleeding is very heavy and leads to severe anaemia, threatening life. There is anovulation in the first few years after menarche and is usually the likely cause of excessive bleeding. Therefore this problem occurs much more commonly in the young teenagers. Only 15% of cycles are ovulatory in the first year after menarche, increasing to 75% cycles in the first 5 years and to 95% by 10 years.

**Pathogenesis** As ovulation does not occur, the endometrium continues to be stimulated by unopposed estrogen. When menstruation eventually occurs, the bleeding tends to be excessive and prolonged. Each episode is usually separated by several weeks of amenorrhea. This can be a recurrent problem until the cycles become regular. Girls might present with mild variety, where there is no anaemia but some others may present with signs of mild or moderate anaemia or in the most severe situation, with profuse prolonged bleeding with severe anaemia, sometimes resulting in hypovolemic shock.

**Investigations** Adolescents with bleeding need to be evaluated for heavy bleeding including idiopathic thrombocytopenia, other bleeding dyscrasias, coagulation disorders, hypothyroidism or feminising ovarian tumour or leiomyoma of uterus. Tuberculosis should also be considered in these girls.

#### Treatment

Hormone therapy needs to be avoided unless essential. If necessary, progestogens are given. Genital tuberculosis also needs to be considered in non-responders.

### Amenorrhea

**A girl who does not menstruate by 16 years** is believed to be having primary amenorrhea. The basic fact that amenorrhea could be because of a fault in the axis from the hypothalamus to the endometrium needs to be given consideration. However menstrual irregularities are common occurrence during adolescence, especially in the first 2–3 years after menarche. So girls too get bouts of 2–3 months amenorrhea. Prolonged amenorrhea, however, is not normal and can be associated with significant medical morbidity, which differs depending on whether the adolescent is estrogen-deficient or estrogen-replete. The details of amenorrhea are dealt with in Chapter 16.

## Abdominal Pain

Abdominal pain in an adolescent girl is a common problem, a cause of hospital admission and parental anxiety.

**Causes** While cyclical pain during menstruation is dysmenorrhea, there are other common gynecological conditions which cause acute/chronic abdominal pain in adolescents.These are discussed in the following sections.

**Causes of Abdominal Pain in Adolescents**

1. Congenital anomalies of the genital tract
2. Rupture of functional ovarian cyst
3. Pelvic inflammatory disease (PID)
4. Tubo-ovarian torsion
5. Endometriosis
6. Genital neoplasms

## Congenital Anomalies of the Genital Tract

Adolescent girls with congenital abnormalities of genital tract may present with acute or chronic abdominal pain. An imperforate hymen, transverse vaginal septum or vaginal agenesis may not be detected until medical attention is sought because of abdominal pain which is due to collection of blood in vagina, uterus or both and salpinx also. It could also be because of a rudimentary horn which is not communicating with the uterine horn which has an open cervix. These conditions are dealt with in more detail in Chapter 5.

## Rupture of Functional Ovarian Cyst

With the onset of puberty, physiological hormonal changes lead to maturation of the internal reproductive organs. Cystic ovaries are frequently seen in adolescents because of the presence of developed follicles in the ovaries. Rupture of follicular or corpus luteal cyst may occur during midcycle and may cause acute abdominal pain. Figures 6.3 and 6.4 show simple follicular cysts.

## Sexually Transmitted Diseases

STDs continue to be major health risks for adolescents. Their sexual experience, risk taking behaviour and immature reproductive system put them at greater risk not only for acquiring sexually transmitted infections, but also for morbidity which follows such diseases. From a biological perspective, the cervix in the physically mature woman provides defence against ascending infection and subsequent PID. Cervical mucus production and humoral immunity starts when ovulation begins, thus potentiating the risk of such complications in the adolescents.

### Vaginal infection

A normal estrogen effect sometimes leads to excessive discharge. The girl presents with leucorrhea, a whitish mucoid discharge. Assurance is the only therapy.

*Trichomonas vaginalis*, candidiasis and bacterial vaginosis are the three usual disease conditions responsible for vaginal discharge. These are dealt with in more detail in Chapter 9.

### HIV infection

The risk of acquiring HIV is higher in those adolescents who engage in unprotected sex, have multiple sexual partners, share drug-injecting equipment and have sex with a 'high risk' person. Poverty, social and cultural barriers and the lack or inadequacy of health care service for adolescents further potentiate the problems. The implications for teenage girls being infected with HIV are serious. When these individuals become mothers they may infect their babies via vertical transmission. There are reports of increased progression rate of cervical intraepithelial neoplasm (CIN) in immunocompromised women.

### Pelvic inflammatory disease

Adolescents between the ages of 15 and 19 years are a high-risk group for PID; impaired immune host defence is frequently cited as a risk factor for this age group. PID results from infection of uterus, Fallopian tubes, ovaries, the pelvic peritoneum, vascular structures and the connective tissue. The Fallopian tubes are common sites for primary infection. It is described more fully in Chapter 12.

## Tubo-ovarian Torsion

Torsion of the enlarged cystic ovary with the Fallopian tube within the twist in adolescents may lead to acute abdomen with severe lower abdominal pain.

## Endometriosis

It is uncommon in adolescents as it is supposed to be a disease of women of reproductive life. It may also cause abdominal pain as well as spasmodic/congestive dysmenorrhea.

## Neoplasms

### Ovarian tumours

Ovarian tumours are the most common genital tract tumours in adolescents but they constitute no more than 1% of all tumours of girls under 16 years of age. Of all the tumours, more than one-third are malignant. In an adolescent girl with neoplasm of the ovary, abdominal pain is usually the presenting symptom. It may present as acute due to torsion or haemorrhage. In others, there may be a long history of intermittent pain followed by a more persistent severe ache leading to surgery. Nausea, vomiting, abdominal enlargement, diarrhea, constipation, urinary symptoms and vaginal bleeding are other presenting symptoms. However one-third of the masses of the ovary could be non-neoplastic. The corpus luteum normally does not exceed 4 cm in diameter, and cysts larger than this are referred to as corpus luteum cysts. Persistent cysts will continue to secrete progesterone and therefore are associated with delayed menstruation. They are prone to rupture giving rise to intratumour bleeding and may present as acute abdomen.

The most common benign ovarian tumour during adolescence is **teratoma** which is usually small, unilateral (bilateral in 10–15%). **Mucinous cystadenoma** (Fig. 6.5) another common benign neoplasm, is also found in late adolescence. **Serous cystadenoma** is occasionally found in adolescence.

Functioning tumours of endocrine significance which arise from specific gonadal stromal elements in childhood usually take the form of **granulosa-theca cell tumours**. Precocious puberty is the presenting symptom in 70% of girls with this tumour.

Malignant ovarian tumours in adolescence are more likely to be of germ cell origin than the epithelial tumour found in elderly. The common malignant tumours found in adolescents are dysgerminoma, endodermal sinus tumour, malignant teratoma, embryonal carcinoma, primary ovarian choriocarcinoma and mixed germ cell tumour, all of which necessitate surgery and very often chemotherapy. Prognosis is usually good with long-term survival, good quality of life and fertility.

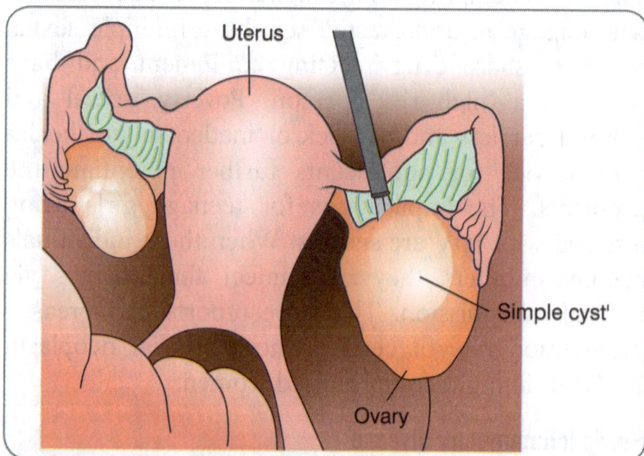


**Fig. 6.3** Simple follicular cyst

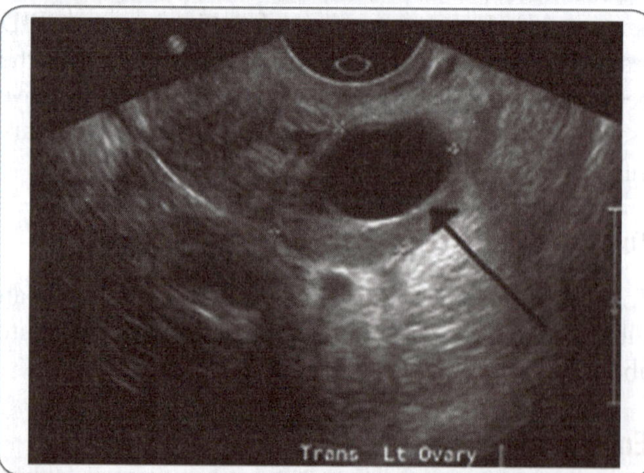


**Fig. 6.4** A 2 cm left ovarian cyst as seen on ultrasound (*Source:* Wikimedia)

### Dysgerminoma

It is the most common malignant ovarian tumour in adolescents (Fig. 6.6). It is usually unilateral and grows rapidly to a considerable size. The prognosis for girls with dysgerminoma is good. Overall 5 year survival rate of 85% to 90% has been reported.

### Endodermal sinus tumour

Also known as yolk sac tumour (Fig. 6.7), this is the second most common ovarian tumour in this age

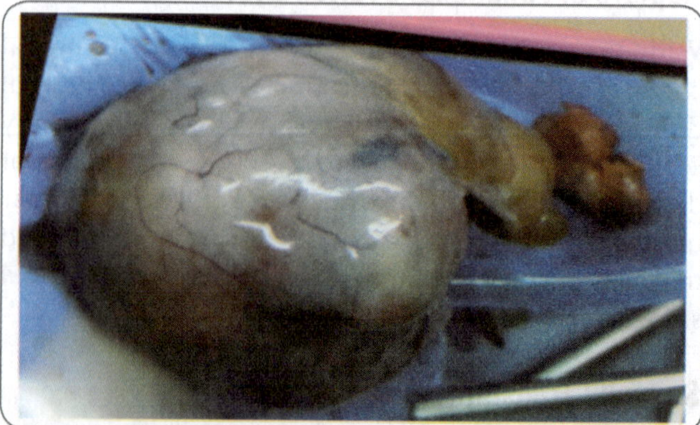

**Fig. 6.5** Ovarian cyst (*Source:* Dr Samundeshwari Mahesh, Consultant Radiologist, Apollo Hospitals, Chennai)

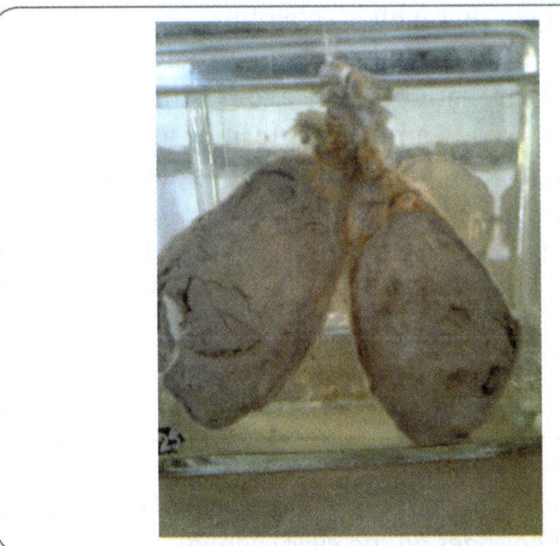

**Fig. 6.6** Dysgerminoma (*Source:* Wikimedia)

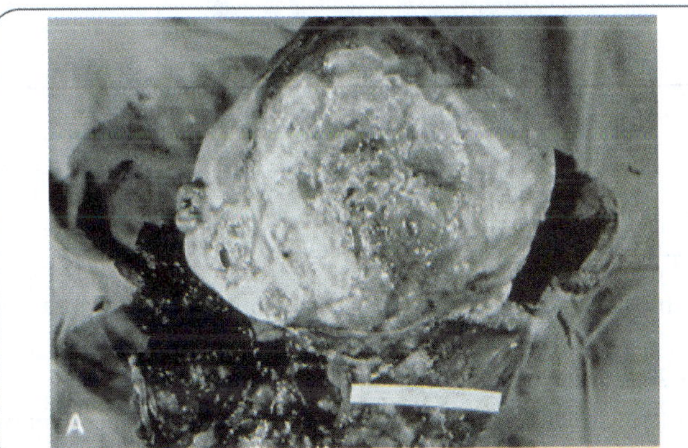


**Fig. 6.7** Yolk sac (endodermal sinus) tumour. (*Source:* ©Breen, J, Denehy, T, et al, Glob. libr. women's med.)

group. It is an extremely aggressive malignant tumour. The tumour is found almost exclusively in teenagers, the median age of presentation being 19 years.

### Teratoma

In girls, teratomas are benign, but two forms of malignant teratomas do exist. The most common is the immature teratoma which occurs most frequently in the first two decades of life. Approximately 8% of all ovarian tumours in children under 15 years are immature teratomas.

### Cervical intraepithelial neoplasia and carcinoma cervix

Cervical screening programmes aim to reduce death from cervical cancer. National recommendations for cervical screening programmes have varied. Screening from age 21 years has been suggested in view of early sexual activity. Vaccine is being advocated for prevention. However controversies continue because of various reasons.

Despite the challenges associated with a new cancer diagnosis, adolescents and parents value the opportunity to discuss fertility concerns in adolescent girls with cancers. Preservation options in adolescents with cancers during adolescence, especially cancers related to genital system must be discussed. Providers play an important role in addressing various issues. Efforts must be made to incorporate fertility preservation discussions into the cancer care for all adolescents, with attention paid to their unique needs.

## Polycystic Ovarian Syndrome

Polycystic ovarian syndrome (PCOS), characterised by hyperandrogenism and chronic anovulation with polycystic ovaries, is probably the most common endocrine disorder that can occur at any age, with risks for metabolic/cardiovascular disorders.This is discussed in greater detail in Chapter 14.

## Genital Prolapse

Congenital cervico-uterine prolapse is uncommon. Usually, it is just elongation of the cervix. Therapy is essentially surgery. Amputation of cervix is needed in cases of elongation of cervix. Sling surgery in cases of cervico-uterine prolapse is the recommended surgery.

## Genetic Problems

Turner's syndrome, Klinefelter's syndrome are some of the conditions and they are dealt with in detail in Chapter 5.

Adolescents might present with a varied clinical picture due to genetic disorders. The 46XY female in essence neither has ovarian tissue nor a uterus but the gonadal tissue tends to be testicular in nature. Genetic females, 46XX have two *AR* genes and can manifest as minimally affected female but they are carriers for *AR* gene abnormalities. The defect of the Y-chromosome or more specifically, *SRY* gene plays a major role in androgen insensitivity syndrome (AIS). Depending on various factors, manifestation could be either complete or partial.The incidence of disorders of sexual development is around 25%. **Pseudohermaphroditism** reflects mismatch of genetic and phenotypic types. When both ovarian and testicular tissues are present in the same individual, they are known as true hermaphrodites. The most common karyotype in true hermaphroditism is 46 XX. In this condition there is unilateral ovotestis with contralateral ovary or testis, or bilateral ovotestes. The other common karyotype is 46XX/46XY.

Gonadectomy may be deferred until adulthood due to the low risk of malignancy.

## Miscellaneous

### Toxic shock syndrome

Toxic shock syndrome (TSS) received much publicity in the early 1980s as a disease that was occurring in young women primarily in association with one brand of tampon.

Knowledge on which absolute guidelines to patients could be based on is insufficient, but it is suggested that patients (a) avoid superabsorbent tampons, (b) use tampons intermittently and use pads at night, (c) change tampons every 4 to 6 hours, and especially (d) remove tampons and call a physician if vomiting, diarrhea, rash, or fever occurs.

***Case study***

*A 16-year-old unmarried girl comes with a history of profuse bleeding during periods lasting for even up to 10 days. She is anaemic without any signs of failure. She gives history of recurrent episodes during every period.*

*a) What is this condition known as?*

*b) What is the probable etiology?*

*c) How is this condition managed?*

## RECAP

- Adolescent gynecology remains an area to which greater attention should be given if we are to protect and promote the health of teenagers.
- Gynecological problems in teenagers need to be sensitively dealt with. Adolescence, the transitional period from childhood to adult autonomy, psychosexual development with acquisition of secondary sexual characteristics and adult reproductive capacities, is a crucial period of human life.
- Adolescents have increased risk of health as well as social aspects alike and the price for the transformation to industrialisation, urbanisation and social uplift is added.
- Adolescent girl herself is a child, since she has not completed her own growth and development. Pregnancy and contraceptives affect occurrence of gynecological disorders in adolescents. So sexual education and creating awareness about use of contraceptives will go a long way in prevention of unintended teenage pregnancy and sexually transmitted diseases.
- She is not yet ready for motherhood and complications like anaemia, preeclampsia, preterm labour and fetal growth restriction are more often seen in teenage pregnancy; therefore teenage pregnancy leads to morbidity to both mother and child, and so adolescent pregnancy should be prevented.
- Contraceptive use needs to be encouraged.
- However it is essential to create awareness about associated morbidities, such as PID, menstrual disorders, infertility, obesity, etc.
- There should be awareness about gynecological disorders in these young girls as some of these disorders may have life-threatening effect on them or may have devastating effect on their future fertility and childbearing.
- For protecting and promoting the health of teenagers, they need to be encouraged to come forward and communicate their anxiety and problems.

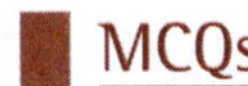

## REVIEW QUESTIONS

### Long-Answer Questions

1. What are the common neoplasms of genital tract during adolescence ?Write treatment of any one.

### Short-Answer Questions

1. Congenital uterine prolapse
2. Puberty menorrhagia

## MCQs

**1. Chromosomal pattern in Turner syndrome is?**
a) 46, XX
b) 45, XO
c) 47 XXX
d) 47 XYY

**2. PCOS and PCO are synonymous?**
a) True
b) False

**3. Stage I dysgerminoma in an adolescent girl is best treated by**
a) Radiotherapy
b) Chemotherapy
c) Surgery
d) All of above

### Further Reading

Bertelloni, S., Dati, E., Baroncelli, G., Hiort, O. Hormonal management of complete androgen insensitivity syndrome from adolescent onward. Horm Res Paediatr. 2011;76:428–33.

Fruzzetti F, Ghiadoni L, Virdis A, De Negri F, Perini D, Bucci F, Giannarelli C, Gadducci A, Taddei S.Adolescents with classical polycystic ovary syndrome have alterations in the surrogate markers of cardiovasculardisease but not in the endothelialfunction. The possible benefits of metformin.J PediatrAdolesc Gynecol. 2016; 24: S1083-3188(16)30001-8.

Golden NH, Carlson JL. The pathophysiology of amenorrhea in the adolescent. Ann N Y Acad Sci. 2008;1135:163–78.

Kim HJ, Lee DY, Yoon BK, et al. Uterine development after estrogen replacement therapy in women with different etiologies of primary hypogonadism. Journal of pediatric and adolescent gynecology. 2016; 29(4):344–47.

Mauldon D. Delayed puberty and menstrual irregularities. In: Emans SJ, Laufer MR, Goldstein DP, editorss. Pediatric and adolescent gynecology.Philadelphia: Lippincott-Raven; 2016.

Sanfilippo JS.The multi facets of androgen insensitivity syndrome.Northe American society for pediatric and adolescent gynecology, 2016. Available at: https://www.researchgate.net/journal/10833188_Journal_of_Pediatric_and_Adolescent_Gynecology

Agenesis of vagina, Transverse vaginal septum, Imperforate hymen. Available at: www.slideshare.net

Causes of Primary amenorrhoea. Available at: www.teluguone.com

Klinefelter syndrome. Available at: www.philipcaruso-story.com

Ovarian cyst, Malignant tumour. Available at: www.mayoclinic.org

Polycystic ovary. Available at: www.medicinenet.com

Precocious Puberty. Available at: www.slideshare.net

Turner syndrome. Available at: www.slideplayer.com

# CHAPTER 7

# Abnormal Uterine Bleeding

## AT A GLANCE

- Etiology
  - Organic Causes
  - Dysfunctional Uterine Bleeding (DUB)
- PALM-COEIN Classification
  - Structural Lesions
  - Non-structural Lesions
- Examination of the Patient
  - History
  - General Examination
- Pathophysiology
  - Endometrial Hyperplasia
  - Anovulatory DUB
  - Ovulatory DUB
- Investigations
- Diagnosis
  - Differential Diagnosis
- Treatment
  - General Measures
  - Pictorial Blood Assessment Chart (PBAC) Scoring
  - Definitive Treatment
  - Medical Management
  - Surgical Management

Abnormal Uterine Bleeding (AUB) is a common symptom seen among women attending gynecology clinics. Women suffer from it from menarche to menopause and it has a negative effect on the physical and mental health. It occurs more in the teenage and perimenopausal age group.

**Definition** Any bleeding from the uterus which is abnormal in frequency, flow and duration, effecting a change in the quantity of blood loss is known as AUB.

**Any deviation in the hypothalamo-pituitary–ovarian axis or defect in hemostasis in the endometrium can result in AUB.**

**Incidence** The reported incidence varies widely between 9–18% to 10–30%. In India, the reported prevalence is around 17.9%.

The normal menstrual events are described in Chapter 4. To summarise:

**Normal Menstrual Cycle**

| | Normal range | Average |
|---|---|---|
| Frequency | 21–35 days | 28 ± 7 days |
| Duration | 2–8 days | 5 ± 3 days |
| Volume of blood loss | 20–80 mL | 50 ± 30 mL |

Normally the bleeding gets arrested by three ways:
- Hemostasis by platelet plugs and clot formation
- Vasoconstriction which is mediated by $PGF_{2\alpha}$, $PGE_2$, $PGI_2$ and thromboxane
- Re-epithelialisation and repair of the vessels

Previously, certain descriptive terms were used to describe the abnormal bleeding pattern.

**Menorrhagia**—cyclical bleeding with increased blood loss (prolonged and/or profuse)

**Polymenorrhea**—frequent cycles with normal blood loss

**Polymenorrhagia**—frequent cycles with increased blood loss

**Metrorrhagia**—acyclical intermenstrual bleeding

**Oligomenorrhea**—infrequent cycles

**Hypomenorrhea**—cyclical but reduced blood loss

All these terms have been replaced by FIGO (International Federation of Gynecology and Obstetrics) with just two terms:
- Heavy menstrual Bleeding (HMB)
- Inter-menstrual Bleeding (IMB)

## ETIOLOGY

AUB is broadly categorised into that due to **organic causes** and that due to **dysfunctional uterine bleeding**.

### Organic Causes

The organic causes of AUB are listed in Table 7.1.

Table 7.1 Organic causes of AUB

| Cause | Conditions |
|---|---|
| **Pelvic pathology (Genital tract)** | |
| Pregnancy-related | • Implantation bleed<br>• Ectopic<br>• Abortion<br>• Gestational trophoblastic disease<br>• Delayed involution (infection) after abortion or delivery |
| Congenital | • Uterus didelphys<br>• Uterus bicornuate |
| Infections | • Acute:<br>1. Salpingo-oophoritis<br>2. Pelvic peritonitis and cellulitis<br>• Chronic:<br>1. Pelvic inflammatory disease and pelvic adhesions<br>2. TB endometritis<br>3. Chronic cervicitis with cellulitis (chlamydial infection)—metrorrhagia and postcoital bleeding |
| Iatrogenic | • IUCD<br>• Post-tubal sterilisation<br>• Progestogen-only pills<br>• Irregular use of pills containing hormones / break through bleeding |
| Benign pathology | • Leiomyoma of uterus<br>• Endometrial / endocervical polyps<br>• Adenomyosis<br>• Endometriosis<br>• Arterio-venous malformation in the uterus<br>• Hormone-producing ovarian tumours (Estrogen-producing ovarian tumours) |
| Malignancy | • Cancer endometrium due to increased bleeding surface<br>• Cancer cervix<br>• Generalised myohyperplasia<br>• Previous DVT (deep vein thrombosis) |
| **General causes** | |
| Coagulation defects | • Thrombocytopenic purpura<br>• Aplastic anaemia<br>• Leukemia<br>• von Willebrand's disease |
| Endocrine dysfunction | • Hypothyroidism<br>• Early stages of acromegaly<br>• Alteration of metabolism of estrogen |

## Dysfunctional Uterine Bleeding (DUB)

**Definition** If there is no general or pelvic pathology, it is designated as **dysfunctional uterine bleeding.** The causes of DUB are listed in Table 7.2.

The International Federation of Gynecology and Obstetrics (FIGO) has classified AUB based on etiopathogenesis. There are nine main categories which are arranged according to the acronym **PALM-COEIN** (pronounced 'palm–koin') (Fig. 7.1).

Table 7.2 Causes of DUB

| Cause | Effect |
|---|---|
| • Anovulatory | • Metropathia hemorrhagica<br>• Threshold bleeding |
| • Ovulatory | Irregular ripening } Luteal<br>Irregular shedding } phase defect<br>Idiopathic menorrhagia—alteration in the ratio of prostaglandin |

## PALM-COEIN CLASSIFICATION

### Structural Lesions

**Polyps (AUB-P)**—Endometrial and/or endocervical canal.

**Adenomyosis (AUB-A)**—Presence of endometrial tissue in the myometrium at least 2.5 mm beneath the endomyometrial interface.

**Leiomyoma (AUB-L)**

- Submucous myoma AUB-L (0,1,2)
- Others

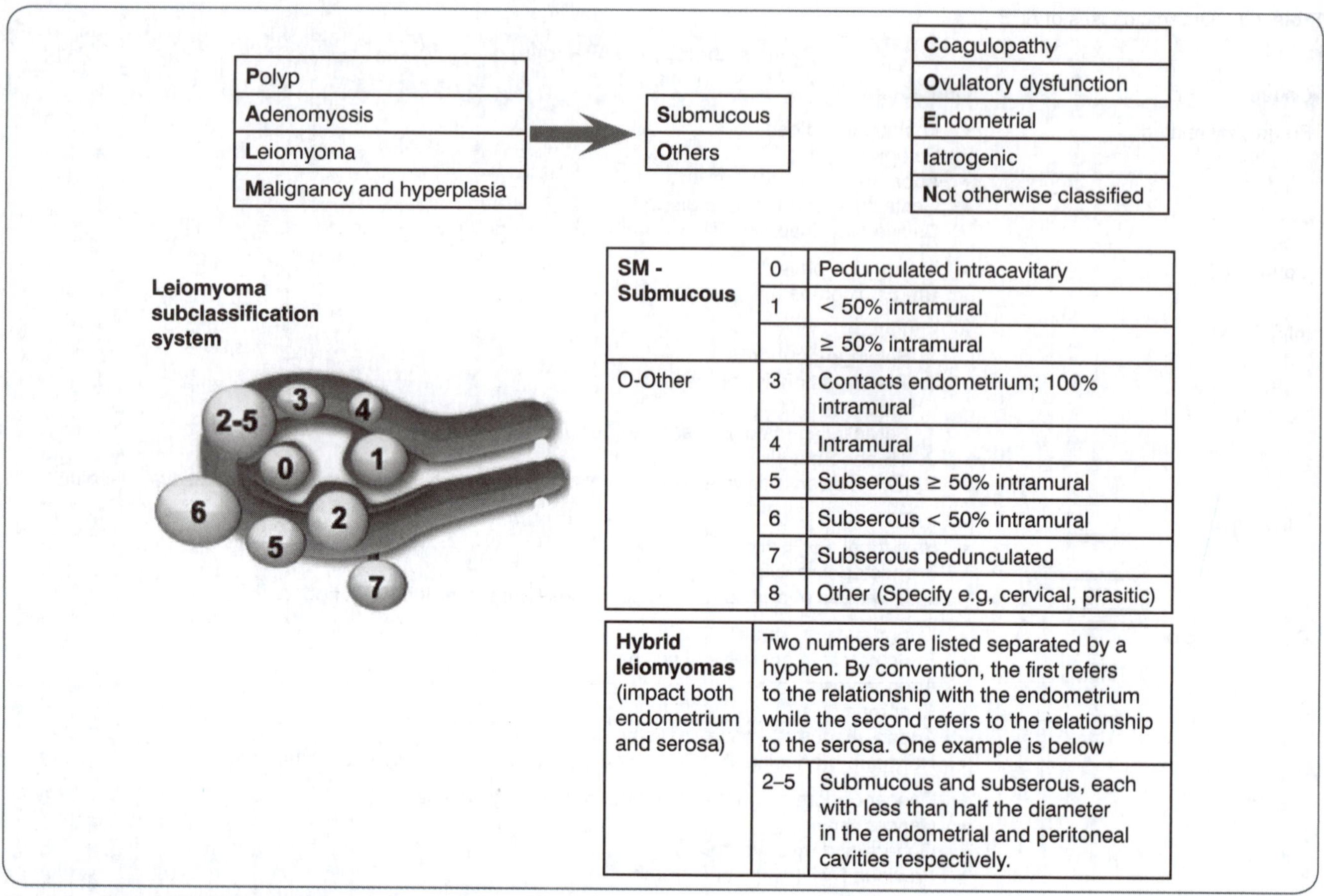


**Fig. 7.1** FIGO PALM-COEIN classification for AUB

- Intramural AUB-L (3,4)
- Subserous AUB-L (5, 6, 7)
- Cervical fibroids and other extrauterine myoma AUB-L (8)

**Malignancy and hyperplasia (AUB-M)**—Premalignant hyperplastic and malignant lesions

## Non-structural Lesions

**Coagulopathy (AUB-C)**

- Inherited (e.g., von Willibrand's disease)
- Acquired (e.g., idiopathic thrombocytopenia)

**Ovulatory dysfunction (AUB-O)**—Can be HMB or oligomenorrhea

**Endometrial (AUB-E)**—Disorder of mechanisms regulating endometrial hemostasis which may be due to endometrial inflammation or infection.

**Iatrogenic (AUB-I)**

- Medicated or inert intrauterine systems
- Use of single or combined gonadal steroid therapy (EPA)
- Use of drugs that interfere with dopamine metabolism or anticoagulant drugs

**Not classified (AUB-N)**—Rare or ill-defined conditions

- Chronic endometritis
- Arterio-venous malformations
- Myometrical hypertrophy
- Other disorders not yet identified

# EXAMINATION OF THE PATIENT

A detailed history, clinical examination and basic investigations are usually sufficient to diagnose AUB and assign a PALM-COEIN category.

## History

1. **Age** Age of the patient is important as AUB can occur at any age. In the adolescents, it will be more of puberty menorrhagia and anovulatory type of bleeding (See Chapter 6 for adolescent menstrual problems). Anovulatory bleeding can

again be expected in the perimenopausal age group.

2. **Menstrual history** A detailed menstrual history with reference to the following would serve as a guide for proceeding further:
   a. Age at menarche
   b. Regularity of menstrual cycle
   c. Frequency of menses
   d. Duration of flow
   e. Volume of blood loss/cycle
   f. Nature of associated pain (dysmenorrhea)
      - Congestive
      - Spasmodic
   g. Last menstrual period
   h. Duration of the present complaint
3. **Marital/Sexual history** Number of years of married life, frequency of coitus.
4. Dyspareunia
5. Postcoital bleeding
6. Parity
7. **Vaginal discharge**
   - Duration of the vaginal discharge
   - Nature of the discharge (profuse/scanty)
   - Frequency of the discharge (present always/ occasionally)
   - Colour
   - Volume (scanty/copious)
   - Foul-smelling
   - Blood-stained, etc.
8. History of recent abortion, IUCD insertion , use of hormone therapy
9. Symptoms of hypo/hyperthyroidism
10. Renal/Liver disorders
11. Symptoms of bleeding disorders

## General Examination

- **Vital signs** Pulse and BP are recorded along with examination of cardiovascular and respiratory systems. Presence of pallor must be noted.
- **Body mass index** needs to be calculated and is more relevant when thyroid disorders or PCOS is suspected.
- Any thyroid enlargement is to be noted.
- Similarly bruising, petechiae in the skin should arouse the suspicion of underlying coagulation disorder. Presence of hirsutism and acanthosis nigricans would alert to the possibility of PCOS (See Chapter14).
- **Abdominal examination** shall reveal the presence of scars, mass (leiomyoma), organomegaly and also ascites.
- A detailed **gynecological examination** should be done as detailed below:
  - Local examination of vulva, anus
  - Speculum examination of the vagina and cervix. A Pap smear should be taken to screen for any cervical pathology.
  - Bimanual pelvic examination is then done to assess the size and mobility of the uterus, tenderness, adnexal masses and/or adnexal tenderness.

  **Rectal examination** is done whenever indicated.

# PATHOPHYSIOLOGY

## Endometrial Hyperplasia

Endometrial hyperplasia (EH) is a pathological condition characterised by hyperplastic changes in endometrial glandular and stromal structures lining the uterine cavity. EH is one of the most common causes of abnormal uterine bleeding (AUB). Though it is not malignant as such, in some it can develop into endometrial carcinoma, if left untreated. EH usually results from excess of estrogen with low levels of progesterone. WHO classified EH as follows (1994) and it is still being followed widely.

### World Health Organisation 1994 classification

1. Simple hyperplasia
2. Complex hyperplasia
3. Simple hyperplasia with atypia
4. Complex hyperplasia with atypia

### New WHO 2014 classification of endometrial hyperplasia

1. Non-atypical endometrial hyperplasia (benign hyperplasia)
2. Atypical endometrial hyperplasia or endometrial intraepithelial neoplasia (EIN)/well differentiated carcinoma.

The various investigations, diagnosis and management are described in relevant chapters.

## Anovulatory DUB

Anovulatory bleeding is seen in a vast majority of AUB. Understanding the pathophysiology of this condition would help in arriving at the appropriate diagnosis and management.

### Metropathia hemorrhagica

This is seen in adolescent girls and perimenopausal women in whom the menstrual cycles are anovulatory. There is a period of amenorrhea followed by profuse, prolonged and painless bleeding. As there is no ovulation, there is no corpus luteum. Endometrium is initially proliferative and becomes hyperplastic due to unopposed estrogen action.

Histopathological examination of endometrium reveals cystic, irregularly dilated glands with hyperplastic stroma, increased vascularisation, infarction and thrombosis. This appearance is known as **'Swiss-cheese appearance'.**

### Threshold bleeding

This is often seen in perimenopausal women. The estrogen level is low due to insufficient development of ovarian follicles. There is also very low or absent progestogens and PGF2α and thromboxane. All these result in profuse bleeding with short cycles. Combination pills containing estrogen and progesterone will help these women.

## Ovulatory DUB

This consists of luteal phase defect which in turn comprises irregular ripening and irregular shedding and idiopathic menorrhagia which is due to alteration in the ratio of prostaglandin (PG).

### Idiopathic menorrhagia

This condition is believed to be due to disordered PG production in the endometrium. In some women, though they produce normal amount of progesterone, there is an alteration in the production of PGE and PGF2α, though they produce normal amount of progesterone. Apart from alteration in the PG, there is also increased fibrinolytic activity and decrease in thromboxane production. These changes result in HMB in spite of ovulation. The condition responds to treatment with antifibrinolytics like tranexemic acid and PG synthetase inhibitors like Indomethacin and Ibuprofen.

### Luteal phase defect

This could manifest itself in two ways—irregular ripening or irregular shedding.

- **Irregular ripening** Irregular ripening manifests as premenstrual spotting or polymenorrhea. This is due to corpus luteum insufficiency and **it results in decreased secretion of estrogen and progesterone in the second half of the cycle.** The low estrogen and progesterone levels are insufficient to support the endometrium. Though the luteal phase is short, endometrium shows irregular ripening.
- **Irregular shedding** Contrary to the previous condition described, in irregular shedding, there is **persistent progesterone secretion during menstruation.** This is usually associated with persistent corpus luteum. As a result of this, the luteal phase is prolonged. The patient usually comes with the complaint of postmenstrual spotting.

## INVESTIGATIONS

The following are the main investigations to be carried out for AUB.

- CBC and hemoglobin—to assess the severity of anaemia
- Pregnancy test (serum β-hCG)
- Coagulation studies (PT, INR, aPTT)—when bleeding disorder is suspected
- Thyroid function tests (if needed)
- Testing for von Willebrand disease (if suspected)
- Ultrasonography—transvaginal ultrasound (Fig. 7.2) for diagnosis of structural lesions and measurement of endometrial thickness
- **Saline infusion sonography or sonohysterography (SIS)**—for diagnosing intracavitary lesions
- **Hysteroscopy**—for diagnosing intracavitary lesions as well as for removing polyps (Fig. 7.3) and endometrial biopsy
- **MRI**—may be rarely indicated
- **Endometrial sampling** This is done to study the endometrium histopathologically with sampling devices like **pipelle** (Fig. 7.4) and **vabra aspirator.**

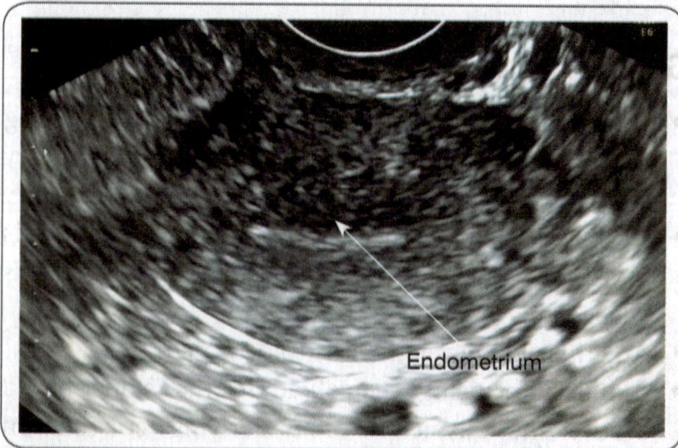


**Fig. 7.2** Transvaginal ultrasound showing the endometrium (*Source:* Dr Narassa Narayani, Consultant Obstetrician and Gynecologist, The Apollo Medical Centre, Chennai)

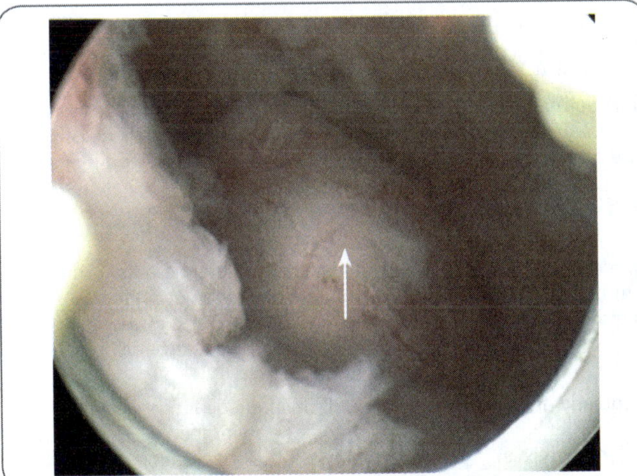

**Fig. 7.3** Hysteroscopy showing a polyp (*Source:* Wikimedia)

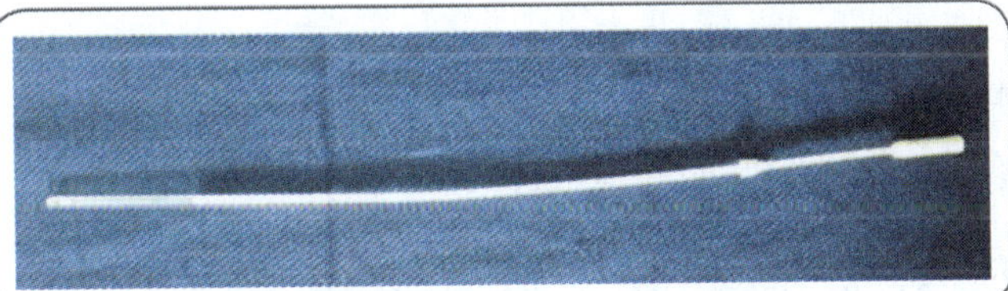

**Fig. 7.4** Pipelle curette

As cervical dilatation is not required it can be done as an office procedure.

- **Dilatation and curettage**— was once very popular and a must-do investigation. This has largely been replaced by pipelle and other office aspiration techniques. It is still being used when a large area needs to be curetted. Moreover, apart from being a diagnostic procedure done to rule out premalignant and malignant conditions of the endometrium, it may be therapeutic in reducing the blood loss in some patients with HMB.

## DIAGNOSIS

The criteria listed in Table 7.3 will be useful in arriving at a diagnosis of AUB.

### Differential Diagnosis

The differential diagnosis of AUB are listed in Table 7.4.

## TREATMENT

### General Measures

1. Correction of anaemia may require oral iron / IV iron preparations, packed cell transfusion depending on the severity and simultaneous treatment of the cause.
2. Life style modification, weight reduction, diet and exercises.
3. Maintaining a menstrual calendar (Fig. 7.5).

### Pictorial Blood Assessment Chart (PBAC) Scoring

This is a user-controlled, user-friendly method (Fig. 7.6) to assess the blood loss during menstrual cycle, particularly in heavy menstrual bleed. It consists of diagrams depicting light, moderate and heavy soiling of sanitary pads or tampons. The chart is also designed to mark the clot passed and flooding. Depending on the type and nature of the flow and clots, a score is assigned to each of the criteria. The woman is asked to maintain the chart during the periods and the physician reviews it at the end of the periods.

### Definitive Treatment

**Structural lesions** The treatment of structural lesions, namely polyp, adenomyosis and leiomyoma, and malignancy of the uterus (PALM) are described in Chapters 9, 10 and 21 respectively.

**Non-structural lesions** Treatment of non-structural lesions depends on the following:

- Age
- Parity
- Patient's wish to preserve the uterus and preserve fertility
- Previous episodes
- Acute or chronic and severity of blood loss
- Co-morbid conditions and family history of gynecological malignancy

### Medical Management

**Medical management is the first line of therapy after excluding malignancy and significant structural causes in both acute and chronic bleeding.**

**Other co-morbid conditions, particularly anaemia, should be effectively treated.**

#### Treatment of acute bleeding

Acute bleeding can be defined as an episode of bleeding marked by sufficient blood loss that requires immediate intervention.

- Admission
- *Conjugated equine estrogen* 25 mg IV × 4-hourly until bleeding reduces. Progestins are added later for 10 days.

**Table 7.3** Criteria for diagnosing AUB

| Pathological condition | Symptoms | Signs | Appearance in imaging |
|---|---|---|---|
| Polyp | • Prolonged uncontrolled bleeding<br>• Intermenstrual bleeding<br>• Anaemia<br>• Infertility<br>• Postcoital bleeding<br>• Postmenopausal bleeding | • Uterus usually normal in size.<br>• If enlarged os may be patulous.<br>• Polyp may be protruding through the os. | • Endometrium may be thickened.<br>• Saline Infusion Sonography (SIS) – Intracavitary mass outlined by fluid. |
| Adenomyosis | • Heavy menstrual bleeding<br>• Dysmenorrhea | • Uterus enlarged uniformly up to 12 weeks size or may be globular.<br>• Tenderness may be present. | • Thickening of uterine mass which may be asymmetrical in focal disease or uniform.<br>• Heterogeneous texture of endometrium. |
| Leiomyoma | Submucous<br>• Prolonged, uncontrolled bleeding<br>• Inter menstrual bleeding<br>Intramural<br>• Variable amount of heavy menstrual bleeding<br>Subserous<br>• May be asymptomatic | • Uterus is irregularly enlarged. Firm.<br>• Movement of the cervix is transmitted to the swelling. | • Well-defined solid masses with a whorled appearance.<br>• May show degeneration |
| Malignancy | • Postmenopausal bleeding<br>• Irregular bleeding at perimenopause | • Uterus normal in size or slightly enlarged | • Thickened endometrium<br>• Irregular endometrial lining<br>• Loss of endomyometrial junction |
| Coagulopathy | • Puberty menorrhagia<br>• History suggestive of bleeding diathesis<br>• Family history | • Uterus normal in size<br>• Easy bruisability, petechiae | • Normal study<br>• Hemorrhagic cysts in the ovary may be present |
| Ovulatory disorders | • Oligomenorrhea<br>• Hirsutism and signs of insulin resistance | • Uterus normal in size | • Polycystic ovaries<br>• Thickened endometrium |
| Endometrial disorders | • Intermenstrual spotting<br>• Prolonged Spotting | • Uterus normal in size | • Fluid in endometrial cavity |
| Iatrogenic | • History of medication (anticoagulants, tamoxifen, atipsychotics and steroids)<br>• IUCD insertion | • Uterus normal in size | • Presence of IUCD |
| Not classified | • Heavy menstrual bleeding | • Uterus normal in size/slightly enlarged | • Doppler for arterio-venous malformations (AVM) |

**Table 7.4** Differential diagnosis of AUB

| Differential diagnosis of AUB |
|---|
| Abortions<br>Ectopic pregnancy<br>Gestational trophoblastic disease<br>Drug intake including contraceptives, hormonal preparations<br>Blood dyscrasias<br>Cervical cancer<br>Uterine cancer<br>Adnexal pathology<br>Cervicitis<br>Vaginitis<br>Hypothyroidism<br>Hyperthyroidism<br>Hyperprolactinemia |

- *High-dose OCP* Initially two tablets of OCP containing 35 mg of ethinyl estradiol (EE) are given for 5 days and then tapered to 1 tab/day for 15 days. Antiemetics are needed when estrogen is given in large doses.
- *High dose progestin*
  - Norethisterone (19 norethisterone derivatives)—10 mg 3–4 times/day
  - Medroxyprogesterone acetate*—20 mg 3–4 times/day
  - Megestrol acetate—20–60 mg twice daily
  - Progestins should be tapered gradually
  - Tranexamic acid 1000 mg IV/oral 3–4 times/day

Medical treatment of chronic AUB includes non-hormonal and hormonal therapy.

### *Non-hormonal treatment*

The usual first line of management of AUB is non-hormonal method. The drugs used and their dosage are given in Table 7.5.

The other drugs used when appropriate for the underlying pathology are:

*To reduce size of myomas and reduce HMB

**Menstrual Calendar**

| Month/Date | | | | | | | | | | | | | | | | | | | | | | | | | | | | | | | | | | | | | | |
|---|---|---|---|---|---|---|---|---|---|---|---|---|---|---|---|---|---|---|---|---|---|---|---|---|---|---|---|---|---|---|---|---|---|---|---|---|---|---|
| Day of cycle | 1 | 2 | 3 | 4 | 5 | 6 | 7 | 8 | 9 | 10 | 11 | 12 | 13 | 14 | 15 | 16 | 17 | 18 | 19 | 20 | 21 | 22 | 23 | 24 | 25 | 26 | 27 | 28 | 29 | 30 | 31 | 32 | 33 | 34 | 35 | 36 | 37 | 38 |
| Information of menstrual cycle | | | | | | | | | | | | | | | | | | | | | | | | | | | | | | | | | | | | | | |
| Period | | | | | | | | | | | | | | | | | | | | | | | | | | | | | | | | | | | | | | |
| Ovulation period | | | | | | | | | | | | | | | | | | | | | | | | | | | | | | | | | | | | | | |
| Fertile days | | | | | | | | | | | | | | | | | | | | | | | | | | | | | | | | | | | | | | |
| Brown discharge | | | | | | | | | | | | | | | | | | | | | | | | | | | | | | | | | | | | | | |
| Unprotected sex | | | | | | | | | | | | | | | | | | | | | | | | | | | | | | | | | | | | | | |
| | | | | | | | | | | | | | | | | | | | | | | | | | | | | | | | | | | | | | | |
| Emotions | | | | | | | | | | | | | | | | | | | | | | | | | | | | | | | | | | | | | | |
| Stress | | | | | | | | | | | | | | | | | | | | | | | | | | | | | | | | | | | | | | |
| Conflict | | | | | | | | | | | | | | | | | | | | | | | | | | | | | | | | | | | | | | |
| Depression | | | | | | | | | | | | | | | | | | | | | | | | | | | | | | | | | | | | | | |
| Super 8 day | | | | | | | | | | | | | | | | | | | | | | | | | | | | | | | | | | | | | | |
| Physical symptoms | | | | | | | | | | | | | | | | | | | | | | | | | | | | | | | | | | | | | | |
| Breast conden | | | | | | | | | | | | | | | | | | | | | | | | | | | | | | | | | | | | | | |
| Abdominal pain | | | | | | | | | | | | | | | | | | | | | | | | | | | | | | | | | | | | | | |
| Weakness | | | | | | | | | | | | | | | | | | | | | | | | | | | | | | | | | | | | | | |
| Headache | | | | | | | | | | | | | | | | | | | | | | | | | | | | | | | | | | | | | | |
| Cramps | | | | | | | | | | | | | | | | | | | | | | | | | | | | | | | | | | | | | | |
| Contraception | | | | | | | | | | | | | | | | | | | | | | | | | | | | | | | | | | | | | | |
| Pills | | | | | | | | | | | | | | | | | | | | | | | | | | | | | | | | | | | | | | |
| Condom | | | | | | | | | | | | | | | | | | | | | | | | | | | | | | | | | | | | | | |
| Emergency contraception | | | | | | | | | | | | | | | | | | | | | | | | | | | | | | | | | | | | | | |

**Fig. 7.5** Menstrual calendar

**PBAC SCORING**

| Name of Patient | Days | | | | | | | Score |
|---|---|---|---|---|---|---|---|---|
| Sanitary pads | 1 | 2 | 3 | 4 | 5 | 6 | 7 | |
| | | | | | | | | |
| | | | | | | | | |
| | | | | | | | | |
| **Tampons** | | | | | | | | |
| | | | | | | | | |
| | | | | | | | | |
| | | | | | | | | |
| **Clots/Flooding** | | | | | | | | |
| 1 Point | For each small clot | | | | | | | |
| 5 Point | For each large clot | | | | | | | |
| 5 Point | For each episode of flooding | | | | | | | |

**For sanitary pads**
1 = Lightly stained
5 = Moderately stained
20 = Completely stained

**For tampoons**
1 = Lightly stained
5 = Moderately stained
10 = Completely stained

**For clots/flooding**
Each small clot = 1 point
Each large clot = 5 points
Each episode of flooding = 5 points

**Fig. 7.6** PBAC scoring

- Desmopressin to treat abnormal uterine bleeding in patients with coagulation defects. It transiently elevates factor VIII and von Willebrand factor.
- Anti-tuberculous drugs for T.B. of endometrium.

**Table 7.5** Non-hormonal drugs for treatment of AUB

| Category of the drug | Name of the drug | Dose |
|---|---|---|
| Antifibrinolytics | Tranexamic acid 1 g | 3–4 times/for 3–5 days |
| NSAIDs* | Mefenamic acid 500 mg | 3 times/day × for 4–5 days |
| SERMs** | Ormeloxifene 60 mg | Twice a week for 12 weeks |
| SPRMs*** | Mifipristone 2.5–25 mg/day<br>Ulipristal acetate 10–20 mg<br>Telapristone and Asoprisnil | For 3 months<br>For 3 months<br>Under study |

*Non-steroidal Anti-inflammatory Drug
**Selective Estrogen Receptor Modulators
*** Selective Progesterone Receptor Modulators

### *Hormonal treatment*

Table 7.6 lists the hormonal drugs used in the treatment of AUB.

**Progestogens** Oral progestogens are used to arrest bleeding and to regulate menstrual cycle. While arresting bleeding, the drug should be started with higher doses, tapered gradually and then maintained for a total duration of 21 days.

Table 7.6 Hormonal drugs for treatment of AUB

| Category of the drug | Name of the drug | Dose |
|---|---|---|
| Progestogens (oral) | Medroxyprogesterone acetate | 10 mg (O) × 3–4 times a day. To be gradually tapered. |
| | 19 nortesterone derivatives like Norethisterone, Norethindrone | 10–20 mg/day to start with and tapered to 15 mg/day, 10 mg/day and maintained at 5–10 mg/day for a total of three weeks. |
| | Cyclical progestogens | 5–10 mg/day from D15 to D25 |
| Progestogens (injectable) | Depot medroxyprogesterone acetate | 150 mg IM |
| Estrogens | Ethinyl estradiol | 50 mcg/day × 5 days |
| | Conjugated equine estrogen | 25 mg IV × 6-hourly |
| Combined oral pills | Ethinyl estradiol | 20 or 30 mcg along with 50–75 mcg or progestogens from day 5 of the menstrual cycle for 21 days |
| Danazol (rarely used) | | 100–200 mg/day |
| GnRH analogues | Goserelin | 3.6 mg IM/month |
| | Leuprolide | 3.75 mg IM/month |
| Levonorgestrel-releasing intrauterine systems | | Releases 20 mcg/day |

Two tablets of medroxyprogesterone acetate (10 mg tab) derivative is given 3–4 times/day and then tapered. 19-nortestosterone derivatives like Norethisterone and Norethindrone are effective in arresting the bleeding. They are given in doses of 10–20 mg/day to start with and tapered to 15 mg/day, 10 mg/day and maintained at 5–10 mg/day for a total of three weeks. After withdrawal bleeding, the same drug is used from day 5 to 25 in 5–10 mg doses daily for 3–6 cycles.

For shortened cycles, cyclical progestogens of 5–10 mg/day can be used from day 15 to day 25.

**Injectable progesterones** Depot medroxyprogesterone acetate 150 mg IM. But bleeding may be irregular and unpredictable.

**Levonorgestrel-releasing intrauterine system** (LNG-IUS) (Fig. 7.7) is effective in both structural and non-structural lesions of AUB. It delivers 20 mcg/day of progesterone and reduces bleeding by causing glandular atrophy and stromal decidualisation.

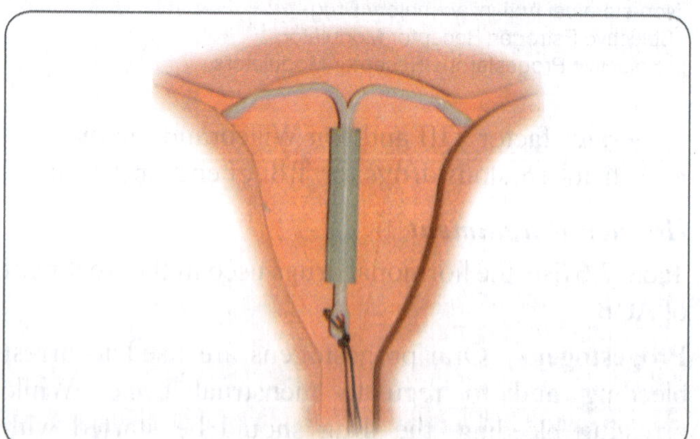

**Fig. 7.7** Levonorgestrel-releasing intrauterine system (*Source:* Wikipedia)

**Estrogens** They are rarely used and are useful in controlling bleeding when AUB is due to atrophic endometrium. Ethinyl estradiol 50 mcg/day × 5 days or conjugated equine estrogen 25 mg IV × 6-hourly are some of the therapeutic options available.

**Combined oral pills** These are widely used to control bleeding and to regularise the cycle. Incidentally it also relieves pain. Ethinyl estradiol 20 or 30 mcg along with 50–75 mcg or progestogens (like levonorgestrel, norethisterone, etc.) are in use. They are given from day 5 of the menstrual cycle for 21 days for 3–6 cycles.

**Danazol** This is rarely used. The dose is 100–200 mg/day for 3 months.

**GnRH analogues** These are used prior to surgical procedures like (AUB-L and AUB-E) leiomyoma and endometrial ablation. The following are some commonly used GnRH analogues.

Goserelin—3.6 mg IM/month
Leoprolide—3.75 mg IM/month

## Surgical Management

**Indications** Surgery is indicated in

- women who do not respond to medical management or
- when women do not prefer the continuous use of hormones

The conservative surgical techniques include

- Endometrial ablation
- Myomectomy
- Uterine artery embolisation
- Hysterectomy

### Endometrial ablation

This is done in women who would prefer to preserve the uterus, or who are at high risk for hysterectomy.

**Contraindications** This procedure is contraindicated in women who desire fertility or in those with suspected malignancy, pre-malignant lesions and large myomas.

Endometrium is resected or destroyed, which results in amenorrhea.

- The **first-generation ablation techniques** like endometrial laser ablation, transcervical endometrial resection and roller ball electrocoagulation have been replaced, since these techniques require hysteroscopy and there are risks of perforation and fluid overload.
- The **second-generation ablation techniques** are preferred and the available techniques are:
  - Thermal balloon ablation (Fig. 7.8).
  - Microwave ablation
  - Hydrotherm ablation
  - Impedance-controlled electrocoagulation (Radio frequency-induced ablation)
  - Laser interstitial therapy

### Myomectomy

If the size of the submucous myoma is less than 4 cm, myomectomy can be done through hysteroscope. Myomectomy can also be done through laparoscope or by laparotomy. In case of fibroid polyp, myomectomy could also be done as a vaginal procedure.

**Uterine artery embolisation** This is an image-guided minimally invasive procedure where the blood supply to the fibroid is blocked. It is useful in A.V. malformation in the uterus.

**Magnetic resonance guided focused ultrasound surgery (MRgFUS)** This can be used in leiomyoma where the energy focused on multiple focal points in leiomyoma results in coagulative necrosis.

### Hysterectomy

This procedure is indicated in women with premalignant lesions, failed hormonal or ablation procedures or with

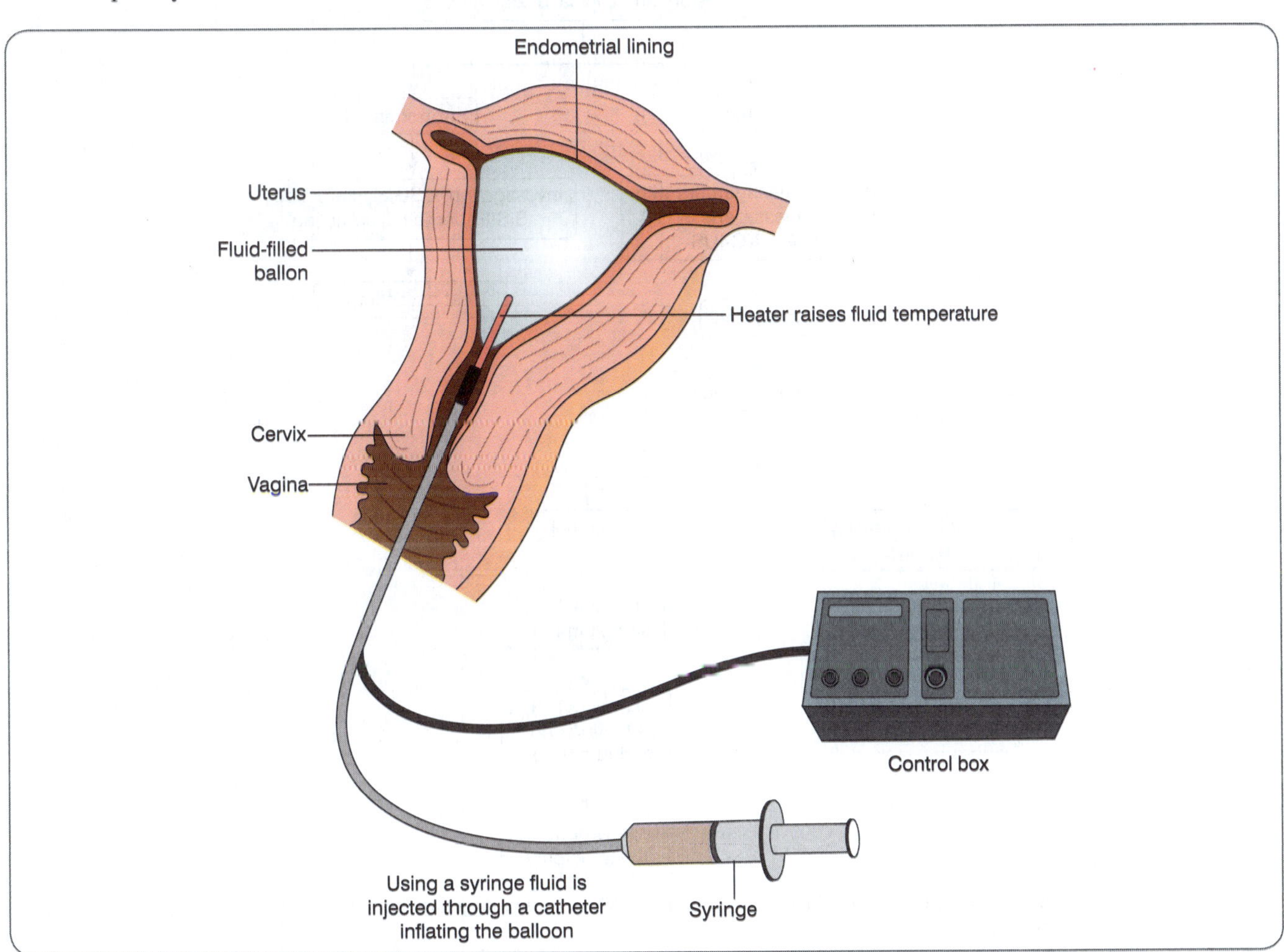


**Fig. 7.8** Thermal balloon ablation technique

associated adrenal pathology. Hysterectomy can be done by vaginal route or by laparoscopy or by laparotomy.

The algorithms in Figs. 7.9 and 7.10 can be used in the investigation and management of AUB.

Presents with features of AUB
History and clinical examination
Investigations: USG-ET, SIS, hysteroscopy, endometrial sampling
Simple hyperplasia. No evidence of malignancy
Atypical hyperplasia
Malignancy
Low-dose OC pills
Hysterectomy
Treat accordingly

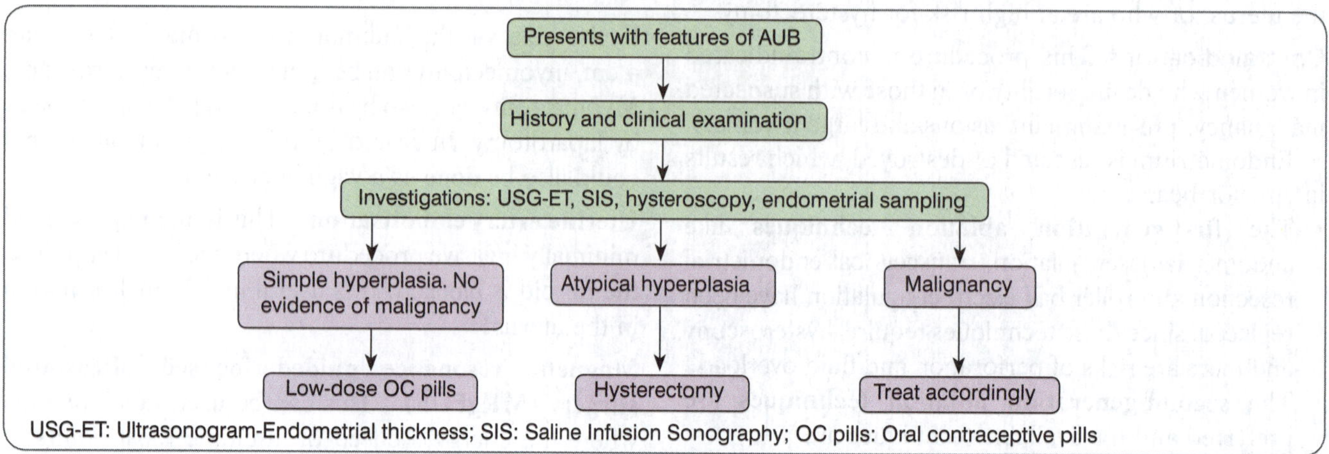

USG-ET: Ultrasonogram-Endometrial thickness; SIS: Saline Infusion Sonography; OC pills: Oral contraceptive pills

**Fig. 7.9** AUB in perimenopausal age group

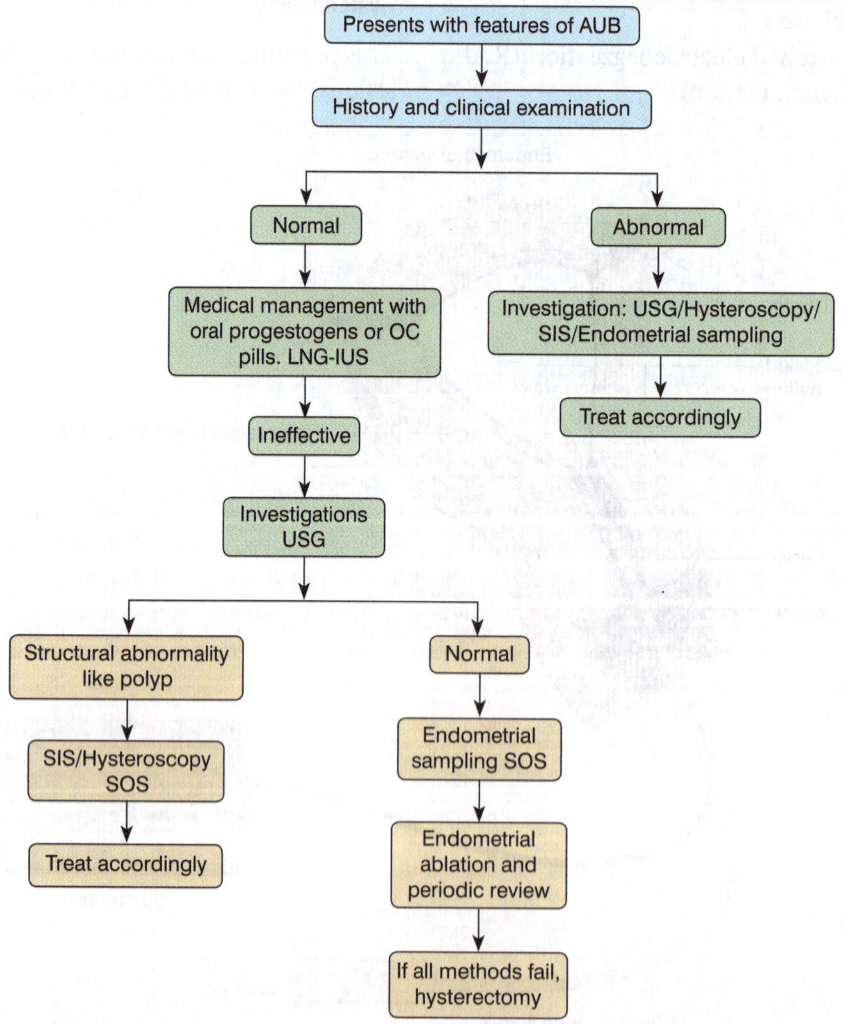

Presents with features of AUB
History and clinical examination
Normal
Abnormal
Medical management with oral progestogens or OC pills. LNG-IUS
Investigation: USG/Hysteroscopy/ SIS/Endometrial sampling
Treat accordingly
Ineffective
Investigations USG
Structural abnormality like polyp
Normal
SIS/Hysteroscopy SOS
Treat accordingly
Endometrial sampling SOS
Endometrial ablation and periodic review
If all methods fail, hysterectomy

USG: Ultrasonography; SIS: Saline Infusion Sonography; LNG-IUS: Levonorgestrel Intrauterine System; OC Pills: Oral contraceptive pills

**Fig. 7.10** AUB in reproductive age group

***Case study***

*A 43-year-old woman with 2 live children presents with a history of profuse and continuous bleeding PV for 20 days. The bleeding is associated with passage of clots and mild abdominal pain. She is having this complaint for the past 6 months. Her previous cycles were regular with normal flow. There was no history of using hormonal preparations or using IUCD.*

*a) What is your probable diagnosis?*

*b) Discuss the relevant investigations required?*

*c) What are the various management options available?*

## RECAP

- Any bleeding from the uterus which is abnormal in frequency, flow and duration effecting a change in the quantity of blood loss is known as AUB.
- AUB is broadly categorised into those due to organic causes and dysfunctional uterine bleeding.
- Organic causes include pelvic pathology (genital tract) including pregnancy-related complications, congenital pathology, infections, chronic conditions like PID, iatrogenic causes like IUCD, benign pathology, malignancy, generalised myohyperplasia and previous DVT.
- General causes include coagulation defects and endocrine dysfunction.
- If there is no general or pelvic pathology, it is designated as dysfunctional uterine bleeding which could be either due to anovulatory or ovulatory cause.
- International Federation of Gynecology and Obstetrics (FIGO) has classified AUB based on etiopathogenesis known as PALM-COEIN.
- A detailed history, clinical examination and basic investigations are usually sufficient to diagnose AUB and assign a PALM-COEIN category.
- Investigations include CBC and hemoglobin, pregnancy test (serum β-hCG), coagulation studies, thyroid function tests (if needed), testing for von Willibrand disease if suspected, ultrasonography, saline infusion sonography or sonohysterography, hysteroscopy and MRI.
- Endometrial sampling by dilatation and curettage are done when indicated.
- Differential diagnosis includes abortions, ectopic pregnancy, gestational trophoblastic disease, drug intake including contraceptives and hormonal preparations, blood dyscrasias, cervical cancer, uterine cancer, adnexal pathology, cervicitis, vaginitis, hypothyroidism, hyperthyroidism and hyperprolactinemia.
- Treatment consists of general measures like correction of anaemia, life style modification, weight reduction, diet and exercises and maintaining menstrual calendar.
- Medical management is the first line of therapy after excluding malignancy and significant structural causes in both acute and chronic bleeding.
- Conjugated equine estrogen, high dose OCP, high dose progestin, tranexamic acid
- Medical treatment of chronic AUB includes non-hormonal and hormonal therapy.
- Non-hormonal therapy includes those using antifibrinolytics, NSAIDS, SERMs and SPRMs.
- Hormonal treatment includes progestogens, LNG-IUS, estrogen, combined oral pills, danazol and GnRH agonists.
- Surgical management consists of conservative surgery like endometrial ablation and myomectomy, uterine artery embolisation and magnetic resonance guided focused ultrasound surgery.
- Hysterectomy is the final option.

# REVIEW QUESTIONS

**Long-answer questions**

1. Define Abnormal Uterine Bleeding. What is the current FIGO classification?
2. Discuss the medical management options for chronic AUB.

## MCQs

1. **Metropathia hemorrhagica is a condition occurring in women**
   a) When the menstrual cycles are anovulatory
   b) When the menstrual cycles are ovulatory
   c) When the endometrium is atrophic
   d) In early weeks of pregnancy
2. **Idiopathic menorrhagia is due to**
   a) Disordered progesterone production in the endometrium
   b) Disordered prostaglandin production in the endometrium
   c) Disordered estrogen production in the endometrium
   d) None of the above
3. **In the treatment of acute bleeding, conjugated equine estrogen is generally given in the dose of:**
   a) 25 mg orally × $4^{th}$ hrly until bleeding reduces
   b) 125 mg IV × $4^{th}$ hrly until bleeding reduces
   c) 250 mg IV × $4^{th}$ hrly until bleeding reduces
   d) 25 mg IV × $4^{th}$ hrly until bleeding reduces
4. **Levonorgestrel-releasing intrauterine systems (LNG-IUS) reduces bleeding by**
   a) Glandular atrophy and stromal decidualisation
   b) Increasing progesterone receptors
   c) Increasing estrogen receptors
   d) By all the three mechanisms

**Further Reading**

American College of Obstetricians and Gynecologists ACOG Committee opinion No. 357: Management of acute abnormal uterine bleeding in nonpregnant reproductive aged women. Obstet Gynecol. 2013; 127(4):891–6.

Murro, MG, Critchley HO, Broder MS, Fraser IS. FIGO working group on menstrual disorder. FIGO classification system (PALM-COEIN) for causes of abnormal uterine bleeding in non gravid women of reproductive age. Intl J Gynecol Obstet. 2011; 113:3–13.

Sharma A, Dogra Y. Trends of AUB in tertiary centre of Shimla hills. J of Midlife Health. 2013; 4:67–8.

# Benign Diseases of the Vulva and Vagina

**At a Glance**

**Benign Diseases of the Vulva**
1. Maldevelopment and Abnormalities
2. Injuries to the Vulva
3. Hemangiomas
4. Dermatologic Disorders
5. Inflammation of the Vulva
6. Pyogenic Diseases
7. Viral Infections
8. Fungal Infections
9. Parasitic Infections
10. Cysts of the Vulva
11. Ulcerations of the Vulva
12. Elephantiasis of the Vulva
13. Dystrophies of the Vulva

**Diseases of the Vagina**
1. Leucorrhea
   **Vaginitis**
   Types of Vaginitis Based on Causative Organisms
2. Vaginal Ulcers
3. Vaginal Cysts

The anatomy of the vulva has been described in detail in Chapter 3. The vulval skin is responsive to hormonal stimulation. Vulvitis is fairly common because of the presence of the vulval hair follicles and glands, and their exposure to urinary and fecal soiling.

## BENIGN DISEASES OF THE VULVA

The vulval diseases will be discussed under the following headings:

1. Maldevelopment and abnormalities
2. Injuries to the vulva
3. Hemangiomas
4. Dermatologic disorders
5. Inflammation of the vulva
6. Pyogenic diseases
7. Viral infections
8. Fungal infections
9. Parasitic infections
10. Cysts of the vulva
11. Ulcerations of the vulva
12. Elephantiasis of the vulva
13. Dystrophies of the vulva

The International Society for the Study of Vulvovaginal Diseases (ISSVD) classifies benign diseases of the vulva and vagina as shown in Table 8.1. The classification in 2006 and subsequent years is too elaborate to be considered here.

Atrophy of the vulva may also occur.

### 1. MALDEVELOPMENT AND ABNORMALITIES

#### Hypoplasia

Scanty pubic hair and small labia minora constitute hypoplasia of the vulva. It is present in young girls only, and resembles the atrophy of the external genitalia seen in postmenopausal women. Hypertrophy of the clitoris and labia minora may be seen in sexual precocity or in the adreno-genital syndrome, though this is rare.

#### Labial adhesions (Vulvar synechia)

These are sometimes encountered in infants. The fusion (Fig. 8.1) is often considered an adhesion caused by low-grade infection in the early weeks of life. Dysuria in these children may cause anxiety to the mother. The recommended treatment is gentle separation of the fused labia. This can also be done by gentle pressure with a probe. Secondary adhesions can occur due to the purulent copious discharge in vulvo-vaginitis. This, however, occurs after the first year of life. In rare cases, absence of the mons pubis or total aplasia of the vulva may be encountered.

**Table 8.1** ISSVD Classification of 1987 of benign diseases of the vulva and vagina

| Inflammatory diseases | Blistering diseases | Pigmentary changes | Benign tumours, hamartomas, and cysts | Congenital malformations |
|---|---|---|---|---|
| Lichen sclerosus | Familial benign chronic pemphigus (Hailey–Hailey disease) | Acanthosis nigricans | Mucous cysts | Ambiguous external genitalia |
| Squamous cell hyperplasia (with and without atypia) | Bullous pemphigoid | Lentigo, lentiginosis, and benign vulvar melanosis | Bartholin and Skene duct cysts | Congenital labial hypertrophy |
| Lichen simplex chronicus (localised neurodermatitis) | Cicatricial pemphigoid | Melanocytic nevus | Epidermal inclusion cyst | Labial adhesions |
| Primary irritant dermatitis | Pemphigus vulgaris | Postinflammatory hyperpigmentation | Seborrheic keratosis | |
| Intertrigo | Erythema multiforme | Postinflammatory hypopigmentation | Acrochordon (fibroepithelial polyp) | |
| Allergic contact dermatitis | Epidermolysis bullosa | Vitiligo | Fibroma, fibromyoma, and dermatofibroma | |
| Fixed drug eruption | | Vulvar melanosis | Lipoma | |
| Atopic dermatitis | | | Hidradenoma | |
| Seborrheic dermatitis | | | Syringoma | |
| Psoriasis | | | Hemangioma | |
| Reiter disease | | | Lymphangioma | |
| Lichen planus | | | Angiokeratoma | |
| Lupus erythematosus | | | Pyogenic granuloma | |
| Darier disease | | | Endometriosis | |
| Aphthosis and Behçet's disease | | | Heterotopic sebaceous glands and sebaceous gland hyperplasia | |
| Pyoderma gangrenosum | | | Papillomatosis (papillary vulvar hirsutism) | |
| Crohn disease | | | Schwannoma | |
| Hidradenitis suppurativa | | | | |
| Fox–Fordyce disease | | | | |
| Plasma cell vulvitis | | | | |
| Vulvar vestibulitis | | | | |

(*Source:* http://emedicine.medscape.com/article/264648-overview; The current classification in 2006 and subsequent years is too elaborate to be considered here.)

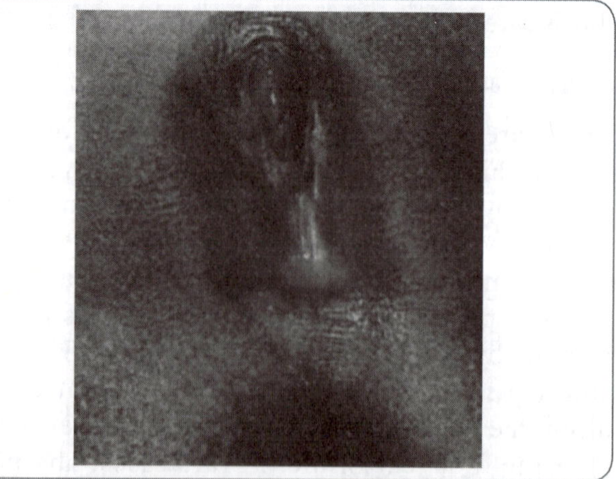

**Fig. 8.1** Labial adhesion (*Source:* ©Syed-Ansari, T, Murray, P, et al, Glob. libr. women's med.)

### Imperforate hymen

This is discussed in Chapter 5.

## 2. INJURIES TO THE VULVA

These may be caused by coitus, automobile accidents and injuries. Sometimes multiple small **lacerations** lead to moderate bleeding which may cause anxiety, but the bleeding usually stops spontaneously in a few minutes or with firm pressure. Severe injuries occur in a **tear of the hymen** involving a branch of vaginal artery, which requires careful visualisation of the hymen and suturing under general anesthesia.

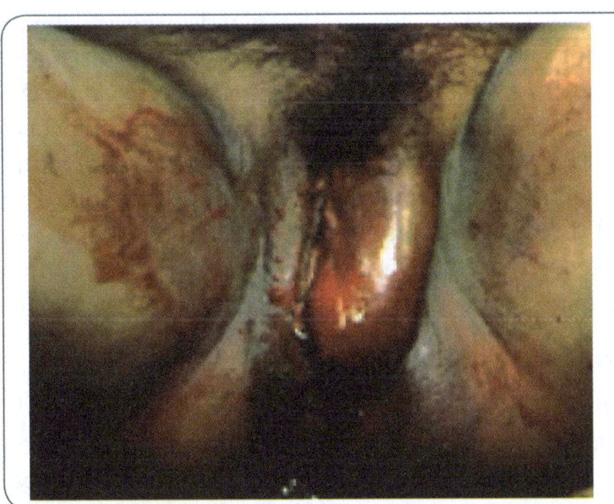

**Fig. 8.2** Hematoma of the vulva (*Source:* Dr. M.D. Mazumdar, reproduced with permission.)

### Hematoma

A hematoma (Fig. 8.2) may occur over the vulva and perineum due to inadequate hemostasis during perineorrhaphy or episiotomy suturing. Hematomas on the vulva can also result from accidents, rupture of a varicose vein or after enucleation of Bartholin's cyst. Sometimes bull-gore injuries also cause vulval hematoma. Vulval hematomas require evacuation under general anesthesia and securing of the bleeding points.

### Varicosities of the vulva

These involve one or more veins. They may be aggravated in pregnancy. In the non-pregnant woman, varicose veins in the vulva are uncommon and treatment is seldom necessary.

## 3. HEMANGIOMAS

### Granuloma pyogenicum

This is usually single, raised and dull red in colour, rarely exceeding 2 cm in diameter. It is considered a variant of capillary hemangioma. It is significant because it tends to bleed easily when traumatised. A wide excision is essential to alleviate symptoms and to rule out malignancy.

### Senile hemangioma

Usually multiple, small, dark blue papules are discovered incidentally in older patients. They remain asymptomatic and require excision only if they bleed repeatedly.

### Hemangiomas in children

These are usually diagnosed in the first few months of life and may vary in size. They tend to be elevated, bright or dark red depending on their size and the thickness of the overlying skin. They usually remain static or regress without treatment after two years of age. Larger ones may require a dermatologist's intervention.

### Lymphangioma

These are tumours of the lymphatic vessels. It is difficult to differentiate them from hemangiomas. Two types of lymphangiomas are encountered: lymphangioma simplex which appears as small, soft, solitary or multiple nodules over the labia majora and lymphangioma cavernosum which causes diffuse enlargement of one side of the vulva. Lymphangiomas are usually asymptomatic but occasionally cause pruritus which necessitates excision of the affected skin.

## 4. DERMATOLOGIC DISORDERS

### Contact dermatitis

This is an inflammatory response of the vulval tissues to agents which may either cause local irritation or be sensitive upon contact, for example pessaries, condoms, creams, detergents or drugs used locally.

### Disseminated lupus erythematosus

It may manifest as recurrent ulcerations of the mucous membranes of the mouth and the vulvo-vaginal area.

### Pemphigus vulgaris

Its first evidence may be bullous eruptions of apparently normal skin and the mucous membrane of the vulva.

### Psoriasis

This is a chronic relapsing skin condition which affects the scalp, the extensor surface of the extremities, trunk and vulva. The lesions in the vulva appear typically erythematous and resemble a fungus infection, but do not have the silver scaly crusts that are seen in other parts of the body.

### Intertrigo

This is an inflammatory reaction involving the genitocrural folds of the skin under the abdominal panniculus. It is common in obese patients and results from the persistent moisture of skin surfaces. Measures that promote dryness, for example, absorbent garments and dusting powder may be helpful.

### Vitiligo

This is a pigmentary deficiency, which remains asymptomatic. No treatment is required.

### Crohn's disease of the vulva

Among dermatological conditions associated with Crohn's disease of the vulva, contiguous perineal lesions are common. The lesions consist of indolent undermined ulcers showing granulomatous inflammation on microscopic examination. In the majority, these may be associated with local abscess, fistula and fissure. Some of these lesions may have gastrointestinal involvement or may be a precursor of gastrointestinal disorder. Patients with Crohn's disease usually have normal immunoglobulins and complement components.

 **Treatment**

Though the treatment is usually medical with drugs like metronidazole (20 mg/kg/day) and systemic steroids, occasionally surgical therapy may be required.

## 5. INFLAMMATION OF THE VULVA

**Vulvitis** or inflammation of the vulva may cause swelling, redness, severe tenderness and exudation. The patient usually complains of burning and itching. As a result of scratching, extensive excoriations may develop over the vulva.

Vulvitis may be due to infection and infestation with pyogenic organisms, viruses, fungi, parasites and protozoa.

## 6. PYOGENIC DISEASES

### Erysipelas

This is a rare spreading erythematous lesion of the skin caused by β-hemolytic streptococci. It is amenable to systemic broad-spectrum antibiotics.

### Gonorrheal vulvo-vaginitis

This is caused by *N. gonorrhoeae*. It is a sexually transmitted disease. Non-venereal inoculation is possible in children before puberty. Inflammation of Skene's glands, Bartholin's glands (the vestibular glands) and the cervix occurs along with a discharge of purulent material. The diagnosis is through the demonstration of intracellular gram-negative diplococci from the smear. The treatment is with long-acting penicillin; for those allergic to it, Inj. Ceftrioxone 250 mg IM single dose along with T.Azithromycin 1 g can be used. In case of Azithromycin allergy, T.Doxycycline 100 mg bd for seven days can be used.

### Abscess of Bartholin's gland

Bartholinitis and Bartholin's abscess are mostly caused by gonococcal infection and are rarely caused by other pyogenic organisms such as *E. coli*. Clinical manifestations are fever, pain and general malaise. **The posterior part of the labium is red, swollen and warm**. Extreme tenderness is present over the tense Bartholin's abscess. An appropriate administration of antibiotics is required followed by surgical incision of the abscess.

## 7. VIRAL INFECTIONS

### Condylomata acuminata

Papillary warty growths found in the anogenital region may simulate syphilitic condylomata. They may become exuberant and coalesce. They are generally seen in pregnant women (Fig. 8.3).

### Human papilloma viruses (HPV)

These are generally associated with benign skin and anogenital warts. Because several types of skin cancers were found to contain HPV-DNA, it has been speculated that certain types of HPV could be specifically associated with cancers. Although HPV-DNAs are not isolated from most skin cancers, they are often isolated from penile cancers, vulval

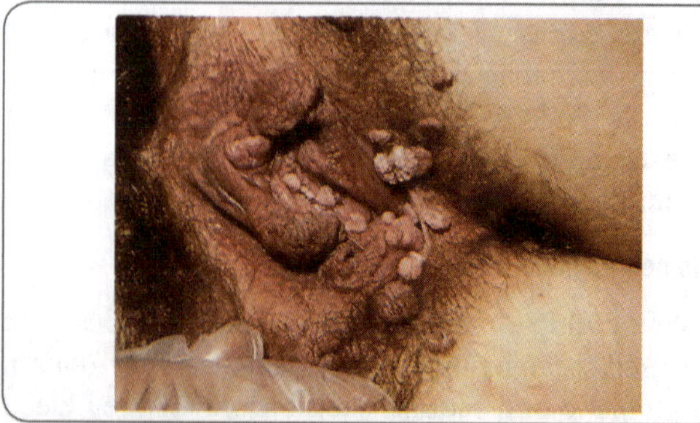

**Fig. 8.3** Condyloma acuminata (*Source:* Wikimedia)

cancers and anogenital Bowen's diseases. Human papilloma viruses may play a role in this malignant transformation.

*Types*

A number of HPV types have been identified by investigations of which the **oncogenic HPV type 16 was found to be present in subclinical HPV lesions of the vulva**. Medium- and high-risk HPV 18, 31 and 33 types were found to be frequently associated with high-grade cervical dysplastic lesions and carcinoma.

 **Treatment**

A wide range of treatment is used for the anogenital warts; podophyllin 20% was the most common first line treatment. Cryotherapy has become the choice of treatment recently.

### Herpes simplex

This condition is **caused by the herpes virus hominis type 2**. It produces painful vulvo-vaginitis and urethritis with vesicles, pain, itching, dysuria, vaginal discharge and a low-grade fever. The regional lymph nodes may be enlarged. Scraping and biopsy may reveal a homogeneous ground-glass appearance of cellular nuclei with numerous small intracellular, scattered, basophilic particles and acidophilic inclusions. **The cytologic smears show multi-nucleated giant cells often mistaken for malignant cells**. Cultures from the vesicles or serologic tests establish the diagnosis.

 **Treatment**

The treatment is symptomatic and analgesics are used to alleviate the pain. Acyclovir 200 mg 5 times a day orally for 5 days is extremely useful in this condition.

### Herpes zoster

This presents as a unilateral painful lesion consisting of vesicular eruptions over the vulval skin, along the course of one or more sensory nerves. The causative agent is Varicella zoster. The vesicles may rupture and heal with a dried-up crust. This scab ultimately separates. Secondary infection and ulceration should be prevented.

### Molluscum contagiosum

In this condition, the lesion is dome-shaped, often umbilicated and varies in size up to 1 cm. The lesions are often multiple and mildly contagious. Histologically, numerous inclusion bodies (molluscum bodies) are seen in the cytoplasm of cells. Each lesion is treated by cautery, freezing or curettage.

### Behcet's syndrome

This is a rare ulcerative disorder. The etiologic agent is probably a virus. The ulcerations are often recurrent involving the vulva and the mouth and are refractory.

## 8. FUNGAL INFECTIONS

### Tinea cruris

Fungal infections of the genitocrural area are more common in men than in women. Tinea cruris is a superficial fungal infection. Initially the lesions are erythematous, dry, scaly areas which coalesce. There is scratching and severe itching. The diagnosis is based on microscopic examination and culture.

### Tinea versicolor

They are usually multiple lesions, red, brown or yellow and occasionally involve the skin of the vulva. The treatment is with selenium sulphide.

### Candida albicans

Fungal infections of the vulva due to Candida albicans is associated with vaginitis and is described in the section on diseases of the vagina in this.chapter. Diabetic vulvitis is usually complicated by candidiasis.

## 9. PARASITIC INFECTIONS

### Scabies

This is caused by *Sarcoptes scabies*. It induces intractable itching and excoriation of the skin. It is found in those from a poor socio-economic environment and with poor hygiene. The diagnosis is made by the characteristic appearance of the lesion and by removing the parasite from the burrow.

 **Treatment**

The treatment consists of the application of 25% benzyl benzoate emulsion for the entire body below the neck. All the family members have to be treated simultaneously to prevent reinfection.

### Pediculosis pubis

The crab louse (*Phthirus pubis*) is transmitted through sexual contact or from infected clothing. The infection causes intense itching around the anus and pubis. Minute pale brown insects may be seen attached to the hair follicles.

### Treatment

The treatment is with 1% gamma benzene hexachloride cream (Lorexane), repeated after an interval of four days, if necessary.

### Enterobiasis

Vulvitis from pinworms is common in children. Nocturnal perianal and vulval itching due to this infestation can be eradicated by piperazine therapy.

### Schistosomiasis (Bilharziasis)

A schistosoma infection of the vulval area is often associated with extensive infection of the urinary bladder. This infection is common in Egypt, Central America and South America. Multiple nodules appear on the vulva involving the skin of the mons pubis or the labia majora. Histologically there is accumulation of schistosome ova surrounded by a granulomatous inflammatory reaction consisting of large numbers of foreign body giant cells. The surgical excision of a nodule establishes the diagnosis after which systemic treatment may be given with antimony compounds.

### Protozoa

Vulvitis due to *Trichomonas vaginalis*, a protozoan flagellate, is described under vaginitis in this chapter.

## 10. CYSTS OF THE VULVA

### Bartholin's cyst

This common cyst is caused by occlusion of the duct of the Bartholin's gland by fibrous tissue (Fig. 8.4). The duct of the gland may be traumatised or cut during a mediolateral episiotomy. **This cyst should be regarded as a retention cyst**. These cysts are adherent to the skin of the inner surface of the labium minus. They are treated by marsupialisation.

### Sebaceous cysts

This is a retention cyst of the vulva occurring on the clitoris, the medial and lateral aspects of the vulva and the outer aspects of the labia majora.

### Post-traumatic cysts

Small implantation dermoids are seen in old perineal tears.

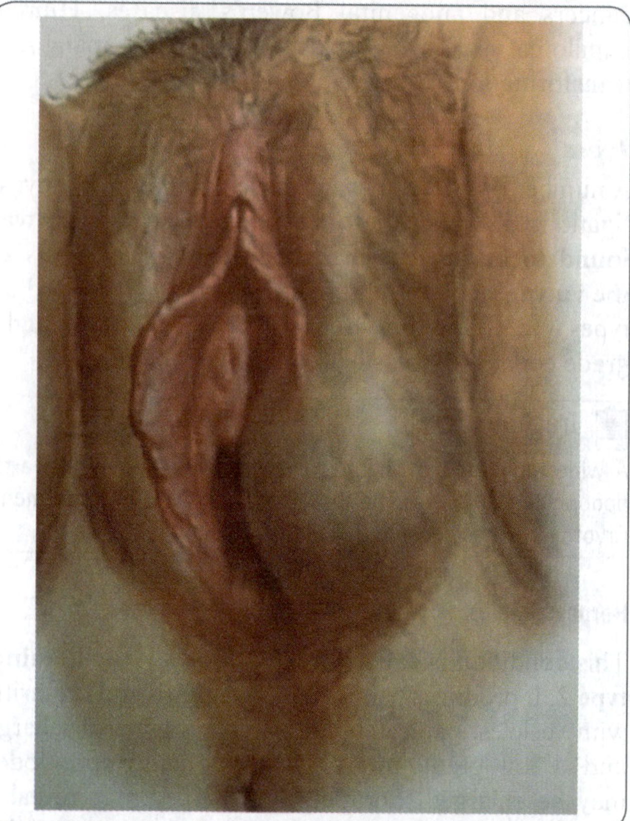

**Fig. 8.4** Bartholin's cyst (*Source:* Omicsonline)

### Dysontogenetic cysts

These are formed by a displaced paramesonephric (Müllerian) or mesonephric (Wolffian) epithelium. The cysts occur on the clitoris, the hymen or the labia minora.

### Papillary cysts

A few cases of papilliferous cysts have been reported which are histologically identical to a papillary serous cystadenoma of the ovary.

### Endometriotic cysts

These cysts, though rare, may sometimes be found on the labia majora, perineum or mons veneris, and are due to endometriosis. They are likely to be caused by lymphatic permeation rather than by implantation.

## 11. ULCERATIONS OF THE VULVA

**Causes**

Vulval ulcerations could be

1. **Traumatic**, due to infected perineal tears seen in the puerperium.

2. Due to **sexually transmitted diseases** such as syphilis, lymphogranuloma, granuloma inguinale and herpes genitalis (discussed earlier).
3. Due to **tuberculosis** of the vulva in which a rare ulcerative lesion is seen in cases of advanced genital tuberculosis.
4. Due to **malignant ulcers** (mainly epidermoid carcinoma) which will be discussed subsequently.

## 12. ELEPHANTIASIS OF THE VULVA

This condition is seen mainly in the tropics, including India, and is due to a lymphatic obstruction in the vulva caused by filariasis and rarely by tuberculosis or lymphogranuloma. Very large tumours of this type may be seen involving the vulva in some endemic areas (Fig. 8.5). The section presents a waxy appearance and histologically shows a marked hyperplasia of the papillae of the skin with a thickening of the cutis. Surgical excision is necessary for cosmetic and other reasons.

## 13. DYSTROPHIES OF THE VULVA

Vulval dystrophies comprise a confusing variety of atrophic and hypertrophic conditions caused by a number of stimuli. The lesions are characterised by shrinking, whitening or reddening exclusive to the skin of the vulva. These include

- kraurosis
- ichthyosis
- lichen sclerosus
- leukoplakia
- leukokeratosis
- neuro-dermatitis
- Bowen's disease
- hyperplastic vulvitis

These lesions do not have a uniform microscopic appearance.

Management of vulval dystrophy is dependent on the type and severity of symptoms. The main symptoms of vulval dystrophy are chronic itching, burning, pain and superficial dyspareunia. The pruritis is often worse at night and can cause insomnia, if severe. The presence of vulval discharge or bleeding suggests infection or malignant ulceration. A thorough systemic examination and local inspection of the vulva, perianal area, vagina and cervix is very essential. Bimanual pelvic examination should also be done unless the vulva is very sensitive.

### Lichen sclerosus (LS)

This condition occurs frequently in postmenopausal women. **This is a systemic atrophic dystrophy apart from its occurring over the vulva and perineum**. The affected areas appear whitish and glistening with clear margins (Fig. 8.6). The shiny papery skin has a **'cigarette-paper' appearance**. During the acute phase, these areas may be red and purple. The affected area on the vulva extends to encircle the anus in a figure of eight fashion causing involutional adhesion of labia minora to the labia majora, thus burying the clitoris and causing shrinkage of the introitus. The leading symptom is intense itching. If secondary infection occurs, ulceration and contractures may follow resulting in dyspareunia and dysuria. Histologically there is a

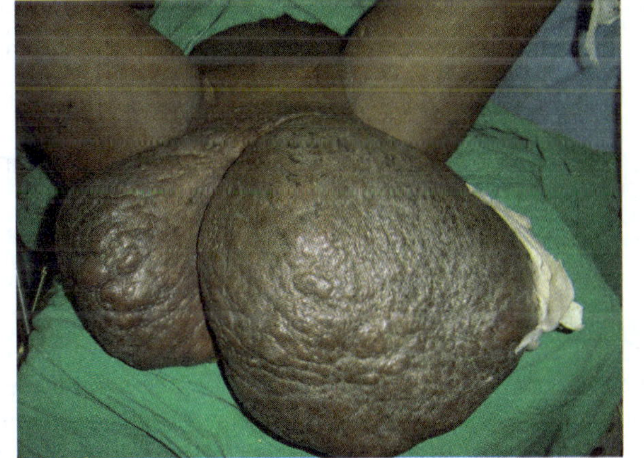

**Fig. 8.5** Elephantiasis of the vulva (*Source:* Chintamani et al; Journal of Medical Case Reports. 2010;4:369.)

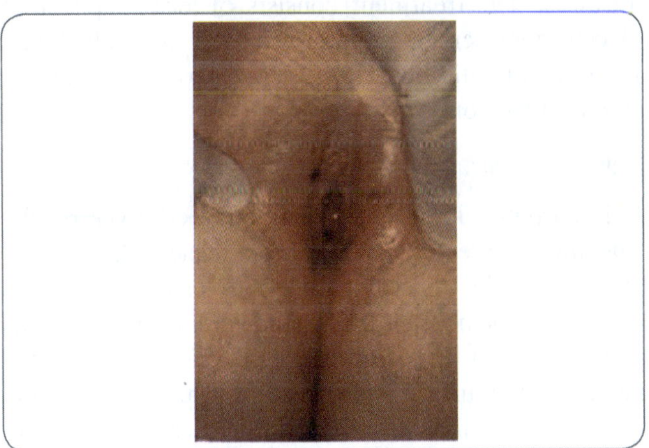

**Fig. 8.6** Lichen sclerosus of the vulva. Note the shiny papery skin. (*Source:* Syed-Ansari, T, Murray, P, et al, Glob. libr. women's med.)

thin inactive epithelium and loss of elastic tissue. At times, hyperkeratosis may also be seen. The cause of this condition is not known.

**Diagnosis** Areas of dysplasia or malignancy may develop in this lesion. Biopsy is essential to diagnose the skin lesion and exclude dysplasia or frank neoplasia. Colposcopy is of limited value for assessment but it will indicate suspicious areas from where biopsies could be taken.

### Treatment

Both atrophic and hypertrophic lesions are treated in the same manner. Deodorants, detergents, perfumed soaps and some talcum powders may aggravate the condition. Better personal hygiene and using cotton underwear would reduce the vulval moisture. Oral antihistamines and topical antipruritic agents may help in relieving itching. A local application of estrogen cream is recommended. Estrogen may have little effect or no direct effect on the epidermis but improves the vascularity of the underlying dermis. Topical corticosteroid such as 1% hydrocorticosterone aqueous cream or ointment has a beneficial effect in hypertrophic lesions. In atrophic histologic lesions, treatment with an androgenic steroid is found to be more useful, for example testosterone propionate ointment 2% twice daily for 3 to 4 weeks. Oral retinoids or Vitamin A analogues have also been used for this condition.

**Surgical therapy** for LS of the vulva has also been reported in those not responding to clinical treatment. Cryosurgery, laser ablation, or simple vulvectomy, though rarely, are the surgical methods followed.

### Primary atrophy of the vulva (kraurosis)

This is a progressive type of atrophy of the skin of the vulva. There is thinning and fibrosis of the vulval skin, especially the epidermis, causing stenosis of the vaginal introitus. The treatment consists of local application of estrogenic cream or oral estrogen in small doses. If severe pruritis occurs, it is advisable to perform a simple vulvectomy.

### Leukoplakia vulva

It is currently known as **squamous cell hyperplasia.** The affected area of the vulva has a thickened, hard and indurated skin consisting of white patches scattered irregularly, mainly over the labia majora. It rarely extends to the perineum. The skin cracks easily due to the increased keratin on the surface. Apart from this hyperkeratinisation of the epidermis, the other pathological changes are marked epithelial hyperplasia of the rete malpighii and chronic inflammatory cells infiltrating upper layer of the corium, which is devoid of elastic tissue, and evidence of hyaline degeneration of the collagen.

Symptoms of leukoplakia are pruritus, severe discomfort and discharge. **Topical corticosteroids is the main therapy for squamous cell hyperplasia.**

### Paget's disease

The extramammary form of Paget's disease of the vulva is rare. The histogenesis of this condition is controversial. It occurs predominantly in post-menopausal women. The clinical manifestations consist of varying degrees of pruritus, burning and tingling of the involved vulval areas. The lesion often has a mottled whitish appearance. The histologic picture shows little or no alteration of the general pattern of maturation of the epidermis. Superficial keratinisation is present. The epidermis contains distinctive clear cells **(Paget's cells)** which are large, round or oval and have a pale cytoplasm. The diagnosis is confirmed by histology.

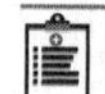

### Treatment

Paget's disease of the vulva is treated by surgical excision.

### Pruritus vulva

Pruritus vulva or itching mainly localised to the vulval region is seen in several gynaecological conditions. This requires detailed investigation and therapy.

**Causes**

The causes of pruritus vulvae are:

1. Vaginal discharge due to trichomonal or monilial vaginitis.
2. Dermatological conditions affecting the vulva such as tinea, scabies, pediculosis, contact dermatitis, chemicals, psoriasis, kraurosis and lichen sclerosis.
3. Precancerous and malignant conditions such as leukoplakic vulvitis, Bowen's disease, Paget's disease and carcinoma of the vulva.
4. General diseases such as diabetes and jaundice.
5. Deficiency states due to hypovitaminosis A and estrogen deficiency in postmenopausal women.
6. Psychogenic causes, when all other organic causes are ruled out.

### Treatment

The treatment depends on the cause. Strict personal hygiene and avoiding local irritants and allergens (including synthetic underclothing) is a useful prophylactic measure. Diabetes has to be tested for and ruled out. Vaginitis and local parasitic and fungal infestations, if present, should be appropriately treated.

If the cause is allergy, oral and local antihistamines are used. Hydrocortisone 1% ointment gives symptomatic relief. In estrogen deficiency states, estrogenic cream is applied locally. If the condition is secondary to leukoplakia, Bowen's disease or Paget's disease, surgical excision is necessary.

## DISEASES OF THE VAGINA

The vagina is a tubular canal connecting the uterus and the vulva. It is related anteriorly to the urethra and the bladder and posteriorly to the perineal body (separating it from the anal canal), the rectum and the pouch of Douglas. The detailed anatomy of the vagina has been described in Chapter 3.

The vaginal epithelium shows changes depending on the age and the phases of the menstrual and reproductive cycles. During childhood and following menopause, the vaginal epithelium is thin. During the reproductive age, it becomes thick and multilayered and the superficial cornified cells are enriched with glycogen. The vaginal pH is maintained around 4.5. This acid medium is not favourable for the growth of pathogenic organisms. During the reproductive years, the vaginal flora consists of Döderlein bacilli, which are predominantly lactobacilli. These bacilli help in converting the glycogen from exfoliated epithelial cells to lactic acid and this acid maintains the vaginal pH around 4.5, thereby preventing the growth of pathogenic organisms. Because of its protective function, the Döderlein bacillus is considered a **vaginal policeman**.

### 1. LEUCORRHEA

Literally, leucorrhea means white discharge. It includes conditions when the vaginal discharge is excessive and associated with or without any obvious local pathology. In practice, all excessive vaginal discharge, white, purulent, yellowish or watery, but not bloodstained, is labelled leucorrhea.

***Etiology*** The causes of leucorrhea may be physiological or pathological. The physiological causes are

- puberty (due to increased vascularity),
- ovulation (due to increased cervical mucus),
- the premenstrual period (owing to the increased secretion of the endometrial glands)
- pregnancy (increased vascularity).

The pathological causes are several general or local conditions. In severe anemia, congestive cardiac failure, debilitating diseases and ascites the patient may complain of leucorrhea, but examination of the vagina and discharge shows no obvious local pathology requiring specific treatment for this complaint.

The local **causes** of leucorrhea are the following:

1. ***Pelvic tumours*** such as fibroids, ovarian neoplasms and PID, which may cause excessive discharge due to the increased blood supply to the pelvic organs.
2. ***Cervical lesions*** which occur as a result of excessive mucus discharge from the endocervical glands in chronic endocervicitis, cervical erosion, polypi and ectropion. The patient complains of excessive mucoid discharge or 'mucorrhea'. Cervical erosion is a misnomer as strictly speaking there is no erosion or ulcer; the thick multilayered squamous epithelium is replaced by a single-layered columnar epithelium.
3. ***Vaginitis***, which may be *specific* due to infections caused by sexually transmitted diseases (STD) such as gonorrhea, protozoal organisms such as *Trichomonas vaginalis*, and fungi such as *Candida albicans*; or non-specific due to infection by mixed organisms such as streptococcus, staphylococcus, *Hemophilus vaginalis*, *E. coli* or anaerobes. This latter condition is seen in women using pessaries, tampons and other foreign bodies and chemicals, and in postmenopausal women.
4. In severe anemia, congestive cardiac failure, debilitating diseases and ascites, the patient may complain of leucorrhea, but examination of the vagina and discharge shows no obvious local pathology requiring specific treatment for this complaint.

#### Vaginitis

Vaginitis is an important cause of leucorrhea and is therefore considered in detail below:

#### Types of Vaginitis Based on Causative Organisms

##### a. Gonococcal vulvo-vaginitis

In the reproductive age, *N. gonorrhoeae* mainly causes Bartholinitis, urethritis and cervicitis besides salpingitis but no vaginitis because the thickness and acid medium of the vagina protects the woman against *N. gonorrhoeae*. In children and menopausal women in whom the vaginal epithelium is thin, gonococcal organisms can easily attack the vaginal mucosa to cause vaginitis. Since it is sexually transmitted, the source of infection must be traced and the carrier treated. The purulent discharge on examination with Gram stain will show gram-negative intracellular diplococci. Preparation of a culture may be helpful.

### Treatment

The current CDC recommendation for gonococcal infections is:

- Ceftriaxone 250 mg IM in a single dose plus Azithromycin 1 g oral in a single dose
- Alternate regimen where Ceftriaxone is not available: Cefixime 400 mg oral as a single dose plus Azithromycin 1 g oral in a single dose

### b. Vaginitis due to *Chlamydia trachomatis*

This is another STD which causes vaginitis and urethritis. The patient complains of dysuria and mucopurulent discharge. It is seen in 25–40% of the female partners of men suffering from non-gonococcal urethritis. The smear is negative with Gram stain but with special cytological staining (like Giemsa), tissue culture and serological tests, diagnosis is possible.

### Treatment

The patient and her sexual partner are treated with Doxycycline 100 mg orally twice daily for seven days.

### c. Trichomoniasis

Perhaps the most common and the most important cause of vaginitis in the reproductive age is vaginal trichomoniasis. It is caused by *Trichomonas vaginalis*, a flagellated protozoan organism which is about 10 $\mu$m long and 7 $\mu$m in width (or slightly larger than a leucocyte) and is an anaerobe (Fig. 8.7). It is actively motile. Sexual intercourse is the main means of transmission of this organism and it is hence considered an STD. Men harbour it in the urethra and prostate.

*T. vaginalis* causes a profuse, thin, frothy, yellowish or greenish discharge (due to the myeloperoxide pigment of the polymorphonuclear leucocytes) containing thousands of polymorphs per mm$^3$.

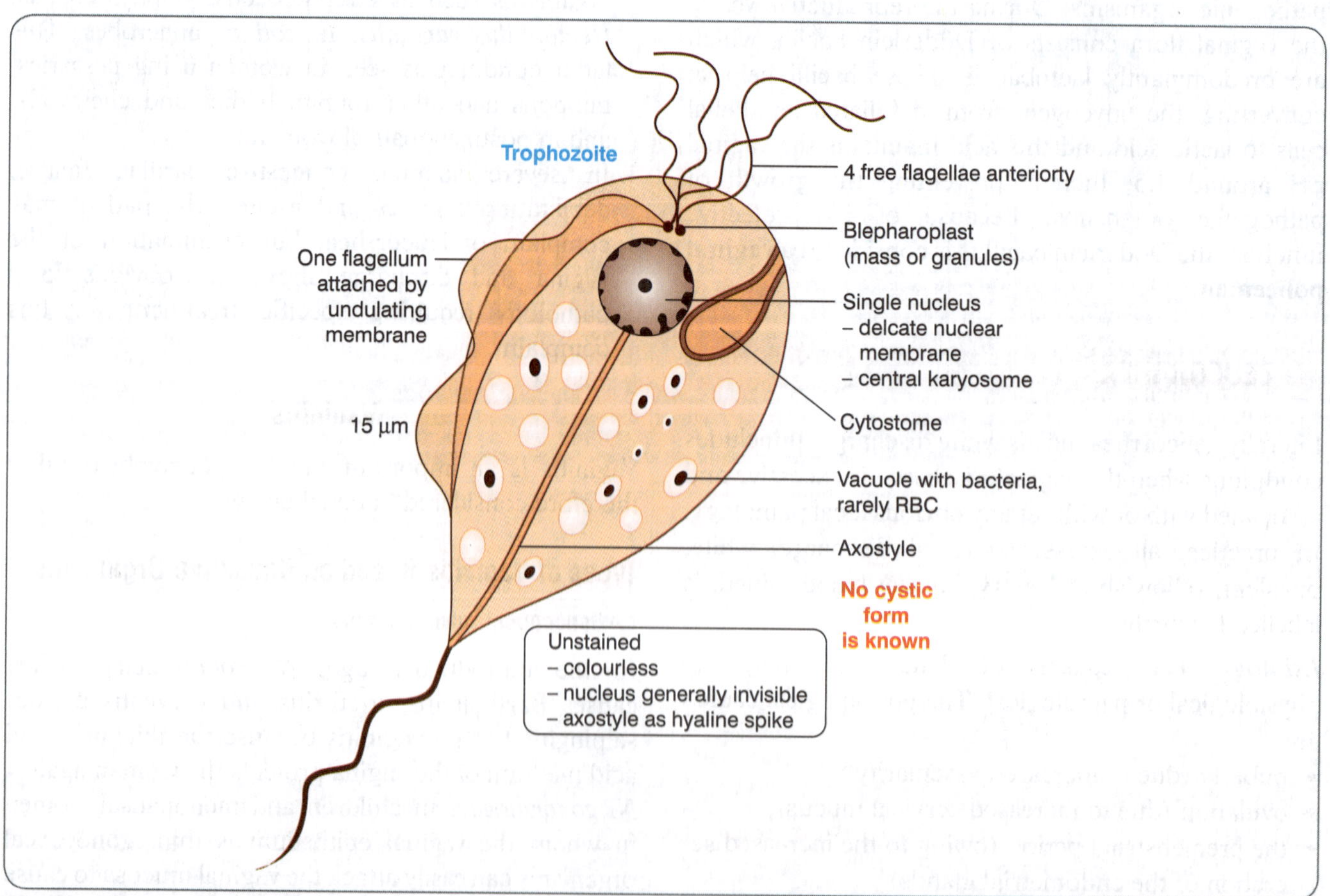

**Fig. 8.7** *Trichomonas vaginalis*

Discharge caused by *T. vaginalis* is
- profuse
- thin
- frothy
- yellowish or greenish

The vaginal walls including the portio vaginalis are tender and congested. There is associated dysuria and pruritus. The pH of the discharge is over 5. A saline wet mount shows motile trichomonads in over 80% of cases. It can also be grown in culture in over 90% of them and is useful in smear-negative patients.

### Treatment

The treatment consists of oral administration of metronidazole or tinidazole 2 g in a single dose for both partners. Alternatively metronidazole 200 mg thrice daily for a week is effective. Failures are due to re-infection especially after the menstrual periods.

#### d. Candidiasis

This is caused by a gram-positive fungus, *Candida albicans*, often seen in the anogenital region (Fig. 8.8). It is transmitted through sexual contact. Other factors which promote its growth are
- diabetes (the fungus thrives in the presence of glucose)
- pregnancy (due to the favourable acid medium in the vagina)
- oral contraceptives
- antibiotics or corticosteroids
- debility and immunosuppression.

There is marked pruritus with vulvitis and a scanty, curdy, white, odourless discharge (Fig. 8.9). The speculum examination shows a reddish congested vaginal wall with cheesy white patches. On removing these white patches, one finds petechial areas. The pH is less than 4.5. The diagnosis is made by direct microscopic examination of the discharge with Gram stain or with 10% KOH solution. The fungus can also be grown in Sabouraud's or Nickerson's media in selected cases.

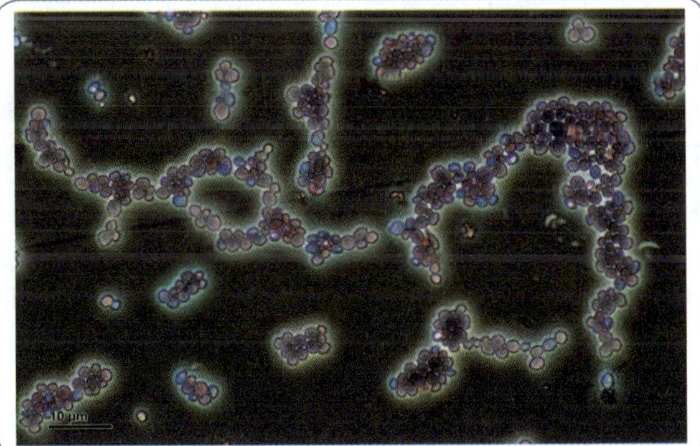

**Fig. 8.8** *Candida albicans* (*Source:* Wikimedia)

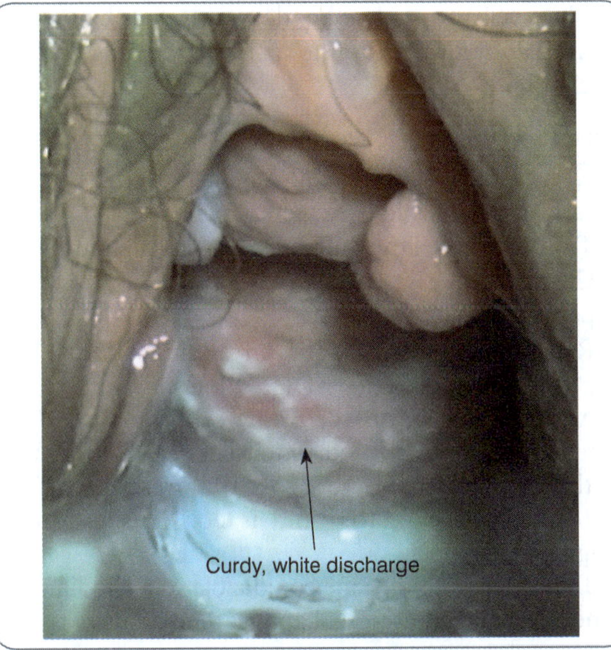

**Fig. 8.9** Candidiasis (*Source:* Wikimedia)

The treatment consists of Nystatin 20–200 mg (100,000 to 1,000,000 units) intravaginally daily for two weeks. In recurrent candidiasis, Ketoconazole 200 mg orally daily for five days or a single dose of fluconazole 150 mg each orally for both partners is recommended.

#### e. Bacterial vaginosis (BV)

Bacterial vaginosis (BV) is a disease due to imbalance of the commensal bacteria in the vagina. The common symptoms are malodourous vaginal discharge which is white or grey in colour, burning micturition and mild itching that can occur sometimes.

The most common infecting organism is *Gardnerella vaginalis*. BV is more frequently seen in women who douch themselves and is also a risk factor for pelvic inflammatory disease, HIV and STD.

It is diagnosed by the **whiff test** which is performed by adding potassium hydroxide to the vaginal discharge in a slide or test tube; if a characteristic fishy odour is emanated, it is considered a positive test for BV.

Clue cells can also be demonstrated by adding sodium chloride solution to a slide containing vaginal discharge.

*Amsel's criteria*

In clinical practice BV can be diagnosed using the Amsel's criteria which are the following:

1. Thin, white, yellow, homogeneous discharge
2. Clue cells (Fig. 8.10) on microscopy
3. pH of vaginal fluid >4.5
4. Release of a fishy odour on adding alkali—10% potassium hydroxide (KOH) solution.

At least three of the four criteria should be present for a confirmed diagnosis. A modification of the Amsel's criteria accepts the presence of two instead of three factors and is considered equally diagnostic.

Treatment is with metronidazole or clindamycin either orally or as a vaginal application.

### f. Vaginitis in extremes of age

This may be of two kinds:

i. **Vulvo-vaginitis in children**, may be due to *N. gonorrhoeae* but is often due to *E. coli*, staphylococci and others. It may be caused by contamination from extraneous sources—from an adult or another child, by the use of infected clothes or the insertion of a foreign body in the vagina.

The vulva is reddish with a purulent or bloodstained discharge and the child may be seen constantly scratching the external genitals.

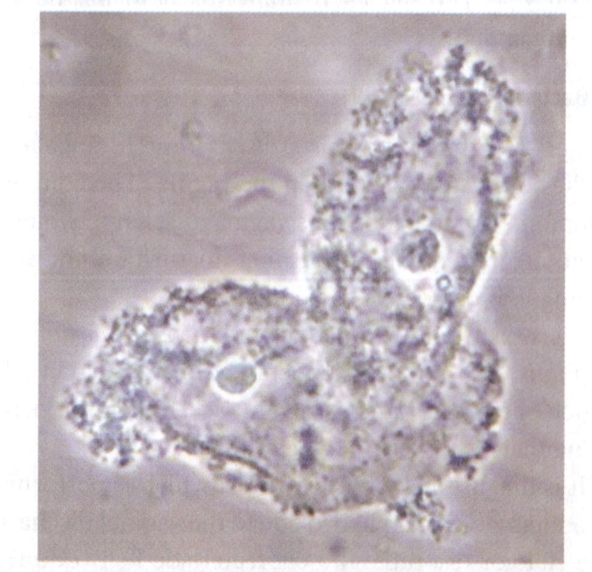

**Fig. 8.10** Clue cell (*Source:* Wikimedia)

Examination under anaesthesia is needed to detect (and remove) any foreign body besides obtaining the smear for investigation and treatment.

Local estrogenic cream and specific chemotherapy (depending on the organisms) are useful.

ii **Senile vaginitis** Due to estrogen deficiency, the thin atrophic vagina may be infected by mixed pathogens, *N. gonorrheae* or even *T. vaginalis*. There is bloodstained discharge from the inflamed vagina. Vulvitis too is present because of the pruritus. Sometimes a forgotten pessary may be the cause.

In these cases, the smear has to be examined for the causative organism. Malignancy has to be ruled out by examination of these patients under anesthesia. Foreign body if any has to be removed. When the discharge is foul-smelling, an infected malignant growth from the cervix or rarely a pyometra may have to be ruled out.

#### Treatment

The treatment consists of small doses of estrogens. Local estrogenic cream and any specific antibiotics depending on the organism have to be administered. **Douches are contraindicated.** In vaginitis, strong antiseptic solutions should never be used for cleaning the vagina. **Non-irritant normal saline or plain water is useful for vaginal irrigation.**

Leucorrhea due to cervical polyps, a foreign body, chemicals, contraceptive creams and urinary fistulae are all secondary, and the treatment depends on the cause.

## 2. VAGINAL ULCERS

Ulcers in the vagina may be due to different factors:

- venereal ulcers
- tuberculous ulcers
- amoebic ulceration
- traumatic ulcers due to radiation
- chemicals or a long-retained vaginal pessary
- trophic ulcers of the vagina as seen in genital prolapse
- malignant ulcers

### a. Venereal ulcers or ulcers due to STD

Primary chancre of the vagina is extremely rare. The vagina may be involved along with vulval lesions in STD as in LGV and granuloma inguinale.

In donovanosis or granuloma inguinale, the causative agent is *Calymmatobacterium granulomatis*, a gram-negative pleomorphic non-motile organism. Primarily, the chronic vulval ulceration may involve the vagina or the cervix, though primary vaginal and cervical ulcerations are also known. The tissue smear from the ulcer when Leishman-stained shows the Donovan bodies. The biopsy helps to distinguish it from carcinoma which it closely resembles.

### Treatment

The current CDC recommendation is azithromycin. Alternate regimens include doxycycline, ciprofloxacin, erythromycin base and trimethoprim-sulfamethoxazole. All antibiotics should be given for at least a 3-week course and continued until reepithelialisation of the ulcer occurs and all signs of the disease have resolved.

#### b. Tuberculous ulceration of the vagina

This is rare and is mostly seen in the late stages of genital tuberculosis after the endometrium and cervix are involved.

#### c. Amoebic ulceration of the vagina

This is seen in the tropics and is associated with a bloodstained discharge. It appears as a shallow ulcer with serpiginous margins and is covered with slough. A wet smear from the ulcer for microscopic examination confirms the diagnosis because actively motile amoebae are seen. It responds to oral metronidazole.

#### d. Ulceration due to radiation

Ulceration due to radiation is painful, associated with discharge and takes several weeks to heal. Chemicals such as potassium permanganate cause severe ulceration. Ulcers resulting from long-retained pessaries are usually seen in the upper part of the vagina and give rise to vaginal discharge. They heal, after removal of the foreign body, with a local application of antiseptic cream and small doses of oral estrogens, if the patient is postmenopausal.

#### e. Vaginal ulcers due to exposure

Ulcers of the vagina due to longstanding exposure of the vaginal wall as seen in cases of genital prolapse require careful attention with local applications of acriflavine glycerine and oral estrogens in small doses (or vaginal estrogenic cream). Once the edema has subsided, the prolapse has to be reduced. In suspected cases, a biopsy of the ulcer is indicated to rule out malignancy.

Vaginal scars may be seen due to childbirth trauma following a forceps delivery, inflammatory lesions, or chemicals. Acquired vaginal atresia of traumatic origin is also known.

## 3. VAGINAL CYSTS

The most common vaginal cyst is the one arising from Gartner's duct or the remnants of the mesonephric duct. It may be seen as a tense cystic irreducible swelling of variable size (1–6 cm in diameter) in the anterolateral wall of the vagina along the course of the duct from the vaginal fornix to a point just lateral to the urethra.

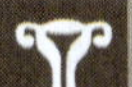

### Clinical Importance

When the cyst of Gartner's duct is seen in the lower part of the vagina, and protrudes at the vulva, it has to be distinguished from a cystocele where the bladder swelling is reducible and there is associated genital prolapse.

The cysts of Gartner's duct (Fig. 8.11) are mostly asymptomatic and rarely assume a size likely to interfere with intercourse or with parturition at which point they will need excision. Microscopically, they are lined by cubical or flattened epithelium and contain clear serous fluid.

Small implantation cysts or dermoids may be seen rarely in the lower third of the vagina following the repair of the perineal tears or episiotomy during parturition.

Occasionally a myoma may arise from the muscle of the vaginal wall. Endometriosis of the rectovaginal septum may rarely spread down to the posterior vaginal fornix and present as a tender reddish swelling which becomes tense with menstruation and sometimes ulcerates to simulate cancer. A biopsy confirms the diagnosis.

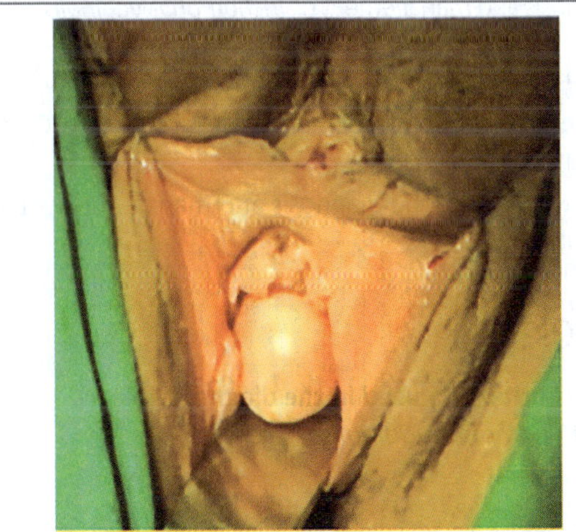

**Fig. 8.11** A cyst of Gartner's duct (*Source:* Chandrasekhar V, Rao JVN (2017)/J Anesth Crit Care; Open Access Vol. No. 7(3): 00259.)

**Case study**

*A 30-year-old lady presents with history of swelling over the vulva for the past 4–5 days. She also gives history of dyspareunia and pain during walking. The swelling is gradually increasing in size. She complains of three similar episodes earlier.*

*a) What is the most probable diagnosis?*

*b) How would you manage this condition if this is the first episode?*

*What would be your management option when it is recurrent as in this woman?*

## RECAP

- Pruritis vulva is a common complaint.
- This could be due to vaginal discharge, dermatological conditions affecting the vulva (scabies, pediculosis), precancerous and malignant conditions (leukoplakic vulvitis), general diseases (diabetes and jaundice), deficiency states (hypovitaminosis A and estrogen deficiency) and psychogenic causes.
- Diseases of the vagina are leucorrhea, vaginitis, gonococcal vulvo-vaginitis, trichomoniasis.
- Treatment of trichomoniasis is oral administration of metronidazole or tinidazole 2 g in a single dose for both partners.
- Alternatively metronidazole 200 mg thrice daily for a week is effective.
- Candidiasis could be due to diabetes, pregnancy (due to the favourable acid medium in the vagina), oral contraceptives, antibiotics or corticosteroids, debility and immunosuppression.
- The treatment consists of Nystatin 20–200 mg (100,000 to 1,000,000 units) intravaginally daily for two weeks.
- Bacterial Vaginosis (BV)—The diagnostic tests are Whiff test and demonstration of clue cells.
- Amsel criteria is a diagnostic criteria for BV.
- Gartner's cyst, the most common vaginal cyst, is the one arising from Gartner's duct.

## REVIEW QUESTIONS

### Long-answer Question

1. What are the various causes of leucorrhea? Discuss the etiology, diagnosis and management of *Trichomonas vaginalis*.

### Short-answer Questions

1. Write briefly about Gartner's cyst (cyst of the Gartner's duct).
2. Write briefly on the diagnosis and management of lichen sclerosis.

### MCQs

**1. Amsel criteria is used in the diagnosis of**

a) *Trichomonas vaginalis*
b) Candidal vaginitis
c) Bacterial vaginosis
d) Paget's disease of the vulva

**2. Lichen sclerosis is more frequently seen in**

a) Premenarcheal girls
b) Postmenopausal women
c) Women between 30–40 years of age
d) Pregnant women

**3. Gartner's duct is the remnant of**

a) Mesonephric duct
b) Wolffian duct
c) Urogenital ridge
d) Round ligament

# Benign and Premalignant Lesions of the Cervix

## At a Glance


Anatomy and Histology of Cervix
**Types of Lesions in the Cervix**
A. Inflammatory Lesions
Cervicitis
Gonorrhea
Chronic Cervicitis
Endocervicitis
Ectropion/Ectopy
B. Benign Tumours
Condyloma Acuminata
Cervical Polyps
Cervical Endometriosis
Squamous Papilloma
Nabothian Follicles and Cysts
C. Premalignant Lesions of the Cervix
Human Papilloma Virus (HPV)
**VIA and VILI**
Pathophysiological Basis of VIA
Pathophysiological Basis of VILI
**Conventional (Pap) Test and Liquid-Based Cytology (LBC)**
Technique of Taking the Smear
Liquid-Based Cytology (LBC)
Interpretation of Pap Smear / LBC (Bethesda System 2001)
**HPV Testing**
Method of Collection
Recent Developments
Recommendations for Screening Programme in India
Intrepretation Done as per IFCPC Recommedations
Diagnosis of Precancerous Lesion
Histopathology of Low-Grade Lesion—CIN 1
CIN2/Moderate Dysplasia
Treatment of Preinvasive Lesion
Prevention


The cervix could be the seat of both benign and premalignant lesions. The advantage of cervical lesions are that they are easily visible, can be subjected to mass screening even in resource-poor settings and even the premalignant lesions take a long time to develop into malignant lesions. However, a clear knowledge of the cervix from the clinical point of view is essential for a better comprehension of these lesions.

## ANATOMY AND HISTOLOGY OF CERVIX

The cervix consists of two parts, ecto- and endo-cervix.

- The **ectocervix** is covered by stratified squamous epithelium which is made of four layers—superficial, intermediate, parabasal and basal layers. The basal layer is separated from the underlying stroma by the basement membrane. The HPV virus gains entry into the cervix through the micro-aberrations in the basal layer following coitarche.
- The **endocervical canal** is lined by a single layer of tall columnar cells with basal nuclei. These columnar cells invaginate into the cervical stroma to a depth of 5–8 mm. These blind invaginations are known as **endocervical glands** or more correctly **endocervical crypts**.
- At the level of the external os, the stratified squamous epithelium of the ectocervix meets the columnar cells of the endocervix. This is known as the **new squamo-columnar junction (SCJ)** (Fig. 9.1b).
- The **old SCJ** (Fig. 9.1a) represents the limit of the columnar cells that has spread out on to the ectocervix during puberty and pregnancy (conditions that are associated with high circulating levels of sex steroids). **Old SCJ is identified by the presence of Nabothian cyst, follicle and crypt openings**.
- The area between the old and new SCJ is known as **transformation zone (TZ)** (Fig. 9.1c). This is a zone of constant mitotic activity where metaplasia is constantly taking place.

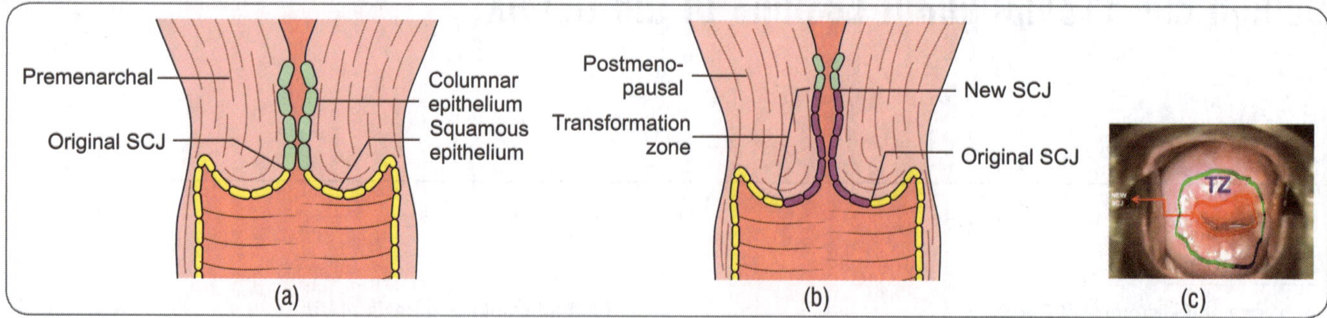


**Fig. 9.1** Figure showing old SCJ (green line), new SCJ (red line) and transformation zone

## TYPES OF LESIONS IN THE CERVIX

Lesions of the cervix could be of the following types.
A Inflammatory
B Benign
C Malignant

## A. INFLAMMATORY LESIONS

### Cervicitis

**Definition** Inflammation of the cervix is known as cervicitis.

**Causes** The causes of cervicitis could be classified as

- Specific
- Non-specific

**Specific causes**

- Bacterial infection—gonorrhea, chlamydia, syphilis, tuberculosis, donovanosis, actinomycosis.
- Viral infection—herpes simplex virus, human papilloma virus, cytomegalovirus.
- Fungal infection—80–95% due to *Candida albicans*.
- Parasitic infection—trichomoniasis, schistosomiasis, amebiasis, pinworm infection, and hydatid disease.
- Systemic inflammatory diseases that can manifest as inflammatory cervicitis—polyarthritis nodosa and Bechet's syndrome.

**Non-specific causes**

- Chemotherapy, radiation, intrauterine device and localised lesions like cervical endometriosis.
- Forgotten foreign bodies like vaginal pessaries, tampons, barrier contraceptive devices, chemicals in douches or contraceptive creams, and allergens like latex.

Cervicitis may ascend and cause endometritis and pelvic inflammatory disease (PID).

**Symptoms and signs**

- Discharge and discomfort are the common symptoms of cervical lesions; careful physical and speculum examination is **necessary** to establish the diagnosis. Other symptoms are **intermenstrual bleeding** or **postcoital spotting**.
- It can also present with **dyspareunia**, vulvar and/or vaginal irritation as **cervicovaginitis** along with urethritis, dysuria and pelvic inflammatory disease.

**Examination** Findings will include

- Profuse foul-smelling purulent or mucopurulent frothy vaginal discharge (Fig. 9.2).
- The cervix bleeds on touch of a swab due to congestion and edema.

The colour of the discharge gives a clue about the causative organism.

- When the infection is caused by ***Candida,*** the discharge is white curdy plaques or flakes adherent to the vagina and cervix.
- In **trichomonal infection,** the discharge is yellowish green and frothy in nature. The cervix is red and swollen—**strawberry cervix**—due to increased terminal vasculature. On histopathological examination it appears as edema of the stroma along with neutrophilic infiltration.

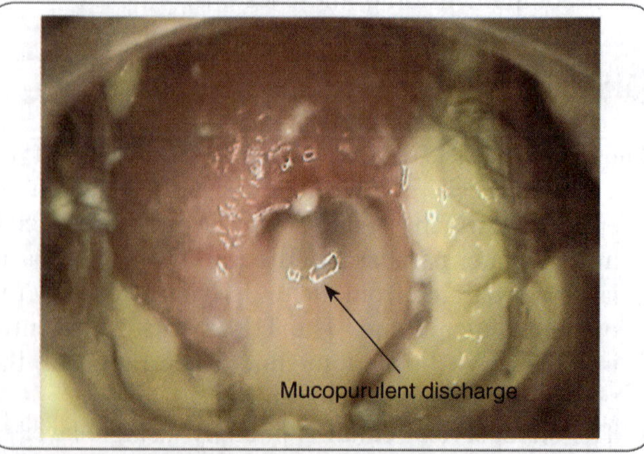


**Fig. 9.2** Mucopurulent discharge caused by cervicitis

- Yet another common infection in the sexually active population is by ***Chlamydia trachomatis***.

### Diagnosis

- Clinical findings
- Testing for vaginitis and STDs

Findings that suggest a specific cause or other disorders include the following:

- Fever—PID
- Cervical motion tenderness—PID
- Vesicles, vulvar or vaginal pain, and/or ulceration—HSV infection
- Punctate hemorrhages (strawberry spots)—trichomoniasis

## Gonorrhea

Gonorrhea is a sexually transmitted bacterial infection. The causative organism is *Neisseria gonorrhoeae* which is a gram-negative diplococcus.

**Diagnosis** Microscopy, culture or nucleic acid amplification tests are the techniques used for diagnosis.

Gonorrhea is diagnosed when gonococci are detected via microscopic examination using Gram stain or culture.

- **Gram stain** is sensitive and specific for gonorrhea.
- **Culture** is sensitive and specific, but because gonococci are fragile and fastidious, samples taken using a swab need to be rapidly plated on an appropriate medium (e.g., modified Thayer-Martin) and transported to the laboratory in a $CO_2$-containing environment.

### Treatment

Treatment consists of the following:

- *Chlamydial infection* Azithromycin 1 g po once or with doxycycline 100 mg po bid for 7 days.
- *Gonorrhea* Ceftriaxone 250 mg IM once plus azithromycin 1 g po once (due to emerging resistance of *N. gonorrhoeae* to cephalosporins).

Once the cause or causes are identified based on the results of microbiological testing, subsequent treatment is adjusted accordingly.

**If cervicitis persists despite this treatment, reinfection with chlamydiae and *N. gonorrhoeae* should be ruled out.**

### Follow-up

- If the cause is a bacterial STD, sex partners should be tested and treated simultaneously. Women should abstain from sexual intercourse until the infection has been eliminated from them and their sex partners.
- **All women with confirmed chlamydial infection or gonorrhea should be tested between 3 and 6 months after treatment because reinfection is common.**

## Chronic Cervicitis

Chronic cervicitis is the chronic or persistent inflammation of the cervix.

If acute cervicitis is left untreated, it may persist resulting in chronic cervicitis.

**Signs and symptoms** In a majority of women, no signs and symptoms of chronic cervicitis are noted. In others, the following signs and symptoms may be seen.

- Swelling and redness of the cervix
- Ulceration
- Abnormal vaginal discharge
- Increased frequency of urination
- Itching in the genital area
- Pain during intercourse
- Pressure in the pelvis

### Diagnosis

- Complete medical history with physical examination
- Speculum and pelvic examination
- Urineanalysis
- Pap smear examination
- Tissue biopsy (definitive diagnosis)

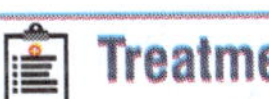

### Treatment

The treatment of chronic cervicitis depends on the cause of the inflammation. The treatment may include:

- **Symptomatic treatment** of the signs and symptoms, if the cause is due to a non-infectious agent.
- **Surgical treatment** for chronic cervicitis, which may include cryotherapy.
- **Antibiotic medication**, in the case of a bacterial infection.
- **Antiviral medication**, in the case of a viral infection.
- **Avoiding sexual intercourse** until the treatment is completed; generally, treating the partner is also important (when the cause is from a sexually transmitted infection).

## Endocervicitis

**Endocervicitis** is the inflammation of the lining of the uterine cervix.

**Pathogenesis** Normally the endocervical canal is lined by columnar cells and extends between the external and internal os. This single layer of columnar cells are thrown into a number of folds called plicae. A vertical fold is present on the anterior and posterior cervical walls; from these, oblique folds radiate. These folds are known as arbor vitae uteri or plicae palmatae. This intrinsic structure makes it prone for infection.

## Ectropion/Ectopy

Obstetric trauma causes unilateral/bilateral, symmetrical/asymmetrical cervical tear which causes eversion of the endocervical canal exposing the entire delicate single layer of columnar cells into the vagina. This is commonly described as Ectropion (Fig. 9.3).

This single layer is converted into stratified squamous epithelium by squamous metaplasia.

When there is high circulating levels of estrogen or sex steroids in the body as during puberty and pregnancy, the columnar cells which were confined to the endocervical canal come out onto the ectocervix giving it a red angry look. This was known as **erosion** but the term has become obsolete. It has been replaced with the term **Ectopy**. This being a physiological event, it needs no treatment.

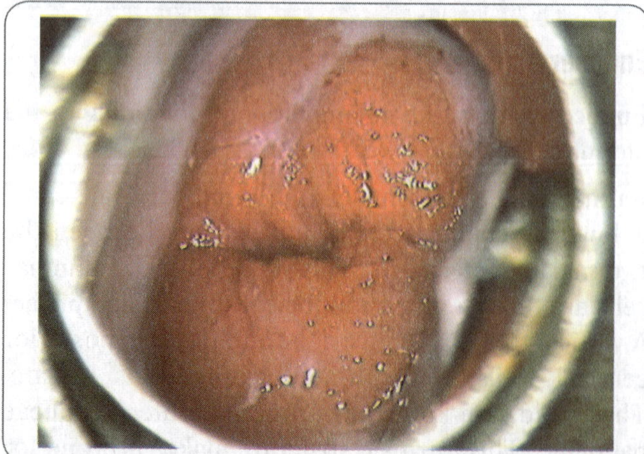

Fig. 9.3 Ectropion

## B. BENIGN TUMOURS

## Condyloma Acuminata

Usually they appear as single or multiple, clearly delineated, elevated, white velvety patches on the cervix and at times extend onto the vagina as well, and can vary in size and shape.

**Etiology** Condylomata are (Fig. 9.4) most commonly associated with HPV types 6, 11.

**Diagnosis**

1. **Colposcopy** The colposcope is a manual binocular stereoscopic microscope with which the cervix is visualised at magnification that varies from 6× to 40×. Digital video colposcope has the great benefit of recording and storage of all data using software in a computer.

   Small lesions may only be apparent through colposcope and after acetic acid application they assume a very dense white colour. The lesions can cause postcoital bleeding as they are delicate and friable and often raising the doubt of cancer. When a patient has vulvar warts, one has to thoroughly inspect the entire vagina and cervix for subclinical or clinically apparent condylomata.
2. **Biopsy** Thorough evaluation of these lesions requires colposcopy-directed biopsy of the lesion.

### Treatment

The treatment for warts differs according to their location—excision with the use of biopsy forceps, cryocautery, diathermy, LEEP, or laser according to the size and location of the lesion as well as the availability of these modalities.

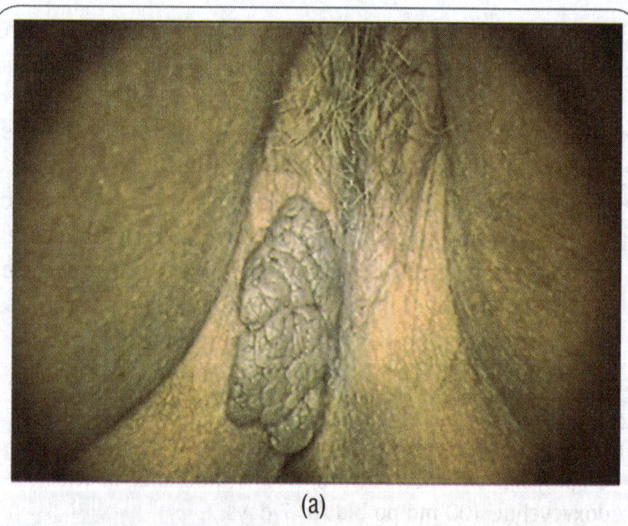

(a)

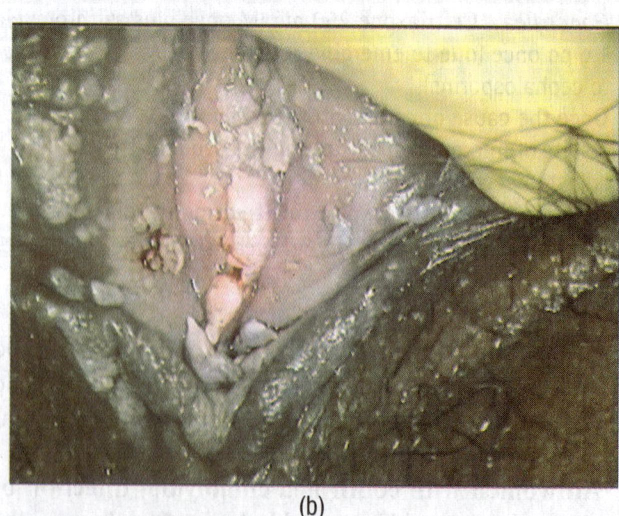

(b)

Fig. 9.4 (a) Condyloma vulva; (b) Condyloma vagina

**Treatment for Warts**

- Excision with the use of biopsy forceps
- Cryocautery
- Diathermy
- LEEP
- Laser

## Cervical Polyps

Cervical polyps are common finger-like projections/ growths that can arise from the ectocervix or are seen projecting through the endocervical canal (Fig. 9.5).

**Symptoms** Most often they are asymptomatic, but can cause menorrhagia and intermenstrual, postcoital or postmenopausal bleeding. The discharge is usually thick white vaginal or yellowish discharge.They are benign.

**Examination** Cervical polyps can be seen at speculum examination as red or purple projections from the cervical canal. On vaginal examination, they are felt as thick fleshy projections. When the pedicle of the polyp is long and narrow, they can be easily twisted off their base. If the pedicle is thick and vascular, it is advisable to suture the pedicle prior to removal of the polyp. Histopathologic evaluation of the polyp is mandatory.

## Cervical Endometriosis

The cervix is regarded as a rare site for endometriosis. Cervical endometriosis could be due to pelvic endometriosis biopsy, loop excision procedures, and laser treatments to the cervix.

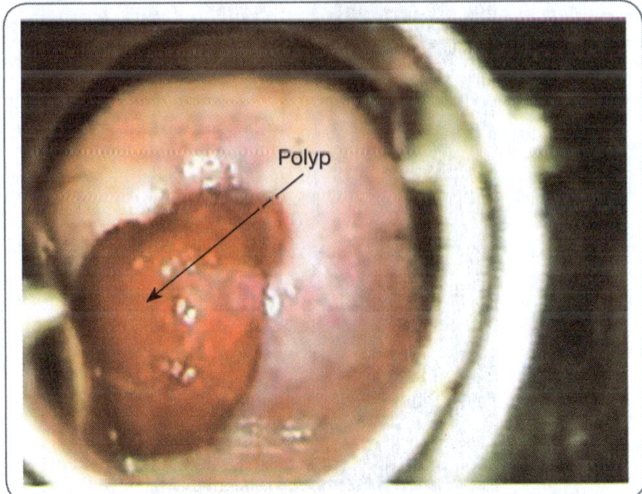


**Fig. 9.5** Endocervical polyp protruding through external os

**Symptoms** It may present as postcoital, intermenstrual bleeding, dyspareunia or discharge, and pelvic pain is usually predominant.

**Differential diagnosis** The colour of these lesions are often mistaken for gestational trophoblastic disease which should be ruled out.

**Treatment**

Excision biopsy of the nodule and where it is not possible, medical management of endometriosis has to be followed.

## Squamous Papilloma

These are often seen in cases of long-standing prolapsed uterus and in cases of obstetric trauma and hence thought to be related to local irritation or scarring. They are usually small and less than 1 cm. It can be anywhere on the cervix. Treatment consists of excision of the papilloma.

## Nabothian Follicles and Cysts

These are common findings in the cervix and are described as pimples on the cervix (Fig. 9.6). They are actually retention cysts when the crypt opening of the endocervical glands gets sealed off by accumulation of yellow mucus. When these follicles undergo cystic changes, they develop a smooth glistening bluish or whitish hue known as nabothian cyst. Usually these are small (less than 0.5 cm), and cysts up to 5 cm or greater in diameter have been seen.They may be single/multiple and temporary in nature. Once they rupture and empty their content, they vanish. A majority of nabothian cysts, therefore, require no treatment.

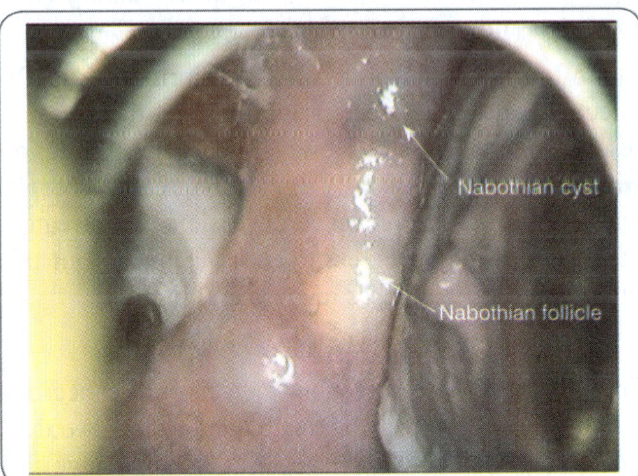


**Fig. 9.6** Nabothian cyst and Nabothian follicle

## C. PREMALIGNANT LESIONS OF THE CERVIX

A thorough knowledge of the premalignant lesions is mandatory to reduce the incidence of cancer cervix. **Human papilloma virus (HPV) has been identified as the etiological agent for premalignant and malignant lesions of the cervix.**

### Human Papilloma Virus (HPV)

Human papilloma virus (HPV) is the most common viral infection of the reproductive tract. Most sexually active women and men will be infected at some point in their lives and some may be repeatedly infected.

The peak time for acquiring infection for both women and men is shortly after becoming sexually active.

#### Transmission

- HPV is sexually transmitted, but **penetrative sex is not required for transmission.**
- Skin-to-skin genital, oral–genital, and digital–genital contact are well-recognised modes of transmission.
- Non-cancer causing types of HPV (especially types 6 and 11) can cause ano-genital warts and it can also be transmitted from the mother to the baby by vertical transmission and can cause recurrent respiratory papillomatosis in the newborn.

**Incubation** The incubation period of HPV infection ranges from 3 weeks to 8 months for warts; it ranges from 7–15 years for cervical intraepithelial neoplasia (CIN) and 20 years for cancer cervix. 90% would clear the infection within 2 years and in the remaining 10%, it persists and progresses to cancer cervix.

**Signs and symptoms** The majority of HPV infections do not cause symptoms or disease and resolve spontaneously. However, persistent infection with specific types of HPV (most frequently types 16 and 18) may lead to precancerous lesions. If untreated, these lesions may progress to cervical cancer, but this progression usually takes many years.

#### Detecting HPV Infection

***Screening*** When screening detects pre-cancerous lesions, these can easily be treated and cancer avoided. Screening can also detect cancer at an early stage and treatment has a high potential for cure.

> **Clinical Importance**
>
> Because pre-cancerous lesions take many years to develop, screening is recommended for every woman aged 30–49 years at least once in a lifetime and ideally more frequently.

***Methods of detection***

- Visual inspection with acetic acid (VIA)
- Conventional (Pap) test and liquid-based cytology (LBC)
- HPV testing for high-risk HPV types

### VIA and VILI

**Visual inspection with acetic acid (VIA)** can be done with the naked eye or with low magnification of 6× when it is called Visual Inspection with Acetic Acid with Magnification (VIAM) (Fig. 9.7).

**Visual inspection with Lugol's iodine (VILI),** also known as **Schiller's test,** uses Lugol's iodine instead of acetic acid.

### Pathophysiological Basis of VIA

On application of 3–5% acetic acid,

- Normal squamous epithelium appears pink
- Columnar epithelium appears red
- Due to the reflection of light from the underlying stroma, which is rich in blood vessels

#### Effects of acetic acid

1. Acetic acid coagulates mucus, and allows a better view of the cervix.

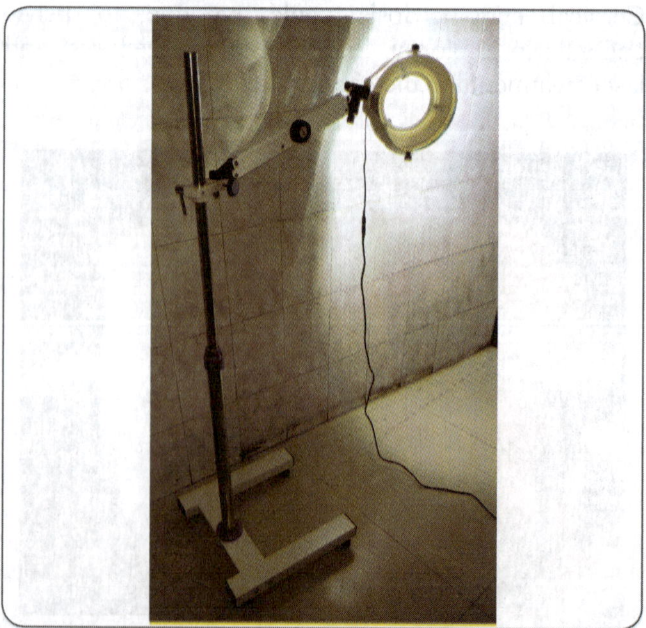

**Fig. 9.7** Mounted magnifying glass with illumination

2. Acetic acid causes dehydration of the cells and coagulation of cellular proteins, thereby reducing the transparency of the epithelium—allows a better recognition of dysplastic epithelium.

## Pathophysiological Basis of VILI

The stratified squamous epithelium with glycogen-laden superficial cells stains mahogany brown after application of iodine.

Columnar epithelium does not take up iodine as the epithelial cells do not contain glycogen, and so remains unstained.

Areas of CIN and invasive cancer do not take up iodine and appear as thick mustard-yellow or saffron-coloured areas.

### Interpretation of the results

*VIA- and VILI-negative*

On application of acetic acid, there will be no aceto-white area or very faint aceto-white lesion.

When Lugol's iodine is applied, the squamous epithelium turns mahogany brown or black and the columnar epithelium does not undergo any colour change.

When a cervix exhibits these changes, it is considered as VIA- and VILI-negative (Fig. 9.8).

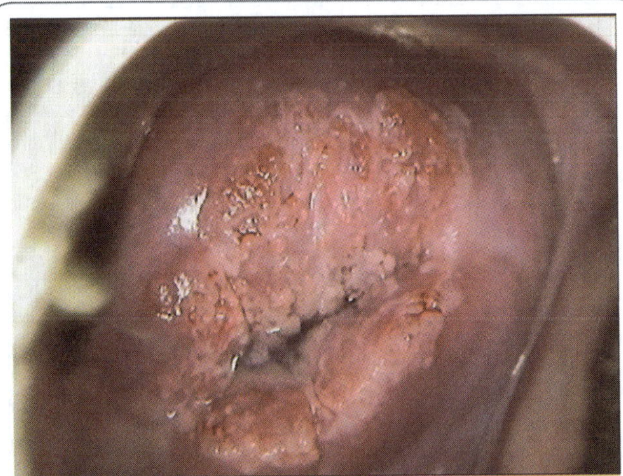

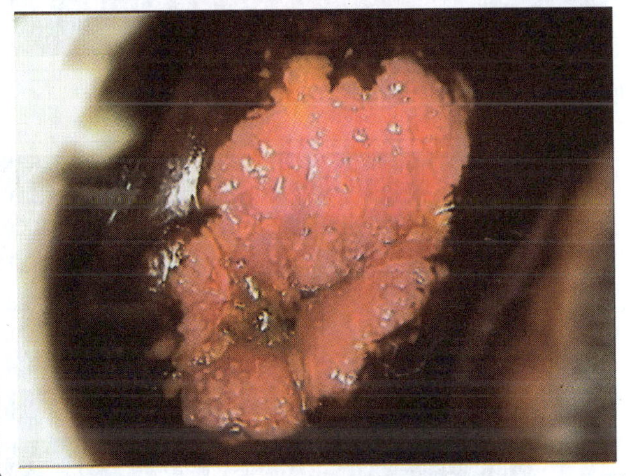

**Fig. 9.8** VIA- and VILI-negative cervix (Note in the first image that there is no aceto-white area after application of acetic acid)

*VIA- and VILI-positive*

When application of acetic acid shows well-defined, dense, (opaque/dull or oyster white) aceto-white areas, it is considered as VIA-positive (Fig. 9.9).

A positive VILI test will show any of the following changes:

1. Entire cervix turns bright yellow.
2. Dense, thick, bright, mustard-yellow or saffron-yellow areas with or without raised margins are seen in the transformation zone, close to or abutting the squamocolumnar junction or close to the os if the squamocolumnar junction is not seen.

*VIA and VILI suspicious of cancer*

Clinically visible frank, nodular, irregular, ulceroproliferative growth is visible on the cervix, which bleeds on touch and which turns densely aceto-white and mustard yellow (Fig. 9.10).

**Advantages of Visual Methods**

- Simple
- Inexpensive
- Low-technology method
- Possible with the existing infrastructure
- Does not require laboratory set-up
- Short learning curve
- Results available immediately
- Further diagnostic investigations and treatment can be planned
- Multiple visits to hospital avoided
- Cost-effective

## Conventional (Pap) Test and Liquid-Based Cytology (LBC)

The spatula which is being used for collecting cells from the transformation zone was introduced by

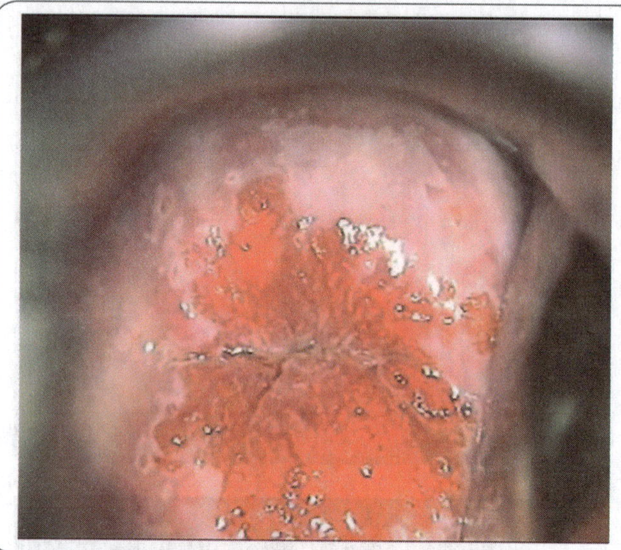

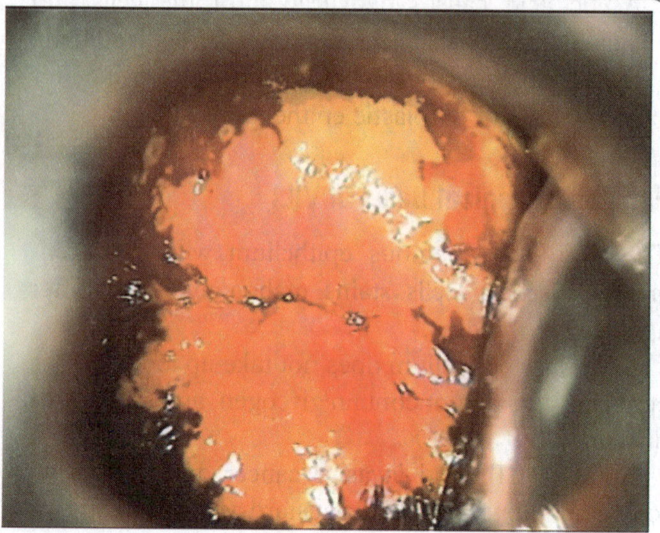

Fig. 9.9 VIA- and VILI-positive cervix

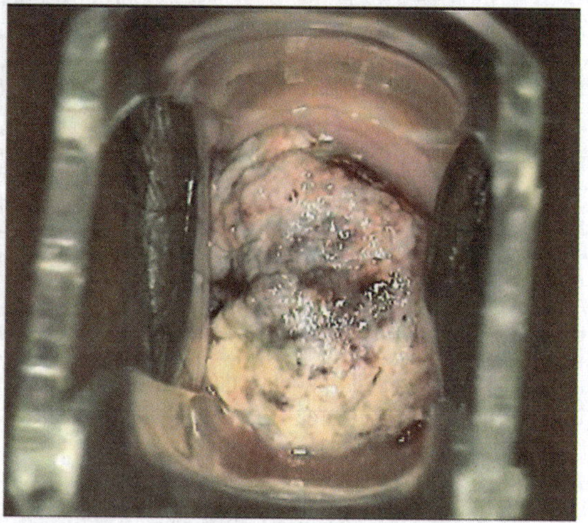

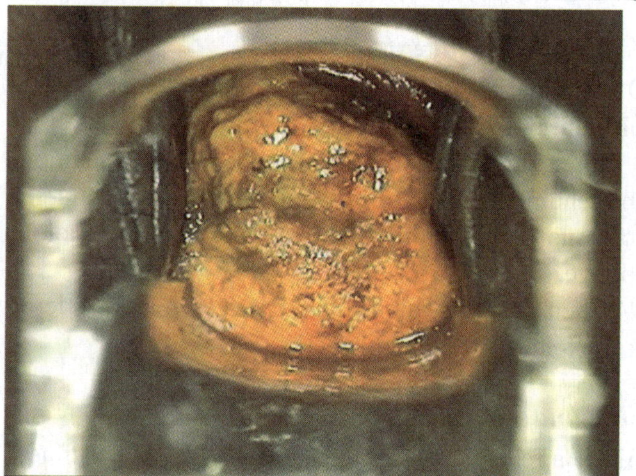

Fig. 9.10 VIA and VILI suspicious of cancer

gynecologist Ernest Ayre and is known as Ayre's spatula.

## Technique of Taking the Smear

Combined use of Ayre spatula with endocervical brush gives good yield of cells for sampling.

- Insert the endocervical brush ensuring that the lower row of bristles are seen as shown in (Fig. 9.11). This is to ensure that the endometrial cavity is not entered.
- The endocervical brush is rotated five times clockwise and the sample is smeared onto a slide.
- The short arm of the Ayre's spatula (Fig. 9.12) is fixed at the external os and the long arm sweeps over the external surface of the cervix five times.

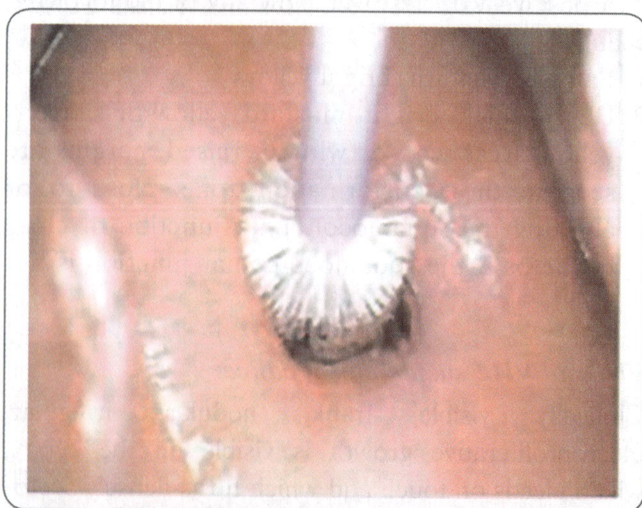

Fig. 9.11 Endocervical brush

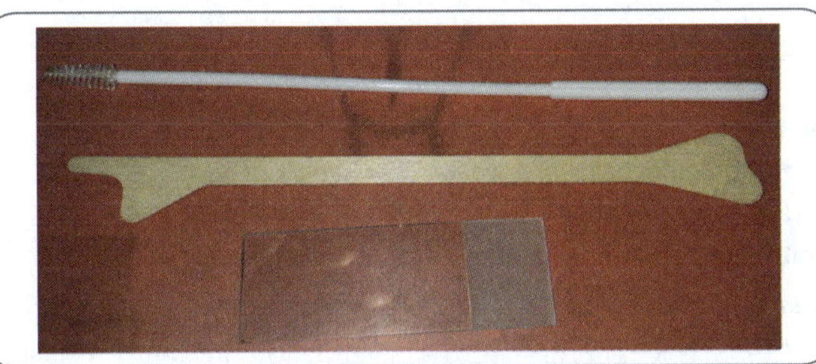

Fig. 9.12 Ayre's spatula and endocervical brush

- The material collected is smeared onto a slide and both the slides are fixed in absolute alcohol and transported to a lab is a Koplick's jar.

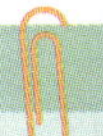

### Disadvantages of Conventional Pap Smear

- Poor sampling
- Inadequate sampling
- Improper fixation of the slide
- Uneven distribution of cells
- Plenty of artifacts

## Liquid-Based Cytology (LBC)

This technique eliminates all the disadvantages of a Pap smear. The sample is collected by a cervical broom device (Fig. 9.13). The sample is placed in a bottle containing the fixative. After processing in the lab, the cervical cells are examined in the usual way.

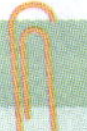

### Advantages of LBC

- Better sample
- Artifacts removed
- Better diagnosis
- Remaining fluid can be used for HPV testing

### Interpretation of Pap smear / LBC (Bethesda system 2001)

The interpretation of Pap smear or LBC is given in Table 9.1.

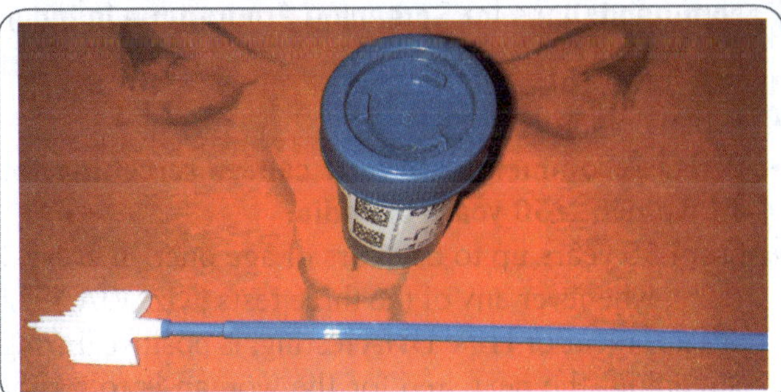

Fig. 9.13 Cervical broom

## HPV testing

HPV infection has been found to be the causative factor in cancer cervix. The era of evidence-based medicine requires the identification of the etiologic agents.

Tests for HPV have become more accurate, objective and reproducible, but its limitations are that it is a time-consuming, laborious procedure requiring sophisticated laboratory, and is very expensive. It is not recommended before the age of 30 as the prevalence of transient HPV infection is very high.

**Currently, 3 tests** are available.

1. Hybrid capture II test.
2. Polymerase chain reaction (PCR)
3. In-situ hybridisation

## Method of Collection

The remaining processed sample from LBC can be used for HPV DNA testing using hybrid capture II test.

PCR has become a standard, non-invasive method for determining the presence of a cervical HPV infection. The sensitivity of PCR is very high.

**In both the tests, the results are reported as "not detected" or as "detected". The specific serotype(s) cannot be reported.** .

**In situ hybridisation** applies hybridisation techniques to the intact DNA of infected cells. The process is performed using a microscope.

## Recent Developments

### 1. Care HPV test

This is a recently developed, simple, affordable, accurate HPV test. It is a signal amplification, rapid test. Since the results are available in 3 hours, the patient need not come again for getting the results. It has been field-tested and found to be a useful test in low-resource settings.

### 2. HPV E6/E7 mRNA testing

- HPV E6/E7 oncoproteins mediate the development of cervical cancer. Their overexpression, which can be measured as E6/E7 messenger RNA (mRNA) transcripts, is associated with a significantly increased risk of CIN and cervical cancer.
- A single positive mRNA result may be more predictive of a persistent infection than a DNA test and is a potential marker for the identification of women at risk of developing cervical carcinoma.

**Table 9.1** Interpretation of Pap smear or LBC

**SPECIMEN TYPE**

*Indicate conventional smear (Pap smear) vs. liquid-based preparation vs. other*

**Specimen adequacy**
- *Satisfactory for evaluation (describe presence of absence of endocervical/transformation zone component and any other quality indicators, e.g., partially obscuring blood, inflammation, etc.)*
- Unsatisfactory for evaluation . . . *(specify reason)*
  - Specimen rejected/not processed *(specify reason)*
  - Specimen processed and examined, but unsatisfactory for evaluation of epithelial abnormality because of *(specify reason)*

**General categorisation *(optional)***
- Negative for Intraepithelial Lesion or Malignancy
- Other: See Interpretation/Result *(e.g., endometrial cells in a women ≥ 45 years of age)*
- Epithelial Cell Abnormality: See Interpretation/Result *(Specify 'squamous' or 'glandular' as appropriate)*

**Interpretation/result**

**Negative for intraepithelial lesion or malignancy**
*(When there is no cellular evidence of neoplasia, state this in the General Categorsation above and/or in the Interpretation/Result section of the report–whether or not there are organisms or other non-neoplastic findings)*
- Non-neoplastic cellular variations
  - Squamous metaplasia
  - Keratotic changes
  - Tubal metaplasia
  - Atrophy
  - Pregnancy-associated changes
- Reactive cellular changes associated with:
  - Inflammation (includes typical repair)
    - Lymphocytic (follicular) cervicitis
  - Radiation
  - Intrauterine contraceptive device (IUD)
- Glandular cells status post hysterectomy

*Organisms*
- *Trichomonas vaginalis*
- Fungal organisms morphologically consistent with Candida spp.
- Shift in flora suggestive of bacterial vaginosis
- Bacteria morphologically consistent with *Actiomyces spp.*
- Cellular changes consistent with herpes simplex virus
- Cellular changes consistent with cytomegalovirus

**Other**
- Endometrial cells *(in a woman ≥ 45 years of age)* *(Specify if "negative for squamous intracepithelial lesion")*

**Epithelial cell abnormalities**

*Squamous cell*
- Atypical squamous cells
  - of undetermined significance (ASC-US)
  - cannot exclude HSIL (ASC-H)
- Low-grade squamous intraepithelial lesion (LSIL) *(encompassing: HPV/mild dysplasia/CIN-1)*
- High-grade squamous intraepithelial lesion (HSIL) *(encompassing: moderate and severe dysplasia, CIS; CIN-2 and CIN-3)*
  - with features suspicious for invasion *(if invasion is suspected)*
- Squamous cell carcinoma

*Glandular cell*
- Atypical
  - endocervial cells *(NOS or specify in comments)*
  - endometrial cells *(NOS or specify in comments)*
  - glandular cells *(NOS or specify in comments)*
- Atypical
  - endocervial cells, favor neoplastic
  - glandular cells, favor neoplastic
- Endocervical adenocarcinoma in situ
- Adenocarcinoma
  - endocervial
  - endometrial
  - extrauterime
  - not otherwise specified (NOS)

**Other malignant neoplasms: *(Specify)***

**Adjunctive testing**
*Provide a brief description of the test method(s) and report the result so that it is easily understood by the clirrician.*

**Computer-assisted interpretation of cervical cytology**
If case examined by an automated device, specify device and result Educational notes and comments appended to cytology Reports (Optional)

Suggestions should be concise and consistent with clinical follow-up guidelines published by professional organisations (references to retevant publications may be included).

### Uses of HPV testing

1. Primary screening modality in future.
2. It has high Positive Predictive Value.
3. When the Pap smear report is ASCUS or LSIL, HPV DNA testing is done to detect the presence or absence of high-risk HPV.
4. It is used as a test to confirm the success of treatment.
5. When combined with Pap smear, it is known as HPV co-test.The main purpose of HPV cotesting is to increase the screening interval from 3 years to 5 years.

## Recommendations for Screening Programme in India

- VIA and VILI
- Papanicolaou (**Pap**) smear.
- **WHO recommends cervical cancer screening for all women ≥30 years in India.**
- From 30 years up to 65 years of age once in every 3 years, whenever any of the three tests , viz. VIA,VILI or Pap smear or HPV DNA testing, is positive during screening, the next step for the woman is to go for colposcopy.

**Table 9.2** IFCPC Nomenclature (2011)

| 2011 IFCPC Noemenclature[1]<br>Accepted in Rio World Congress, July 5, 2011; Nomenclature Committee Chairman: Jacob Mostein MD | | | |
|---|---|---|---|
| **2011 IFCPC colposcopic terminology of the cervix[1]** | | | |
| General assessment | | • Adequate/inadequate for the reason ... (i.e., cervix obscured by inflammation, bleeding, scar)<br>• Squamo-columnar junction visibility: completely visible, partially visible, not visible<br>• Transformation zone types 1, 2, 3 | |
| Normal colposcopic findings | | Original squamous epithelium:<br>• Mature<br>• Atrophic<br>Columnar epithelium<br>• Ectopy<br>Metaplastic squamous epithelium<br>• Nabothian cysts<br>• Crypt (gland) openings<br>Deciduosis in pregnancy | |
| Abnormal colposoopic findings | General principles | Location of the lesion: Inside or outside the T-zone,<br>Location of the lesion by clock position<br>Size of the lesion: Number of cervical quadrants the lesion covers,<br>Size of the lesion in percentage of cervix | |
| | Grade 1 (Minor) | Thin aceto-white epithelium<br>Irregular, geographic border | Fine mosaic<br>Fine punctuation |
| | Grade 2 (Major) | Dense aceto-white epithelium, rapid appearance of aceto whitening, cuffed crypt (gland) openings | Coarse mosaic, coarse punctuation, sharp border, inner border sign, ridge sign |
| | Non-specific | Leukoplakia (keratosis, hyperkeratosis), Erosion<br>Lugol's staining (Schiller's test): stained/non-stained | |
| Suspicious for invasion | | Atypical vessels<br>Additional signs: fragile vessels, irregular surface, exophytic lesion, necrosis, ulceration (necrotic), tumour/gross neoplasm | |
| Miscellaneous finding | | Congenital transformation zone, Condyloma, Polyp (Ectocervical/endocervical) Inflammation, | Stenosis, congenital anomaly, post treatment consequence, endometriosis |

## Intrepretation Done as Per IFCPC Recommedations

Table 9.2 gives the interpretation as per IFCPC recommendations.

## DIAGNOSIS OF PRECANCEROUS LESION

This is done by endocervical curetting and colposcopic-directed biopsy. Colposcopy-directed biopsy is better than four-quadrant biopsy or random biopsy as it would provide more accurate diagnosis.

### Histopathology of Low-Grade Lesion—CIN 1

- **Koilocytes** are (Fig. 9.14) those cells with nuclear enlargement, irregular **("raisinoid")** nuclear membranes, perinuclear halos, and bi- and multi-nucleation which are the hallmarks of HPV infection.
- Disturbed structural organisation of the epithelium in the lower third.

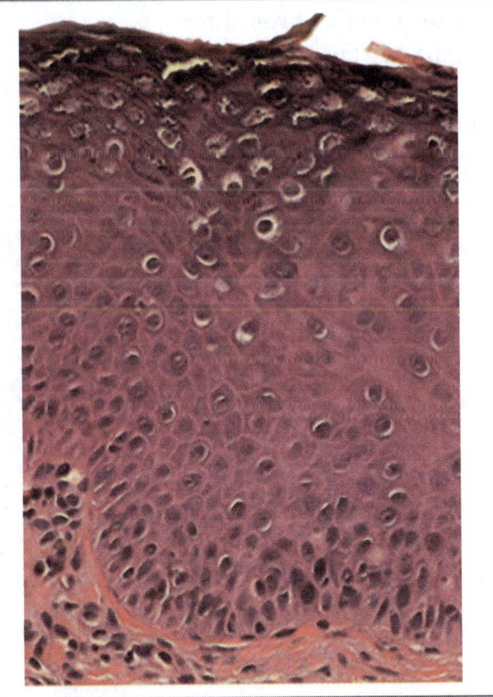

**Fig. 9.14** Koilocytes

### CIN 2/Moderate Dysplasia

- Marked koilocytosis
- Disturbed structural organisation of the epithelium in the lower half
- Microinvasive squamous carcinoma

### Treatment of Preinvasive Lesion

The purpose of treating precancerous lesions is to destroy the affected areas and thereby reduce the mortality and morbidity associated with cancer cervix.

Cervical intraepithelial neoplasia (CIN) is a premalignant lesion that is diagnosed by histology as CIN 1, CIN 2, or CIN 3. If left untreated, CIN 2 or CIN 3 (collectively referred to as CIN 2+) can progress to cervical cancer.

CIN 1 is considered as a transient tissue reaction to HPV infection. In view of low progression, it can be observed and treated accordingly.

CIN 2 and CIN 3 (Figs. 9.15 and 9.16) indicate persistent HPV infection that is more likely to progress. Treatment consists of **ablation or excision** of the abnormal transformation zone. In the ablative procedure, the entire transformation zone is destroyed in vivo, i.e., no tissue specimen is available for histopathological correlation whereas in the second method, the transformation zone is excised in toto, and this provides sample for tissue diagnosis.

**Ablative/destructive procedure**

- Cryocautery (Fig. 9.17)
- Cold coagulation (currently known as thermal coagulation)
- Laser vapourisation

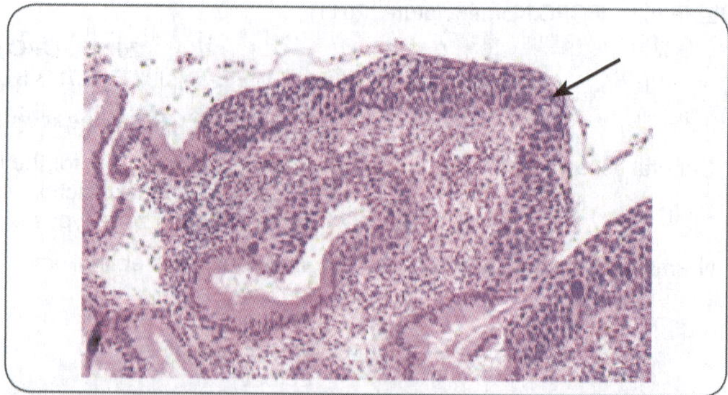

**Fig. 9.16** Full thickness disorganised epithelium involving the endocervical gland

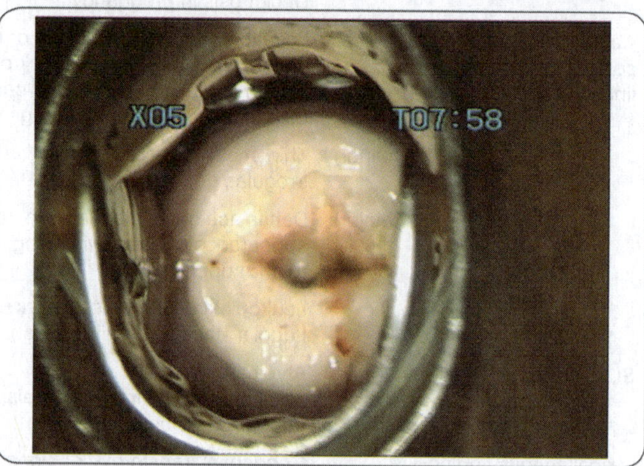


**Fig. 9.17** Cervix following cryocautery

**Excisional method**

- **L**arge **L**oop **E**xcision of the **T**ransformation **Z**one (LLETZ)
- Conisation—Surgical cone biopsy commonly known as cold knife conisation (CKC)
- Simple hysterectomy

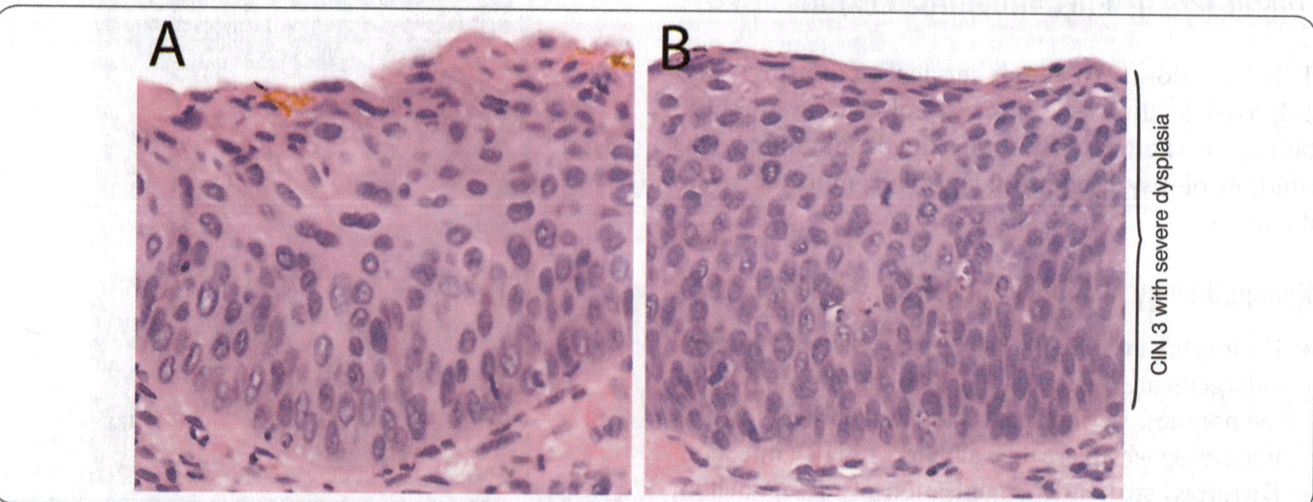


**Fig. 9.15** CIN 3 showing severe dysplasia

### Cryotherapy

- Ideally suited for small and low-grade lesions.
- The cryotherapy technique uses a cryoprobe with a tip made of highly conductive metal. Nitrous oxide ($N_2O$) or carbon dioxide ($CO_2$) are used. The temperature at the core of the tissue ice ball is around –20°C.
- This leads to cell death known as **cryonecrosis.**

### Cold coagulation

Cold coagulation uses much lesser current than electrodiathermy. Hence it was previously known as cold coagulation. Currently it is described as **thermocoagulation**.

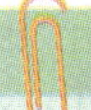

#### Advantages of Cold Coagulation

1. All grades of CIN can be treated in the outpatient clinic since it requires no anaesthesia
2. Safe, efficient,with a very low morbidity rate.
3. High success rate (CIN 2 and 3 — 96.5–99%) without affecting fertility

### Laser vapouristion

Here carbon dioxide laser is used to produce energy beam which causes intracellular water content to boil and vapourise to form a shallow crater at the point of contact.

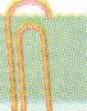

#### Advantages of Laser Vapourisation

- Precision and good control of depth
- Good haemostasis
- Excellent healing
- Treatment of choice when the premalignant lesion extends on to vagina.

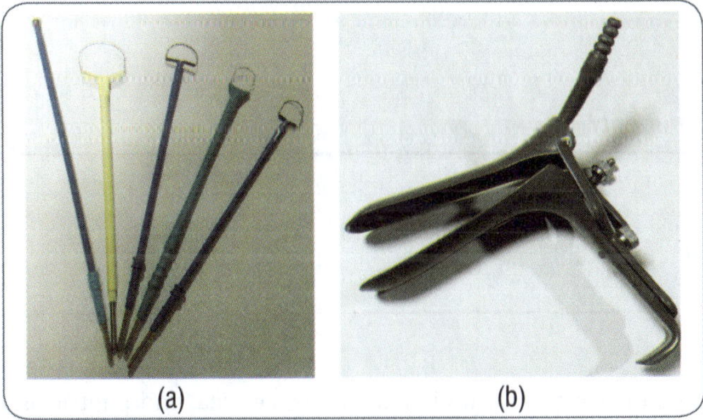

(a) (b)

**Fig. 9.18** (a) Loops of varying size; (b) Speculum with smoke vent

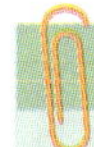

#### Disadvantages of Laser Vapourisation

- Costly equipment
- Has a long learning curve

### Large loop excision of the transformation zone (LLETZ)

This is also known as Loop Electrosurgical Excision Procedure (LEEP).

Loops of varying sizes are available (Fig. 9.18a), which can be fitted to the cautery pen. A speculum with smoke vent (Fig. 9.18b) is used in the procedure. A blend monopolar current of 35–50 watts is used to remove a cylindrical piece of tissue from the cervix.

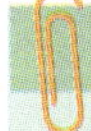

#### Advantage of LLETZ

- The ease of the technique and its efficacy has made it a popular procedure.

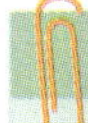

#### Disadvantage of LLETZ

- Long-term cervical morphological changes like stenosis, dysmenorrhea, cervical incompetence, pregnancy complications such as miscarriage, and premature labour may result.

### Cold knife conisation (CKC)

This refers to the excision of a cone-shaped portion of the cervix surrounding the endocervical canal and including the entire transformation zone with a cold knife blade (Figs. 9.19 and 9.20).

- The goal of cone biopsy is to remove the entire transformation zone.
- The size and shape of the cone biopsy should be tailored to the individual situation and based upon findings.

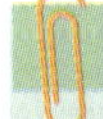

#### Advantage of CKC

- Preservation of histological characteristics without any thermal damage to the specimen.

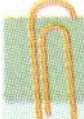

#### Disadvantages of CKC

- Cervical stenosis
- Increased pregnancy wastage
- Inadequate colposcopy on follow-up
- Possibility of recurrent disease due to incomplete excision

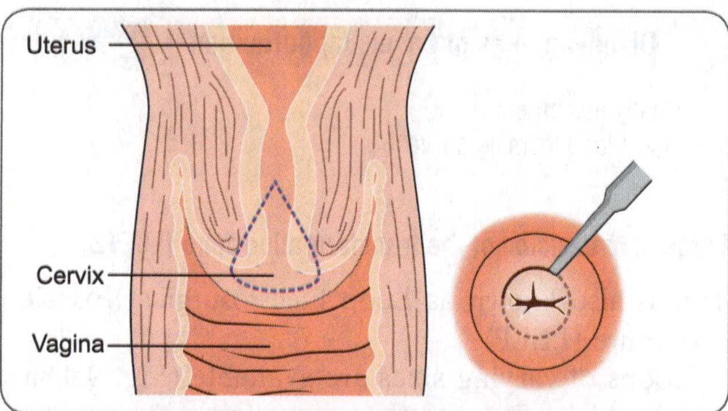


**Fig. 9.19** Diagrammatic representation of incision for cervical cone and the area of tissue that would be removed

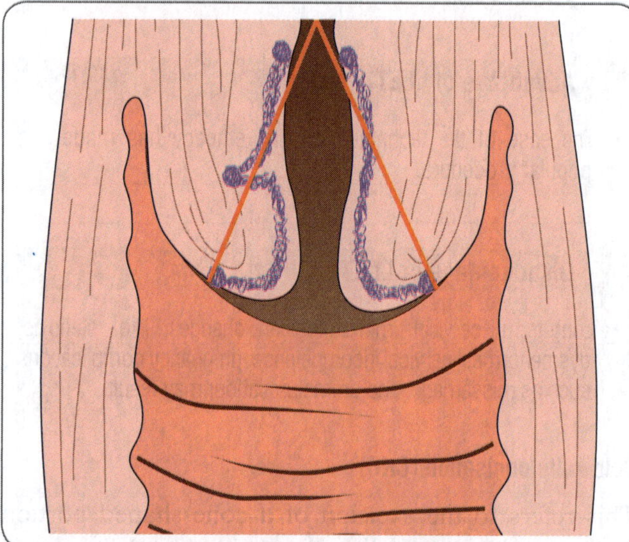

**Fig. 9.20** Incomplete excision leading to recurrence

### Simple hysterectomy

This is indicated in women who have associated conditions like fibroid, adnexal mass, endometriosis, uterovaginal prolapse and recurrence of CIN or when there is vaginal extension of the cervical lesion.

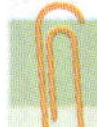

**Follow-up for Pre-invasive Lesions**

- There is a need for follow-up up to 10 years after treatment of pre-invasive lesions. Annual monitoring of these women by HPV testing and Pap smear is mandatory.

## Prevention

### Vaccines

Primary prevention in the form of vaccination is available since 2007. They are prophylactic vaccines and are prepared from **virus-like particles (VLPs)** which do not contain any live biological product or DNA, so they are non-infectious. The vaccines are produced by recombinant technology.

Whereas **quadrivalent vaccine- QHPV** is against **HPV types 6, 11, 16**, and **18, bivalent vaccine-BHPV** is **against HPV types 16**, and **18. 9-valent HPV vaccine** Nona vaccine **against HPV 6, 11, 16, 18, 31, 33, 45, 52, 58** is also available.

**Age** It is recommended from 10–12 years of age up to 26 years of age.

**Dosage** Both the vaccines are given in three doses at 0, 2 and 6 months. It is mandatory to continue cytological screening for cancer cervix in spite of vaccination.

***Case study***

*A 35-year-old woman with three living children presents with history of excessive vaginal discharge and dyspareunia for the past three months. She also has increased frequency of micturition. Examination revealed red and minimally ulcerated cervix.*

*a) What is the probable diagnosis?*

*b) What investigations would confirm the diagnosis?*

*c) What are the different treatment modalities available for this patient?*

## RECAP

- Cervicitis could be classified as specific and non-specific.
- Non-specific causes include chemotherapy, radiation, intrauterine device and localised lesions like cervical endometriosis.
- Symptoms and signs include discharge and discomfort and need careful physical and speculum examination to establish the diagnosis.

- Colour of the discharge gives a clue about the causative organism.
- Diagnosis is by microscopy, culture, or nucleic acid amplification tests.
- Human papilloma virus (HPV) is the most common viral infection of the reproductive tract.
- HPV is sexually transmitted, but penetrative sex is not required for transmission. Skin-to-skin genital, oral-genital, and digital-genital contact is a well-recognised mode of transmission.
- Non-cancer causing types of HPV (especially types 6 and 11) can cause ano-genital warts and it can also be transmitted from the mother to the baby by vertical transmission and can cause recurrent respiratory papillomatosis in the newborn.
- The majority of HPV infections do not cause symptoms or disease and resolve spontaneously. However, persistent infection with specific types of HPV (most frequently types 16 and 18) may lead to precancerous lesions
- Methods of detection are visual inspection with acetic acid (VIA), Conventional (Pap) test and liquid-based cytology (LBC) and HPV testing for high-risk HPV types.
- Recommendations for screening programme in India includes VIA & VILI, Papanicolaou (Pap) smear. From 30 years up to 65 years of age once in every 3 years. Whenever any of the three tests , viz. VIA,VILI or Pap smear or HPV DNA testing is positive during screening, the next step for the woman is to go for colposcopy.
- Diagnosis of precancerous lesion is done by endocervical curetting and colposcopic directed biopsy.
- Colposcopy directed biopsy is better than four quadrant biopsy or random biopsy as it would provide more accurate diagnosis.
- Treatmentof preinvasive lesion- CIN1 is considered as a transient tissue reaction to HPV infection. In view of low progression, it can be observed and treated accordingly.
- CIN 2 and CIN 3 indicate persistent HPV infection and is more likely to progress. Treatment consists of ablation or excision of the abnormal transformation zone.
- Ablative/destructive procedures available are cryocautery, cold coagulation currently known as thermal coagulation and laser vapourisation.
- Excisional Methods include **L**arge **L**oop **E**xcision of the **T**ransformation **Z**one ( LLETZ), Conisation - Surgical cone biopsy commonly known as cold knife conisation (CKC) and simple hysterectomy.
- Primary prevention in the form of vaccination is available.
- The available vaccines are quadrivalent vaccine (QHPV) is against HPV types 6, 11, 16, and 18, bivalent vaccine (BHPV) is against HPV types 16, and 18. 9-valent HPV vaccine, Nona vaccine against HPV 6,11,16,18,31,33,45,52,58 is also available.

## REVIEW QUESTIONS

### Long-Answer Questions

1. What are the excisional methods available for treating preinvasive lesions?
2. Describe the technique, advantage and disadvantage of Large Loop Excison of Transformation Zone (LLETZ).

### Short-Answer Questions

1. Describe the characteristics of VIA- and VILI-positive lesion. What are the advantages of visual methods of screening?
2. Write briefly about ectropion.

### MCQs

**1. Quadrivalent vaccine- (QHPV) is effective against**
   a) HPV types 7,10,14,18
   b) HPV types 16, 18, 31, 33
   c) HPV types 6, 11, 16, 18
   d) HPV types 31,33,45,52

**2. Full thickness disorganised epithelium involving the endocervical gland is seen in**
   a) CIN-3/Severe dysplasia
   b) CIN-2/Moderate dysplasia
   c) CIN-1/Low-grade lesion
   d) Gonorrhea

**3. At the level of the external os, the stratified squamous epithelium of the ectocervix meets the columnar cells of the endocervix. This is known as**
   a) Old squamo columnar junction (SCJ)
   b) New squamo columnar junction (SCJ)
   c) Transformation zone
   d) Isthmus of the uterus

**4. Cervical broom is used for collecting samples for**
   a) Conventional Pap test
   b) Visual inspection with Lugol's iodine (VILI)
   c) Visual inspection with acetic acid (VIA)
   d) Liquid-based cytology

# Chapter 10

# Benign Diseases of the Uterus

## At a Glance


Endometrial Polyps
- Types
- Incidence
- Pathogenesis
- Risk Factors
- Signs and Symptoms
- Diagnosis
- Management

Adenomyosis
- Types
- Pathogenesis
- Risk Factors
- Signs and Symptoms
- Diagnosis
- Management

Fibroid Uterus
- Incidence
- Etiology
- Risk Factors
- Histopathology
- Clinical Classification
- Vascular Supply
- Complications
- Symptoms of Fibroid
- Signs of Fibroid
- Differential Diagnosis
- Investigations
- Management

Endometrial Tuberculosis (TB)
- Pathogenesis
- Signs and Symptoms
- Investigations
- Management


Benign diseases of the uterus are frequently seen in women of all ages. The common symptom of these conditions is menstrual disturbance. With the routine use of ultrasound, the diagnosis is made early and with greater amount of accuracy. This has reduced the complications associated with the disease and its management.

Benign diseases of the uterus are very often considered synonymous with fibroid uterus. Though fibroid uterus is a common benign uterine tumour, there are other benign conditions which can arise in the uterus. The most common presenting symptom of these diseases is abnormal uterine bleeding, but they may also be asymptomatic and be diagnosed accidentally during imaging for some other condition.

The common benign diseases of the uterus are:

1. Endometrial polyps
2. Adenomyosis
3. Fibroid uterus (leiomyoma)
4. Endometrial tuberculosis

## ENDOMETRIAL POLYPS

An endometrial polyp (Fig. 10.1) is a mass arising from the inner lining of the uterus.

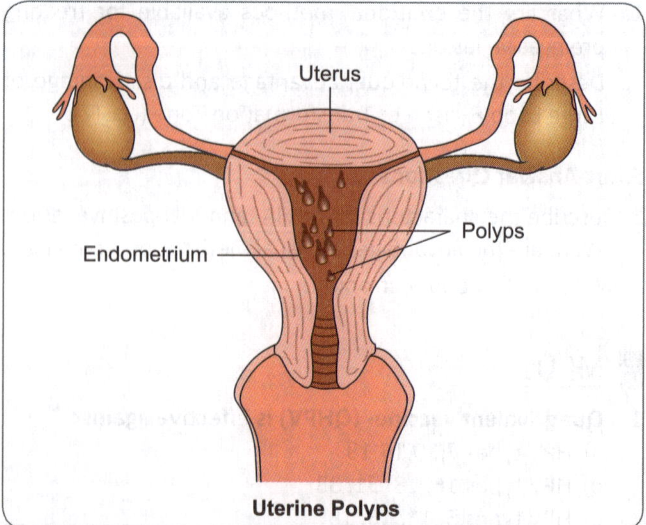


Fig. 10.1 Uterine polyps

## Types

- When the polyp is attached to the uterus by a stalk, it is called **pedunculated polyp.**
- When no stalk is present, it is known as **sessile polyp**.

Pedunculated polyps are usually seen protruding through the cervix into the vagina. Polyps may be very small (few mm) to fairly large size (few cm).

## Incidence

The exact incidence of polyp is not known but it ranges from 5–8% in the general population to about 10–30% in those women with abnormal uterine bleeding.

## Pathogenesis

The polyp is comprised of endometrial glands and fibrous stroma with a surface epithelial covering.

Estrogen and progesterone are believed to elongate the endometrial glands, stroma and the spiral arteries resulting in the formation of polyps.

## Risk factors

Polyps are more frequently seen in women in the older age group, obese women and those on tamoxifen. Oral contraceptive pills appear to offer some protection against formation of polyps.

## Signs and Symptoms

- In most of the women the polyps are **asymptomatic** and are found mainly during ultrasound examination, particularly transvaginal sonography.
- **Menstrual irregularity** This is the most common symptom associated with polyps. It could be irregular menstrual bleeding or profuse bleeding or menorrhagia, intermenstrual bleeding or postmenopausal bleeding.
- **Infertility** Polyps identified near the tubal ostia in infertile women could be a cause for infertility since they block sperm migration.

## Diagnosis

The diagnosis is confirmed by transvaginal sonography (TVS), sonosalpingography (SIS) and hysteroscopy.

- In **TVS**, the polyp appears as a non-specific thickening or as a round or elongated focal mass within the cavity (Fig. 10.2).

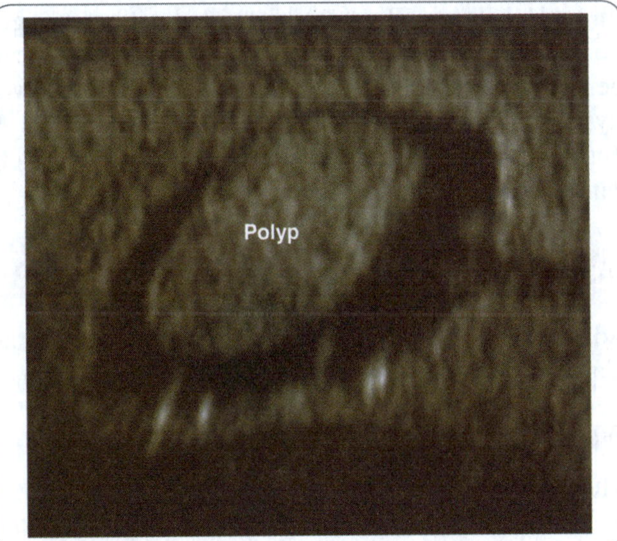


**Fig. 10.2** Endometrial polyp seen in sonography (*Source:* Wikipedia)

- Both **SIS and hysteroscopy** are better in identifying endometrial polyps. In SIS, the polyps appear as echogenic, smooth intracavitary lesions with thin pedicle or broad base (Fig. 10.3).
- **Hysteroscopy** can be used not only to identify an endometrial polyp with certainty but also for removal of the same.

## Management

Polyps, particularly the symptomatic ones, need to be removed and subjected to histopathological examination. Polyps which are seen protruding

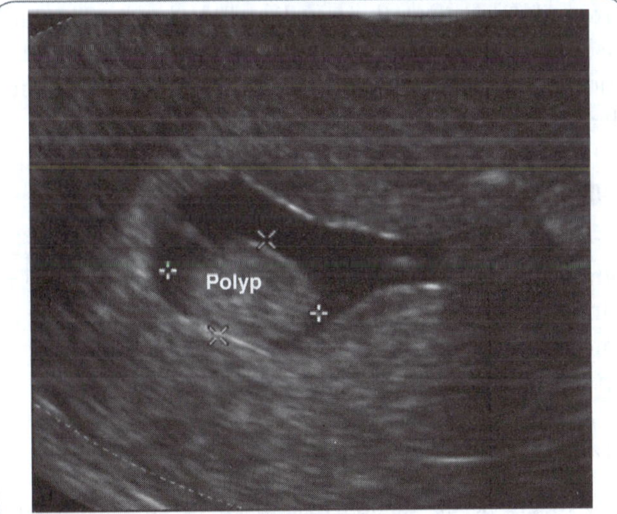


**Fig. 10.3** Saline infusion sonography of endometrial polyp (*Source:* NIH/Khan F, et al; Ann Saudi Med; 2011)

through the cervical os can be twisted with a sponge-holding forceps and removed. The sessile polyps can be removed by dilatation and curettage. **However hysteroscopic visualisation and polypectomy is a better way of treating the polyps since it effectively removes all the polyps under vision.**

## ADENOMYOSIS

Adenomyosis is a condition in which the endometrial glands are seen invading the myometrial tissue.

### Types

There are two types of adenomyosis.

- When the endometrial glands are scattered throughout the myometrium, it is known as **diffuse adenomyosis.**
- When they are restricted to few areas, it is known as **focal adenomyosis** or **adenomyoma.**

**The endometrial glands found within the myometrium are from the basalis layer.** Hence, they do not undergo the cyclical changes during menstruation and therefore the hemorrhage within the foci is minimal. The reported incidence of this condition from hysterectomy specimens varies from 20 to 60%.

### Pathogenesis

Adenomyosis is believed to develop by the invagination of the basalis layer into the myometrium.

### Risk Factors

Adenomyosis is more often seen in women in the 40s and 50s age group. Parous women are more often affected than their nulliparous sisters. They are also associated with leiomyomas, endometriosis and endometrial cancer. Women who are on tamoxifen therapy are at risk of developing adenomyosis.

### Signs and Symptoms

Menorrhagia and dysmenorrhea are common symptoms. About 10% women have dyspareunia. On clinical examination, the uterus is usually found to be smooth-surfaced and regular. It is enlarged but mostly up to the size of a 12-week pregnant uterus.

### Diagnosis

The diagnosis of adenomyosis used to be retrospective following hysterectomy. With the introduction of TVS (Fig. 10.4), the diagnosis is more often made prior to surgery.

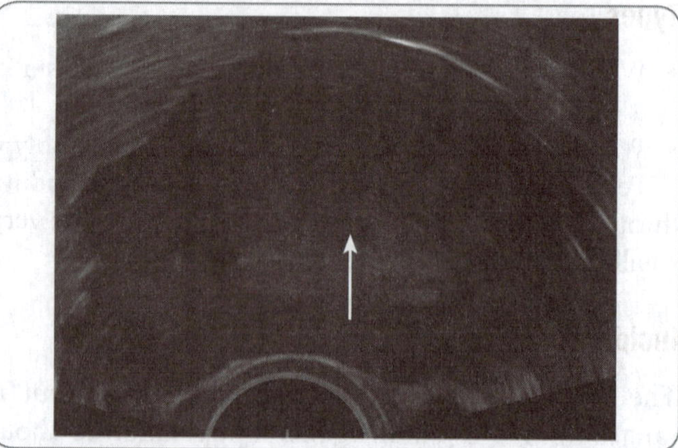

**Fig. 10.4** Transvaginal sonography of adenomyosis. Endometrium (shown by arrow) is seen as hyperechoic area in the middle, with linear striations extending upwards from it. (*Source:* Wikimedia)

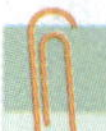

**Characteristics of Adenomyosis in TVS**

1. Difference in the myometrial wall thickness.
2. Small myometrial hypoechoic areas depicting cystic glands.
3. Striated projection from the endometrium into the myometrium.

Magnetic resonance imaging (MRI) has a better diagnostic potential compared to TVS (Fig. 10.5).

### Management

#### Medical management

NSAIDs are often the first line of management. They reduce the pain associated with adenomyosis.

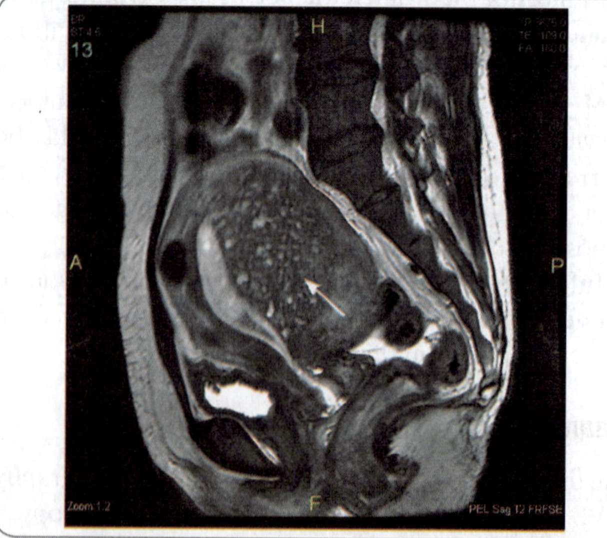


**Fig. 10.5** Magnetic resonance imaging showing uterus with adenomyosis (shown by arrow) in the posterior wall (*Source:* Wikimedia)

Combined oral contraceptives and progestin-only pills have also been tried to induce endometrial atrophy and to decrease endometrial prostaglandin production. Levonorgestrel-releasing intrauterine system (LNG-IUS) has also been found to be effective in the management of adenomyosis. GnRH agonists and danazol have also been tried for the relief of symptoms associated with adenomyosis.

### Surgical management

#### *Uterus-sparing procedures*

**Uterine artery embolisation (UAE)** In this procedure, the uterine arteries are blocked under radiological guidance. This procedure is successful when it is a focal adenomysis.

**Resection of focal adenomyosis** This is another procedure in which the adenomyoma is resected either through a hysteroscope or by open surgical method. However complete eradication of diffuse adenomysis is problematic.

**Ablations** Non-hysteroscopic procedures like high-energy radiofrequency ablation, thermal balloon ablation, cryo-endometrial ablation and microwave ablation are some of the other methods used in the management of adenomyosis with variable results.

#### *Procedures where uterus is removed*

**Hysterectomy** This has been the main surgical therapy prior to the introduction of uterus-sparing procedures. Even today, hysterectomy remains the final treatment for women in whom other treatment modalities are unsuccessful. However even after hysterectomy, pelvic pain may persist in about 20% women.

Hysterectomy could be done by the abdominal route or by laparoscopic method (Fig. 10.6). The postoperative specimen of the uterus (Fig. 10.7) shows a typical endometrial tissue invading the myometrium.

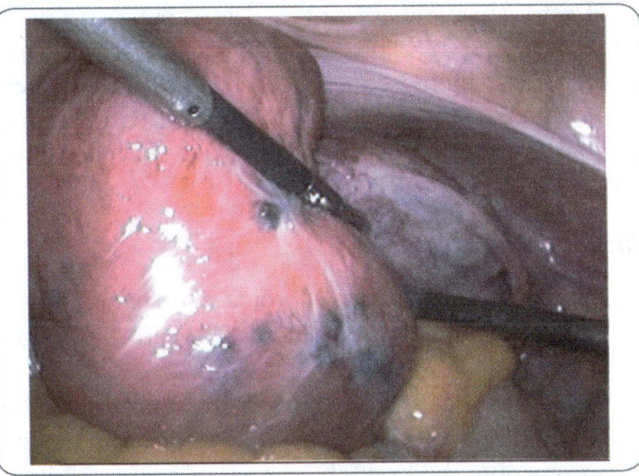

**Fig. 10.6** Adenomysis seen during laparoscopy (*Source:* Wikimedia)

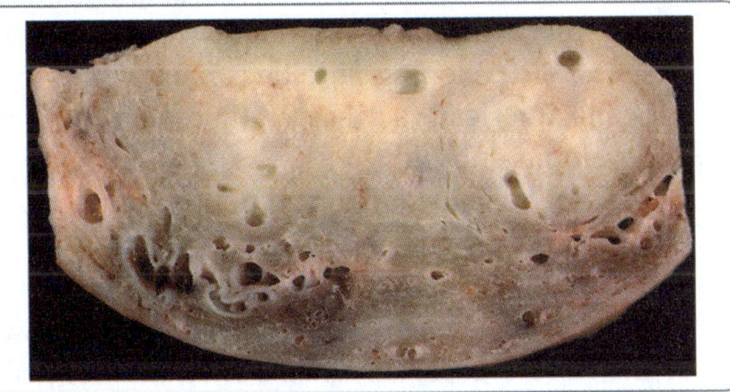

**Fig. 10.7** Cut section showing endometrial tissue in the myometrium (*Source:* Wikimedia)

## FIBROID UTERUS

It is the most common benign disease of the uterus in the reproductive age group. The term fibroid is inaccurate as it arises from the smooth muscle cell (myocyte). A fibroid also contains varying amounts of elastic collagen and extracellular matrix protein and so it is more accurate to call it leiomyoma or myoma.

### Incidence

The true incidence of fibroid in the general female population is unknown because 50% of fibroids are asymptomatic. The risk of developing a fibroid over 45 years of age is greater than 60%. The incidence in the perimenopausal age group is greater than 60% and the reported incidence varies from 30% to 70%. A histological study detected fibroids in 77% of hysterectomy specimens. It is detected clinically in 33% of patients and by ultrasound examination in 50% of patients.

### Etiology

The precise etiology of fibroids is unknown. The most frequent cytogenetic studies are translocations involving chromosomes 7 and 14 and deletion in chromosome 7.

Once the fibroid tumour has been initiated, growth of the tumour is dependent on estrogen and progesterone. Circulating levels of estrogen and progesterone are not high in patients with fibroids. Fibroids have raised local estrogen relative to normal myometrium due to increased fibroid expression of aromatase enzyme. There is also increased estrogen receptor level. There is increased responsiveness to estrogen compared to normal myometrial cells. Progesterone receptor levels are increased in myometrium.

## Risk factors

1. The precise etiology of fibroids remains unknown.
2. Early menarche leads to increased years of estrogen exposure.
3. Elevated BMI results in increased conversion of androgen to estrogen and decreased hepatic protection by sex hormone binding globulin (SHBG).
4. Tamoxifen increases the risk of developing fibroid.
5. When there are affected family members, the chances of developing fibroids is more.
6. African–American race has a 5 times increased risk of developing fibroid.
7. PCOS due to anovulation and unopposed estrogen increases the risk.
8. Age is the most common risk factor.
9. Hormone replacement therapy increases the growth of the fibroid especially in the first six months of therapy due to failure of normal postmenopausal regression.
10. The risk is decreased in the postmenopausal women due to hypoestrogenism.
11. Similarly high parity decreases the risk for fibroids.
12. Combined contraceptive pill decreases the risk since exposure to estrogen is opposed by progesterone.
13. Smoking also decreases the risk for fibroid.

### Risk Factors for Fibroids

**Increased risk**

1. Etiology of fibroids unknown.
2. Early menarche
3. Elevated BMI
4. Tamoxifen
5. Family history
6. African–American race at 5 times increased risk
7. PCOS
8. Age
9. Hormone replacement therapy

**Decreased risk**

1. Hypoestrogenism (postmenopausal women).
2. High parity
3. Combined contraceptive pill
4. Smoking

## Histopathology

### Gross appearance

Fibroids are well circumscribed and round or oval shaped. They are firm, fibrous and pearly white in appearance.

A cut section of a fibroid shows a white whorled appearance. It may be single or multiple. Tiny seedling fibroids are commonly seen in association with large tumours accounting for their recurrence. The fibroid has a pseudocapsule which consists of connective tissue fixing the tumour to the myometrium. The blood vessels to the fibroid lie in the capsule and send radial branches to the substance of the fibroid.

### Microscopic appearance

Under a microscope, interlacing smooth muscle bundles with smooth muscle cell proliferation are seen. There is variable amount of fibrous tissue.

## Clinical Classification

The fibroids are commonly classified as
1. Subserous
2. Intramural
3. Submucosal

Figure 10.8 shows the various types of fibroids.

### Subserous fibroids

Subserous fibroids grow outwards from the uterine surface and reach very large size. They are covered

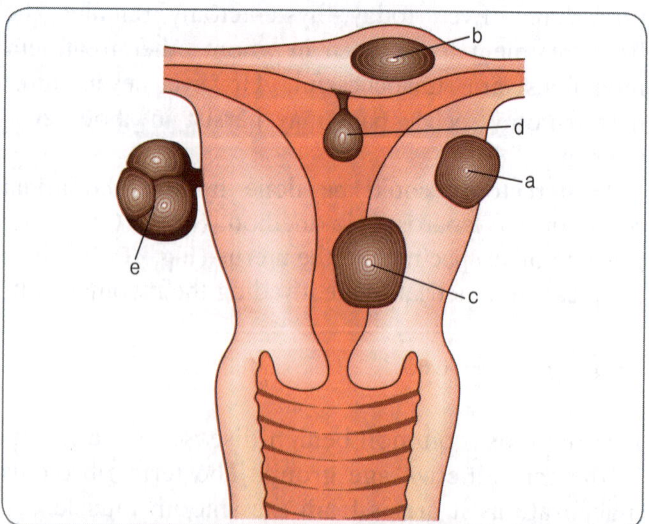


**Fig. 10.8** Schematic drawing of various types of uterine fibroids: a=subserosal fibroids, b=intramural fibroids, c=submucosal fibroid, d=pedunculated submucosal fibroid, e=pedunculated subserosal

with peritoneum. They may be **sessile** or **pedunculated** (Fig. 10.9). **Torsion is a complication of pedunculated fibroid**. Sessile fibroids projecting from the fundal region may get attached to the omentum or bowel rarely due to coexisting infection. If it derives its blood supply from the omentum or bowl it may get detached to become a **parasitic fibroid**.

### Intramural fibroids

They lie within the wall of the uterus. It is necessary for **50% of fibroid mass to be within the uterine wall to be called intramural fibroid.** In a few cases, it may project into the uterine cavity or outside the serosal layer. The pseudocapsule which is a thin layer of connective tissue separates the fibroid from the adjacent myometrium. This allows for the easy cleavage of fibroid during myomectomy (Fig. 10.10).

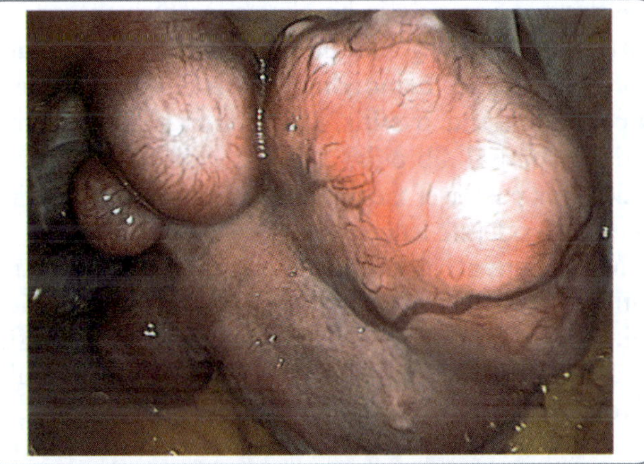

**Fig. 10.9** Subserous fibroids as seen by laparoscopy (*Source:* Dr. Girija Wagh, Professor, Obstetrics & Gynecology, Bharati Vidyapeeth University Medical College)

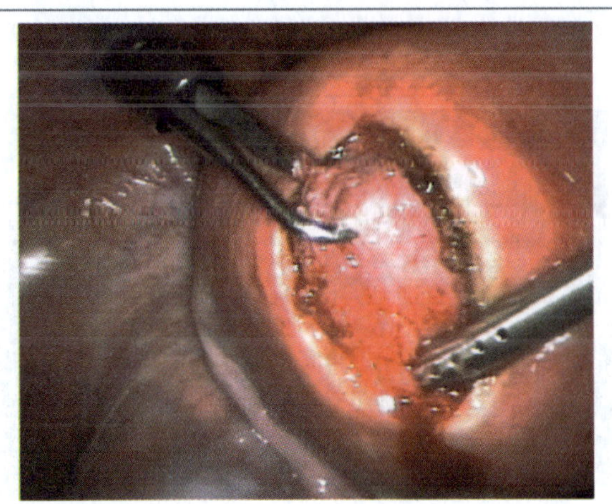

**Fig. 10.10** Intramural fibroid during laparoscopic surgery (*Source:* Wikimedia)

### Submucosal fibroids

Submucosal fibroids (Fig. 10.11) are less common.

#### *Types of submucosal fibroids*

Type 0: Pedunculated—lie entirely within the uterine cavity.
Type I: Sessile—more the 50% in the uterine cavity.
Type II: Sessile—less than 50% in the uterine cavity.
Uterus is not usually enlarged.

### Broad ligament fibroid

This is the most common solid tumour of the broad ligament. Broad ligament fibroid may arise from the uterus and invade the broad ligament when it is called **pseudobroad ligament fibroid** or it may arise from the broad ligament itself, when it is called **true broad ligament fibroid**. The two types are differentiated by their relationship to the ureter. If the ureters are medial to the fibroid, it is a true broad ligament fibroid, and when the ureters are lateral to the fibroid, it is a pseudo broad ligament fibroid.

### Cervical fibroid

Overall, cervical fibroids account for 1–4% of fibroids. They are usually single. A cervical fibroid may be central, anterior or posterior or may grow laterally. Its close proximity to the bladder and ureters greatly complicates surgery. Its impaction on the pelvis causes urinary retention and ureteric obstruction. During labour, it can prevent the descent of the fetal head and cause obstructed labour. If it is on the anterior surface of the uterus, it may complicate caesarean section.

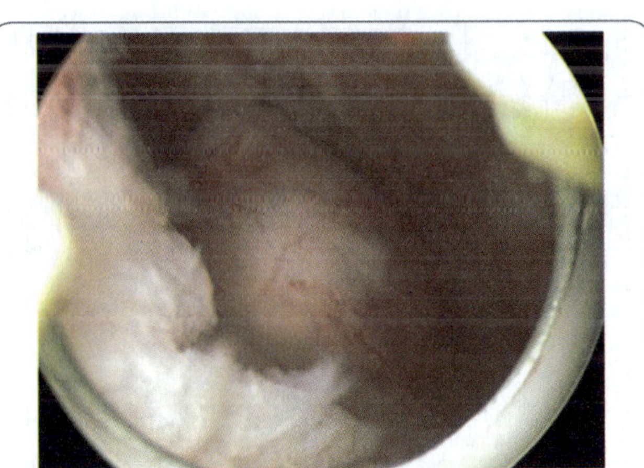

**Fig. 10.11** Submucosal fibroid seen through hysteroscope (*Source:* Wikimedia)

## Vascular Supply

A single large artery usually provides the major blood supply to the fibroid, sending small nutrient arteries to penetrate the capsule.

## Complications

### Degeneration

Degeneration occurs when fibroids outgrow their blood supply. These are a common consequence of

- rapid growth
- pregnancy
- trauma
- postmenopausal atrophy.

Two-thirds of all fibroids show some form of degeneration, mildest being hyaline degeneration (65%). Some of the types of degeneration are as follows:

#### *Hyaline degeneration*

The term hyaline refers to the cytoplasm becoming glassy and homogeneous. This is a focal degeneration and is the mildest form of degeneration accounting for 65% of all forms.

#### *Myxomatous degeneration*

It is generally considered uncommon. Excessive mucus is noticed in this type of degeneration. Acute myxomatous degeneration accounts for 15%.

#### *Calcareous degeneration*

It usually occurs in older patients with longstanding fibroids. Phosphates and carbonates are deposited along the periphery of the blood vessels (Fig. 10.12).

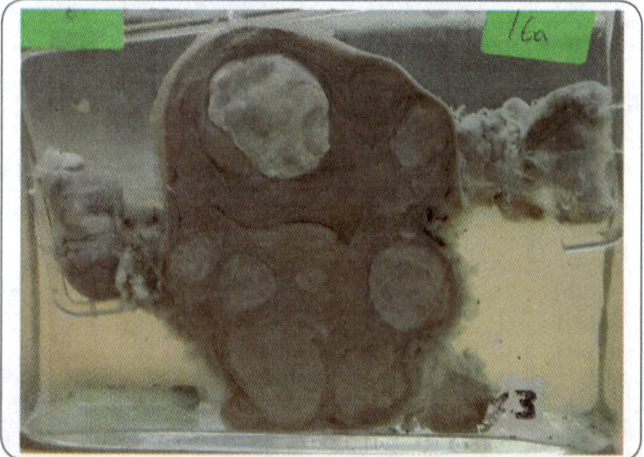

**Fig. 10.12** Multiple uterine leiomyoma with calcification (*Source:* Wikimedia)

They are like tombstones in graveyards and are commonly seen in subserous fibroids.

**Calcareous and red degeneration account for 10% of all forms of degeneration.**

#### *Red degeneration*

It is otherwise known as **carneous degeneration**. It occurs when a fibroid outgrows its blood supply and is commonly seen in pregnancy especially in the mid-trimester. It may also occur in the non-pregnant state.

**Symptoms** It presents with severe abdominal pain, fever and constitutional symptoms. Fibroids become tense and tender. It occurs in 8% of fibroids complicating pregnancy although the prevalence is 3% of all uterine leiomyomas. It is the hemorrhagic infarction of fibroids. It is due to venous obstruction at the periphery of the fibroid. The tumour becomes purple red in color (Fig. 10.13) and develops a fishy odour. It is an aseptic condition. Diagnosis is by clinical assessment and by ultrasound. **Red degeneration should be differentiated from accidental hemorrhage, twisted ovarian cyst, appendicitis and pyelitis.** It is common in subserous and intramural fibroids. Patients complain of acute abdominal pain over the tumour with fever and vomiting. There is moderate leucocytosis and raised ESR.

**Management** of red degeneration is conservative. Patient is advised bed rest. Analgesics are given to relieve pain. IV fluids are given. The acute symptoms subside in 3–10 days and pregnancy proceeds uneventfully. Myomectomy is contraindicated.

### Sarcomatous changes

This is a very rare complication of fibroid uterus occurring only in 0.2 to 0.5% of cases. It is rare before the age of 40 years. There is a 3% risk of developing endometrial carcinoma and is more common in

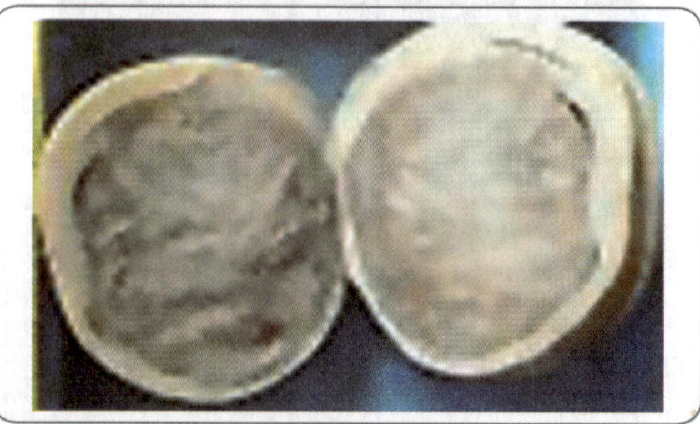

**Fig. 10.13** Red degeneration in a large fibroid (*Source:* Wikimedia)

postmenopausal women. Whenever there is abdominal pain, tenderness and sudden increase in size and bleeding pervaginum in a postmenopausal woman, this condition should be thought of.

### Torsion

Rarely subserous pedunculated fibroids may undergo torsion. Torsion usually occurs in the pedicle at the site of its attachment to the uterus. Torsion of pedunculated myoma presents mostly as acute abdomen and needs intervention and removal of the tumour. It can also occur during pregnancy.

### Infection

Submucous fibroid polyps usually get infected when they protrude through the dilated cervix or into the vagina. This produces bloodstained profuse purulent vaginal discharge. Infection is more common in the puerperium. Such symptomatic fibroids can usually be removed vaginally under antibiotic cover.

### Capsular hemorrhage

This is a rare condition due to rupture of large veins on the surface of subserous myoma. The treatment is immediate laparotomy and either myomectomy or hysterectomy. Blood transfusion will be needed to replace the lost blood.

### Inversion of the uterus

This occurs with submucous fundal fibroid polyp.

## Symptoms of Fibroid

### Abnormal uterine bleeding (AUB)

Abnormal uterine bleeding is the most common symptom associated with uterine fibroids and is experienced by 30% of the patients. AUB can be life-threatening since it may cause

- acute blood loss
- hemorrhage
- symptomatic anemia requiring hospitalisation and emergency blood transfusions.

Symptoms are more common in intramural and submucosal fibroids.

The various theories postulated to explain menorrhagia in fibroids are

- Increase in endometrial surface
- Increased vascularity of uterus
- Vascular congestion caused by compression of venous drainage by the fibroid
- Abnormal uterine contractility
- Dysregulation of growth factors causing disordered angiogenesis of uterine vasculature
- PID causing polymenorrhagia
- Ulceration of submucous fibroids causing metrorrhagia

### Dysmenorrhea

Secondary dysmenorrhea of congestive type is a usual symptom due to increased vascularity and venous stasis. The uterus may attempt to expel a large submucous myoma causing spasmodic dysmenorrhea.

### Pelvic pain

Fibroids usually do not give rise to pain. When fibroids are associated with pain or discomfort, it is usually described as pressure or a dragging sensation. Acute pain in fibroids may be due to

- Torsion
- Red degeneration
- Hemorrhage or
- Sarcoma.

Pain is experienced as heaviness of lower abdomen. Associated endometriosis can also give rise to pain.

### Pressure symptoms

Fibroids can cause pelvic pressure due to physical pressure.

- **Anterior fibroids** can cause bladder symptoms varying from urinary frequency to difficulty in emptying of bladder and occasionally urinary obstruction. Urinary obstruction can produce hydronephrosis and hydroureter ultimately leading to obstructive uropathy.
- **Posterior fibroids** can exert pressure on the rectum producing
  - constipation
  - tenesmus or
  - low back pain
- **Cervical fibroids** cause obstruction to micturition and may cause acute retention of urine.
- **Broad ligament** fibroids can cause hydronepherosis and hydroureter on the ipsilateral side, which is reversible after their removal.

### Fibroids and sexual functions

The relationship between fibroids and dyspareunia is well-documented.

### Infertility and miscarriage

Fibroids are the underlying cause in only 2–3% of infertility.

### Abdominal lump

A large fibroid may be noted as an abdominal tumour. A pedunculated fibroid is felt separately from the uterus and is very often mistaken for an ovarian tumour.

### Vaginal discharge

This is common with pedunculated submucous fibroid protruding through the cervical canal or into the vagina.

## Signs of Fibroid

Fibroids present as follows:
- abdominal lump
- firm in consistency
- bosselated surface
- well-defined margins
- non-tender
- midline suprapubic masses
- side-to-side mobility

Bimanual pelvic examination reveals an enlarged uterus. It may be uniform or irregular depending on the number of fibroids. The cervical movement will be transmitted to the uterine mass.

Broad ligament fibroid pushes the uterus to the opposite side and is felt in the adnexal region and hence has to be differentiated from an ovarian tumour.

Cervical fibroids can be felt on pelvic examination producing thinning and stretching of cervical lips. The normal sized uterus is pushed into the abdomen to give a **"lantern on St.Paul's cathedral"** appearance. Fibroid polyp dilates the cervical canal and descends into the vagina.

## Differential Diagnosis

1. **Pregnancy** Serum beta hCG and ultrasonogram confirm pregnancy.
2. **Hematometra/Pyometra** This occurs secondary to cervical stenosis or Müllerian anomalies. Ultrasound confirms the diagnosis.
3. **Adenomyosis** The signs and symptoms are similar to fibroid uterus. However, in adenomyosis the uterus is uniformly enlarged to 12–14 weeks size. It is tender on palpation. Ultrasound, MRI and histopathological examination confirm the diagnosis.
4. **Endometrial polyp** There are no definite differentiating signs and symptoms. Sonohysterography shows a well-circumscribed isoechoic polypoid mass with stalk.
5. **Bicornuate uterus** HSG, hysteroscopy and ultrasound can diagnose this condition.
6. **Benign ovarian tumour** A subserous or pedunculated fibroid may be mistaken for a benign ovarian tumour. AUB which is usually present in fibroid is generally absent in benign tumours of ovary. Ultrasound and MRI can usually diagnose this condition but sometimes laparotomy may be required.
7. **Malignant ovarian tumour** Clinical signs like rapid growth associated with weight loss and ascites along with ultrasound and MRI can diagnose the condition.
8. **Myomatous polyp** This condition can be mistaken for cervical cancer or products of conception.
9. **Ectopic pregnancy** Chronic ectopic pregnancy can mimic a fibroid. Ultrasound will help in the diagnosis.
10. **Chronic inversion of uterus** Clinical examination for the presence of cervical rim, sounding of uterus, ultrasonography and laparoscopy may all be required to differentiate these two conditions.
11. Pelvic kidney
12. Endometrial carcinoma
13. Endometriosis
14. Inflammatory mass
15. Sarcoma of the uterus

## Investigations

The required investigation depends on the presenting complaints. The routine investigations are
- Hemoglobin and CBC.
- Blood grouping and typing.
- **Ultrasonography** It not only confirms the diagnosis but also gives the number, size and location of fibroids (Fig. 10.14) with an accuracy of 80%. This process is also known as fibroid mapping.
- **Sonosalpingography** This is a technique where under ultrasound guidance,sterile saline is instilled into the uterine cavity. This enables better visualisation of intrauterine pathology (Fig. 10.15).
- **Hysterosalpingogram (HSG)** In addition to identifying intrauterine pathology, HSG also delineates the patency of tubes.
- **Endometrial sampling** This is indicated in women with menstrual abnormalities, thickened endometrium diagnosed by ultrasonogram and postmenopausal bleeding.
- **3D Ultrasound** This can also help in management. Doppler study may be required as a predictor of

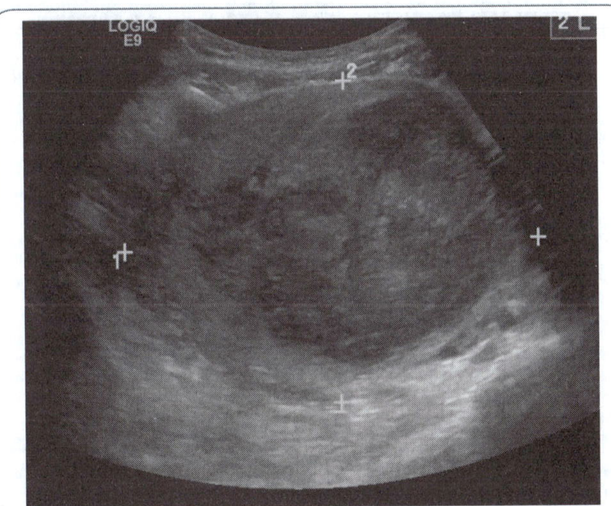

**Fig. 10.14** A very large (9 cm) fibroid of the uterus (*Source:* Wikimedia)

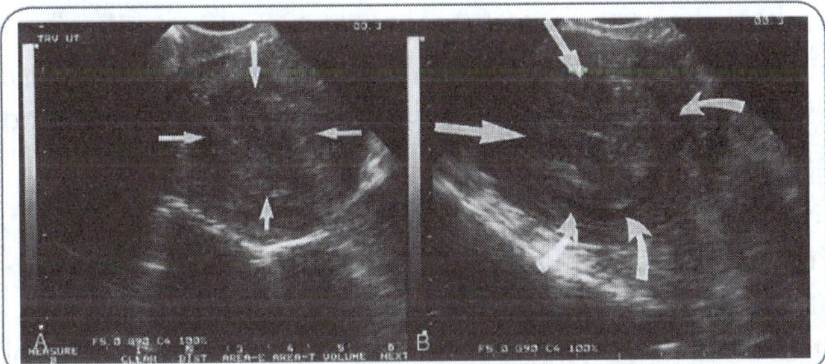

**Fig. 10.15** Submucous leiomyoma after saline infusion sonography (*Source:* ©Cohen, L, Valle, R, Glob. libr. women's med. Reproduced with permission.)

response to GnRH treatment and also in cases where blood flow to the tumour needs to be assessed.

- **MRI** This is an excellent imaging modality.
- **Laparoscopy** Diagnostic laparoscopy can be used when the uterine size is not more than twelve weeks. It is particularly useful when fibroids are associated with infertility, endometriosis and pelvic adhesions.

## Management

### General management

Since leiomyoma is associated with vaginal bleeding, most of the patients would be anaemic. This has to be treated appropriately. Pain symptoms, if any, should be treated.

### Expectant management

50% of the fibroids are asymptomatic. Small and asymptomatic fibroids do not require surgical or medical interference. They can be observed every 6 months provided there is no other endometrial pathology.

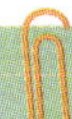

**Indications for Interference in Asymptomatic Fibroid**

Fibroids more than 12 weeks size
Rapidly growing fibroids
Subserous pedunculated fibroids prone to torsion
Where fibroid could be the cause for infertility
Unexplained recurrent abortion
When the nature of the fibroid is doubtful

### Medical management of symptomatic fibroids

- **Iron therapy** for correction of anaemia.
- **Tranexamic acid** could be used when the blood loss is less. It is given as 650 mg tablets two tablets three times daily for 5 days.
- **GnRH Analogues** These drugs reduce the size of the fibroid. The GnRH agonist leupride acetate is approved for short-term preoperative treatment.
- The other group of drugs which are being tried include the following.
  - **Antiprogesterone therapy** RU486
  - **Selective Estrogen Receptor Modulator (SERM)**
  - **Selective progesterone receptor modulator (SPRM)** Ulipristol acetate 5–10 mg / day for 3 months.

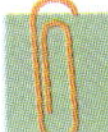

**Benefits and Limitations on the Use of GnRH Agonists**

1. Reduction in size of the fibroid and uterine volume
2. Correction of preoperative iron deficiency anemia
3. Reduced intraoperative blood loss
4. Laparoscopic myomectomy, vaginal hysterectomy and hysteroscopic procedures are more feasible.

### Non-surgical option for management of fibroids

#### *Uterine fibroid embolisation (UFE) or uterine artery embolisation (UAE)*

This is a minimally invasive therapy for symptomatic fibroid,which was first reported in 1995. The technique involves injecting embolising agents (spheres or beads) through the femoral artery under radiological guidance. This will reduce or completely block blood supply to the fibroid ultimately shrinking the fibroid.

#### *Magnetic resonance guided focused ultrasound surgery (MRgFUS)*

This is a treatment for uterine fibroids.

Exabilate 2000 [Insigntec Inc.] Harfa, Isreal, is the first MRgFUS device. Magnetic resonance imaging offers anatomical, functional and thermal guidance during delivery of the focused ultrasound beam.

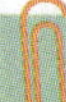

**Limitations**

1. Multiple small fibroids
2. Too big >10 cm
3. Too posterior
4. Abdominal wall scarring
5. Calcified fibroid
6. Degenerated fibroid
7. Intervening bowel loops

## Minimally invasive treatment option for uterine fibroids

Minimally invasive gynecological surgery (MIGS) broadens the clinician's therapeutic options for the treatment of fibroids.

### *Laparoscopic myolysis*

This is an optional surgery using NdYAG laser, cryo probe or diathermy to coagulate a subserous fibroid in multiparous women.

### *Hysteroscopy*

Hysteroscopy is an integral part of both diagnosis and treatment. Submucosal fibroids are most amenable to hysteroscopic surgical approach (*see* Fig. 10.11).

### *Laparoscopic myomectomy*

Laparoscopic myomectomy is done for women desiring future childbearing. But today many women desire uterine preservation even if they have completed their family indications.

## Surgical treatment

### 1. *Myomectomy*

For women desiring pregnancy, myomectomy is the treatment option (Fig. 10.16), but the recurrence rate following myomectomy is 60% and it occurs in 3–5 years. Abdominal myomectomy is chosen when the option of laparoscopic or hysteroscopic hysterectomy is not feasible and when other pelvic or abdominal pathology co-exist.

**Abdominal myomectomy** After opening the abdomen through a lower right paramedian or transverse incision, the size, position and number of myoma are noted. The condition of the tubes and the ovaries is taken note of. The surgeon has to then decide on the ideal site over the uterus where a

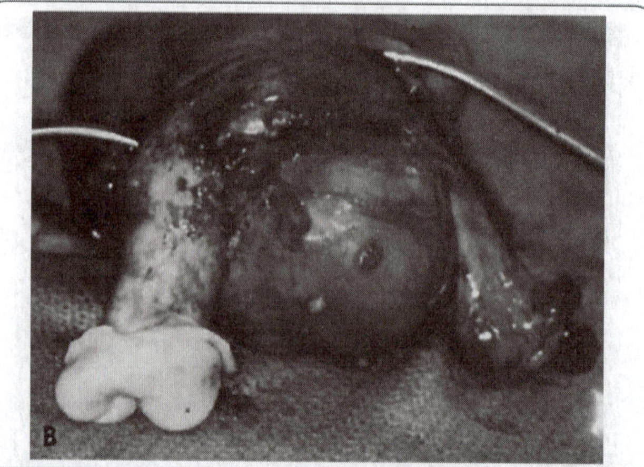


**Fig. 10.16** Myomectomy of a posterior wall fibroid (*Source:* Neuwirth, R, Moritz, J, Glob. libr. women's med.)

myomectomy incision could be placed to enucleate the tumours. The line of incision is preferably made on the anterior wall of the uterus to reduce adhesions as far as possible. When many fibroids in close proximity need to be excised, they can be enucleated from through one incision.

**Hemorrhage during surgery** The principal risk is hemorrhage during the operation; the blood loss is limited by

- Myometrial vasopressin injection and the use of cautery for enucleation.
- The use of Bonney's myomectomy clamp placed as a tourniquet at the level of the internal os on the ovarian vessels.
- After the enucleation of all myoma, the clamps are released, and the hemostasis is confirmed.
- If there is marked myohyperplasia, it could be trimmed. The cavities are obliterated by tiers of catgut sutures.

Myomectomy in conjunction with a cesarean section is contraindicated due to the difficulty in controlling blood loss.

### Complications

***Minor complications*** These include postoperative fever, infection, wound hematoma and wound separation. Release of prostaglandins and cytokines due to tissue damage is the probable cause for postoperative fever which can be managed by NSAID drugs.

***Major complications***

- **Hemorrhage** Major complications include hemorrhage requiring blood transfusion. Hemorrhage could be due to bladder or ureteric injury, or bowel injury. Hemorrhage could also necessitate switching over from a laparoscopic procedure to abdominal hysterectomy. Ureteric and bladder injury occur in 1–3% of cases and bowel injury occurs in 1% of cases. Average blood loss in 200–800 mL with 2–28% of patients requiring transfusion.

- **Postoperative adhesions** Adhesions between the uterus and bowel, adnexa and other structures occur in 90% of cases. Adhesions are more common with incision in the posterior wall of the uterus and abdominal myomectomy.

**During pregnancy, the fear of rupture of uterus in the third trimester should be borne in mind. If the endometrial cavity was entered, caesarean section should be resorted to.**

***Recurrence*** Whereas the recurrence rate for myomectomy by laparotomy ranges from 5.7 to 11.1% at the end of five years, the reoperation rates for the same period is from 4.3 to 16.8%.

### *2. Hysterectomy*

Abdominal, vaginal or laparoscopic hysterectomy is the definitive surgical procedure for fibroid uterus and it is indicated in women over 40 years of age, who have completed their families and in whom there is associated pelvic pathology or malignancy.

***Complications***

- Mortality 0.32 per 1000 procedures
- Hemorrhage
- Postsurgical infection
- DVT
- Pulmonary embolism
- Injury to surrounding pelvic organ and structure

## ENDOMETRIAL TUBERCULOSIS (TB)

In areas where pulmonary TB is common, genital TB has a higher prevalence. Very often, genital TB is secondary to pulmonary TB. It usually occurs in young women between 20 and 40 years of age, frequently diagnosed during investigations for infertility. Though the exact incidence is not definitely known, it is expected to be approximately around 19% in India.

### Pathogenesis

As stated earlier, genital TB is usually secondary to TB elsewhere in the body, mainly the lungs, but could also be from the kidney, GIT or other areas. It spreads by the hematogenous route or lymphatic route or by direct spread.

#### Hematogenous spread

After the TB bacilli affect the lungs, the spread through the bloodstream occurs within few hours.

#### Lymphatic spread

This method of spread is less common and occurs when the primary lesion is in the abdominal cavity. It can also occur in those who drink unpasteurised milk obtained from cattle affected by TB.

#### Direct spread

Direct spread to the genital organs could occur from the bladder, rectum, intestine, etc.

Since the endometrium is shed every month, spread of this disease is rare. Hence the myometrium is also spared.

### Signs and Symptoms

The common symptoms resemble the general symptoms of pulmonary TB, such as low-grade fever and malaise. There is persistent lower abdominal pain with menstrual abnormalities like profuse bleeding during periods, scanty bleeding or amenorrhea. Since the disease affects younger women, infertility is frequently seen in these affected women and very often it is during investigation for infertility that endometrial TB is diagnosed.

### Investigations

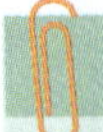

**Common Investigations for Endometrial TB**

- Complete blood count
- Chest X-ray
- Tuberculin test
- Endometrial curettage
- Histological examination
- Polymerase chain reaction

**Endometrial biopsy** still has a role in the diagnosis of endometrial TB. It should be performed in the premenstrual phase of the cycle. Histopathological examination will reveal small tubercles scattered throughout the endometrium (Fig. 10.17).

**X-Ray of chest** will show the presence of pulmonary TB.

**Ultrasonography** may not give much information in endometrial TB but it can demonstrate other affected organs, if any, in the pelvis like hydrosalpinx or pelvic mass.

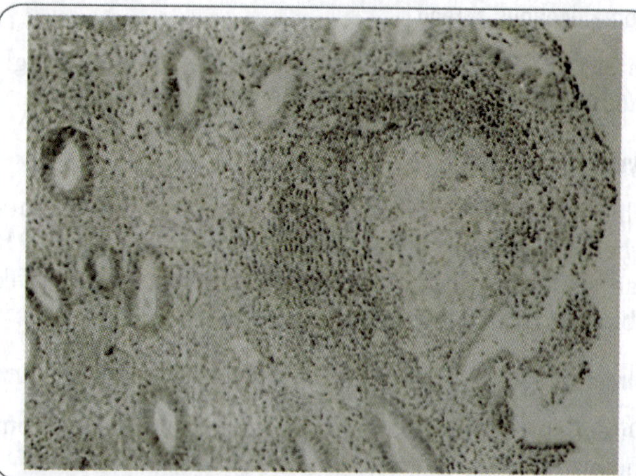

**Fig. 10.17** Tuberculous endometritis (*Source:* Varma, T, Glob. libr. women's med.)

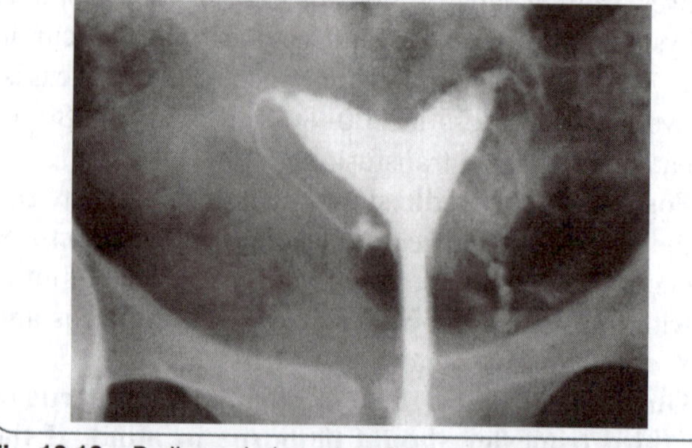

**Fig. 10.18** Radiograph demonstrating lymphatic extravasation, a deformed uterine cavity, and a narrow-rigid Fallopian tube with a dilated and closed fimbrial end on the right side (*Source:* Varma, T, Glob. libr. women's med.)

**Hysterosalpingography** is better avoided when there is suspicion of TB. However during investigation for infertility, HSG might reveal the appearance as shown in Fig. 10.18.

**Polymerase chain reaction** has not been found to be very effective in the diagnosis of genital TB.

## Management

The aims of the treatment are to achieve TB cure, to prevent the long-term sequelae and to restore normal anatomy if it has been distorted.

**As per the Revised National Tuberculosis Control Programme (RNTCP) and Directly Observed Treatment Short course (DOTS) strategy, the first line of treatment is 2RHZE/4RHE.**

It indicates two months of treatment with Rifampicin(R), Isoniazid(H), Pyrazinamide(Z), Ethambutol(E) followed by four months of treatment with RHE. All drugs are given three times a week as per the dosage schedule given below.

Rifampicin 450 mg
Isoniazid 600 mg
Pyrazinamide 1500 mg
Ethambutol 1200 mg

(Patients weighing more than 60 kg are given an additional 150 mg of Rifampicin)

***Case study***

*A 25-year-old woman comes with complaints of profuse bleeding PV during her menstrual cycle associated with severe abdominal pain for the past 1 year. Her cycles are regular. She had one vaginal delivery four years back. She is not on any contraception. She was found to be anaemic and her uterus enlarged to 14–16 weeks size. Both adnexae were normal.*

*a) What is your tentative diagnosis?*
*b) What investigations are required to confirm the diagnosis?*
*c) What are the management options available?*

## RECAP

- The common benign diseases of the uterus are endometrial polyps, adenomyosis and fibroid uterus (leiomyoma).
- An endometrial polyp is a mass arising from the inner lining of the uterus. When it is attached to the uterus by a stalk, it is called pedunculated polyp and when no stalk is present, it is known as sessile polyp.
- The diagnosis is confirmed by transvaginal sonography (TVS), sonosalpingography (SIS) and hysteroscopy.
- Polyps which are seen protruding through the cervical os can be twisted with a sponge-holding forceps and removed.

- Sessile polyps can be removed by dilatation and curettage. Hysteroscopic visualisation and polypectomy is a better way of treating the polyps.
- Adenomyosis is a condition in which the endometrial glands are seen invading the myometrial tissue.
- Adenomyosis is more often seen in women in the 40s and 50s age group.
- Parous women are more often affected than their nulliparous sisters.
- They are also associated with leiomyomas, endometriosis and endometrial cancer.
- Women who are on tamoxifen therapy are at risk of developing adenomyosis.
- Endometritis and abortion are other known risk factors.
- Menorrhagia and dysmenorrhea are common symptoms.
- Diagnosis is by transvaginal sonography (TVS) and magnetic resonance imaging (MRI).
- NSAIDs are often the first line of management.
- Combined oral contraceptives and progestin-only pills have also been tried to induce endometrial atrophy and to decrease endometrial prostaglandin production.
- Levonorgestrel-releasing intrauterine system (LNG-IUS) has also been found to be effective in the treatment of adenomyosis.
- GnRH agonists and danazol have also been tried in the relief of symptoms associated with adenomyosis.
- Uterus-sparing procedures include uterine artery embolisation (UAE), resection of focal adenomysis.
- Non-hysteroscopic procedures include high-energy radiofrequency ablation, thermal balloon ablation, cryo-endometrial ablation and microwave ablation
- Hysterectomy
- Fibroid uterus is the most common benign disease of the uterus in women in the reproductive age group.
- Risk factors are early menarche, elevated BMI, tamoxifen, family history, African–American race, PCOS, high parity, age, hormone replacement therapy.
- Combined contraceptive pill decreases the risk since exposure to estrogen is opposed by progesterone.
- Smoking also decreases the risk for fibroids.
- The fibroids are commonly classified as subserous, intramural and submucous fibroids.
- Secondary changes include hyaline degeneration, myxomatous degeneration, calcareous degeneration, red degeneration, sarcomatous changes.
- Complications of fibroids are torsion, infection, capsular hemorrhage, inversion, endometrial carcinoma.
- Symptoms of fibroids are abnormal uterine bleeding, chronic pelvic pain, pressure symptoms, abdominal lump, vaginal discharge, infertility and recurrent abortion.
- Fibroids present as abdominal lump are firm in consistency with bosselated surface; the margins are well defined and are non-tender.
- Bimanual pelvic examination reveals an enlarged uterus. It may be uniform or irregular depending on the number of fibroids. The cervical movement will be transmitted to the uterine mass.
- 50% of the fibroids are asymptomatic. Small and asymptomatic fibroids do not require surgical or medical interference.
- Medical management is by the use of GnRH analogues, antiprogesterone therapy, selective estrogen receptor modulator (SERM), selective progesterone receptor modulator (SPRM).
- Non-surgical options for management of fibroids are uterine fibroid embolisation (UFE) or uterine artery embolisation (UAE), magnetic resonance guided focused ultrasound surgery (MRgFUS).
- Minimally invasive treatment options for uterine fibroids include laparoscopic myolysis, hysteroscopy and laparoscopic myomectomy.
- Surgical treatment includes myomectomy and hysterectomy.
- In areas where pulmonary TB is common, genital TB (endometrial tuberculosis) has a higher prevalence. Very often, genital TB is secondary to pulmonary TB.
- It usually occurs in young women between 20 and 40 years of age.
- It spreads by the hematogenous route or lymphatic route or by direct spread.
- The common symptoms resemble the general symptoms of pulmonary TB, such as low-grade fever and malaise.
- Persistent lower abdominal pains with menstrual abnormalities like profuse bleeding during periods or scanty bleeding during periods or amenorrhea are other common symptoms.

- Since the disease affects younger women, infertility is frequently seen in these affected women and very often it is during investigation for infertility that endometrial TB is diagnosed.
- Investigation is by complete blood count, chest X-Ray, tuberculin test, endometrial curettage, histological examination and polymerase chain reaction.
- Management is as per the Revised National Tuberculosis Control Programme (RNTCP) and Directly Observed Treatment Short course (DOTS) strategy, the first line of treatment is 2RHZE/4RHE, which indicates two months of treatment with Rifampicim (R), Isoniazid (H), Pyrazinamide (Z), Ethambutol (E) followed by four months of treatment with RHE.

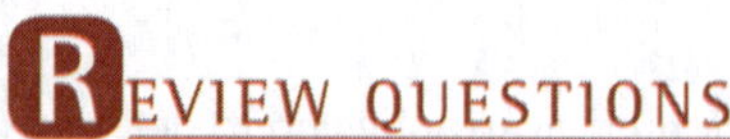

## REVIEW QUESTIONS

### Long-answer Question

1. Discuss the secondary changes in leiomyoma. How will you manage red degeneration of fibroid?

### Short-answer Questions

1. Describe the pathogenesis and mode of spread of endometrial tuberculosis. What is its first line of management as per Revised National Tuberculosis Control Programme (RNTCP) and Directly Observed Treatment Short course (DOTS) strategy?
2. Describe the risk factors and signs and symptoms of adenomyosis. Enumerate the characteristics of Adenomyosis observed using transvaginal sonography (TVS).

### MCQs

**1. Adenomyoma is also known as**

a) Focal adenomyosis
b) Diffuse adenomyosis
c) Leiomyoma
d) Endometrioma

**2. Endometrial polyps arise from the**

a) Endocervix
b) Ectocervix
c) Inner lining of the uterus
d) Myometrium

**3. Endometrial tuberculosis spreads by**

a) Only hematogenous spread
b) Both hematogenous and lymphatic spread
c) Only direct spread
d) By hematogenous, lymphatic and direct spread

**4. Laprascopic myolysis uses**

a) NdYAG laser
b) Instillation of saline into the fibroid
c) Instillation of drugs into the fibroid
d) Open laparotomy technique

### Further Reading

Green TH. Gynecology. 3rd ed. Boston: Little Brown;1977. 381 p.

Hawkins J and Bourne G.Shaw's Textbook of Gynecology. 9th ed. London: Churchill Livingstone; 1977.

Novak ER. *Novak's Textbook of* Gynecology, 15th edn. Baltimore: Lippincott, Williams and Wilkins.

Parsons L and Ulefelder H.An Atlas of Pelvic Operations. London: WB Saunders; 1968. p. 70.

RockJA, Murphy AA and JonesHWJR. Female Reproductive Surgery. Baltimore: Williams and Wilkins;1992.

William's Gynecology, 2nd ed.

CHAPTER 11

# Benign Tumours of the Ovary and Fallopian Tube

**AT A GLANCE**


Classification of Ovarian Tumours
Distribution of Ovarian Tumours
1. Non-neoplastic or Functional Cysts of the Ovary
   i) Follicular Cysts
   ii) Corpus Luteum Cysts
   iii) Theca Lutein Cysts
2. Endometrial Cysts or Endometrioma
3. Ovarian Neoplasms
   Epithelial Tumours
4. Mucinous Tumours
5. Brenner Tumour
6. Stromal Tumours
   Thecomas
   Fibromas
7. Germ Cell Tumours
   Teratomas
Clinical Features and Diagnosis of Benign Ovarian Tumours
   Menstrual Symptoms
   Abdominal Examination
   Pelvic Examination
   Rectal Examination
Investigations
Differential Diagnosis
Complications
   Torsion
   Infection
   Rupture
Management
   Expectant Management
   Surgery
Paraovarian Cysts
Benign Pathology of Fallopian Tube
   Hydrosalpinx
   Benign Neoplasms


## INTRODUCTION

No other organ in the body gives rise to such diverse and interesting types of tumours as the ovary. As the histogenesis of these tumours is not clearly understood, there is no unanimity regarding their classification. To complicate matters, there are some functional ovarian cysts or swellings which may at times be clinically mistaken for neoplastic tumours.

***Incidence*** Ovarian tumours form about 1–2 per cent of all gynecological admissions. One of every four ovarian tumours is malignant. In India, ovarian cancer is the second most common malignancy of the female genital tract after cancer of the cervix. Ovarian neoplasms may be seen at any age, though the chances of their being malignant are high when seen in a postmenopausal woman.

## CLASSIFICATION OF OVARIAN TUMOURS

Ovarian tumours may be classified according to their clinical features (cystic or solid; benign or malignant), histogenesis (arising from epithelial, connective tissue, or embryonic cells), or histologic patterns (Table 11.1). The most commonly accepted classification is the WHO-sponsored International Histologic Classification of Ovarian Tumours (Serov, Scully and Sobin, 1973).

## DISTRIBUTION OF OVARIAN TUMOURS

Table 11.2 shows the distribution of various ovarian tumours.

The benign ovarian tumours are the following.

1. Functional cysts
2. Endometrioma
3. Serous cystadenoma
4. Mucinous cystadenoma and
5. Brenner tumour
6. Stromal tumours
7. Germ cell tumours

## 1. NON-NEOPLASTIC OR FUNCTIONAL CYSTS OF THE OVARY

These include follicular cysts, corpus luteum cysts, theca lutein cysts, and endometrial cysts or endometriomas.

**Table 11.1** Histologic classification of ovarian tumours

1. Epithelial tumours
   a. Serous tumours
      i. benign
      ii. borderline malignancy
      iii. malignant
   b. Mucinous tumours
      i. benign
      ii. borderline malignancy
      iii. malignant
   c. Endometroid
      i. benign
      ii. borderline malignancy
      iii. malignant
   d. Clear-cell or mesonephroid
   e. Brenner tumours
      i. benign
      ii. borderline malignancy
      iii. malignant
   f. Mixed epithelial tumours
   g. Undifferentiated
   h. Unclassified
2. Gonadal stromal or sex-cord tumours
   a. Granulosa cell tumours
      i. Granulosa cell tumours
      ii. Theca cell tumours
   b. Fibroma, sarcoma
   c. Androblastoma
   d. Gynandroblastoma
   e. Unclassified
3. Lipid or lipoid-cell tumours
4. Germ cell tumours
   a. Dysgerminoma
   b. Endodermal sinus tumours
   c. Embryonal carcinoma
   d. Polyembryoma
   e. Choriocarcinoma
   f. Teratoma
      i. immature
      ii. mature (solid/cystic)
      iii. monodermal
      iv. mixed
5. Gonadoblastoma—pure or mixed
6. Unclassified
7. Secondary or metastatic tumours

**Table 11.2** Distribution of ovarian tumours

| Tumour type | Percentage distribution |
|---|---|
| Serous tumours | 35–50% |
| Mucinous group | 25% |
| Germ cell tumours | 15% |
| Stromal cell tumours | 5–10% |
| Endometroid | 3% |
| Mesonephroid | 1% |
| Metastatic tumours | about 2% |
| Unclassified | 2–3% |

These mostly physiological cysts are at times mistaken for ovarian tumours and vice versa.

## i) Follicular Cysts

These are often seen in association with the anovulatory type of dysfunctional uterine bleeding where the Graafian follicle fails to rupture and the cyst (about 5 cm in diameter) may remain active without regressing normally (Fig. 11.1). The cyst fluid is rich is estrogen. Its rupture can create sharp, severe pain on the side of the ovary on which the cyst appears. About a fourth of women with this type of cyst experience pain. These cysts subside in 3–4 weeks and the ovary returns to its normal size.

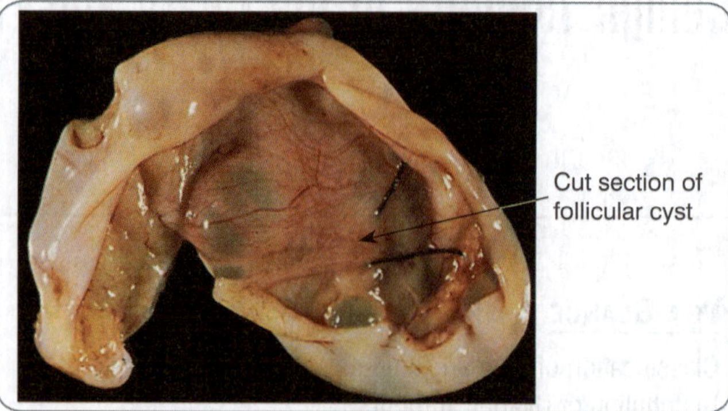


**Fig. 11.1** Follicular cyst of the ovary (Courtesy of AFIP and PathologyOutlines.com. Reproduced with premission)

## ii) Corpus Luteum Cysts

After the egg is released from the follicle, the ruptured follicle becomes a corpus luteum. In the absence of pregnancy, the corpus luteum usually disappears. But sometimes there is hemorrhage into the corpus luteum, and it becomes a corpus luteum cyst (Fig. 11.2). It is transient though in rare cases, it may rupture, simulating a ruptured tubal pregnancy. A persisting corpus luteum may sometimes give rise to a delayed onset of periods and to prolonged menstrual flow.

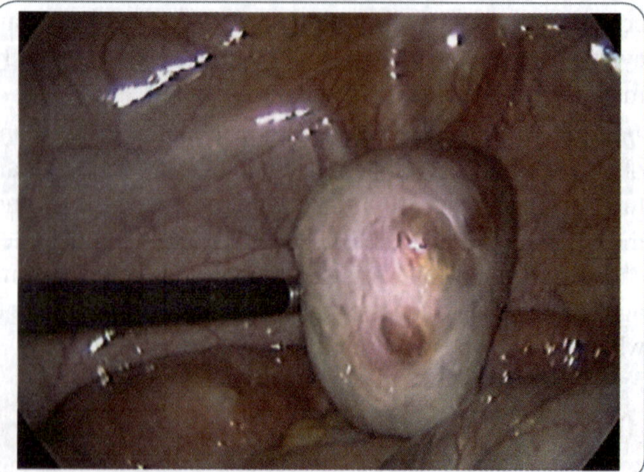

**Fig. 11.2** Corpus luteal cyst visualised through laparoscope (*Source:* © Roy Patankar/Lapsuregeon.com. Reproduced with permission)

### iii) Theca Lutein Cysts

These are seen in cases of trophoblastic tumour such as the hydatidiform mole and choriocarcinoma in response to the large amounts of chorionic gonadotropins produced in these conditions. Such cysts may also be caused by the hyperstimulation of the ovaries by the pituitary gonadotropins (Fig. 11.3). They may be unilateral or bilateral and resolve spontaneously over a few weeks after the source of β-hCG is removed.

## 2. ENDOMETRIAL CYSTS OR ENDOMETRIOMA

Ovarian endometriosis resulting in bilateral endometrial or chocolate cysts is not rare but the typical symptomatology with acquired dysmenorrhea and clinical findings help in its diagnosis (*see* Chapter 15).

All these functional cysts are not more than 5–6 cm in diameter except the theca lutein cysts which may grow larger. Whereas the follicular and corpus luteum cysts are unilateral, theca lutein cysts and endometrial cysts are often bilateral. Functional cysts (except the endometrial cysts) resolve over time. It is therefore necessary to review the cases suspected to be having functional cysts after 3–4 cycles. If it is neoplastic, the tumour will either be stationary or grow larger, whereas the functional ones will subside. Careful history-taking and clinical findings, including imaging modalities like ultrasound and laparoscopy, are useful in deciding doubtful cases.

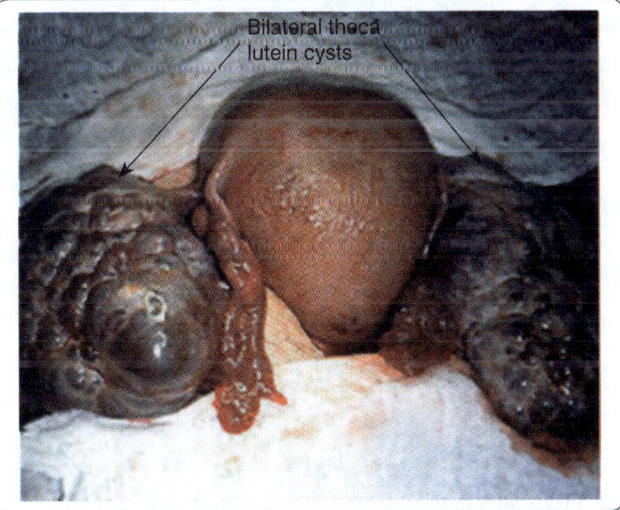


**Fig. 11.3** Large bilateral theca lutein cysts (*Source:* Radiology Key/© Michael Peterson)

## 3. OVARIAN NEOPLASMS

### Epithelial Tumours

#### Serous tumours

These are the most common tumours of the ovary and most of them are cystic.

1. Typically, a **simple ovarian cystoma** is about 15–20 cm in diameter, unilateral, smooth, thin-walled, and contains a serous fluid. The lining epithelium is low cuboidal. As it is pedunculated and freely mobile, the tumour is likely to undergo torsion.
2. **Serous cystadenomas** are often **bilateral, moderate in size and mostly unilocular**, containing a thin straw-coloured serous fluid. The cyst wall shows numerous papillary projections. Sometimes these papillary growths are seen on the outer surface of the tumour. Microscopically, the cyst wall and the papillary growths are lined by a single layer of low cuboidal, non-mucus-secreting cells (Fig. 11.4). Sometimes they are atypical, multilayered with mitosis to suggest borderline malignancy as there is no stromal involvement. Some cases of serous cystadenoma, of the benign or malignant variety, show calcium deposits in the stroma of the papillary growths to form calcified granules called **psammoma bodies** (*psammos* is Greek for "sand").

## 4. MUCINOUS TUMOURS

A **mucinous cystadenoma** is a common benign tumour of the ovary. It is mostly **unilateral, multiloculated and contains a sticky mucinous fluid**. Though mostly moderate in size, if left untreated it may reach enormous proportions, and the largest on record is 149 kg. Under the microscope the lining epithelium

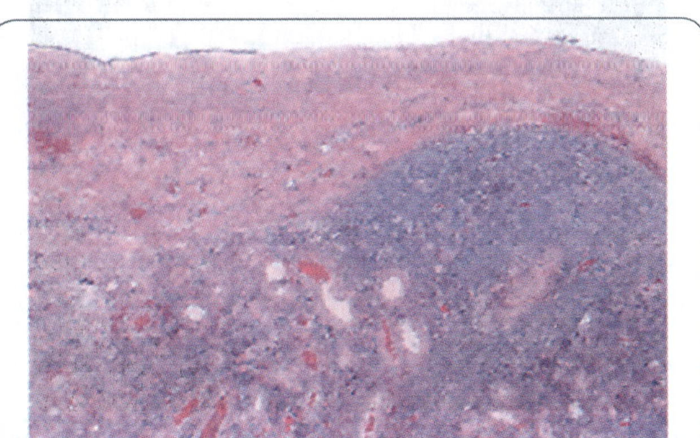

**Fig. 11.4** Serous cystadenoma (*Source:* Wikipedia)

is tall columnar with a pale cytoplasm and with all the basal nuclei arranged in a uniform row. About 5 per cent of these tumours are bilateral and show malignant characteristics on clinical and microscopic examination and are designated mucinous cystadenocarcinoma.

When the mucin in this tumour spills into the peritoneal cavity usually due to rupture of the tumour, it can lead to mucinous ascites, a condition known as **pseudomyxoma peritonei**. This can produce pressure symptoms on the peritoneal viscera and if left untreated or undiagnosed could even be fatal. This is more common with the malignant counterpart, mucinous cystadenocarcinoma. A mucocele of the appendix may also give rise to pseudomyxoma peritonei.

## 5. BRENNER TUMOUR

This is a rare **unilateral solid tumour** seen in postmenopausal women. The tumours are well-encapsulated, benign and resemble fibromas but show small cystic spaces (Fig. 11.5). Microscopically, epithelial cell collections similar to Walthard cell nests are scattered in a dense fibrous tissue stroma. These **epithelial cells are grooved like coffee beans** (Fig. 11.6). Malignancy is rare. Occasionally they may be associated with postmenopausal bleeding due to the functioning stroma. Like fibroma, some of these benign tumours may be associated with ascites.

## 6. STROMAL TUMOURS

These tumours arise from the stroma or the primitive mesenchyma of the ovary. When the stromal cells differentiate into epithelioid cells of the granulosa or the theca cell type, they are called granulosa-theca cell tumours which are the most frequent in this group. The same tumour may show either granulosa or thecal elements or both. Some of the tumours in this group are mainly fibromatous, and are called fibromas. Rarely, the mesenchyma may differentiate into the Sertoli or Leydig cell types as in androblastoma. **Broadly, the granulosa-theca cell tumours are considered feminising tumours, the androblastomas masculinising and fibromas endocrinologically inactive.**

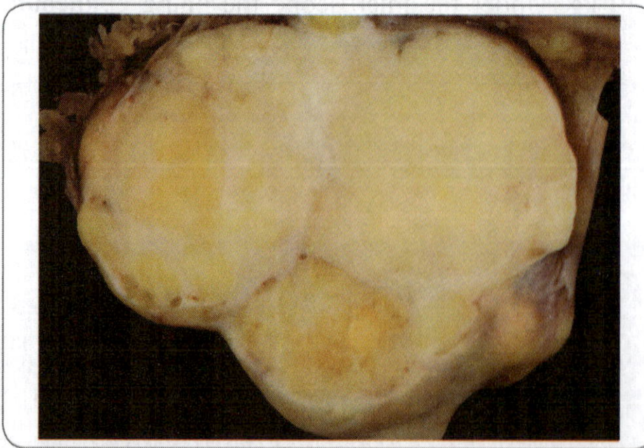

**Fig. 11.5** Brenner tumour gross appearance (*Source:* Wikipedia ©Ed Uthman)

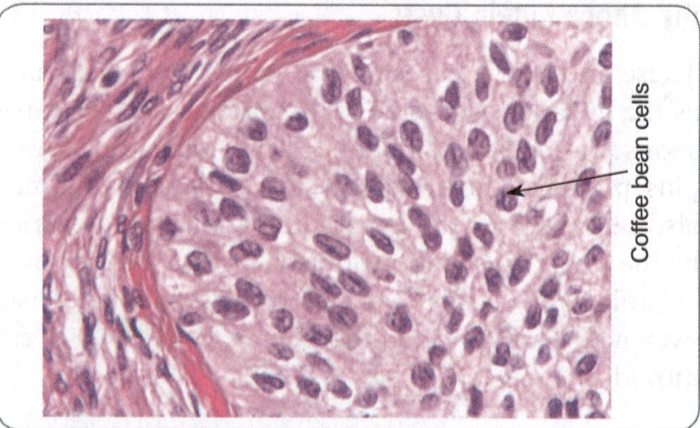


**Fig. 11.6** High magnification micrograph of a Brenner tumour showing the characteristic coffee bean nuclei. H&E stain. (*Source:* Wikimedia)

### Thecomas

Theca cell tumours are rare, **unilateral solid tumours** seen after menopause. On microscopy, one finds spindle-shaped fat-laden epithelioid cells (Fig. 11.7). The tumour is intensely estrogenic and when luteinised, gives rise to endometrial secretory hypertrophy due to the progestogens. The endocrine effects are often similar to those in a granulosa cell tumour. As stated earlier, the same tumour may show a mixture of both

**Fig. 11.7** HPE low-magnification micrograph of a thecoma showing compression of the ovarian cortex (right of image) (*Source:* Wikipedia/© 2011 Michael Bonert)

granulosa and thecal elements. In rare cases, the thecoma may be androgenic due to the progesterone being converted to androgens in these cells.

### Fibromas

These are solid benign tumours (Fig. 11.8). Usually **unilateral, a fibroma may vary in size from a small asymptomatic nodule in the ovary to a large-sized heavy pedunculated tumour**. In a section, it resembles a myoma presenting a whorled appearance with hyalinisation or calcification in areas. On microscopic examination it shows a network of closely packed spindle cells of uniform appearance (Fig. 11.9).

When this benign fibroma is associated with ascites and hydrothorax, it is called **Meig's syndrome.** This is often mistaken for a malignancy but on removal of the tumour, there is a dramatic disappearance of the fluid from the abdomen and the chest within a week.

## 7. GERM CELL TUMOURS

Histogenetically, these tumours arise from the germ cells of the undifferentiated gonad. Teratoma, dysgerminoma, choriocarcinoma, embryonal carcinoma and endodermal sinus tumour form the group of germ cell tumours. Of these, teratomas and dysgerminomas are relatively common.

### Teratomas

The teratoma arises from the totipotent cells of the primitive gonad and differentiates into any of thc cmbryonic germ cell layers: the ectoderm, the mesoderm and the endoderm. The structures may be well-differentiated, and mature or immature. The teratomas may be clinically solid or cystic, the latter being more common.

#### Mature cystic teratomas

These are also called **dermoid cysts** of the ovary and form 10–15 per cent of all ovarian tumours. They are seen during reproductive life and are **bilateral in 25 per cent** of cases. Moderate in size, well-encapsulated and freely mobile (pedunculated), these tumours show on section, fatty sebaceous material, matted hair and a raised solid area or 'embryonic node' in the cyst wall with teeth or cartilage (Figs. 11.10 and 11.11).

On microscopic examination, the cyst wall reveals skin, hair, sebaceous glands, teeth, bone, cartilage, gastrointestinal mucosa and thyroid tissue. **As these structures are derived from all the three germinal layers, the term 'dermoid cyst' is a misnomer**. In about one per cent, they may turn malignant, mostly giving rise to squamous cell carcinoma.

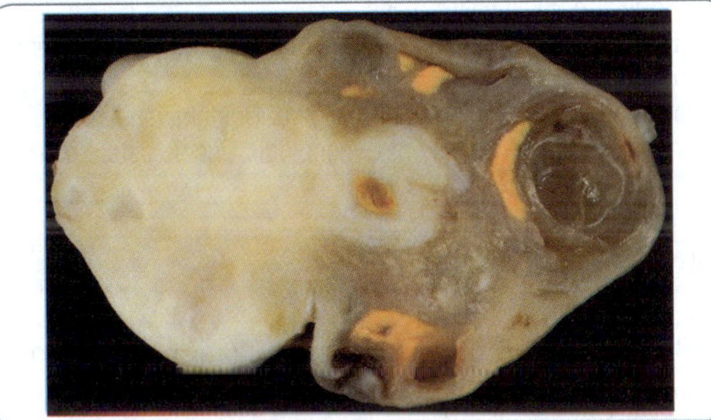

**Fig. 11.8** Cut section of fibroma of the ovary (*Source:* Wikipedia)

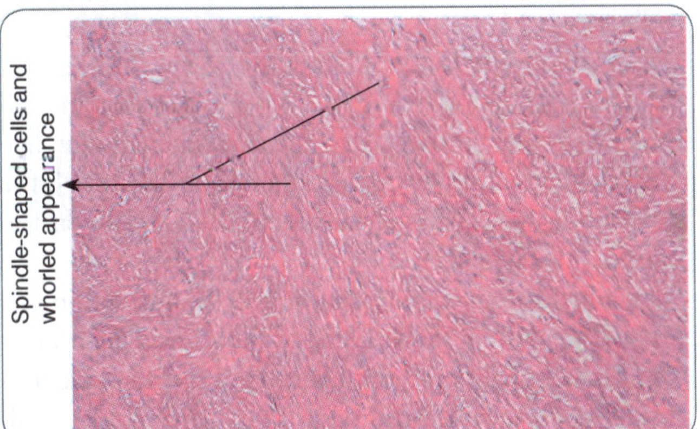


**Fig. 11.9** Fibroma of the ovary: Histopathology (*Source:* Wikimedia/©Ed Uthman)

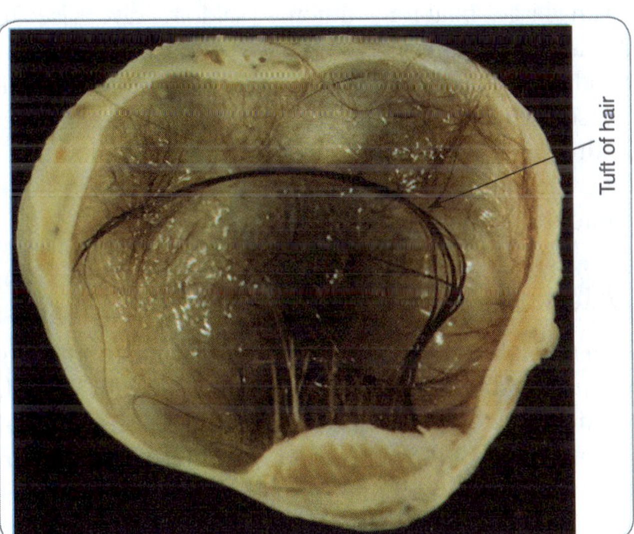


**Fig. 11.10** Mature cystic teratoma of ovary (*Source:* Wikipedia/©Ed Uthman)

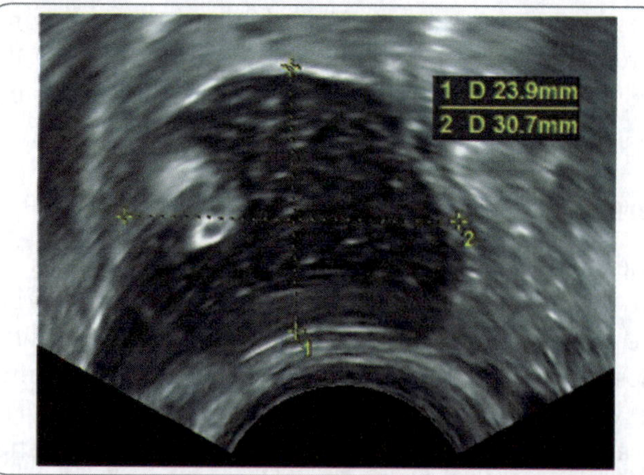


**Fig. 11.11** Ultrasonogram of dermoid cyst (*Source:* Häggström, Mikael. "Medical gallery of Mikael Häggström 2014". WikiJournal of Medicine 1 (2).)

## CLINICAL FEATURES AND DIAGNOSIS OF BENIGN OVARIAN TUMOURS

Most benign ovarian tumours are asymptomatic. As stated earlier, with small cystic tumours, the functional cysts have to be ruled out by reviewing the patient after four cycles.

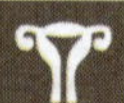

**Clinical Importance**

If the adnexal tumour persists or increases in size, or if in a postmenopausal woman it is 5 cm or more in size, it is likely to be an ovarian neoplasm.

### Menstrual Symptoms

Even large bilateral tumours seldom give rise to menstrual disturbances except in the rare hormone-producing varieties. If it is a feminising tumour it will cause menorrhagia or postmenopausal bleeding; if androgenic, there will be amenorrhea and hirsutism. The pressure symptoms are noted only with the large tumours.

### Abdominal Examination

In a typical case, the patient presents with a uniformly enlarged abdominal swelling often smooth-walled, cystic and with well-defined upper and lateral boundaries. **The lower border is not felt except when the tumour is small and has a long pedicle.** Unless it fills the whole abdomen, the tumour has considerable mobility. In a cystadenoma a fluid thrill can be elicited. The presence of ascites is not diagnostic of malignancy when there is a unilateral solid tumour like a fibroma.

### Pelvic Examination

The uterus will be pushed to one side by the ovarian tumour, the lower pole of which may be felt through one of the lateral fornices. The movement of the tumour per abdomen is not transmitted to the cervix.

### Rectal Examination

This is carried out routinely as the presence of any nodules in the pouch of Douglas suggests malignancy.

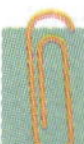

**Guidelines for Referral of Newly Diagnosed Pelvic Mass to Gynecologic Oncologist**

**Premenopausal woman (<50 years)**
- Very elevated CA 125 level
- Ascites
- Evidence of abdominal or distant metastasis (by examination or imaging study)

**Postmenopausal woman (≥50 years)**
- Elevated CA 125 level
- Ascites
- Nodular or fixed pelvic mass
- Evidence of abdominal or distant metastasis (by examination or imaging study)

[Compiled from the American College of Obstetricians and Gynecologists and Society of Gynecologic Oncologists, 2011]

## INVESTIGATIONS

- Routine blood and urine investigations need to be done in all these women.
- A serum CA 125 assay is not indicated in all premenopausal women when an ultrasonographic diagnosis of a simple ovarian cyst has been made (RCOG Green top guidelines No. 62).
- Lactate dehydrogenase (LDH), α-fetoprotein and hCG should be measured in all women under age 40 with a complex ovarian mass because of the possibility of germ cell tumours (RCOG Green top guidelines No. 62).
- An ultrasonographic examination of the abdomen/pelvis definitely helps identify the uterus separately and gives additional information about the side and size of the ovarian tumour, the nature of cyst wall, its contents, vascularity (with colour doppler flow), and the presence of ascites, if any. Transvaginal

ultrasound is better than transabdominal route, if the tumour is not very large.

- In the hormone-producing tumours, vaginal cytology, endometrial histology and hormonal assays are useful.
- In case of doubt, examination under anesthesia and laparoscopy are helpful.

Table 11.3 lists the rules to classify masses as benign or malignant.

## DIFFERENTIAL DIAGNOSIS

In the differential diagnosis of small to moderate-sized tumours, one has to rule out

- myoma of the uterus,
- uterine pregnancy
- extra-uterine gestation
- distended bladder
- hydrosalpinx
- hydronephrosis
- mesenteric cyst
- tuberculous encysted ascites

Ascites may be mistaken for a large ovarian cystadenoma. In an ovarian tumour, there is dullness over the tumour with resonance on the flanks whereas with ascites, there is dullness over the flanks and resonance in the middle. A shifting dullness may also be elicited in cases of ascites.

## COMPLICATIONS

### Torsion

The most common complication is torsion or **axial rotation**. This is likely to occur in small to moderate-sized neoplasms which are freely mobile and pedunculated like simple serous cysts, pedunculated cystadenomas (not more than 10–15 cm diameter) and cystic teratomas, as the pedicle is twisted twice or even thrice. There is venous congestion with some hemorrhage in the tumour giving rise to increased tension of its contents. The patient complains of sudden, extremely severe pain over the tumour which becomes more tense but the general condition is not alarming as in a ruptured ectopic gestation, as there is no intraperitoneal hemorrhage or shock. If it goes undiagnosed or untreated, the twisted ovarian tumour may adhere to the surrounding structures and may get infected later.

**Table 11.3** IOTA Group ultrasound 'rules' to classify masses as benign (B-rules) or malignant (M-rules)

| B-rules | M-rules |
|---|---|
| Unilocular cysts | Irregular solid tumour |
| Presence of solid components where the largest solid component < 7 mm | Ascites |
| Presence of acoustic shadowing on ultrasound imaging | At least four papillary structures on ultrasound imaging |
| Smooth multilocular tumour with a largest diameter < 100 mm | Irregular multilocular solid tumour with largest diameter ≥ 100 mm |
| No blood flow | Very strong blood flow |

IOTA = International Ovarian Tumor Analysis
*Source:* RCOG Green Top Guidelines, No. 62

### Infection

An infection of the tumour from the adjacent bowel may give rise to pain, fever and sometimes discharge of its contents into the adherent rectum.

### Rupture

The rupture of the cyst is rarely spontaneous but is often traumatic due to direct violence over the abdomen. The symptoms depend on the nature of its contents. It may lead to irritant peritonitis in dermoid cysts or to **pseudomyxoma peritonei** in a mucinous cystadenoma.

## MANAGEMENT

### Expectant Management

Benign ovarian tumours of size < 50 mm, generally resolve within 3–4 menstrual cycles. But where the diameter of the ovarian cyst is between 50–70 mm, a conservative approach could be adapted if she would come for annual USG follow-up. **The use of combined oral pills is no more considered a treatment option in functional ovarian cysts as the pill does not promote resolution of the cyst.**

### Surgery

#### Indications

In postmenopausal women with persistent ovarian cysts of 10 cm or more or with cysts of less than 10 cm size but with increasing CA 125 level, surgical intervention is required. Similarly in premenopausal women, persistent simple ovarian cysts larger than

10 cm (particularly if symptomatic) and complex ovarian cysts (complex ovarian cysts are ovarian cysts containing both fluid and solid material like dermoid cyst) should be surgically removed. Similarly, where the ovarian cysts persist or increase in size, it would require surgical intervention.

Though surgical intervention could be by **laparotomy** or **laparoscopic approach**, the latter is preferred for elective surgical intervention due to its lower postoperative morbidity and hospital stay. However, it needs a skilled and experienced laparoscopic surgeon. In the presence of a large ovarian mass with solid components, laparotomy would be a better choice. **Due to its high recurrence rate, aspiration of cysts is not recommended either by abdominal or vaginal route.** During laparotomy or laparoscopy, all precautions should be taken to avoid spillage of the contents of the cyst. In spite of all this, the need for removal of the ovary(ies) should be discussed with the patient preoperatively. In older parous women, total hysterectomy with bilateral salpingo-oophorectomy may be considered if so desired by the patient. In a twisted ovarian tumour, on laparotomy, the twisted pedicle is unwound, clamped and the tumour removed. The tumour is cut open and the opposite ovary is also examined before closing the abdomen.

- In granulosa cell tumours, if the patient is young, conservative surgery is performed.
- In older women, a total hysterectomy with bilateral salpingo-oophorectomy may be considered due to the increased risk of granulosa cell carcinoma.
- If the patient is pregnant, the ovarian tumour should be removed after the fourth month of gestation. If left alone, there is a risk of torsion or its impaction in the pelvis, causing dystocia.

## PARAOVARIAN CYSTS

These mostly non-neoplastic cyts are **distended remnants of either paramesonephric ducts or mesothelial inclusion cysts**. The cysts are usually small, about 3 cm in size and are mostly asymptomatic. The diagnosis is often incidental either during an ultrasonographic examination for some other reason or during surgery. The symptoms, if they develop, mimic ovarian pathology.

## BENIGN PATHOLOGY OF FALLOPIAN TUBE

### Hydrosalpinx

The most common Fallopian tube pathology is hydrosalpinx. This is usually due to chronic pelvic inflammatory disease (PID). The affected tube is distended with a clear fluid. The fimbria and ostia are obliterated. The tube is very often adherent to the ovary of that side.

The affected woman may be asymptomatic or may have chronic pelvic pain. Very often the diagnosis is made during investigation for infertility.

Management depends on the symptoms and the desire for fertility. In those women where fertility is not of cencern, laparoscopic adhesiolysis and salpingectomy can be done. In those desiring fertility, the outcome depends on the extent of tubal damage. In those with mild tubal damage, laparoscopic neosalpingostomy has been tried with reasonably good outcome.

### Benign Neoplasms

These are very uncommon and consist of tubal leiomyoma and mesothelioma. Mesotheliomas arise in the tubal wall. The leiomyoma arises either from the smooth muscle of the muscularis or from the broad ligament.

**Case study**

*A 30 year-old lady was admitted with severe lower abdominal pain for the past two days. She had fainting attack at home before coming to hospital. The pain has been increasing for the past three months. She also gives history of lower abdominal distension which has been gradually increasing for the past six months.*

*Examination revealed a 20 weeks cystic mass arising from the pelvis and its lower margin was not made out.*

*a) What do you think is the reason for severe abdominal pain and fainting attack?*
*b) What investigation will help you to come to a diagnosis?*
*c) How would you manage this patient?*

## RECAP

- Common benign ovarian tumours are functional cysts, endometriomas, serous cystadenoma, mucinous cystadenoma and mature teratoma.
- Functional cysts are not more than 5–6 cm in diameter except the theca lutein cysts which may grow larger.
- Whereas the follicular and corpus luteum cysts are unilateral, theca lutein cysts and endometrial cysts are often bilateral
- Functional cysts (except the endometrial cysts) resolve over time.
- Serous cystadenomas are often bilateral, moderate in size and mostly unilocular, containing a thin straw-coloured serous fluid.
- A mucinous cystadenoma is mostly unilateral, multiloculated and contains a sticky mucinous fluid.
- Mostly moderate in size, if left untreated, it may reach enormous proportions, and the largest on record is 149 kg.
- Brenner tumour is a rare unilateral solid tumour seen in postmenopausal women.
- The tumours are well-encapsulated, benign and resemble fibromas but show small cystic spaces.
- Thecomas are rare, unilateral solid tumours seen after menopause.
- Fibromas are solid benign tumours. Usually unilateral, they may vary in size from a small asymptomatic nodule in the ovary to a large-sized heavy pedunculated tumour.
- Mature cystic teratomas are also called dermoid cysts of the ovary and form 10–15 per cent of all ovarian tumours.
- They are seen during reproductive life and are bilateral in 25 per cent of cases.
- Moderate in size, well-encapsulated and freely mobile (pedunculated), these tumours show on section, fatty sebaceous material, matted hair and a raised solid area or 'embryonic node' in the cyst wall with teeth or cartilage.
- The patient presents with a uniformly enlarged abdominal swelling often smooth-walled, cystic and with well-defined upper and lateral boundaries.
- The lower border is not felt except when the tumour is small and has a long pedicle.
- On pelvic examination, the uterus will be pushed to one side by the ovarian tumour, the lower pole of which may be felt through one of the lateral fornices.
- Rectal examination is carried out routinely as the presence of any nodule in the pouch of Douglas suggests malignancy.
- In the differential diagnosis of small to moderate-sized tumours, one has to rule out myoma of the uterus, uterine pregnancy, extra-uterine gestation, distended bladder, hydrosalpinx, hydronephrosis, mesenteric cyst and tuberculous encysted ascites.
- The most common complication is torsion or axial rotation.
- This is likely to occur in small to moderate-sized neoplasms which are freely mobile and pedunculated like simple serous cysts, pedunculated cystadenomas (not more than 10–15 cm diameter) and cystic teratomas, as the pedicle is twisted twice or even thrice.
- Benign ovarian tumour of size <50 mm generally resolve within 3–4 menstrual cycles.
- But where the diameter of the ovarian cyst is between 50–70 mm, a conservative approach could be adopted if the patient would come for annual USG follow-up.
- In larger cysts, surgical intervention is preferable.
- Similarly when the ovarian cyst persists or increases in size, surgical intervention would be required.
- The use of combined oral pills is no more considered a treatment option in functional ovarian cysts as the pill does not promote resolution of the cyst.
- Though surgical intervention could be by laparotomy or laparoscopic approach, the latter is preferred for elective surgical intervention due to its lower postoperative morbidity and lesser hospital stay.
- However, it needs a skilled and experienced laparoscopic surgeon.
- In the presence of a large ovarian mass with solid components, laparotomy would be a better choice.
- The need for removal of the ovary(ies) should be discussed with the patient preoperatively.

# REVIEW QUESTIONS

## Long-answer Question

1. What are the common benign ovarian tumours? Discuss the presenting symptoms, diagnosis and management of dermoid cyst.

## Short-answer Questions

1. Briefly discuss theca lutein cyst.
2. What is mucinous cystadenoma? Discuss the complications that can occur if the tumour ruptures and there is intraperitoneal spill.

## MCQs

**1. Mucinous cystadenoma is usually**

a) Bilateral and uniloculated
b) Unilateral and multiloculated
c) Contains clear, serous fluid
d) Contains hair and teeth

**2. Brenner tumours are commonly seen in**

a) Postmenopausal women
b) Premenopausal women
c) Adolescents
d) No specific age group

**3. Meig's syndrome is associated with**

a) Serous cystadenoma
b) Mucinous cystadenoma
c) Thecoma
d) Fibroma

**4. Psammoma bodies are associated with**

a) Mucinous cystadenomas
b) Serous cystadenomas
c) Choriocarcinoma
d) Thecoma

### Further Reading

Hoffman BL, Schorge JO, Schaffer JI, Halvorson LM, Bradshaw KD, Cunningham FG. Williams gynecology. 2nd ed. New York: McGraw-Hill; 2012. 265 p.

# CHAPTER 12

# Pelvic Inflammatory Disease

**AT A GLANCE**


Barriers to Infection
Etiology
Organisms Involved in PID
Pathogenesis
Acute Stage
Chronic Stage
Risk Factors for PID
Clinical Manifestation
Clinical Signs
Differential Diagnosis
Investigations
Laparoscopy
Indications for Laparoscopy in PID
Management
Goals of Management
Management Principles
CDC Guidelines (2015) to Initiate Presumptive Treatment of PID
CDC 2015 Guidelines for Out-Patient Management
Indications for Hospitalisation and Parenteral Therapy
Other Measures
Surgical Intervention
Indications
Follow-up
The Sequelae of PID
Short-Term Sequelae
Long-Term Sequlae
Chronic PID
Prevention


## INTRODUCTION

Pelvic inflammatory disease (PID) is a major health problem both in the developed and developing countries, which causes considerable immediate and long-term morbidity in affected women.

**Definition** PID is the infection and inflammation involving the upper genital tract, namely the uterus, Fallopian tubes and the ovaries, and not related to pregnancy and surgery. It is due to the ascending infection from the vagina and cervix. If untreated, the infection can spread to involve the adjacent pelvic structures and the general peritoneum.

> The term PID should not be used to describe the lower genital tract infections namely vulvitis, vaginitis and cervicitis.

## BARRIERS TO INFECTION

Though there are number of potent pathogenic organisms present in the vagina, normally they do not ascend to the upper genital tract to cause PID. This is due to the presence of barriers which prevent the ascent of organisms from the vagina to the upper genital tract. The barriers are:

- **Vaginal acidity, which** inhibits the growth of the pathogenic organisms.
- The **cervix which** offers a barrier to the ascending micro-organisms by its narrow cervical canal and thick alkaline mucus plug. The ability to prevent the ascent of the infection is at its lowest during ovulation and during menstruation when the mucus plug is absent.
- Normally, **cervical secretions** have a protective and defensive function. Any procedure on the cervix such as dilatation and curettage, and intrauterine contraceptive (IUCD) insertion will disrupt or alter the cervical mucus which will impair the bacteriostatic mechanism and will facilitate the ascent of the organisms from the lower genital tract.

## ETIOLOGY

The disease is often polymicrobial and the infection can be caused by exogenous organisms or endogenous organisms (Table 12.1) present in the vaginal flora.

Table 12.1 Organisms involved in PID

| Sexually transmitted infections | Organisms from the vaginal flora | Rare organisms |
|---|---|---|
| Neisseria gonococci<br>*Chlamydia trachomatis* | **Aerobic organisms**<br>Gram-positive cocci—streptococci, staphylococci<br>Gram-positive rods—*Listeria*<br>Gram-negative—*E. coli, Klebsiella, Enterobacter, Proteus, Salmonella, Pseudomonas, Corynebacterium vaginalis*<br>**Anaerobic organisms**:<br>*Peptococcus, Peptostreptococcus*<br>*Clostridium* species<br>*Bacteroides, Fusobacterium*<br>**Organisms associated with bacterial vaginosis**<br>*Gardnerella vaginalis, Mycoplasma hominis, Mobilincus* | Actinomyces |

## Organisms Involved in PID

The microbiological causes of PID can be divided into:

- Those caused by **sexually transmitted infections (STIs)** such as *Neisseria gonorrhoeae* and *Chlamydia trachomatis*. These organisms can easily penetrate the bacteriostatic action of the cervical mucus.
- Those caused by **endogenous vaginal flora**, the **aerobic** and **anaerobic organisms** and **genital mycoplasmas**. The proteolytic enzymes produced by the anaerobic bacteria, especially those associated with bacterial vaginosis may damage the endocervical mucus barrier allowing the ascent of organisms to the upper genital tract.
- **Actinomycosis** which is a rare cause of PID, and is usually associated with the use of IUCD.

Pathogenic organisms such as gonococci, mycoplasma and other bacterial organisms may be transported to the upper genital tract by the motile vectors such as spermatozoa and trichomonads.

# PATHOGENESIS

Once the organism gains access to the upper genital tract, the infection causes **endometritis** and **endosalpingitis.** During the healing process,they cause fibrosis and morphological damage. In chlamydial PID, the tubal damage is thought to be due to an immune-mediated delayed hypersensitivity.

## Acute Stage

At the stage of endometritis, the patients present with symptoms of irregular vaginal bleeding. Then the infection ascends into the endosalpinx causing mucosal inflammation and edema and produces exudates which leak through the fimbrial end of the tube. This causes inflammation of the other pelvic structures, sticky adhesions between the inflamed tissues. If left untreated, this leads to **salpingo-oophoritis**, **pelvic peritonitis**, and **formation of tubo-ovarian** and **pelvic abscesses.**

## Chronic Stage

The infection can become chronic, where the tube is grossly distorted, with **hydrosalpinx** and **pyosalpinx** formation. There will be mild to dense **peritubal adhesions** to the adjacent structures such as the bowel and ovary (Figs. 12.1 and 12.2).

Untreated severe infection can also lead to **general peritonitis**. Infection caused by *Neisseria gonorrhoeae* and *Chlamydia trachomatis* can also spread to the upper abdomen through the para-colic gutter to cause **peri-hepatic inflammation** presenting with right upper-quadrant pain and pleuritic type of pain. There can also be **systemic spread** with involvement of joints and eyes.

# RISK FACTORS FOR PID

- The risk of acquiring sexually transmitted infection is high in young women with **multiple sexual partners** and in those not using barrier contraceptives.

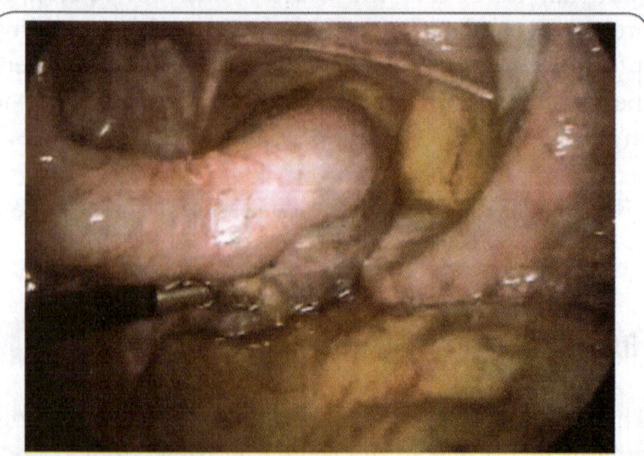

**Fig. 12.1** Laparoscopy picture showing distended and edematous Fallopian tube in PID

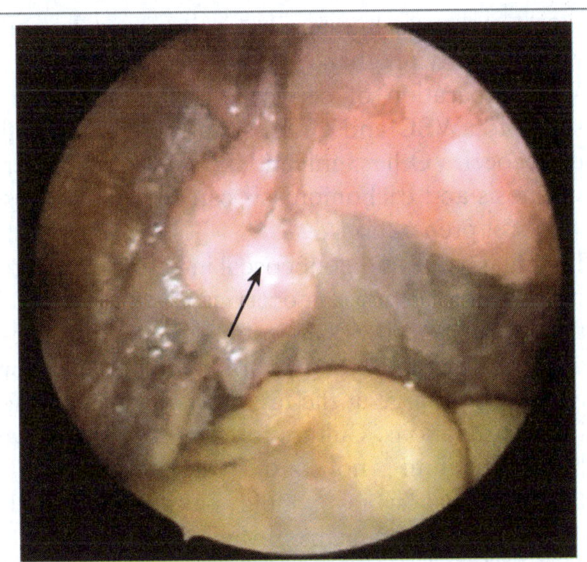

**Fig. 12.2** Picture showing distended Fallopian tube with hydrosalpinx and adhesions between the posterior surface of uterus and the bowel (shown by arrow)

- Young girls have **wide ectropion** which allows easy colonisation of *Chlamydia trachomatis* and *N. gonorrhoeae* organisms.
- Women involved in **high-risk sexual behaviour.**
- In women with **compromised immune status** due to various reasons such as malnutrition, lower socioeconomic status or smoking, the organisms in the normal vaginal flora can get activated and ascend to the upper genital tract to cause infection.
- Procedures that involve the cervix and upper genital tract such as insertion of intrauterine contraceptive device.

## CLINICAL MANIFESTATION

**Symptoms** PID has a wide spectrum of clinical features ranging from no symptoms at all to life-threatening disease.

- In the acute phase of the disease, the patients present with **bilateral lower abdominal pain**, localised to the suprapubic region and both iliac fossae or pelvis. The pelvic pain is continuous, dull in character and is the first symptom of ascending infection. The dull ache becomes severe with palpation, movement and coitus.
- In gonococcal infection, the pain most often starts with menstrual bleeding, is more rapid in onset, has a short history of less than 3 days duration and presents with severe clinical picture.
- The PID caused by *Chlamydia* is often silent and is diagnosed while evaluating cases of infertility.
- In PID caused by anaerobic organisms, there is acute manifestation and the disease is often severe with palpable **adnexal masses**, **abscess** formation and **peritonitis.**
- There is increase in **vaginal discharge** in more than 50% of cases which can be purulent, watery or blood-stained.
- Patients can also present with **abnormal vaginal bleeding**, heavy menstrual bleeding (HMB), irregular bleeding or postcoital bleeding due to severe cervicitis.
- With severe infection, malaise, fever, nausea and vomiting will be present, which may suggest peritonitis.
- There could be **urinary symptoms** with increased frequency and dysuria.
- Patients can also present with **low backache** both in the acute and chronic stage.
- Gonorrhea can also cause **proctitis** and can present with rectal symptoms.
- Pain and discomfort in the right upper quadrant may be a symptom of possible concomitant peri-hepatitis (**Fitz-Hugh–Curtis syndrome**), which is seen in < 5% of cases. Here there is fibrous adhesion between the liver surface and the diaphragm producing violin string adhesions, which may be mistaken for cholecystitis/pleurisy if they are dominant features in the history.
- Once the PID becomes chronic, the predominant symptoms are chronic pelvic pain, congestive dysmenorrhea, dysparuenia and heavy menstrual bleeding. Intermittent acute exacerbations can also occur.

### Clinical Symptoms

| |
|---|
| Bilateral lower abdominal pain |
| Abnormal vaginal discharge |
| Abnormal vaginal bleeding—heavy menstrual bleeding, irregular vaginal bleeding and postcoital bleeding |
| Fever, nausea and vomiting |
| Urinary symptoms |
| Low backache |
| Right upper quadrant pain due to perihepatitis |

## CLINICAL SIGNS

- Patient may be **pyrexial** or **apyrexial**. If pyrexial, a temperature > 38°C with tachycardia is seen in more than one-third of cases, and is most common with gonococcal and anaerobic infections.

- In acute PID, there is **bilateral lower abdominal tenderness** and in the presence of peritonitis, there will be associated abdominal rigidity and guarding.
- On speculum examination, the cervix will appear florid red suggesting cervicitis, and there will be muco-purulent vaginal discharge.
- On bimanual pelvic examination, the movement of the cervix will be painful (**cervical motion tenderness**) and there will be tenderness in the fornices, or uterine tenderness may be present.
- If there is a tubo-ovarian abscess, tender soft mass can be felt in the fornices.
- In the presence of a pelvic abscess, soft, boggy fluctuant swelling can be felt in the POD and can be well appreciated by a rectal examination.
- In cases of chlamydial infection, the disease is often silent and there may not be any demonstrable clinical signs.

## DIFFERENTIAL DIAGNOSIS

In women presenting with the above symptoms and signs, the following differential diagnoses should be considered and necessary investigations should be carried out.

- Acute appendicitis
- Ectopic gestation
- Ruptured corpus luteal cyst
- Endometriosis
- Ovarian pathology such as twisted ovarian cyst, haemorrhage and rupture
- Urinary tract infection
- Diverticulitis

## INVESTIGATIONS

Once a diagnosis of PID is made or suspected clinically, as per the **Centre for Disease Control (CDC)** recommendations, the patients are empirically started on antimicrobial therapy to prevent immediate and long-term complications.

The following investigations are carried out simultaneously. **A positive result will support the diagnosis of PID, but a negative result does not exclude the diagnosis of PID.**

- A complete haemogram for elevated total count.
- An elevated ESR and C-reactive protein.
- Urine analysis and urine culture.
- Urine or serum human chorionic gonadotropin to rule out early pregnancy and its complications.
- Wet preparation of cervical discharge is done in saline for WBC and Gram stain for gram-negative diplococci. Other infections such as bacterial vaginosis and trichomoniasis can also be diagnosed with wet preparations.
- For chlamydial and gonococcal infections, diagnosis is made by testing endocervical swabs by ELISA techniques and by PCR testing. In the absence of cervical discharge, the urethra can be milked down and the discharge at the urethral orifice can be sent for investigations. Culture for gonococci in Thayer-Martin medium is not routinely done.
- High vaginal swabs should be taken for other polymicrobial organisms of vagina.
- Also look for associated infections such as syphilis and HIV.
- USG of abdomen and pelvis will be helpful in the diagnosis of tubo-ovarian abscess, pelvic abscess and hydrosalpinx. USG may also be useful in ruling out ovarian torsion, ectopic gestation and acute appendicitis.

| Investigations |
|---|
| Complete haemogram |
| C-reactive protein |
| Urine analysis and urine culture |
| Wet smear for WBC, trichomoniasis, bacterial vaginosis |
| Endocervical swab for Gram stain, PCR and ELISA technique for chlamydial and gonococcal infection |
| High vaginal swab |
| Tests for syphilis and HIV infections |
| USG of abdomen and pelvis |

## LAPAROSCOPY

Laparoscopy allows direct visualisation of the pelvic structures to confirm the diagnosis. It is also useful for collecting material from the peritoneal cavity for microbiological investigations.

Though it is considered the "Gold standard" for the diagnosis of PID, laparoscopy is not used in routine clinical practice as it is an invasive procedure.

### Indications for Laparoscopy in PID

- Failure to respond to medical treatment
- In the case of doubtful diagnosis—to rule out ectopic pregnancy / appendicitis

- Presence of a pelvic mass which necessitates surgical intervention

## MANAGEMENT

### Goals of Management

- The goals of management are to treat the infection effectively so as to prevent immediate and long-term complications and to preserve fertility.

### Management Principles

- While awaiting the results of microbiological investigations, empirical treatment should be started with antibiotics which are effective against chlamydia, gonococcus, genital mycoplasmas, gram-negative and gram-positive bacteria and the anaerobic organisms related to bacterial vaginosis.
- In clinically suspected cases, antibiotic treatment should not be delayed while waiting for the laboratory investigation results.
- Negative swabs do not exclude PID, therefore, should not influence the decision to treat.
- Contact tracing is vital, and sexual partners should also be treated.
- In those with sexually transmitted infections, referral should be made to a genito-urinary medical clinic for full screening of sexually transmitted infections.

### CDC Guidelines (2015) to Initiate Presumptive Treatment of PID

Because of the difficulty in making a definitive diagnosis and the cause of PID and in order to avoid delay in the treatment, CDC has given recommendations to initiate empirical management of PID (Table 12.2).

**Table 12.2** CDC guidelines for presumptive treatment of PID

| **Criteria for empirical treatment** |
|---|
| When sexually active young women or women at risk of STD experience pelvic or lower abdominal pain. |
| When other causes for lower abdominal pain are unlikely. |
| When one or more of the minimal clinical criteria namely cervical excitation pain or uterine tenderness or bilateral adnexal tenderness are present on pelvic examination. |
| The presence of one or more of the additional criteria will enhance and support the diagnosis of PID. |
| **Additional criteria** |
| Oral temperature >101°F (>38.3°C) |
| Abnormal cervical mucopurulent discharge or cervical friability |
| Presence of abundant numbers of WBC on saline microscopy of vaginal fluid |
| Leucocytosis > 10,000 |
| Elevated erythrocyte sedimentation rate |
| Elevated C-reactive protein |
| Complex mass or abscess by bimanual examination or USG |
| Laboratory documentation of cervical infection with *N. gonorrhoeae* or *C. trachomatis* |
| Definitive diagnosis of PID |
| Endometrial biopsy showing evidence of endometritis |
| Imaging studies (USG/ MRI) showing evidence of thickened fluid-filled tubes, with or without tubo-ovarian complex/abscess |
| Laparoscopic findings being consistent with PID. |

### CDC 2015 Guidelines for Out-Patient Management

In patients with acute PID, out-patient management using intramuscular and oral medication (Table 12.3) can be undertaken if the temperature is < 39°C, abdominal and pelvic findings are minimal, the patient is not toxic and the patient can take oral medication.

Because of the emergence of quinolone-resistant *N. gonorrhoeae*, regimens that include a quinolone agent are no longer routinely recommended for the treatment of PID.

### Indications for Hospitalisation and Parenteral Therapy

In the following situations, hospitalisation is indicated and patients are given parenteral therapy, the recommended regimen for which is listed in Table 12.4.

- Suspected surgical emergencies such as appendicitis or ectopic pregnancy are suspected.
- When the patient cannot follow or tolerate oral medication.
- When the patient is less than 19 years.

**Table 12.3** Recommended intramuscular/oral regimen for out-patient management

| Regimen I | Regimen II | Regimen III |
|---|---|---|
| Ceftriaxone 250 mg IM in a single dose and<br>Tablet Doxycycline 100 mg twice daily for 14 days with<br>Tablet Metronidazole 500 mg twice daily for 14 days. | Cefoxitin 2 g IM in a single dose with 1 g of oral Probenecid.<br>Tablet Doxycycline 100 mg twice daily for 14 days with<br>Tablet Metronidazole 500 mg twice daily for 14 days | Other parenteral third-generation cephalosporin—Cefotaxime<br>Tablet Doxycycline 100 mg twice daily for 14 days with<br>Tablet Metronidazole 500 mg twice daily for 14 days |

**Table 12.4** Recommended parenteral regimens

| Regimen I | Regimen II | Regimen III |
|---|---|---|
| Cefotetan 2 g IV every 12 hours for 72 hours<br>Doxycycline 100 mg orally twice daily for 14 days. | Cefoxitin 2 g IV every 6 hours for 72 hours<br>Doxycycline 100 mg orally twice daily for 14 days | Clindamycin 900 mg IV every 8 hours for 72 hours<br>Gentamicin 2 mg/kg IV/ IM as loading dose followed by 1.5 mg/kg as maintenance dose every 8 hours for 72 hours<br>Followed by oral clindamycin 450 mg four times daily and doxycycline 100 mg twice daily to complete the 14 days course |

- When there is severe abdominal pain, abdominal guarding or rigidity, when rebound tenderness is made out or when there is severe nausea, vomiting, all findings suggestive of peritonitis.
- When there is fever >38.5°C.
- In the presence of tubo-ovarian abscess.
- In the presence of underlying illnesses such as diabetes, HIV or active hepatitis infection.
- When there is no clinical response to oral antimicrobial therapy.
- In the presence of pelvic abscess, following IV clindamycin therapy, either clindamycin 450 mg four times daily or metronidazole 500 mg twice daily should be given along with doxycycline 100 mg twice daily for 14 days.

### Other Measures

- In order to minimise the disease transmission, women should abstain from sexual intercourse until their treatment course is completed and till the male partners have been adequately treated.
- All women treated for PID should be investigated for sexually transmitted infections.

**Managing Male Partners**

All men who have had sexual contact with women who were treated for PID in the last 6 months should be treated presumably for gonococcal and chlamydial infection even if they are asymptomatic.

## SURGICAL INTERVENTION

Though most cases will respond to medical management, in certain situations surgical intervention by laparotomy/laparoscopy would be required.

### Indications

- Whenever the diagnosis is in doubt
- Patient not responding to medical management
- Co-existing conditions such as appendicitis are suspected
- Spreading peritonitis
- In the presence of tubo-ovarian abscess or pelvic mass when there is no response to medical management or the abscess has ruptured, surgical drainage should be carried out. Pelvic abscess can also be drained through an incision in the pouch of Douglas (colpotomy).

## FOLLOW-UP

Follow-up is mandatory in all women who were treated for acute PID.

- In order to confirm clinical improvement, patients on out-patient regimen should be reviewed in 72 hours. If 'there is no clinical improvement in 72 hours, the patient should be admitted and the diagnosis is reviewed; if necessary, laparoscopy should be carried out. The antibiotic regimen should also be reassessed.
- If the PID was due to STI infections, patients should be reviewed at 3 months and investigations are carried out to confirm clearance of the disease.

## THE SEQUELAE OF PID

PID can lead to short-term complications and long-term sequelae. The short-term complications are acute, can lead to considerable morbidity and even mortality. The short-term and long-term complications/sequelae of PID are listed in Table 12.5.

### Short-Term Sequelae

#### Fitz-Hugh–Curtis syndrome

In women with gonococcal and chlamydial infections, along the para-colic gutters the infection can spread to the perihepatic region causing perihepatitis and can form adhesions between the anterior surface of the

Table 12.5 Sequelae of PID

| Immediate sequelae | Long-term sequelae |
|---|---|
| Fitz-Hugh–Curtis syndrome | Infertility due to tubal occlusion |
| Tubo-ovarian abscess | Ectopic pregnancy |
| Pelvic abscess | Chronic pelvic pain |
| Septicaemia | Chronic infection |
| Mortality | Acute exacerbations |

liver and the parietal wall. The adhesions are called **violin string adhesions**. The condition is seen in <5% of cases diagnosed with PID. The patients present with pain and discomfort in the right upper quadrant and can be mistaken for cholecystitis/pleurisy if they are dominant features in the history. In 50% of cases, bilirubin and liver enzymes may be elevated. Fig. 12.3 shows adhesions between the liver and the parietal wall (Fitz-Hugh–Curtis syndrome).

### Tubo-ovarian abscess

A tubo-ovarian abscess is the most serious immediate complication of PID. Initial management includes bed rest, support, and use of broad-spectrum antibiotics. If there is no response within 72 hours, or T-O mass is large, > 8 cms or bilateral, less likely to respond, then surgical intervention would be required.

### Pelvic abscess

In untreated PID and in those caused by anaerobic organisms, patients can develop pelvic abscess which collects in the pouch of Douglas. The clinical manifestation is acute with high temperature with features of peritonitis. It is a life-threatening condition.

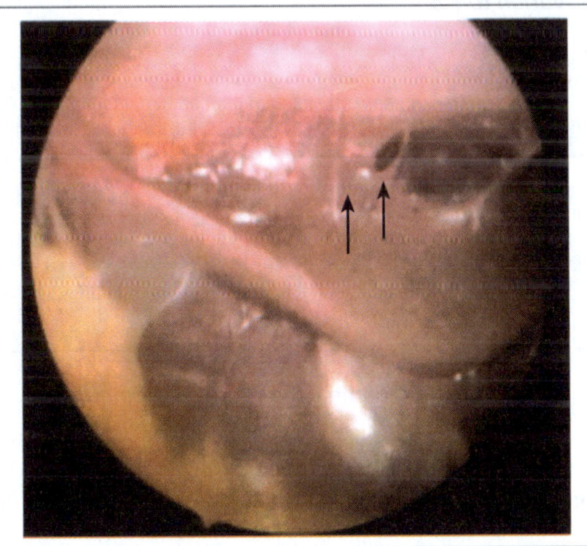

**Fig. 12.3** Adhesions between the liver and the parietal wall (Fitz-Hugh–Curtis syndrome)

If the pelvic abscess ruptures, it can lead to general peritonitis with the associated morbidity and mortality.

## Long-Term Sequlae

Women with PID are at increased risk of chronic PID with exacerbations, chronic pelvic pain, ectopic pregnancy and infertility.

### Infertility

PID is the most important cause of tubal block leading to infertility. **After one episode of PID, approximately 12% of women become infertile because of tubal block, 25% after two episodes and 50% after three or more episodes of infection.**

### Ectopic pregnancy

Because of the endosalpingitis associated with PID, there is increased risk of ectopic gestation. After one episode of PID, a woman's risk of ectopic pregnancy increases seven-fold compared to the woman who never suffered from PID.

### Recurrent PID

As the epithelium is already damaged, it is easily invaded by the vaginal flora, or infection can be transmitted from the male partner. Therefore it is important to take urethral culture from the male partner and treat even if they are asymptomatic.

### Chronic pelvic pain after PID

**Nearly 15–20% of patients suffer from long-term pain** and they become pelvic cripples presenting with chronic pelvic pain, dysmenorrhea and dyspareunia. The chronic pain may be due to adhesion formation or pelvic congestion. Pain may be due to chronic infection with pockets of pus in the pelvis. They can also develop recurrent infections by endogenous or exogenous organisms.

## Chronic PID

An acute PID can become chronic presenting with abnormal vaginal discharge, chronic pelvic pain, backache, heavy menstrual bleeding, congestive dysmenorrhea, and dyspareunia. They can have intermittent acute exacerbations.

### Clinical features

On examination, there will be lower abdominal tenderness, and the uterus will be retroverted, tender and fixed in the pouch of Douglas due to adhesions. Due to the presence of tubo-ovarian mass, hydrosalpinx or pyosalpinx, a tender mass can be felt in the adnexal region. There may be tender nodularity in the pouch of Douglas. Endometriosis also presents with similar signs and symptoms and laparoscopy is a valuable tool in differentiating the two conditions.

### Management

Patients with chronic PID will need surgical intervention. In those presenting with infertility, ART techniques should be offered. In those who have completed the family and in whom the ovaries could not be retained due to complex masses, total hysterectomy with bilateral salpingo-oophorectomy would be required.

## PREVENTION

Prevention should focus on:

- Use of contraceptives
  - Use of barrier contraceptives should be encouraged to reduce the risk of developing PID.
  - Use of oral contraceptives thickens the cervical mucus and reduces menstrual blood loss thereby reducing the risk of PID.
  - IUCD should not be used on high-risk patients
- The importance of sexual monogamy should be emphasised to the public.
- Cervicitis, urethritis and lower genital tract symptoms should be evaluated early and treated effectively.
- At-risk population should be identified, screened and treated to prevent transmission of PID to the general population.
- Sexual contacts should be traced and treated effectively even if they are asymptomatic.
- There should be public education and awareness programmes to reduce the risk of STIs.

**Case study**

*A 24-year-old sexually active nulliparous woman complains of lower abdominal pain and low-grade fever of 4 days duration. Her menstrual period started 5 days earlier and the flow was heavier than usual. There was no abnormal vaginal discharge. She has urinary urgency and frequency. On examination, her temperature was 100° and other vitals were normal. There was tenderness on palpating the lower abdomen. On pelvic examination, the cervix was congested and the uterus and adnexae were very tender. Her pregnancy test was negative.*

- *The most likely diagnosis is acute PID as the patient is having the three important criteria for PID, namely, lower abdominal pain, cervical motion tenderness and adnexal tenderness. She also has fever.*
- *The DD would be acute appendicitis, pyelonephritis, renal colic, ovarian torsion.*
- *What are the investigations to order?*
- *What are the criteria for out-patient management?*
- *What are the criteria for hospitalisation?*
- *What are the sequelae of acute PID?*

## RECAP

- Pelvic inflammatory disease (PID) is the infection involving the upper genital tract, namely the uterus, Fallopian tubes and the ovaries, and which is not related to pregnancy and surgery.
- It is due to the ascending infection from the vagina and cervix.
- PID can be caused by sexually transmitted infections such as gonococcus and chlamydia or by aerobic and anaerobic organisms from the endogenous vaginal flora.
- In women diagnosed or suspected with PID, treatment should be initiated empirically to prevent immediate and long-term complications.

# REVIEW QUESTIONS

### Long-answer questions

Define pelvic inflammatory disease (PID). What are the signs and symptoms of acute PID? Discuss the differential diagnosis of PID.

### Short-answer questions

1. Discuss the recommended parenteral regimens for treating PID.
2. Enumerate the CDC guidelines for presumptive treatment of PID.

## MCQs

1. **A 19-year-old sexually active girl presented with fever of 101°, associated with lower abdominal pain; pelvic examination showed adnexal and right fornix tenderness. A differential diagnosis of PID/ acute appendicitis was made. Her pregnancy test was negative. Which of the following methods will you adopt to make an accurate diagnosis?**
   a) Serial USG
   b) Serial total count and C-reactive protein
   c) Laparoscopy
   d) Observation
2. **Laparoscopy revealed inflammation of the Fallopian tubes. Culture of the discharge will reveal which of the following organisms.**
   a) Gonococci
   b) Chlamydia
   c) Anaerobic organisms
   d) Multiple organisms
3. **A 30-year-old woman presented with features of acute PID. She has been using IUCD for the past 3 years. During laparoscopy, sulphur granules are seen at the fimbria. What are the possible causative organisms?**
   a) *C. trachomatis*
   b) *Actinomyces*
   c) *N. gonorrhoeae*
   d) *Staphylococcus aureus*

CHAPTER 13

# Infertility

**AT A GLANCE**

History
Evaluation for Specific Causes of Female Infertility
1. Ovulatory Dysfunction
2. Tubal Factors
3. Uterine Factors
4. Cervical Factors
5. Immunological Factors
6. Infectious Factors
7. Unexplained Infertility
8. Female Aging
Diagnostic Evaluation of Female Infertility
1. Tests for Ovulation
2. Tests for Tubal Patency
3. Tests for Uterine Factors
4. Test for Cervical Factors
5. Tests for Ovarian Reserve
6. Test for Endometriosis
Treatment of Infertility
I. Treatment of Anovulation
II. Treatment of PCOD
III. Management of Tubal Disease
IV. Treatment of Uterine Factors
Male Infertility
Male History—Key Points
Etiology
Diagnostic Evaluation
Treatment of Male Infertility
1. Intra-uterine Insemination (IUI)
2. Intracytoplasmic Sperm Injection (ICSI)
3. Gametocyte Intra-Fallopian Transfer (GIFT)
4. Zygote Intra-Fallopian Transfer (ZIFT)
5. Microassisted Fertilisation Technique (MAF)
6. Assisted Reproductive Techniques (ART)
7. Surrogacy
8. Gestational Surrogates

## INTRODUCTION

Infertility is a common condition affecting 10–15% of couples of reproductive age. Although the prevalence of infertility is believed to have remained relatively stable during the past 40 years, the demand for infertility evaluation and treatment has increased with advances in infertility treatment.Patients, now have greater hope that medical intervention will help them to achieve their goal.

**Infertility is defined as the inability of a couple to conceive after one year of unprotected intercourse of reasonable frequency.**

Infertility can be subdivided into

- Primary infertility where there is no prior pregnancy
- Secondary infertility referring to infertility following at least one prior conception.

**Fecundablity** is the ability to conceive in a single menstrual cycle and estimated to be 20–25%. In those attempting conception, approximately 50% of women will be pregnant at 3 months,75% at 6 months and more than 85% will be pregnant by 1 year.

Sexually transmitted infections (STI) such as that of *Chlamydia trachomatis* in young women and environmental factors in the case of males have been found to have potential impact on the prevalence of infertility.

Successful conception requires a specific series of complex events:

- Ovulation of competent oocyte
- Ovum pick up by a patent Fallopian tube
- Fertilisation
- Generation of a viable embryo
- Transport of the embryo into the uterine cavity
- Successful implantation of the embryo into the endometrium

In **male factors,** sperm of adequate number and quality must be deposited near the cervix at the time of ovulation. Any defect in one or more of the above essential steps can result in diminished fertility or infertility.

In general, infertility is due to the female factor one-third of the time, due to male factor one-third of the time and due to both the factors in the remaining one-third. Hence it is essential to evaluate both the partners in the management of infertility. The other advantage of having both the partners during the initial consultation is that it gives an opportunity to educate them regarding the normal process of conception.

### Etiology of Infertility

| | |
|---|---|
| Male | 25% |
| Ovulatory | 27% |
| Tubal/Uterine | 22% |
| Unexplained | 17% |

## HISTORY

**Table 13.1** Important points in the history and examination of female patients

| Area of investigation | History |
|---|---|
| Infertility | Duration of infertility<br>Length and type of contraceptive used, if any<br>Previous investigation and treatment for infertility |
| Social history | Occupation<br>Obesity<br>Cigarette smoking<br>Alcohol consumption<br>Caffeine<br>Illicit drugs<br>Cocaine<br>Toxins |
| Sexual | Coital history<br>Frequency and timing of coitus<br>Knowledge about fertile period<br>Dyspareunia, postcoital bleeding |
| Gynecological | Menstrual history<br>Menarche<br>Frequency and duration of periods<br>Dysmenorrhea<br>Menorrhagia<br>Intermenstrual bleeding<br>Hot flashes<br>H/O PID, STD, fibroid, endometriosis, previous abortion, PTL, retained placenta, PPH, D&C, foetal anomalies |
| Medical | Symptoms of thyroid disease or hyperprolactinemia.<br>Symptoms of androgen excess: acne or hirsutism<br>Prior chemotherapy or pelvic irradiation.<br>History of mumps, particularly in men |
| Surgical | Surgery done for ruptured appendicitis or diverticulum, prior uterine surgery |
| Medication/drugs | NSAID |

PID: Pelvic inflammatory disease; STD: Sexually transmitted disease; PTL: Preterm labour; PPH: Postpartum hemorrhage; D&C: Dilatation and curettage

The points requiring particular attention in the history-taking and examination of a female patient are listed in Table 13.1 and the points to be considered in the detailed physical examination of a female patient are listed in Table 13.2.

**Table 13.2** Detailed physical examination of a female patient

| | |
|---|---|
| Female | **General examination**<br>Height,weight, BMI, hirsutism<br>Acne<br>Alopecia<br>Acanthosis nigricans<br>Galactorrhea<br>Thyroid enlargement |
| | **Local examination**<br>State of hymen<br>Labia and clitoris<br>Vagina—presence of rugae<br>Cervix—mucus<br>Enlarged or irregularly shaped uterus, fixed uterus<br>Uterosacral nodularity |

## EVALUATION FOR SPECIFIC CAUSES OF FEMALE INFERTILITY

### 1. Ovulatory Dysfunction

Disturbances in ovulation is the principal factor in approximately 25% of the couples. Ovulation may be disturbed by abnormalities of the hypothalamus, anterior pituitary or ovaries. Thyroid disease and hyperprolactinemia may also contribute to menstrual disturbances.

**A patient's menstrual history is an excellent predictor of regular ovulation.** A woman with regular cyclical menses at an interval of 25–35days and duration of 3–7 days is most likely to have normal ovulation.One of the probable signs of ovulation is **Mittelschmerz** which is midcycle pelvic pain associated with ovulation or by symptoms such as breast tenderness, acne, food cravings and mood changes. Ovulatory cycles are more likely to be associated with dysmenorrhea although severe dysmenorrhea may suggest endometriosis.

WHO classification of ovulatory dysfunction, which is as follows, is a helpful system and based on classification of the pathogenesis of the disorder.

| Group | Type | Percentage | Biochemical changes |
|---|---|---|---|
| 1 | Hypothalamo-pituitary failure/hypogonadohypogonadism | 10% | FSH decreased<br>LH decreased<br>Estrogen—low<br>PRL—normal |
| 2 | Hypothalamo-pituitary dysfunction | 85% | FSH, LH, estrogen—normal |

| 3 | Ovarian failure | 4–5% | FSH increased<br>LH increased<br>Estrogen—low |
|---|---|---|---|

FSH: Follicular stimulating hormone; LH: Luteinising hormone; PRL: Prolactin

### WHO type I (Hypogonadotropic hypogonadal anovulation)

This is a failure of the hypothalamus to produce gonodatropin releasing hormone (GnRH) which regulates the production of gonadotropin from the anterior pituitary. Hence FSH, LH levels are low (<5IU/L), oestrogen levels are low and ultrasound scan of the uterus will reveal a thin or absent endometrial strip. The patient fails to menstruate even after exposure to a short course of progesterone treatment. Acquired GnRH deficiency may arise in anorexia nervosa and in excessive exercise. In Kallman syndrome there is lack of gonadotropin secretion which leads to hypogonadism with anosmia.

A similar situation occurs in cases of hyperprolactinemia, which may be associated with galactorrhea as well as amenorrhea. Hyperprolactinemia can be caused by hypothyroidism wherein high levels of thyrotropin-releasing hormone (TRH) can alter the dopamine-mediated regulation of the anterior pituitary and cause hyperprolactinemia. An MRI may identify larger pituitary adenoma or microadenoma. Some drugs which block the effect of dopamine such as phenothiazine, antipsychotics, metoclopramide can also cause hyperprolactinemia.

Rarely, massive postpartum hemorrhage and prolonged hypotension can lead to pituitary infarction which is known as **Sheehan's syndrome.**

### WHO type II (Normo-gonadotropic, normo-estrogenic anovulation)

This is the most common ovulatory disturbance. These women will have normal oestrogen levels and many are overweight presenting with oligomenorrhea/amenorrhea. USG will reveal the presence of polycystic ovaries in up to 90%. These women menstruate after exposure to a short course of progesterone treatment. The presence of any two of the following triad is sufficient to make the diagnosis of polycystic ovarian syndrome (PCOS) (Society of Obstetricians and Gynaecologists of Canada (SOGC))

1. Oligo-ovulation and/or anovulation
2. USG—polycystic ovaries
3. Clinical and/or biochemical changes—hyperandrogenism

High androgens disturb normal follicular growth and patients may present with irregular or absent menses. The associated signs of androgen excess are hirsutism, acne and enlargement of clitoris. 10–20% of PCOS patients also have associated elevation in prolactin levels. Ovulatory failure may result from 21-hydroxylase deficiency in the adrenal gland leading to elevated 17-hydroxyprogesterone. Other causes of hyperandrogenism such as adrenal tumours and Cushing's syndrome should be assessed and ruled out when androgen levels are high.

Insulin resistance has been well described in PCOS with 3–7 times higher risk of developing type 2 DM in later life; they also have lifetime risk of developing endometrial cancer. Hence menstruation should be induced with progesterone at least 3–4 times/year particularly when endometrial thickness is increased as seen in USG.

### WHO type III (Hyper-gonadotropic, hypoestrogenic anovulation)

These are caused by ovarian failure and consist of about 5% of ovulation disorders. In some patients the presence of Turners 45XO or Turner mosaic (45XO/46XX) should be considered and a karyotype should be performed.

- In the presence of normal karyotype, premature ovarian failure and agenesis of ovaries should be considered.
- Acquired ovarian failure may occur as a result of previous chemo- or radiotherapy for cancer. Screening for antiovarian antibodies may be useful to diagnose autoimmune ovarian failure. If positive, autoimmune disorders including hypothyroidism, adrenal insufficiency, diabetes mellitus and pernicious anaemia should be considered.

## 2. Tubal Factors

Normal tubal function should permit gamete transport, fertilisation and subsequent passage of the embryo to the uterus for implantation. Tubal pathology is a contributory factor in 25–30% of women presenting with infertility. During the past 3 decades, the incidence of infertility caused by damage to the Fallopian tube has increased because of an increased incidence of salphingitis.

**Etiology** The most common cause of tubal pathology is past pelvic infection like genital tuberculosis and sexually transmitted infections such as chlamydial and gonococcal infections.

Genital tuberculosis leads to tubal involvement is about 90%; it results in exosalpingitis, endosalpingitis and perisalpingitis.

Chlamydial infection though asymptomatic can cause more tubal damage especially proximal occlusion of the tube. Proximal tubal occlusion is seen most frequently in pathological conditions like obliterative fibrosis, salpingitis isthmica nodosa (SIN), chronic inflammation and endometriosis.

Gonococcal infection results in distal tubal occlusion and presents as bilateral hydrosalpinx. **Mid-tubal blocks are commonly associated with SIN and previous sterilisation. Distal obstruction is more common than proximal occlusion.**

## 3. Uterine Factors

The uterus not only serves as a conduit for the transfer of sperm from the vagina/cervix into the Fallopian tube, but has the function of nurturing the embryo and carrying the fetus to term. Uterus per se may account for 5% of infertility.

**Uterine Factors**

| Anatomical | Functional |
|---|---|
| Intrauterine adhesions<br>Uterine fibroids<br>Endometrial polyps<br>Uterine malformations<br>Adenomyosis<br>Infections—Tuberculosis | Luteal phase defect<br>Thin non-receptive endometrium |

### i. Intrauterine adhesions (Asherman syndrome)

Intrauterine adhesions may develop after trauma to the basal layer of endometrium. It usually follows endometrial curettage after a spontaneous, incomplete or elective abortion. Any endometrial injury such as myomectomy or caesarean section may result in intrauterine adhesions. Intrauterine adhesions may present as infertility, reduced menstrual bleeding or previous pregnancy loss.

### ii. Uterine myomas

Submucous and large intramural fibroids may affect fertility by distorting the uterine cavity, obstructing the tubal ostia and altering the uterine contractility. Sperm and embryo transport are also affected by associated endometrial thinning.

### iii. Endometrial polyps

Like submucous myoma, larger polyps may interfere with reproduction. Small polyps may be present at the tubal ostia.They usually present with intermenstrual bleeding or heavy bleeding.

### iv. Congenital uterine anomalies

It is the result of an abnormal development of the Müllerian ducts during embryogenesis.The most common anomaly is the septate uterus and is frequently associated with infertility. A septate uterus results from failure of the resorption of the septum between the two uterine horns.The septum can be partial or complete and composed of myometrium or fibrous tissue.

### v. Endometritis

A variety of infectious agents have been implicated in the pathogenesis of chronic endometritis. Tuberculous endometritis is responsible for 3–15% of infertility. Diagnosis is based on histologic examination of an endometrial specimen and typical acid-fast bacilli on culture or PCR. Subtle cause of endometritis is infection with chlamydial trachomatis. Chlamydial trachomatis can be demonstrated only in 20% of the women having chlamydial infections.

## 4. Cervical Factors

The cervix stands as the gatekeeper to the female genital tract. For fertilisation of the ovum to occur in the Fallopian tube, the cervix must permit the sperms to pass through.This is facilitated by the preovulatory mucus which is thin and acellular and renders permissibility to sperms. The cervical cause of infertility is less than 5%.

The cervix could become scarred or stenosed from previous surgery resulting in destruction of the cervical glands or obstruction to the sperms. Presence of antisperm antibodies, both IgG and IgA, in the cervical mucus cause disordinate movements of the spermatozoa thereby making them incapable of penetrating the mucus. Rarely, prenatal exposure to diethylstilbesterol can cause cervical stenosis.

## 5. Immunological Factors

Both sperm-agglutinating and sperm-immobilising antibodies have been found in the serum and cervical mucus, which are mainly IgM and IgG antibodies. Autoimmunity to sperm in semen and serum has been found in some infertile men. These antibodies are treated by corticosteroid therapy and sperm-washing techniques.

### 6. Infectious Factors

Asymptomatic or occult infection of the upper genital tract in both male and female is a cause of infertility. *Ureaplasma urealyticum*, *Mycoplasma hominis* and *Mycoplasma fermentas* are the main organisms. Treatment with doxycycline will help to eradicate these organisms.

### 7. Unexplained Infertility

For some couples, comprehensive evaluation of both partners does not identify the etiology for their infertility. The test results identify a normal semen analysis, evidence of ovulation, a normal uterine cavity and patent Fallopian tube. About 15% of couples come under this category. If laparoscopy is performed, subtle lesions such as pelvic endometriosis and pelvic adhesions may be identified and treated at the same time.

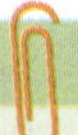

**Contributing Factors to Unexplained Infertility**

Luteal phase defect
Luteinised unruptured follicle syndrome
Minimal endometriosis
Small endometrial polyps

**Endometriosis and unexplained infertility** Prevalance of endometriosis is 33% in infertile women. The reasons for decreased fertility include anatomical distortion, toxic influence of peritoneal fluid, decreased oocyte or embryo quality, defective endometrial receptivity or diminished ovarian reserve.

### 8. Female Aging

Age-related infertility is closely linked to the loss of viable oocytes. At mid-gestation, a normal human female fetus has approximately 7 million oocytes which will decrease to between 1 to 2 million by birth. Ongoing atresia of non-dominant follicles proceeds throughout a woman's reproductive lifespan. Approximately 300,000 follicles are present at puberty and less than 1000 follicles at the onset of menopause. Thus even before menarche, a woman has lost most of her eggs.

With increasing age of the female partner, risks of genetic abnormalities and mitochondrial deletions in the remaining oocytes are increased resulting in decreased pregnancy rates and increased miscarriage rates. **Therefore, if women over age 35 fail to conceive for 6 months, infertility workup for them should be started earlier.** Ovarian reserve can be lost for other reasons also, like heavy smoking, ovarian surgery, chemotherapy or pelvic irradiation. Measurement of FSH and estradiol levels is probably the most cost-effective approach. Figure 13.2 shows a normal ovary with normal follicle on day 12 following menstruation.

## DIAGNOSTIC EVALUATION OF FEMALE INFERTILITY

### 1. Tests for Ovulation

Regularity in menstrual cycles is an index for ovulation; so, women with irregular cycles require tests for confirmation of ovulation and to evaluate the cause of anovulation. Figure 13.1 shows a normal ovary with normal follicle on day 12 following menstruation.

#### Basal body temperature (BBT)

BBT charting (Fig. 13.2) has long been used to identify ovulation. The test requires that a woman's morning oral temperature be graphically charted. Oral temperature is usually 97–98°F during the follicular phase. A postovulatory rise in progesterone increases basal temperature by approximately 0.4–0.8°F. This biphasic temperature pattern is strongly predictive of ovulation. Although it is inexpensive, it is insensitive in some women.

#### Ovulation predictor kits

These kits measure the concentration of luteinising hormone (LH) in urine by calorimetric assays. LH level

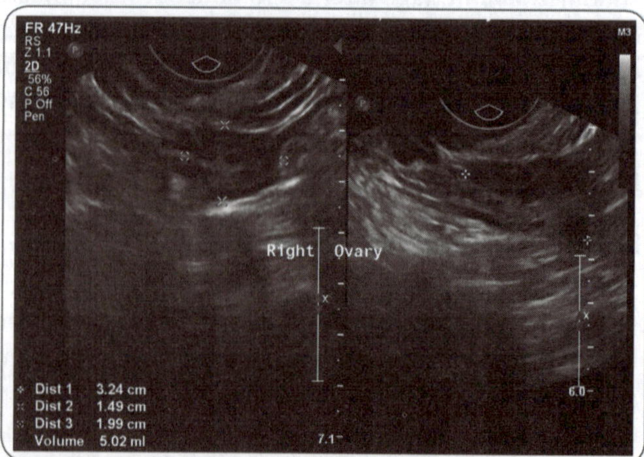


**Fig. 13.1** Normal ovary with normal follicle on day 12 following menstruation (*Source:* Swatee Halbe, Head of the Department of Radiology, Senior Consultant Interventional Radiologist, Apollo Speciality Hospitals, Chennai)

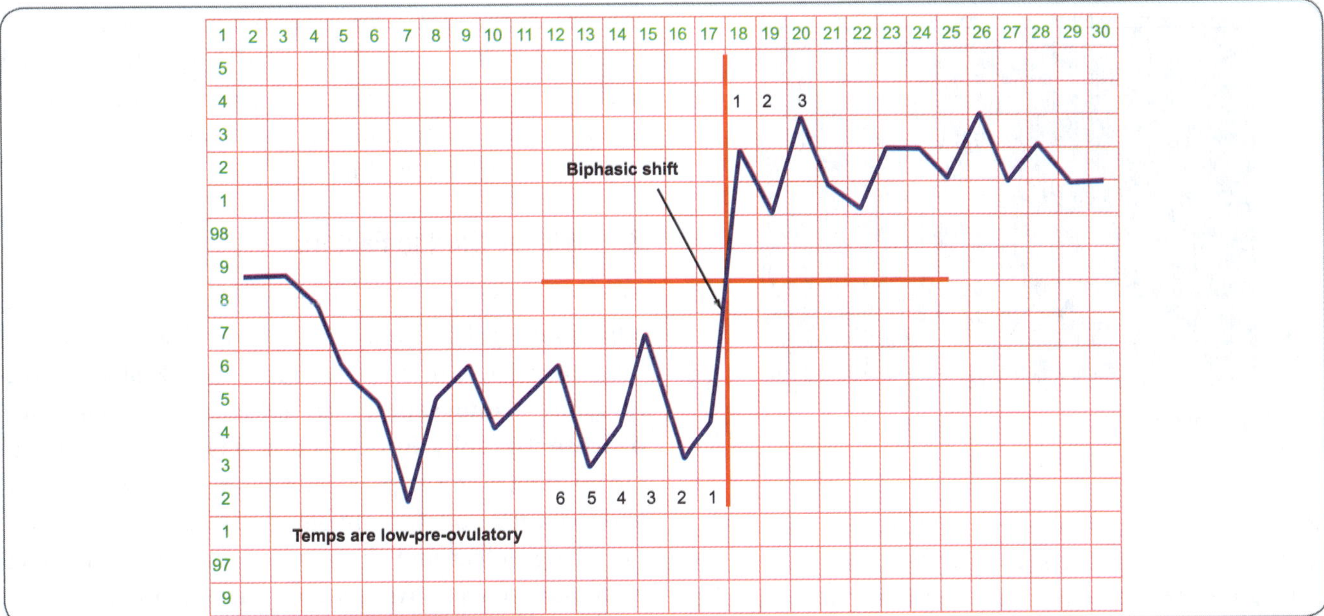


**Fig. 13.2** Basal body temperature chart—ovulatory pattern

of more than 40 milli IU suggest a surge. LH surge spans only 48–50 hours. The testing should be done daily beginning 2–3 days prior to the expected LH surge and should be performed daily. Mostly ovulation will occur the day following the urinary LH peak. This fact is used to determine the optimal time to have intercourse or insemination. Recently several ovulation kits have been developed similar to the pregnancy card test.

### Serum progesterone

In a 28-day cycle, serum is tested on the twenty-first day or 7 days after ovulation. Levels during the follicular phase is less than 2 ng/mL. Values above 4–6 ng/mL can be highly correlated with ovulation and progesterone production by the corpus luteum. A mid-luteal progesterone concentration of more than 9.4 ng/mL is predictive of higher pregnancy rates. Though it predicts ovulation correctly, it is not an absolute indicator of adequate luteal function.

### Endometrial biopsy

Adequate progesterone levels are required for endometrial preparation before implantation. Luteal phase defect (LPD) occurs when suboptimal progesterone production results in inadequate endometrial development. **Hence endometrial biopsy reflects both corpus luteal function and endometrial response.**

**Luteal phase defect (LPD)** is defined as a lag in the histological appearance of the endometrium of greater than 2 days relative to the actual day of the cycle determined retrospectively. This discrepancy in dating is termed as out-of-phase biopsy. LPD in infertile population is between 5 and 10%. It is based on the length of the previous cycle and the timing of the LH surge.

### Sonography

Serial sonographic evaluations can demonstrate the development of a mature antral follicle and its subsequent collapse during ovulation. Ovarian ultrasound to track follicular development rupture and corpus luteum formation may be useful in ovulation induction treatment cycles. Presence of cysts within the ovary in the luteal phase is known as luteinised unruptured follicles (LUF). Scanning in early follicular phase is used in assessing ovarian morphology. **A diagnosis of polycystic ovaries (PCO) (Fig. 13.3) is made if there are at least 12 follicles of 2–9 mm diameter or the ovarian volume is more than 10 cm$^3$.**

## 2. Tests for Tubal Patency

Tubal patency can be assessed by **HSG** (Fig. 13.4), **laparoscopy** and **saline infusion sonography**. The **ideal time to perform the test for tubal patency is the follicular phase of the cycle.** HSG will determine the presence of hydrosalpinx and whether tubal obstruction is complete or partial. If no dye enters the tube during HSG, a proximal tubal

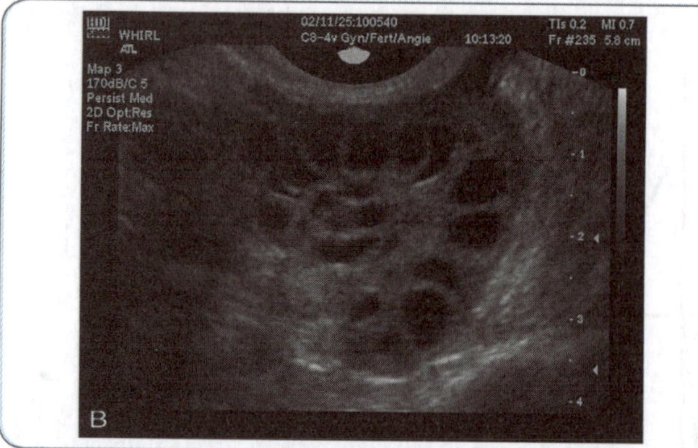


**Fig. 13.3** Polycystic ovary (*Source:* Chizen, D, Pierson, R, Glob. libr. women's med.)

occlusion is likely. However the diagnosis cannot be confirmed because the spasm of the tubes during the procedure may occlude the intramural portion of the tube. In such cases laparoscopy will reveal the patency of the tube. Complete or partial distal tubal block can also be determined by HSG. Laparoscopy determines the size of the hydrosalpinx and thickness of the wall of the tube after distension with dye and the presence and extent of pelvic adhesions. Chromopertubation during laparoscopy confirms the tubal patency. These tests are discussed in Table 13.3.

## 3. Tests for Uterine Factors

Abnormalities of the uterine cavity, intrauterine adhesions, polyps and submucous fibroids can be diagnosed by various methods like **HSG, saline infusion sonography, transvaginal sonography, hydrosonography, hysteroscopy** (Fig. 13.5) and **MRI. Ultrasonography** helps in determining the size, number and location of the myomas. HSG demonstrates the filling defect and this can be confirmed by direct visualisation with hysteroscopy. Hysteroscopy is the best tool to visualise the uterine cavity. Resection of the septum and polypectomy can be done in the same setting. Saline infusion sonography is superior to HSG

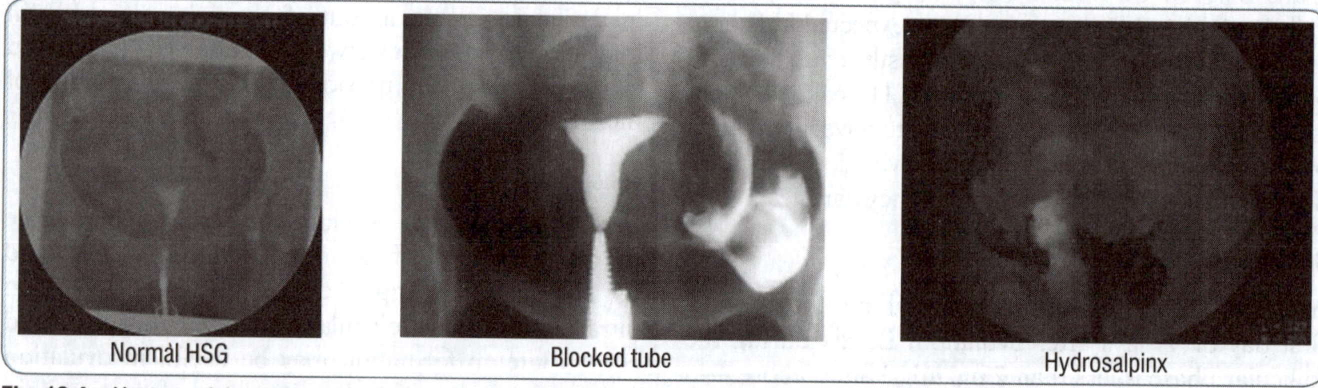


**Fig. 13.4** Hysterosalpingogram (*Source:* Radiopaedia/©Andrew Murphy, Alexandra Stanislavsky et.al.)

**Table 13.3** Test for tubal patency

| Diagnostic technique | Significance |
|---|---|
| **Hysterosalpingography**<br>Injection of radioopaque dye into the uterus followed by X-rays and fluoroscopy | Performed in follicular phase<br>Can visualise uterine septum, polyps, hydrosalpinx and site of tubal block<br>*Contraindicated in active bleeding,*<br>**High sensitivity for diagnosing tubal block* |
| **Saline infusion sonography**<br>Injection of saline into the uterine cavity | Test for tubal patency, differentiates endometrial polyp from submucous fibroid |
| **Transvaginal USG** | Can diagnose tubal block, polyp, septate uterus |
| **Falloposcopy**<br>Flexible microendoscopy of the tube performed along with hysteroscopy | Visualisation of tubal lumen, tubal cannulation under guidance<br>*Not routinely used for tubal patency and hydrosalpinx* |
| Laparoscopy | Tubes—condition of the fimbriae, tubal block, hydrosalpinx, peritubal adhesions<br>Ovaries—Polycystic ovaries, endometriotic cyst, adhesions, tubo-ovarian mass (tuberculosis, PID)<br>Uterus—myomas and uterine anomalies, peritoneal factors, endometriotic deposits in pouch of Douglas, adhesions |

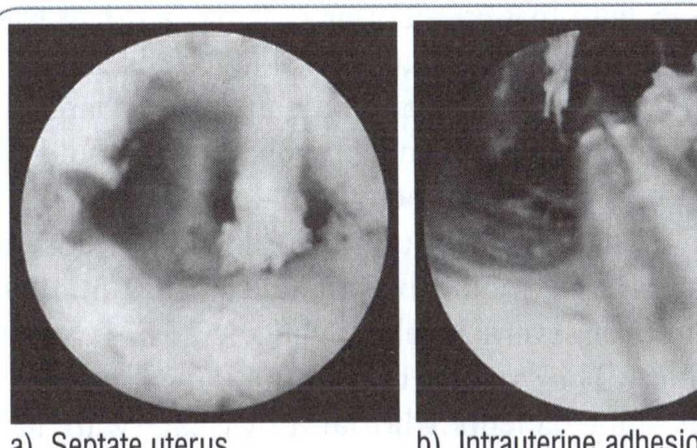


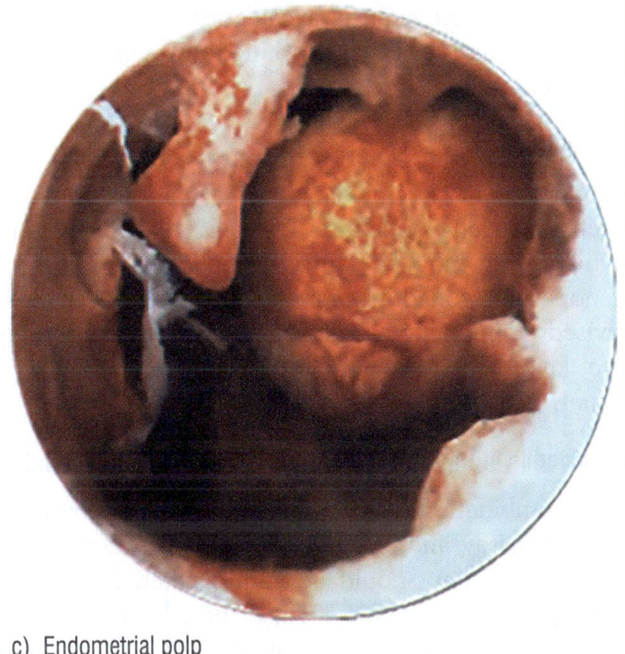


**Fig. 13.5** Uterine cavity: Hysteroscopic view (*Source:* Valle, R, Glob .libr. women' smed.)

in detecting uterine anomalies; it also delineates polyp better than transvaginal sonography (TVS).

#### Markers for receptive endometrium

Recent potential markers for uterine receptivity include osteopontin, cytokines, cell adhesion molecules and L-selectin ligand which have been proposed to mediate embryo attachment.

### 4. Test for Cervical Factors

#### Postcoital test (PCT)

Postcoital test is a subjective test, and is rarely indicated as a necessary part of the infertility investigation. It is done prior to ovulation. A normal PCT is one in which at least 5 motile sperms are visible in normal cervical mucus obtained from the cervical canal.

### 5. Tests for Ovarian Reserve

#### i. FSH

This is a simple and sensitive predictor of ovarian reserve and involves measurement of serum FSH performed on the 3rd day of the cycle. A value of more than 10 milliIU/mL indicates significant loss of ovarian reserve and needs more intense treatment.

#### ii. Estradiol

Estradiol measurement on day 3 decreases the incidence of false-negative results of FSH values alone. A value of more than 80 pg/mL on day 3 is considered abnormal.

#### iii. Anti-Müllerian hormone (AMH)

Anti-Müllerian hormone is the most recent circulating factor being used as a predictor of ovarian reserve. AMH is expressed by the fetal testes during male differentiation to prevent development of the Müllerian system. It is also expressed by granulosa cells of small preantral follicles. It plays a role in recruitment of a dominant follicle. Its expression is independent of cycle stage.Recent studies suggest that AMH levels correlate with ovarian primordial follicle number.

#### iv. Antral follicle count (AFC)

The number of small antral follicles reflects the size of the resting follicular pool. Antral follicles 2 and 10 mm are counted in both ovaries.The total count is between 10 and 20 in a woman of reproductive age. A count of less than10 predicts poor response to gonadotropin stimulation.

### 6. Test for Endometriosis

The gold standard for the diagnosis of endometriosis is visual inspection by laparoscopy preferably with histologic confirmation.

## TREATMENT OF INFERTILITY

### I. Treatment of Anovulation

#### Clomiphene citrate

This is the first line pharmacologic agent for treating women with oligomenorrhea and those with amenorrhea who have sufficient ovarian estrogen production. **The drug is given 50 mg/day for 5 days from the second day to the sixth day of the cycle after the onset**

**of spontaneous menses.** Presumptive evidence of ovulation can be obtained by sustained rise in BBT or measurement of an elevation of serum progesterone level (>3 ng/ml). If ovulation fails to occur with the 50 mg dose, the dosage is increased to 100 mg/day, for 5 days in the next treatment cycle. If ovulation does not occur with 100 mg/day, the dosage is increased to 150 mg in subsequent cycles but for not more than 6 cycles. In anovulatory women who respond to clomiphene, HSG should be performed if pregnancy does not occur after 3 months. The incidence of multiple gestation is 8%.

When the drug is used in normally ovulating women with unexplained infertility, the incidence of twin gestation is 20% and clinical spontaneous abortion is 15–20%. Formation of ovarian cyst is the major side effect of clomiphene citrate treatment. The cysts (5–10 cm) will regress spontaneously without therapy. Prolonged clomiphene therapy can cause estrogen deficiency with menopausal symptoms. Up to 10% of women treated with clomiphene citrate fail to ovulate. The use of dexamethasone may enhance the ovulation-inducing effect of clomiphene in women with elevated levels of DHEAS.

#### Letrozole

Previously, letrozole was an off-label drug and was not recommended for the management of anovulation by the Government of India.

Recently, the Govt. of India has reapproved letrozole for induction of ovulation. Aromatase inhibitors are efficacious as primary agents for ovulation induction. With letrozole, ovulation occurs in 90% of cases with a pregnancy rate of 40–50%. **Letrozole is given 2.5 mg/day for 5 days starting on the second day of the cycle.** The mechanism of action is that of inhibition of E2 production during the 5 days of administration with a negative feedback causing an increase in FSH levels much like the response to clomiphene citrate. Intraovarian androgen levels are also increased, which may enhance FSH sensitivity. Because it is short-acting, the problems of thick cervical mucus or thin endometrium associated with clomiphene citrate and increased incidence of multiple pregnancies are not seen. **It is valuable as second-line therapy in clomiphene citrate failures and in women with side effects or who show poor response to clomiphene.**

### II. Treatment of PCOD

Metformin, a biguanide used to control blood sugar in diabetics, has a role in ovulation induction in women with PCOS with insulin resistance. It has a direct role in inhibiting ovarian androgen steroidogenesis and acts on the endometrium, which are the major mechanisms that help with ovulation and pregnancy. It should be considered in obese women with impaired glucose tolerance or significant insulin resistance. The dose is 1500 mg/day but should be initiated at 500 mg and titrated up over several weeks. Lactic acidosis is a rare complication. The ovulation rate is 60%. In clomiphene citrate-resistant patients who fail to ovulate with 150 mg/day, 25% will respond to clomiphene citrate with metformin. Metformin is a category B substance for pregnancy and can be continued through the first trimester and beyond.

#### Gonadotropins

Gonadotropins are indicated for ovulation induction when estrogen levels are low (E2 < 30 pg/ml). Ovulation is induced with clomiphene and human menopausal gonadotropin (HMG). The patient is advised clomiphene citrate 50–100 mg/day from day 2 to day 6 of the cycle for 5 days. Injection HMG 75 units IM is added on days 3, 5, and 7.

#### Combination of HMG and human chorionic gonadotropin (hCG)

This combination should be preceded by baseline estradiol assay and USG. HMG 150 IU (2 ampoule 75 IU each)/day should be administered for 3 days and estradiol is to be repeated. If there is no response, HMG dosage should be increased by 50% for 3 days. USG should be performed every 2–3 days until the dominant follicle is more than 14 mm. The follicle should be monitored daily until it reaches 20 mm size. The serum E2 level should be 200 pg/mL for a mature follicle.

Following this, hCG 5000 IU IM should be administered to trigger ovulation. This can be followed by natural intercourse or IUI. 7 days later hCG 3000 IU should be administered.

Following this regimen, onset of menses is awaited or urine pregnancy test performed. The pregnancy rates are highest for young women who are hypo-estrogenic with low or normal gonadotropin levels and worse in older women and in those with anovulation with normal estrogen status.

#### *Complication of ovulation-inducing agents*

**Ovarian Hyperstimulation Syndrome (OHSS)** Significant OHSS occurs in 0.5% women receiving gonadotropins. It can be life-threatening causing massive fluid shifts, ascites, pleural effusion, electrolyte disturbances and thromboembolism.The cause may be large cystic ovaries, high E2 levels and ovarian substances (like vascular endothelial growth factor (VEGF)) which increase vascularity and vascular permeability. hCG triggers this syndrome and blood levels of hCG continue to stimulate the ovaries in OHSS.Therefore the syndrome is worse if pregnancy occurs. In the absence of pregnancy, OHSS abates within 1 week. OHSS has been classified into mild, moderate and severe forms.

Treatment of OHSS is largely supportive with judicious use of fluids and prevention of thrombosis. Correction of electrolyte disturbances and maintenance of urine output are important. OHSS can be prevented by avoiding excessive stimulation. GnRH agonist can be used instead of HMG as an ovulation-inducing drug because it is much shorter-acting and, unlike hCG, will clear from the circulation soon after ovulation.

#### GnRH

An alternative to the administration of HMG is GnRH therapy. GnRH is to be administered in a pulsatile manner at intervals of 1–2 hours. It is a peptide and cannot be given orally. It can be given as IV or by SC routes. Ovulation rates are 75–85% and pregnancy rates are 25–30%. The risk of hyperstimulation is greatly reduced (1%) as compared to HMG (20–25%).However the drug is very expensive.

#### Other therapeutic modifications

##### *1. Weight and lifestyle management*

Lifestyle changes in diet and exercise may improve metabolic parameters as well as ovulatory responses.

##### *2. Ovarian electrocauterisation*

In clomiphene-resistant women with PCOS, use of laparoscopic ovarian electrocautery is the alternative to gonadotropin therapy. The major advantage is that it decreases the risk of hyperstimulation and multiple pregnancies.Term pregnancy rate is 5% and the rate of multiple pregnancy is low.

### III. Management of Tubal Disease

Gomel and Winston were the first to employ microsurgery to perform tubocornual anastomosis (Fig. 13.6) for pathologic cornual occlusion and reversal of sterilisation—tubotubal anastomosis—to restore fertility. Microsurgery is performed using operating microscope, specialised instruments and fine suture materials which allows accurate tissue dissection, precise placement of sutures, minimised tissue trauma and restoring anatomical and physiological function of the tube as close to normal as possible.

**Principles of microsurgery**

The following should be strictly observed while performing a microsurgery.

- gentle handling of tissues,

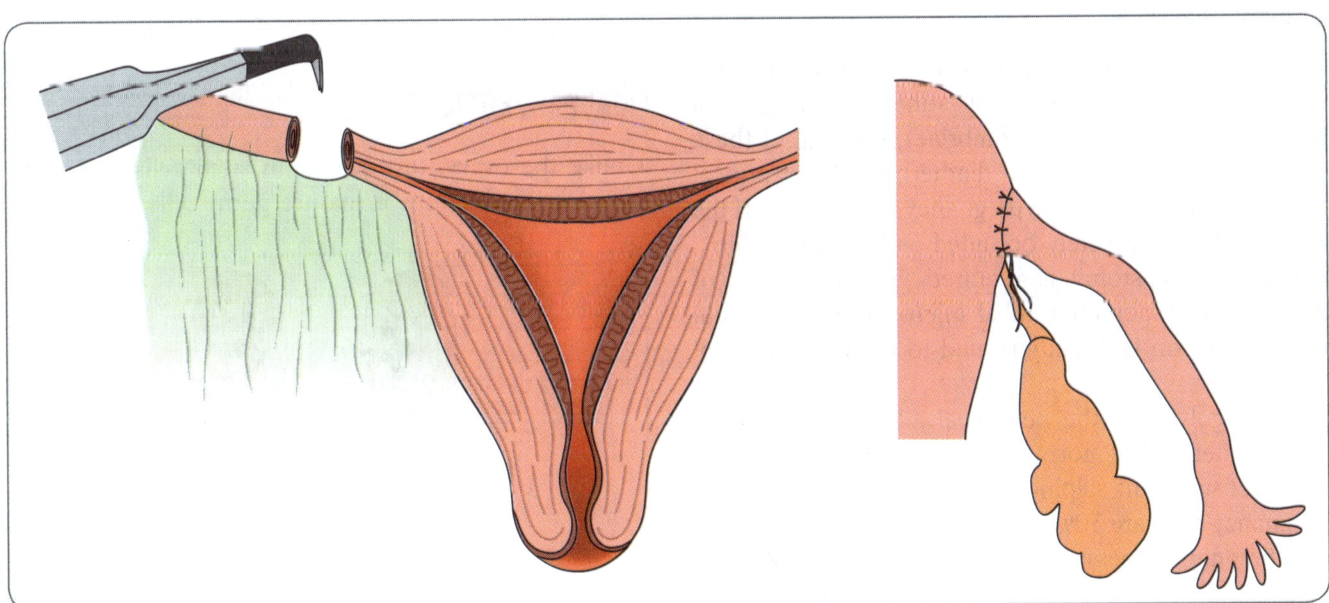

**Fig. 13.6** Tubocornual anastomosis

- continuous irrigation with Ringer lactate containing heparin over the operating site to prevent drying of the tissues and
- meticulous haemostasis by using both monopolar and bipolar cautery.

### A. Proximal tubal occlusion

Microsurgical tubocornual anastomosis gives a term-pregnancy rate of 37–56%.

Tubal implantation has a lower success rate.

Transcervical cannulation using hysteroscopic guidance will help to remove the mucous plugs in the cornual region.

### B. Midtubal block

Tubal sterilisation is the most common cause of midtubal block. About 1% women undergoing surgical sterilisation seek reversal of the procedure. Accidental death of a child, and change in marital and economic status are the most common reasons in our country.

The other causes of midtubal block are tuberculous salpingitis, endometriosis, SIN and tubal pregnancy.

**Laparotomy and microsurgical end-to-end anastomosis has best results and remains a method of choice for reversal of sterilisation and pathological midtubal block.** The anastomosis is done in 2 layers with 8–0 ethilon under magnification.

Success rate depends on the type of anastomosis, length of the tube after reconstruction, interval between sterilisation and reversal surgery.

### C. Distal tubal block

If the fimbriae of the distal end of the tube are normal with only partial occlusion by adhesions or fimbrial bridges (conglutination of fimbriae), removal of these adhesions can be done by diathermy. Microsurgical fimbrioplasty will improve pregnancy rate by 60%. If the distal end is completely occluded as by hydrosalpinx, a cuff salpingostomy is required. The incidence of ectopic pregnancy after tubal microsurgery for distal tubal occlusion is directly related to pre-existing tubal damage.

Salpingolysis of the peritoneal adhesions, with the tubal lumen being normal results in 64% pregnancy rate. But with cuff salpingostomy for hydrosalpinx, the pregnancy rates are 30% with 10% of ectopic pregnancy.

If pregnancy does not occur within 6–12 months after surgery, HSG should be performed. If tubal occlusion recurs, repeat surgical procedure is not advised. Tubal surgeries are contraindicated in tuberculous salpingitis even after completion of ATT. Women with extensive tubal disease will benefit more from an IVF procedure. So the extent and location of the intrinsic and extrinsic tubal disease should be ascertained by HSG and laparoscopy to determine whether IVF or tubal microsurgery offers a better prognosis.

**Treatment of Tubal Occlusion**

**Proximal tubal occlusion**
- Hysteroscopic cannulation
- Microsurgical tubocornual anastomosis

**Midtubal block**
- Isthmo-isthmic anastomosis (Fig. 13.7)
- Isthmo-ampullary anastomosis
- Ampullo-ampullary anastomosis

**Distal tubal occlusion**
- Fimbrioplasty
- Cuff salpingostomy
- Salpingectomy and in vitro fertilisation (IVF)

## IV. Treatment of Uterine Factors

Apart from developmental anomalies, intrauterine adhesions can cause infertility. Hysteroscopic adhesiolysis improves fertility rate. Perioperative antibiotics and postoperative combined OC pills are given to prevent recurrence of adhesion and for rapid proliferation of endometrium at the operative site. In septate uterus, pregnancy rate is low in open metroplasty when compared to hysteroscopic intervention. Pregnancy rate after polypectomy is 78%. The advantage of hysteroscopy is that it can be used for diagnosis and treatment at the same sitting.

## MALE INFERTILITY

Unlike the ovary, testes contain stem cells that allow ongoing production of mature germ cells throughout

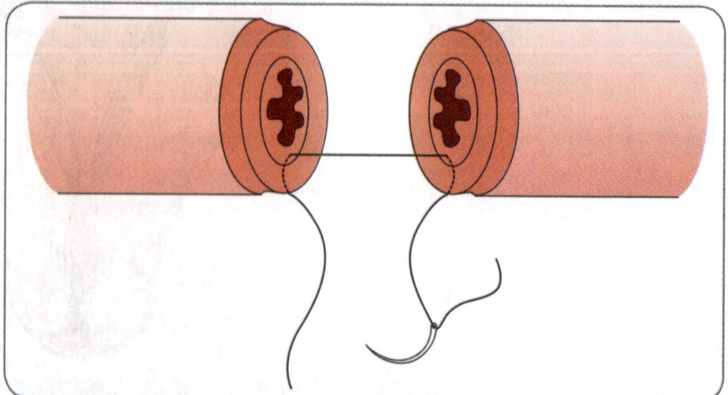

Fig. 13.7 Isthmo-isthmic anastomosis

a male's life. In a fertile male, approximately 100–200 million sperms are produced each day. It takes 70 days for the production of sperms to be complete and a further 12–21 days for the sperms to be transported into the epididymis. Further maturation and development of motility takes place at the epididymis. **Hence the results of a semen analysis reflect events during the past 3 months.**

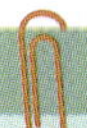

**Causes of Male Infertility**

The causes can roughly be categorised as
- abnormalities of sperm production
- abnormalities of sperm function
- obstruction of the ductal outflow tract.

## Male History—Key Points

- Pubertal development
- Beard growth
- Sexual function
- H/o mumps
- H/o cryptorchidism
- Trauma to testis
- Torsion of testis
- H/o varicocele
- H/o chemotherapy or local radiation therapy
- H/o diabetes and Hypertension
- DRUGS: Cimetidine, tetracycline, anabolic steriods, gentamicin, erythromycin and spironolactone.

### Detailed physical examination of a male patient

| Male partner | Secondary sexual characters<br>Beard growth<br>Axillary and pubic hair<br>Male pattern balding<br>Gynecomastia<br>Local examination<br>Penile urethra<br>Testicular length<br>Testicular mass<br>Epididymis—non-tender and soft<br>Prostate—smooth and non-tender<br>Both vas—palpable pampiniform plexus of veins. |
|---|---|

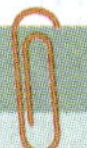

**Factors Responsible for Male Infertility**

1. Disorders of spermatogenesis (50%)
2. Obstruction of the efferent ducts (30%)
3. Disorders of sperm motility (15%)
4. Sexual dysfunction
5. Unexplained (15%)

## Etiology

Male infertility can be subdivided into pretesticular, testicular and post-testicular factors.

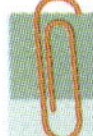

**Factors for Male Infertility**

**Pretesticular (Hormonal)**
- Hypothalamic disorder
- Kallman's syndrome
- Hyperprolactinaemia
- Hypothyroidism
- Diabetes

**Testicular (Primary testicular disorders)**
- Chromosomal defect (Klinefelter syndrome, Kartagener syndrome)
- Cryptorchidism
- Varicocele
- Orchitis (mumps, TB, gonorrhea, trauma)
- Drugs (antihypertensives, calcium channel blockers, spironolactone and cimetidine)

**Post-testicular (Duct obstruction)**
- Congenital absence
- Inflammatory block (gonococcal, tubercular)
- Surgical trauma
- Infections (chlamydia, mycoplasma causing DNA fragmentation of sperms, decreased motility and apoptosis)
- Antibodies to sperms

## Diagnostic Evaluation

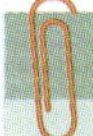

**Diagnostic Evaluation of Male Infertility**

1. Seminal analysis
2. Hormonal evaluation—FSH, LH
3. Sperm penetration test
4. Genetic studies
5. Sperm–cervical mucus contact test
6. USG scrotum
7. Colour flow Doppler
8. Scrotal thermography
9. Vasogram
10. Testicular biopsy

### 1. Semen analysis

The male partner needs to refrain from any sexual activity for at least two days but not more than 10 days before collection. Longer or shorter periods of abstinence may result in a lower sperm count or decreased sperm motility. Samples produced after two days of abstinence will have the greatest forward velocity, **Percentage of live sperm decreases with the increasing abstinence**. There should be no smoking, drinking or drugs during the ten days preceding the sperm collection. The following specific things could affect the quality of sperm sample.

**Semen Analysis—WHO 2010**

| | |
|---|---|
| Volume | >1.5 mL |
| pH | 7.2–7.8 |
| Viscosity | <3 (scale 0–4) |
| Count | >40 million/ejaculate |
| Sperm concentration | 20 million/mL |
| Motility | >50% with progressive motilities |
| Morphology | >30% |
| Viability | >75% |
| WBC | <1 million/mL |
| Round cells | <5 million/mL |

**Medicines** Cimetidine, sulfa, estrogen and testosterone. caffeine, alcohol, cocaine, tobacco and marijuana can interfere with analysis.

Mastrubation is the usual way of semen specimen collection. Any lubricants containing spermicidal agents should not be used. First part of the ejaculate should be collected directly in the sample cup within one hour of ejaculation. The specimen should be kept in plastic bag and kept as close as possible to body temperature.

Abnormal semen pattern and their causes are listed in Table 13.4.

**Table 13.4** Causes of abnormal semen

| Finding | Cause |
|---|---|
| Low semen volume | Ejaculatory dysfunction<br>Retrograde ejaculation<br>Hypogonadism<br>Poor collection technique |
| Acidic semen | Ejaculatory duct obstruction<br>Congenital absence of the vas deferens and/or seminal vesicles |
| Azoospermia or oligospermia | Genetic disorders<br>Endocrine disorders<br>Varicocele<br>Cryptorchidism<br>Infections<br>Exposure to toxins, radiation, medications<br>Genital tract obstruction<br>Idiopathic |
| Decreased motility (Asthenospermia) | Prolonged abstinence<br>Immunologic factors: antisperm antibodies<br>Partial genital tract obstruction<br>Infection<br>Sperm structural defects<br>Idiopathic |
| Abnormal morphology (Teratospermia) | Varicocele<br>Genetic disorder<br>Cryptorchidism<br>Infection<br>Exposure to toxins, radiation, medications<br>Idiopathic |

### 2. Hormonal evaluation

Endocrine evaluation is appropriate for individuals with abnormal sperm concentrations or signs of androgen deficiency.

- Primary hypogonadism shows decreased testosterone, increased FSH and LH.
- Secondary hypogonadism shows low testosterone, FSH and LH.
- A low LH level in the presence of oligospermia and normal testosterone level indicate exogenous steroid use.
- Serum PRL level should be assessed in men with low testosterone level.

### 3. Genetic testing

Genetic abnormalities may affect sperm production or transport. Genetic testing is indicated in men with azoospermia and severe oligospermia. The most common genetic disorder is cystic fibrosis. A karyotype may reveal abnormalities like Klinefelter syndrome (47 XXY) or chromosomal inversion and translocations. Microdeletions of Y chromosome are associated with abnormalities of testicular development and more frequently with spermatogenesis. It has been found that miscarriage rates and pregnancy loss rates are more frequent when the paternal age is more than 40 years.

### 4. Aspirations

In men with azoospermia, if obstruction is suspected, sperms should accumulate just before obstruction, e.g., men with congenital absence of vas or who had vasectomy have a swollen epididymis where constant production of sperm results in a small collection. Percutaneous epididymal sperm aspiration and microsurgical epididymal sperm aspiration procedures can retrieve motile healthy sperm.

### 5. Testicular biposy

It is indicated in azoospermia to distinguish between testicular failure and obstruction in the vas. It also reveals whether the seminiferous tubules are normal but unstimulated by anterior pituitary or are incapable of function due to primary gonadal failure. A biopsy can also diagnose genital TB. Apart from chromosomal and histological study, the testicular tissue provides cryopreservation for ART. The spermatozoa as well as spermatids extracted from the testis can be used for ICSI.

### 6. Ultrasound scanning

Ultrasound scanning of the scrotum detects scrotal volume and hydrocele. Colour flow Doppler and scrotal thermography detect varicocele. Vasogram is useful when normal FSH level is associated with azoospermia.

### 7. Assays of sperm function

**Mannose fluorescent assay** It is a receptor assay based on the ability of the sperm to recognise the zona pellucida of an oocyte; it is dependent on a number of sugars including mannose on the zonal surface.

#### *Hemi-zonal assay*

It is a technique for analysing the sperm's ability to bind to the zona pellucida.

#### *Sperm penetration assay*

A normal sperm is capable of penetrating the zone-free hamster egg showing its fertilising capacity. The test is obsolete.

Sperm agglutination tests, immmobilsation tests and immunoglobulin-specific assays are available to detect immunological defects in the semen.

#### *Sperm cervical mucus contact test*

Equal quantity of semen and mucus is mixed so that there is no interface. In the presence of antibodies, more than 25% sperms show jerky or shaky movements.Cross-checking with donor semen will indicate the source of antibiodies whether it is cervical or seminal antibodies.

#### *Hypo-osmotic swelling test (HOS)*

**This is done in IVF for selecting best sperms for fertilisation.**The sperms are treated with hypo osmotic saline. If the sperm membrane is intact, the sperms swell up and coiling occurs, and these are the best sperms.

## TREATMENT OF MALE INFERTILITY

Management of male infertility begins with sexual education and psychological counselling followed by other medical and surgical means as and when necessary. This is followed by assessment of coital function, semen report and result of postcoital test.

1. Education—sexual counselling
2. Substance abuse—avoidance of tobacco and alcohol
3. Antioxidants,Vit E 100 mg—improve semen parameters
4. Pentoxifylline 400 mg tid—improves sperm motility
5. Reducing heat around the scrotum—Advice to avoiding hot bath and to wearing loose cotton underwear
6. Treating diabetes and thyroid disorders
7. Treating conditions like prostatitis, epididymo-orchitis and STD with antibiotics. Doxycycline100 mg bd for 6 weeks is beneficial for chlamydial infection.
8. Carnitidine 3 g/day for 6 months to prevent sperm DNA damage and to improve quality of sperms.
9. Premature ejaculation—Selective serotonin re-uptake inhibitors—Dapoxetine 30–60 mg 1 hour before sexual act.
10. Hormonal therapy
    i) hCG 3000 IU IM/thrice weekly for 12 weeks.
    ii) FSH—37.5–75 mg subunit thrice a week with follow-up with serum testosterone and semen analysis. It takes 6–9 months to produce normal counts. Pregnancy rate is 40%.
    iii) Testosterone—25–50 mg/day orally improves testicular functions. Higher dose of 100–150 mg/day suppresses spermatogenesis. After 3 months, rebound phenomenon occurs with improved spermatogenesis.
    iv) Clomiphene—25 mg/day for 25 days cyclically for 3–6 cycles. It is recommended for hypogonadal infertility.
    v) GnRH can be used in hypothalamic failure in a dose of 5–20 mcg every two hours. It is usually delivered by subcutaneous pump. Nasal spray is also available.
    vi) Tamoxifen 10 mg/day for 6 months is effective in some men.
    vii) Dexamethasone—0.5 mg/day or 50 mg prednisolone daily for 10 days in each cycle for 3–6 months is recommended in the presence of sperm antibodies. This treatment has a successful pregnancy rate of 25–40%. In prolonged therapy, osteopenia and avascular necrosis of the head of the femur occur. If steroids are contraindicated, anti-inflammatory agents such as naproxen 50 mg bd may lower antibody levels.
    viii) Sildenafil—25–100 mg 1 hour before intercourse improves erectile function. Since ischemic heart disease is reported, it should be prescribed with care. This drug is effective in 50–70%. It is contraindicated in diabetic

retinopathy, patients on antihypertensive drugs and cardiac diseases.

11. Penile implant AMS 700, a 3-piece inflatable penile prosthesis, is now available.
12. Surgical treatment
    - Varicocele—varicocelectomy has no role in improving male infertility.
    - Surgical correction improves the semen quality in 60–70% of undescended testis in childhood.
    - Vasovasal anastomosis and vasoepididymal anastomosis are successful options in obstruction of the vas.
    - Microsurgical vasovasostomy is the treatment of choice for reanastomosis following vasectomy.
13. Artificial insemination with husband's semen for 4 cycles has a success rate of 40% with 10% success per cycle. The results are better if combined with ovulation induction for multiple ovulation.

## 1. Intra-uterine Insemination (IUI)

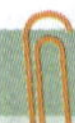

**Indications for IUI**

1. Oligospermia
2. Impotency
3. Premature ejaculation, retrograde ejaculation
4. Hypospadiasis
5. Antisperm antibodies in cervical mucus
6. Unexplained infertility
7. HIV-positive male or female
8. In genetic and chromosomal abnormalities. X-Y fractionation of sperms.

**Indication for IUI with donor semen**

- Azoospermia
- Immunological factors not correctable
- Genetic disease of the husband

## 2. Intracytoplasmic Sperm Injection (ICSI)

Proved successful in case of immobile sperms and decreased sperm count less than 5 million/mL with a pregnancy rate of 30–40%. A single sperm is injected into the cytoplasm of the oocyte which is then incubated overnight.

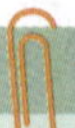

**Indications for ICSI**

1. Sperm count less than 5 million/cc
2. Absent or reduced sperm motility
3. Abnormal sperm morphology
4. Previous IVF failure
5. Unexplained sterility

## 3. Gametocyte Intra-Fallopian Transfer (GIFT)

In this technique, following ovarian stimulation 2 eggs are retrieved and mixed with 50,000 sperms and transferred to each of the Fallopian tubes.

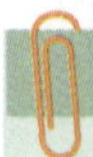

**Indications for GIFT**

1. Unexplained infertility
2. IUI failure
3. Male infertility

Both the tubes must be patent.The results are better with GIFT than IVF. The main disadvantage is that fertilisation cannot be confirmed. Some prefer GIFT for religious reasons.

## 4. Zygote Intra-Fallopian Transfer (ZIFT)

ZIST is similar to GIFT except that the eggs and sperms are combined in the lab, then inserted into the Fallopian tubes at the zygote stage and it requires laparoscopy as in GIFT technique.

## 5. Microassisted Fertilisation Technique (MAF)

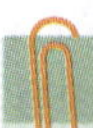

**Indications for MAF**

1. Oligospermia and asthenospermia
2. IVF or GIFT failure due to fertilisation failure
3. Sperm binds to zona pellucida but fails to penetrate due to spermal antibodies or antibodies to zona pellucida.

## 6. Assisted Reproductive Techniques (ART)

ART refers to any fertility treatment in which the gametes (sperms and ova) are manipulated. All fertility procedures that involve manipulation of gametes, zygotes, or embryos to achieve conception are known as ARTs. IVF accounts for more than 99% of all ART procedures. The process of IVF involves ovarian stimulation to produce multiple follicles, retrieval of the oocytes from the ovaries, oocyte fertilisation in vitro in the laboratory, embryo incubation in the laboratory, and transfer of embryos into a woman's uterus through the cervix. The required medications for IVF include gonadotropins to stimulate follicle development, a gonadotropin releasing hormone analogue (agonist or antagonist) to prevent premature ovulation to prevent follicular development, and hCG to initiate the final maturation of oocytes prior to their retrieval.

IVF provides the tools necessary to by-pass the normal mechanisms of gamete transport, fertilisation, and embryo transport. After oocyte retrieval, daily progesterone supplementation is necessary to ensure appropriate secretory changes in the endometrium and to support the potential pregnancy; if conception occurs, supplementation is continued until at least 10 weeks of gestation.

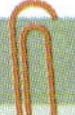

**Indications for ART**

The common indications for ART procedures include the following:
- Abnormal Fallopian tubes: Blocked tubes or absent tubes (surgical removal)
- Endometriosis adversely affecting tubo-ovarian pick-up function or distorting the tubes
- Idiopathic or unexplained infertility
- Male subfertility
- Immunologic infertility
- Failure of ovulation—endometriosis and ovarian cancer

### Investigations prior to ART

- Thyroid function tests, and tests to diagnose diabetes
- Serum FSH on day 3 of cycle. FSH >25 mIU/mL indicates poor prognosis
- Serum estradiol on day 3 of cycle. Serum estradiol >75 pg/mL indicates poor prognosis
- 100 mg CC is administered from day 5 to day 9 and FSH is repeated on day 10. FSH values must be the same as on day 3 of the cycle.
- Tests for chlamydial infection. Serologic evidence of chlamydial infection is associated with reduced birth rates and increased perinatal loss.
- Zona-free hamster oocyte penetration test to assess fertilising capacity of sperm (optional)
- Enhanced sperm penetration test using TEST- yolk buffer
- Testing both partners for antisperm antibodies
- Assess uterine cavity –HSG/hysteroscopy/ transvaginal sonography. Hydrosalpinx reduces IVF success rates by the 50%. Success rate increases after excision of hydrosalpinx.
- Complete seminogram and treatment of male partner prior to ART procedure
- Diagnostic laparoscopy to assess tubal patency and treat any subtle causes of infertility such as lysis of adhesions, treatment of endometriosis, excision of hydrosalpinx or ligation of medial end of the tube.

Success rates with IVF depend on the etiology of infertility and the age of the female partner.The chance of conception with one IVF cycle depends on the number and quality of embryos transferred and can be as high as 40% to 50% with a 30% rate of multiple gestations and at least a 15% rate of spontaneous abortion.

## 7. Surrogacy

This is one of the most expensive ART procedures. Traditional surrogate is a woman who gets artificially inseminated with the father's sperm.She then carries the baby and delivers for the couple. She is the biological mother because her egg was used for fertilisation.

## 8. Gestational Surrogates

Here, eggs and sperm from the couple are fertilised artificially and the embryo is placed in the uterus of the gestational surrogate. She then carries the baby until birth. She does not have genetic ties with the baby. Recently, the Govt. of India has brought in a draft legislation to restrict the use of surrogacy.

Some of the other techniques include the following.
1. Microsurgical epididymal sperm aspiration (MESA)
2. Percutaneous epididymis sperm aspiration (PESA)
3. Epididymal or testicular aspiration
4. IVF

Today, greater number of men and women are seeking infertility treatment due to increased public awareness of infertility and changes in social acceptance of infertility, improvements in availability, range of fertility treatments and improvements in physicians' ability to evaluate and diagnose infertility.While opportunities to prevent infertility are limited,encouragement should be given to the young to engage in safe sexual practices and limit exposure to risk of sexually transmitted infection. For teenage girls, Rubella immunisation programmes and HPV vaccination programmes should be established. It is important to raise public awareness about the decline in fertility beyond 35 years of age and the need for preconceptional folic acid supplementation for women to reduce the risk of neural tubal defects.There is convincing evidence that smoking whether active or passive affects reproductive performance in women and men as well as increases the risk of small-for-gestational-age infants, stillbirth and infant mortality.

**Case study**

*A 35-year-old lady, living with her husband, presents with history of vaginal discharge associated with pruritis and dysuria. She has had similar episodes in the past and was treated symptomatically. But she has been getting this attack frequently. She has one child who is 7 years old. She is planning for her next pregnancy.*

*a) What is the probable diagnosis?*

*b) What investigations are required for confirming the diagnosis?*

*c) How would you manage this patient?*

## RECAP

- The chance of pregnancy in a normal fertile population is 85% after 1 year of unprotected intercourse and 92% after 2 years.
- Couples should be referred only after 1 year of trying unless there is an obvious risk factor for infertility.
- Irregular cycles are suggestive of ovulatory dysfunction—polycystic ovarian syndrome is the most common cause.
- Serum progesterone level >30 nmol/L in the luteal phase of the cycle is indicative of ovulation.
- Unless there is a strong suspicion of pelvic pathology, a hysterosalpingogram is a reasonable first line test of tubal factor infertility.
- Fibroids may be associated with infertility if the cavity of the uterus is distorted. Hysteroscopy or hydrosonography are useful ancillary investigations if uterine abnormality is suspected.
- Tubal patency and morphology of the endosalpinx can be studied by HSG, laparoscopic chromopertubation, Falloposcopy, salpingoscopy.
- The prognosis for fertility after tubal reconstruction depends upon the amount of damage to the tube as well as the site of the obstruction.
- The success rate following reversal of sterilisation is more with isthmo-isthmial anastomosis.
- In women with unexplained infertility, use of controlled ovarian stimulation and intrauterine insemination should be the initial treatment.
- Laparoscopy combined with hysteroscopy forms one set of investigation to detect the cause of female infertility. This is cost-effective and saves time.
- Andrology has expanded into extensive male investigation, and study of the morphology and function of the sperms by adopting techniques such as semen wash, IUI, MAF, MESA, ICSI and IVF.
- For IVF with and without ICSI, the delivery rate per cycle in which ova are retrieved is as high as 50% depending upon the age of the patient.

## REVIEW QUESTIONS

### Long-Answer Question

Define infertility? What are the causes of female infertility? Write the etiology, investigations and management of tubal factor in infertility?

### Short-Answer Questions:

1. What is ovarian hyperstimulation syndrome (OHSS)? Discuss briefly about the diagnosis and management of the same.
2. Enumerate the uterine factors for infertility.

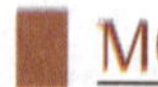

### MCQs

**1. Gonococcal infection is associated with**

a) Proximal tubal occlusion
b) Bilateral hydrosalpinx
c) Salpingitis isthmica nodosa
d) Endometritis

2. **Chlamydial infection is mostly asymptomatic but can cause**
   a) Proximal tubal occlusion
   b) Fimbrial occlusion
   c) Perisalpingitis
   d) Tubo-ovarian mass
3. **The following are the causes of intrauterine adhesions except**
   a) Tuberculous endometritis
   b) Septate uterus
   c) Following vigorous curettage
   d) Intrauterine contraceptive device
4. **The management of tuberculous salpingitis is by**
   a) Tuboplasty
   b) In vitro fertilisation
   c) Antituberculous treatment + In vitro fertilisation
   d) Intrauterine insemination

### Further Reading

Dispiezio sardo a mazzon 1, bramantes et al. Hysteros myomectomy a comprehensive review of surgical techniques-human reproductive update 2008. 14:101:119.

Dubey, AK. Infertility: diagnosis, management and IVF. New Delhi: Jaypee Brothers; 2012.

Gleicher N, Barad D. Unexplained infertility does it really exist? Human reproduction. 2006; 21(8):1951–1955.

Gomel V. Microsurgery in female infertility. 3rd ed. New Delhi: Little Brown & Co.; 1983.

Hoffman BL, Schorge JO, Schaffer JI, Halvorson LM, Bradshaw KD, Cunningham FG. Williams gynecology. 2nd ed. New York: McGraw-Hill; 2012. 265 p.

Hunt RB. Text and atlas of female infertility surgery. 3rd ed. Maryland Heights: Mosby; 2016.

Lentz G, Lobo R, Gershensen D, Katz V. Comprehensive gynecology. 6th ed. Maryland Heights: Mosby; 2012.

Padubitri VG, Daftary S. Shaw's textbook of gynecology. 16th ed. Gurgaon: Elsevier India; 2014.

Rao K. The infertility manual. 2nd ed. New Delhi: Jaypee Brothers; 2005.

Somighind E, Vercellini P, Daguati R, Pasin R, De Giorgio O, Crosignani PG. Fibriods & female reproduction:a critical analysis of the evidence. Human Reproduction Update. 2007, Sep–Oct;13(5):465–76.

Strauss J, Barbieri R. Yen & Jaffe's Reproductive endocrinology. 7th ed. Philadephia: Saunders; 2013.

Tripathy SN.The uterus manual. New Delhi: Jaypee Brothers; 2009.

# Chapter 14

# Polycystic Ovarian Syndrome

## At a Glance

Severe Forms of PCOS
Etiology of PCOS
Pathophysiology
Gonadotropin
Insulin Resistance
Androgens
Sex Hormone Binding Globulin (SHBG)
Anovulation
Signs and Symptoms
Diagnosis
Consequences of Polycystic Ovarian Syndrome
Treatment
Management of Obesity
Treatment of Oligo-ovulation and Anovulation
Management of Hirsutism
Surgery

## INTRODUCTION

PCOS (polycystic ovarian syndrome) is a common endocrinopathy but it is poorly understood. It is a disorder of unexplained hyperandrogenic chronic anovulation and is heterogeneous in etiology. Despite evidence of familial clustering, no clear molecular or genetic mechanism has been identified to explain the vast majority of cases.

PCOS was first diagnosed in situ on the basis of enlarged ovaries by pelvic examination combined with history of amenorrhea and hirsutism. An abnormal morphology was subsequently confirmed. The ovary was viewed as the prime culprit of the syndrome and assays confirming increased androgen excretion and circulating levels appeared to validate this belief. The discovery of hyperinsulinemia and decreased sensitivity to insulin in women with PCOS led to a de-emphasis on the ovary as a diagnostic criterion. This concept was summarised in the 1990 consensus conference of the National Institute of Child Health and Human Development (**NICHD**) and National Institutes of Health (**NIH**) (NIH-NICHD) on PCOS and has been upheld in similar proceedings in recent years.

### Clinical Importance

The criteria for diagnosis of PCOS are hyperandrogenism and oligo-ovulation with the exclusion of other potential causes such as congenital adrenal hyperplasia, Cushing's syndrome and androgen-secreting tumours.

**Incidence** PCOS is the most common endocrine disorder of women in the reproductive age and affects approximately 4–12%. Although symptoms of androgen excess may vary among ethnicities, PCOS appears to equally affect all races and nationalities.

**Definition** The definition of PCOS includes women who are **anovulatory** or have **irregular periods** as well as **hyperandrogenism** (as determined by signs such as hirsutism or elevated levels of androgens, testosterone or dehydroepiandrosterone (DHEA) in the absence of enzymatic disorders) or tumours. This diagnosis does not require findings of polycystic ovaries on ultrasound. A conference in Rotterdam had come up with a new definition in 2004. To include two out of three of the following:

1. Oligo- or anovulation
2. Clinical and/or biochemical signs of hyperandrogenism
3. Polycystic ovaries (with exclusion of related disorders)

**Women with PCOS may have all 3 findings but it requires any two of three to make a diagnosis of PCOS.** 95% of women who have features of anovulation and hyperandrogenism have polycystic ovaries. The diagnosis of PCOS is currently being made on the basis of

- finding enlarged ovaries greater than 10 $cm^3$ and
- the presence of 10 or more peripherally oriented cystic structures (2–8 mm) surrounding a dense stroma. This isolated finding alone should not be

confused with PCOS; it may be a risk factor for other traits of PCOS like insulin resistance and cardiovascular disease.

## SEVERE FORMS OF PCOS

More severe forms of PCOS include

- **Ovarian hyperthecosis** This is a rare condition characterised by nests of luteinised theca cells distributed throughout the ovarian stroma. Affected women exhibit severe **hyperandrogenism** and may occasionally have **frank virilisation** such as clitoromegaly, temporal balding and deepening of voice. They have greater degree of insulin resistance and acanthosis nigricans.
- **Hairan syndrome** (**H**yper**A**ndrogenic **I**nsulin-**R**esistant **A**canthosis **N**igricans) This is uncommon and consists of marked **hyperandrogenism, severe insulin resistance** and **acanthosis nigricans.** It may represent either a variant of PCOS or a distinct genetic syndrome.

## ETIOLOGY OF PCOS

The exact cause of PCOS is unknown. A genetic basis that is both multifactorial and polygenetic is suspected because affected individuals usually have similarly affected sisters and mothers. Autosomal dominant inheritance has been noticed in first-degree male relatives of women with PCOS. Dysregulation of the *CYP11a* gene is seen in patients with PCOS.

## PATHOPHYSIOLOGY

PCOS appears to manifest itself during adolescence and is associated with increased weight gain during puberty. Prior to puberty, there appears to be two periods of increased ovarian growth.

The first is the **adrenarche** in response to increased concentration of circulating androgens and the second is just before and during puberty due to rising gonadotropin (GT) levels and the actions of growth hormone (GH), insulin-like growth factor - 1 (IGF-1) and insulin on the ovary. Obese premenarcheal girls with polycystic ovaries have larger uterine and ovarian volumes than obese postmenarcheal girls with normal ovaries. Obesity leads to hyperinsulinism which causes both hyperandrogenemia and increased IGF-1, which in turn augment the ovarian response to GT.

> **Clinical Importance**
>
> After menarche, it is common for the menstrual cycle to be erratic for several months. If the irregularity persists beyond 2 years, there is a high chance that the adolescent girl has PCOS.

As mentioned above, GT, insulin resistance, androgens and SHBG levels play a role in the development of PCOS. The following description will give an insight into the role of these four factors in the development of PCOS.

### Gonadotropin

Women with PCOS have a normal serum FSH. LH is under the influence of pulsatile release of GnRH. The estradiol should be primed before it becomes responsive to GnRH and LH. But FSH is under the inhibitory effect of inhibin which acts by a negative feedback loop from the ovaries. Therefore in estrogen deficiency such as weight-related amenorrhea, LH secretion is lower than FSH. The midcycle surge that is primed by rising estradiol secretion from the ovary results in a greater release of LH than FSH.

> **Clinical Importance**
>
> - An elevated serum LH (greater than 10 IU/L) in the follicular phase of the cycle suggests PCOS.
> - 40% of patients with elevated serum LH have higher risk of developing infertility. LH–FSH ratios are elevated and rise above 2 : 1 in 60% of patients.

### Insulin Resistance

Insulin resistance is defined as a reduced glucose uptake response to a given amount of insulin.

Both lean and obese women with PCOS are found to be more insulin-resistant. Insulin resistance has been associated with an increase in several disorders including type 2 DM, hypertension, dyslipidemia and cardiovascular disease. **Therefore PCOS is not simply a disorder of short-term consequences such as irregular periods and hirsutism but also one with long-term health sequelae.**

### Androgens

Both insulin and LH stimulate androgen production by ovarian theca cell. The affected ovaries secrete elevated levels of testosterone and androstenedione. Elevated androstenedione levels contribute to an increase in estrone levels through peripheral conversion of androgens to estrogens by aromatase enzyme. Elevated free testosterone levels are noted in 80% women with PCOS and 25–65% have elevated levels of DHEAs. In overweight women, hypersecretion of insulin is the main cause of androgen secretion by the ovaries.

### Sex Hormone Binding Globulin (SHBG)

Women with PCOS have decreased levels of SHBG. The synthesis of SHBG by the liver is suppressed by insulin as well as androgens, steroids and growth hormone. Because of suppressed SHBG production, less circulating androgen is bound and more remains available to bind with androgen receptors. **It is for this reason that some women with PCOS have total testosterone levels in the normal range but will be clinically hyperandrogenic due to elevated free testosterone levels.** Normal female range for total serum testosterone is 0.5–3.5 nmol/L.

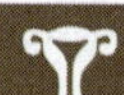

**Clinical Importance**

If the total serum testosterone level is greater than 5 nmol/L, it is necessary to exclude other causes of hyperandrogenemia such as late onset CAH, Cushing's syndrome and androgen-secreting tumours.

There also appears to be an association between low SHBG levels and subsequent development of GDM.

### Anovulation

Hypersecretion of LH has been implicated in menstrual irregularity. Anovulation may result from insulin resistance and some may resume ovulatory cycles when treated with metformin, an insulin sensitiser.

## SIGNS AND SYMPTOMS

Symptoms classically become apparent within a few years of puberty.

- **Menstrual dysfunction** It may range from **amenorrhea** to **oligomenorrhea** to **episodic menometrorrhagia** with **anemia.**
- Oligomenorrhea or amenorrhea with PCOS begins with menarche. Anovulation and elevated androgen levels result in amenorrhea and oligomenorrhea. In women with heavy and unpredictable bleeding due to chronic estrogen exposure, thickened endometrium results from constant mitogenic stimulation of endometrium. This instability of the thickened endometrium results in unpredictable bleeding pattern.
- **Hyperandrogenism** This is manifested by hirsutism, acne or androgenic alopecia. Hirsutism is defined as coarse, dark terminal hairs distributed in a male pattern. Women with PCOS typically report hirsutism beginning in late adolescence or the early 20s.
- **Acanthosis nigricans** This skin condition is characterised by thickened grey-brown velvety plaques seen in flexure areas such as neck, axillae, and crease beneath the breast, waist and groin. These are more often found in obese women with PCOS than in normal-weight women with PCOS (Fig. 14.1).
- **Dyslipidemia** In 70% of women with PCOS, LDL, triglyceride levels and total cholesterol : HDL ratio are elevated.
- **Obesity** The pattern of increased waist circumference and thick subscapular skinfolds are predictors of insulin resistance. Obesity can worsen ovulatory dysfunction, hyperandrogenism and the appearance of acanthosis nigricans (Fig. 14.1). Obstructive sleep apnea is more common in women with PCOS.
- **Infertility** PCOS is the most common cause of infertility in 80–90% of cases.
- **Complications in pregnancy** Gestational diabetes mellitus (GDM), pre-eclampsia (PE), preterm labour (PTL), twins and perinatal mortality (PNM)

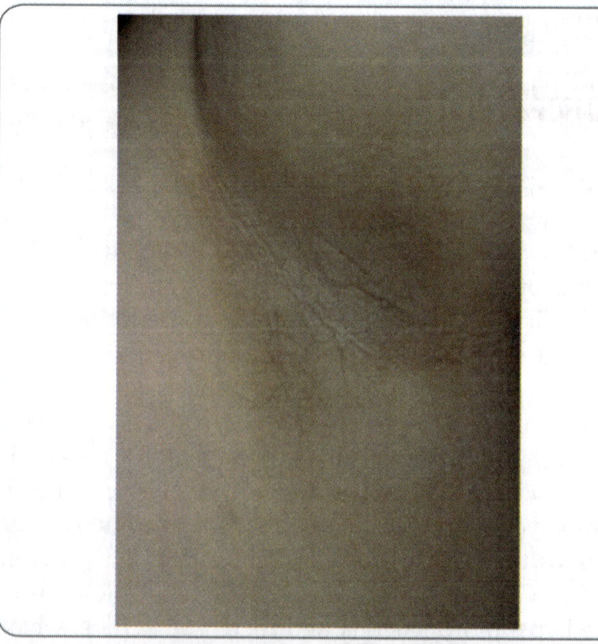

**Fig. 14.1** Acanthosis nigricans (*Source:* Wikimedia)

are some of the complications associated with pregnancy in women with PCOS.

- **Others** Women with PCOS may present with psychosomatic problems such as anxiety, depression and pulmonary conditions.

## DIAGNOSIS

- **TSH and PRL** Hyperprolactinemia leads to anovulation through inhibition of pulsatile secretion of GnRH from the hypothalamus.
- **Testosterone** Free testosterone levels are more sensitive than the total testosterone levels as an indicator of hyperandrogenism. Total testosterone levels remain the best approach to exclude tumour (greater than 200 ng/100 ml).
- Pelvic sonography is to be done to exclude ovarian neoplasm.
- **DHEAs** DHEAs are produced by the adrenal gland and serum DHEAs greater than 700 ng / 100 mL are suggestive of adrenal tumours.
- **Gonadotropin** Both FSH and LH levels are measured to exclude premature ovarian failure (POF) and hypergonadotropic hypogonadism. Serum LH levels are affected by sample timing and use of OC pills and BMI.
- **Insulin resistance** The markers to evaluate insulin resistance are
  - 2 hour GTT
  - Fasting insulin
  - Calculation of ratio of serum glucose to insulin
- **Fasting lipid profile** to evaluate dyslipidemia
- **Endometrial biopsy** Recommended in women older than 35 years with abnormal bleeding and in younger women with anovulatory bleeding refractory to hormonal treatment.
- **USG** PCO increases in volume, number of ripening and atretic follicles, cortical stromal thickness (Fig. 14.2).

**Sonographic Criteria for Polycystic Ovaries**

- More than 12 small cysts (2–9 mm)
- Increased ovarian volume (more than 10 mL)
- Both with increased stromal thickness.

Only one ovary with these findings is sufficient to define PCOS.

Table 14.1 summarises the hormone levels encountered in PCOS and the various conditions associated with it.

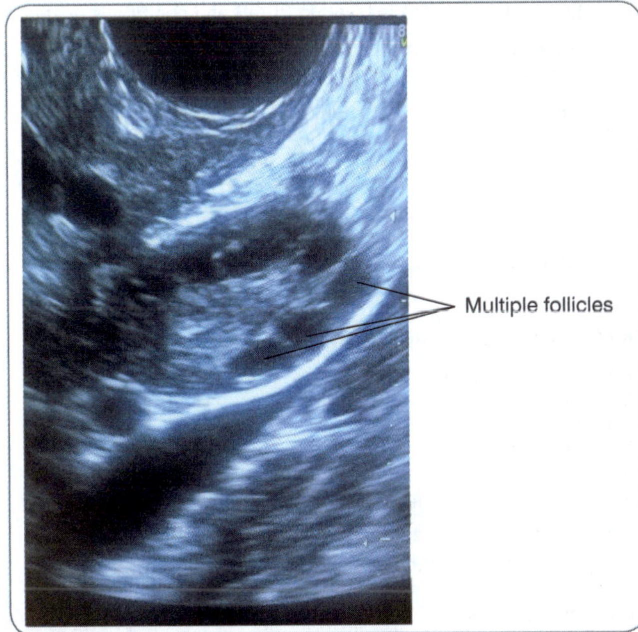


**Fig. 14.2** Ultrasound image showing polycystic ovary (*Source:* Wikimedia)

## CONSEQUENCES OF POLYCYSTIC OVARIAN SYNDROME

PCOS has both long- and short-term consequences (Table 14.2). The long-term consequences have a greater impact on quality of life. It is desirable that those managing PCOS discuss with the patients these consequences as these women should be prepared for lifestyle modifications.

## TREATMENT

The choice of treatment for each symptom of PCOS depends on a woman's need and the severity of endocrine dysfunction.

Thus anovulatory women desiring pregnancy will undergo treatment that is significantly different from that for adolescents with menstrual irregularity and acne.

Women with PCOS with regular cycle intervals (8–12/year) and mild hyperandrogenism need no treatment. **But periodic screening for dyslipidemia and diabetes mellitus is prudent.**

### Management of Obesity

For obese women with PCOS, lifestyle changes focused on diet and exercise should be advocated. **Even weight loss of 5% of body weight can result in restoration of normal**

**Table 14.1** Hormone levels in PCOS and conditions associated with the altered hormone levels

| Follicle-stimulating hormone | Luteinising hormone | Estradiol | Diagnosis |
|---|---|---|---|
| Normal | Elevated | Usually normal | Polycystic ovary syndrome |
| Normal | Low | Low | Weight-related amenorrhea |
| Low | Low | Low | Hypogonadotrophic hypogonadism, functional or organic |
| Elevated | Elevated | Low | If oligomenorrheic or amenorrheic: ovarian failure |
| Elevated | Elevated | High | If mid-cycle, think of mid-cycle surge |

**Table 14.2** Consequences of polycystic ovarian disease

| **Short-term consequences** |
|---|
| Obesity |
| Infertility |
| Irregular menses |
| Abnormal lipid levels |
| Hirsutism/Acne/Androgenic alopecia |
| Glucose intolerance/Acanthosis nigricans |
| **Long-term consequences** |
| Diabetes mellitus |
| Endometrial cancer |
| Cardiovascular disease |

**ovulatory cycles in some women due to reduction in insulin and androgen levels.** Well-balanced hypocaloric diet offers the most benefit for obese PCOS women.

## Treatment of Oligo-ovulation and Anovulation

### Combined Oral Contraceptive (COC) Pills

The first line treatment for menstrual irregularities is COCs which will induce regular cycles and reduce androgen levels by suppressing gonadotropin release. The estrogen component increases sex hormone binding globulin levels and progestin antagonises the endometrial proliferative effect of estrogen thus decreasing the risk of endometrial hyperplasia due to unopposed estrogen. **Hence COCs that contain progestins with fewer androgenic properties are preferred** such as norethindrone, desogestrol or drospirenone.

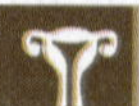 **Clinical Importance**

Before initiating therapy, if a woman's last menses was less than 4 weeks, prior pregnancy test is indicated.

If negative, progesterone is given to produce withdrawal bleed prior to COC pill initiation.

### Cyclic Progestogens

Progesterone withdrawal every 1–3 months is recommended.

### Insulin sensitivity agents

Metformin decreases androgen levels in both lean and obese women leading to increased rates of spontaneous ovulation. Metformin is a category B drug safe to use as an ovulatory induction agent. It can be used alone or with clomiphene. In patients who are clomiphene-resistant, metformin increases the ovulatory response.

**Dose** The typical dosage is 500 mg tid (three times a day) with meals.

**Side effects** A rare adverse side effect is lactic acidosis which is exclusively found in patients with renal insufficiency, liver disease or congestive cardiac failure. More common side effects are gastrointestinal and can be minimised by starting at a low dose and gradually increasing the dose over several weeks to an optimal level.

## Management of Hirsutism

The primary goal is lowering androgen levels to halt further conversion of vellous hairs to terminal ones. Medical therapies will not eliminate abnormal hair growth already present and treatment requires 6–12 months before clinical improvement is apparent. Temporary hair removal methods may be used in the interim.

### For abnormal hair growth

1. **Combined oral contraceptives** Estrogen component of the pills leads to increased sex hormone binding globulin levels; this ensures greater binding of free testosterone thus making it biologically unavailable at the hair follicle.
2. **GnRH antagonists** These effectively lower gonadotropin levels and in turn androgen levels. It is not a preferred long-term treatment method due to associated bone loss and high cost and menopausal side effects.
3. **Eflorithine hydrochloride** This antimetabolite topical cream is applied twice daily to areas of facial hirsutism and requires 4–8 weeks of use for visible results.

4. **Androgen receptor antagonist** None of the antiandrogen agents are approved by FDA for treatment of hyperandrogenism and are used off label. Spironolactone 50–100 mg orally twice daily is a primary antiandrogen and affects hair conversion from vellous to terminal hair by its direct inhibition of 5α-reductase. It is also a potassium-sparing diuretic. Cyprotrone acetate is not approved by FDA.
5. **Hair removal** Depilation and epilation techniques are used for hair removal; lighting hair colour with bleach is an additional cosmetic option.
   - *Depilation* This is hair removal above the skin surface. Topical chemical depilators are available as gel, cream and lotion.
   - *Epilation* It removes the entire hair shaft and root and includes techniques such as plucking, waxing, threading, electrolysis and laser treatment.

### For acne

**Topical treatment** The topical retinoids used are tretinoin and topical benzoyl peroxide.
**Systemic antibiotics** Oral antibiotics—doxycycline and erythromycin—are more effective.

Isoretinoin is highly effective but is teratogenic if taken during the first trimester of prenancy.

## Surgery

The surgery performed to treat PCOS is laparoscopic ovarian drilling (LOD) (Fig. 14.3).

**Indications** The application of LOD appears to be best suited for anovulatory women who are resistant or fail to respond to clomiphene citrate treatment.

The surgery is performed by penetration of the ovarian capsule by diathermy or LOD using either cautery or laser. The technique involves puncture of the capsule with a unipolar coagulating current at about 3–6 different areas to a depth of 4–10 mm.

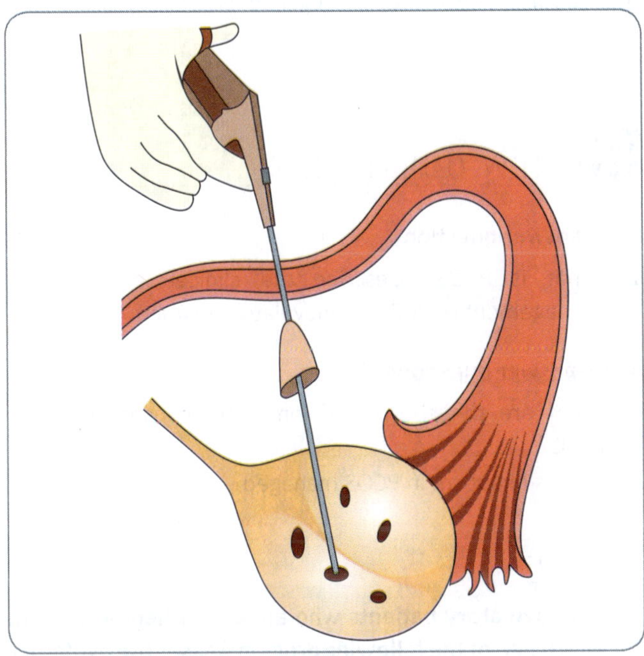

**Fig. 14.3** Laparoscopic ovarian drilling

***Case study***

*A 24-year-old unmarried woman comes with a complaint of amenorrhea for four months. Her periods had been irregular for the past three years. She says that she has put on excessive weight during the last three months. She also gives a history of excessive hair growth in the face. She is planning to get married shortly.*

*a) What is the possible etiology of this condition?*
*b) What are the relevant investigations?*
*c) How would you manage this patient?*
*d) What advice other than medication would you give to this woman?*

## RECAP

- PCOS is the common endocrine disorder in 20–25% of women.
- It is a heterogeneous condition. Diagnosis is made by finding 2 out of the following 3 criteria:
  - Menstrual cycle disturbance

    - Clinical or biochemical hyperandrogenism
    - USG detection of PCO
- Management is symptom-oriented.
- If obese, weight loss improves symptoms. A glucose tolerance test should be performed for women with BMI of >30 kg/m$^2$.
- Menstrual cycle control is achieved by cyclical OCP or progestogens.
- Ovulation induction is done with clomiphene citrate, gonadotropin therapy or laparoscopic ovarian diathermy.
- Hyper-androgenism is managed with OCP containing ethinyl estradiol in combination with cyproterone acetate or drospirenone.
- Alternatives include spironolactone, flutamide and finasteride. All have potential side effects.
- Metformin decreases androgen levels in both lean and obese women leading to increased rates of spontaneous ovulation.

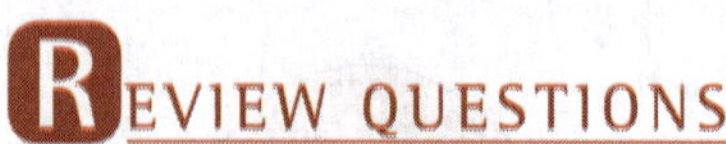


### Long-answer question

1. What is PCOS? Describe the clinical features and management of PCOS in anovulatory women.

### Short-answer questions

1. What are the short- and long-term consequences of PCOS?
2. How is hirsutism in PCOS managed?

## MCQs

1. **In anovulatory patients who are clomiphene-resistant, which one of the following drugs increases the ovulatory response?**
    a) Metformin
    b) Rosiglitazone
    c) Pioglitazone
    d) Dexamethasone
2. **Hyperandrogenism is manifested clinically by the following features except**
    a) Acne
    b) Alopecia
    c) Deepening of voice
    d) Hirsutism
3. **The following are the USG findings of polycystic ovaries except**
    a) Ovarian volume more than 10 mL
    b) Stromal thickness
    c) More than 12 small cysts
    d) Both ovaries have the above features
4. **PCO can also be found in other conditions of androgen excess except**
    a) CAH
    b) Cushing's syndrome
    c) Exogenous use of androgens
    d) Pituitary tumour

### Further Reading

Boomsma CM, Eijkemans MJ, Hughes EG, Visser GH, Fauser BC, Macklon NS. A meta-analysis of pregnancy outcomes in women with polycystic ovary syndrome. Hum Reprod Update. 2006 Nov-Dec;12(6):673–83.

Burgers JA, Fong SL, Louwers YV, Valkenburg O, de Jong FH, Fauser BC, Laven JS. Oligoovulatory and anovulatory cycles in women with polycystic ovary syndrome (PCOS): what's the difference? J Clin Endocrinol Metab. 2010 Dec;95(12):E485–9.

Dunaif A, Insulin resistance and the polycystic ovary syndrome: mechanism and implications for pathogenesis. Endocr Rev. 1997 Dec;18(6):774–800.

Gretchen Lentz Rogerio Lobo David Gershenson Vern Kat. 2012. Comprehensive gynecology. 6th ed. Maryland Heights: Mosby; 2012.

Hoffman, B., Schorge, J., Schaffer, J., Halvorson, L., Bradshaw, K. and Cunningham, F. Williams Gynecology, 2nd edn.

Michelmore KF, Balen AH, Dunger DB, Vessey MP. Polycystic ovaries and associated clinical and biochemical features in young women. Clin Endocrinol (Oxf). 1999 Dec;51(6):779–86.

Shaw R, Luesley D, Monga A. 2011. Gynaecology. 4th ed. London: Churchill Livingstone; 2011.

# CHAPTER 15

# Endometriosis

## At a Glance

Pathogenesis
Epidemiology of Endometriosis
Risk Factors for Developing Endometriosis
Classification/Staging of Endometriosis
Revised American Fertility Society (AFS) Score
Pathology
Possible Sites of Endometriosis
Pathogenic Mechanism of Endometriosis
Ovarian Endometriosis
Endometriosis of the Tubes
Pelvic Endometriosis
Endometriosis of the Rectovaginal Septum
Intestinal Endometriosis
Endometriosis in Unusual Sites
Diagnosis of Endometriosis
Symptomatology
Endometriosis and Infertility
Clinical Examination
Investigations
Differential Diagnosis
Management
Management of Endometriosis in Adolescent Girls
Management of Endometriosis in Infertile Women
Expectant Management
Medical Management
Surgical Management
Management of Moderate or Severe Endometriosis
Effect of Endometriosis on Pregnancy
Effect of Pregnancy on Endometriosis
Medical Therapy for Endometriosis
Mechanism of Action
Drugs Used in Endometriosis
Surgical Therapy

## INTRODUCTION

**Definition** Endometriosis is the presence of functioning endometrial glands and stroma outside the uterine cavity and musculature. The ectopic endometrium functionally responds to ovarian hormones. It is an estrogen-dependent condition. It is one of the most common benign gynecological conditions, **affecting 6–10% of women of reproductive age.**

**Incidence** The prevalence of endometriosis among women presenting with chronic pelvic pain is more than 33% and in women with sub-fertility, it is as high as 30–50%.

Though endometriosis is a disease of the genital tract, almost any organ in the body can be affected. The occurrence of endometriosis outside the pelvis is termed "**extra genital**" or "**extra pelvic" endometriosis**.

## PATHOGENESIS

The exact etiology of endometriosis remains unknown. It is often called **disease of theories**. It is an estrogen-dependent condition and regresses after menopause.

Several theories have been proposed to explain the occurrence of endometriosis.

1. **The implantation or retrograde menstruation theory (Sampson's theory)** Sampson in 1927 hypothesised that the viable endometrial tissue from the uterus is transported in a retrograde fashion through the Fallopian tubes to the pelvic and abdominal organs. When the environment is conducive, endometriosis can develop in the pelvic organs as well as in abdominal organs such as appendix, caecum, colon, etc.
2. **The coelomic cell metaplasia theory (Meyer's theory)** Meyer and Ivanoff hypothesised that the peritoneal cavity contains progenitor cells capable of differentiating into endometrial tissue and the metaplasia of these coelomic epithelium is the origin of endometriosis. This theory explains the occurrence of endometriosis of the rectovaginal septum, the umbilicus and the abdominal viscera.

3. **Immune system dysfunction theory** This theory suggests that there is deficient cell-mediated immune response and there is ineffective clearance of menstrual effluent from the peritoneal cavity by intraperitoneal macrophages. This allows ectopic endometrial cells to proliferate.

   A number of autoimmune disorders such as SLE, hypothyroidism and rheumatoid arthritis have been reported in women with endometriosis.
4. **The dissemination theory (Halban's theory)** The dissemination theory proposes that endometrial tissue can be transported to distal sites through the lymphatics or blood vessels. This theory explains the occurrence of endometriosis at sites such as lungs, pleura, pericardium, liver, CNS and distal cutaneous tissue.
5. **Direct transplantation theory** This theory explains the occurrence of endometriosis in surgical scars. When there is direct inoculation of surgical incisions with endometrial cells, these can be subsequently stimulated by estrogen to produce scar endometriosis.
6. **Genetic predisposition** There is familial predisposition to endometriosis. It has been demonstrated that there is increased incidence of endometriosis among the first-degree relatives compared to the controls.

## EPIDEMIOLOGY OF ENDOMETRIOSIS

Endometriosis is more common in women in the 20–40 age group. 90% of endometriosis occurs in this age group. Adolescent girls with congenital anomalies of the uterus also have a higher predilection for developing endometriosis. Though endometriosis is rare after menopause, reactivation by endogenous hormones or use of exogenous hormones such as in hormone replacement therapy (HRT) can give rise to this condition. The incidence is more common in affluent communities where delayed childbearing and small family size predispose the women to more number of menstrual cycles and uninterrupted ovarian activity. Endometriosis is commonly seen in nulliparous women and in women who have had few children. There is a familial predisposition with a 7% incidence of endometriosis among the first-degree relatives as compared to 1% among the controls.

## RISK FACTORS FOR DEVELOPING ENDOMETRIOSIS

Epidemiological studies have shown various risk factors for the development of endometriosis.

- **Increased risk** is seen in women who had early menarche, shorter menstrual cycle and heavy periods. The risk is high in women with immune disorders and in women having first-degree relatives with endometriosis.
- Factors which facilitate **retrograde flow of menstrual blood** such as, acute retroversion of the uterus, congenital abnormalities of the genital tract with stenosis and atresia of the lower Müllerian tract, haematometra/haematocolpos, and pin hole os also increase the risk.

  **Iatrogenic causes**—the risk is more in when tubal patency tests such as hysterosalpingogram (HSG), and laparoscopy with dye test are performed during the pre-menstrual, menstrual or immediate postmenstrual period; tubal patency tests conducted during these periods carry the risk of transporting the endometrial cells into the peritoneal cavity.

  Whenever surgical procedures such as appendicectomy/cryo or cautery to the cervix are carried out in the pre-menstrual phase, the endometrium can deposit over the raw areas, and may develop as endometriosis at a later date.
- **Reduced risk** may be seen in those with increased parity, who practised prolonged lactation, with healthy vegetable-rich diet and exercise. Risk is also supposed to be low in women with increased BMI.

**Risk Factors for Developing Endometriosis**

| Increased risk | Decreased risk |
|---|---|
| • Early age at menarche<br>• Shorter menstrual cycle<br>• Heavy periods<br>• Müllerian anomalies<br>• Endometriosis in first-degree relatives<br>• Iatrogenic factors<br>• Individuals suffering from immune disorders | • Increased parity<br>• Prolonged Lactation<br>• Exercise<br>• Diet rich in vegetables<br>• Increased BMI |

## CLASSIFICATION/STAGING OF ENDOMETRIOSIS

### Revised American Fertility Society (AFS) Score

Based on the severity of endometriosis at laparoscopy or findings at surgery, the American Society for Reproductive Medicine has classified endometriosis into four stages (Fig. 15.1).

A detailed scoring chart is beyond the scope of this book. However, those interested can refer to the point-

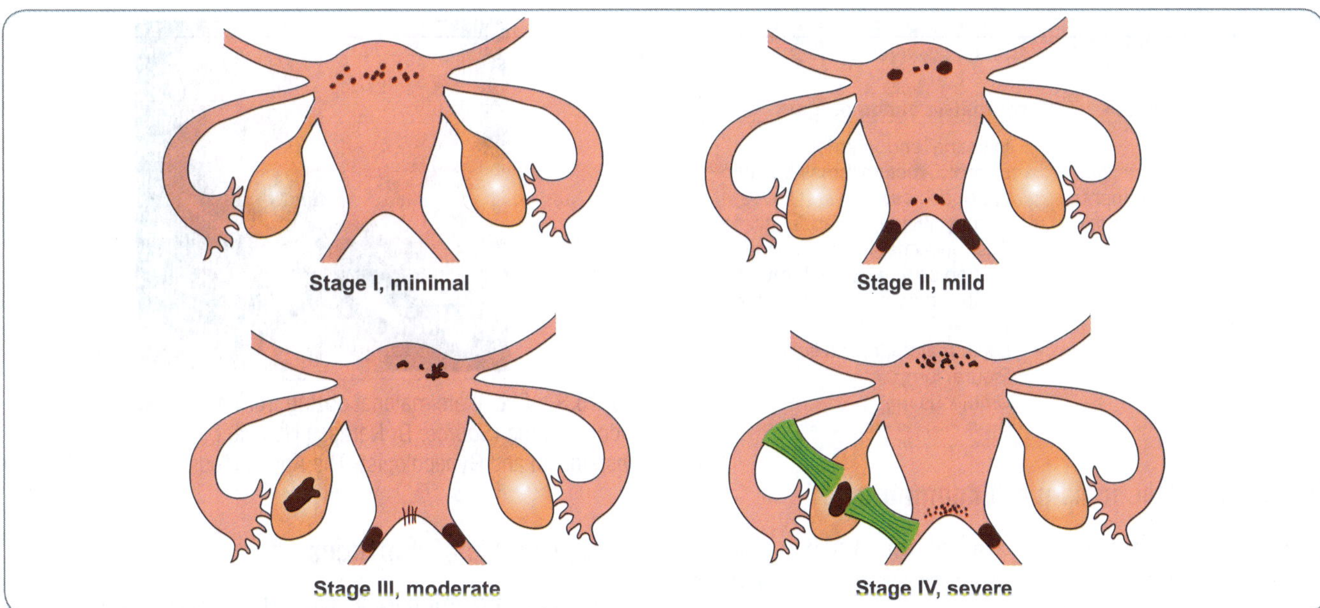


**Fig. 15.1** Classification of endometriosis

wise scoring in the ASRM website, https://www.asrm.org/BOOKLET_Endometriosis/

### *Minimal (Stage I)*

Very few small superficial endometriotic areas scattered over the peritoneum.

### *Mild (Stage II)*

Characterised by scattered superficial implants on structures other than uterus, tubes or ovaries with no associated scarring or significant adhesions and at worst superficial implants on the ovaries.

### *Moderate (Stage III)*

Characterised by multiple implants or small endometriomas less than 2 cm involving one or both ovaries, minimal periovarian or peritubular adhesions, scattered, scarred implants on other structures.

### *Severe (Stage IV)*

Characterised by large ovarian endometriomas, significant tubal or ovarian adhesions, tubal obstruction, obliteration of the cul-de-sac, major uterosacral involvement , significant bowel and urinary tract disease.

## PATHOLOGY

### Possible Sites of Endometriosis

The most commonly affected sites are the pelvic organs and the peritoneum including the ovaries, Fallopian tubes, uterosacral ligaments, ovarian fossa, pouch of Douglas (POD) and rectovaginal septum (Fig. 15.2). Occasionally bladder, bowel and appendix are involved. Extrapelvic location of endometriosis is rare but can occur in upper abdomen, diaphragm, lungs, abdominal wall, umbilicus and scar tissue, etc.

The most common site is the ovary and it is affected in 54% of cases, POD and posterior aspect of broad ligament are affected in 35% of cases and uterosacral ligaments in 28% of cases.

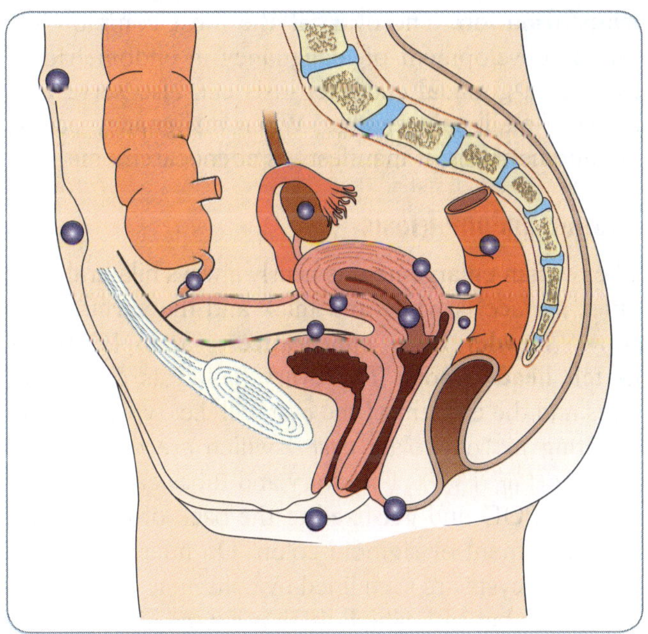

**Fig. 15.2** Common sites of endometriosis

**Sites of Endometriosis**

| Pelvic endometriosis | Extra-pelvic endometriosis |
|---|---|
| • Ovary, tubes<br>• POD<br>• Uterosacral ligaments<br>• Bladder peritoneum<br>• Recto-vaginal septum | • Intestinal endometriosis—sigmoid, rectum, small bowel, appendix, caecum<br>• Urinary system—bladder, ureter<br>• Scar endometriosis—caesarean section scar, myomectomy scar, hysterotomy scar, episiotomy wound<br>• Labia majora, round ligament<br>• Pleura, lung<br>• Umbilicus |

## Pathogenic Mechanism of Endometriosis

Pathologically, both endometrial glands and stroma are present, and the ectopic endometrium responds to estrogen and to a lesser degree to progesterone and is capable of miniature menstruation. The endometriotic tissue responds to both exogenous and endogenous hormones. The lesion promotes a fibrous and fibromuscular tissue reaction which is diffuse and the lesion is not capsulated. When the patient becomes pregnant, the endometriotic lesions show decidual reaction in the stromal cells. The lesion atrophies after menopause.

When there is no outlet for menstrual discharge, blood and the debris collect within the tissue to form a cyst. With continuous absorption of fluid, the blood gets thickened or inspissated and dark-coloured forming the so-called chocolate cyst of the ovary.

The endometriotic areas can also undergo **malignant transformation**. The ovary is the most common site for the development of malignancy in endometriosis. But, extra-gonadal endometriosis can also serve as a focus of malignant change. When malignancy occurs in endometriosis, it manifests as adenocarcinoma.

## Ovarian Endometriosis

The ovarian enlargement is nearly always bilateral. The outer surface is white and thick and the surface may show "**Powder burn appearance**"—multiple "**burnt match head" spots**. The ovary has cysts of varying sizes and the content of the cyst will be typically tarry resulting in "chocolate cysts" which are devoid of a capsule (Fig. 15.3). The ovary and tubes can prolapse into the POD and get fixed to the back of the uterus, broad ligament or sigmoid colon. On microscopy, the chocolate cysts are seen lined by columnar or flattened epithelium beneath which there is a zone of polyhedral cells laden with hemosiderin.

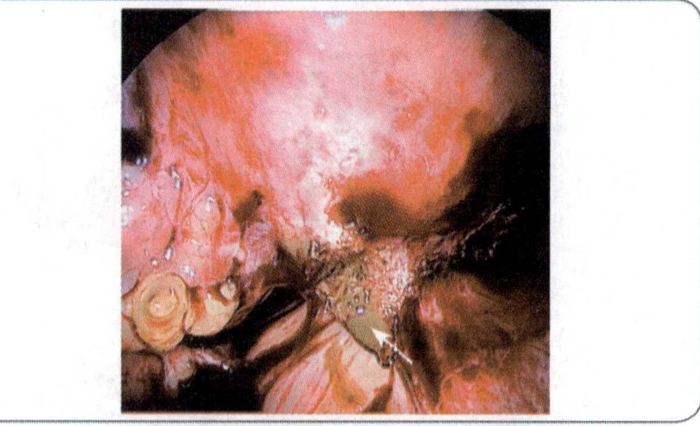

**Fig. 15.3** Chocolate material oozing from mobilised endometrioma (*Source:* Dr Narassa Narayani, Consultant Obstetrician and Gynecologist, The Apollo Medical Centre, Chennai)

## Endometriosis of the Tubes

Peritoneal endometriosis can affect the outer wall of the Fallopian tube. When there is fibrosis, the tubes will become rigid. Endometriosis can also affect the inner wall to result in endosalpingiosis.

## Pelvic Endometriosis

The pelvis is the second most frequent site for endometriosis and involves the POD, uterosacral ligaments, peritoneum covering the posterior wall of the vagina, and the bladder peritoneum. Black spots called **"Powder burn"** lesions can be seen widely scattered or cystic areas can be seen beneath the peritoneum (Fig. 15.4).

## Endometriosis of the Rectovaginal Septum

Endometriosis can infiltrate into the recto-vaginal septum and present as induration in the POD. Papillary excrescences or several blue-domed cysts may be seen

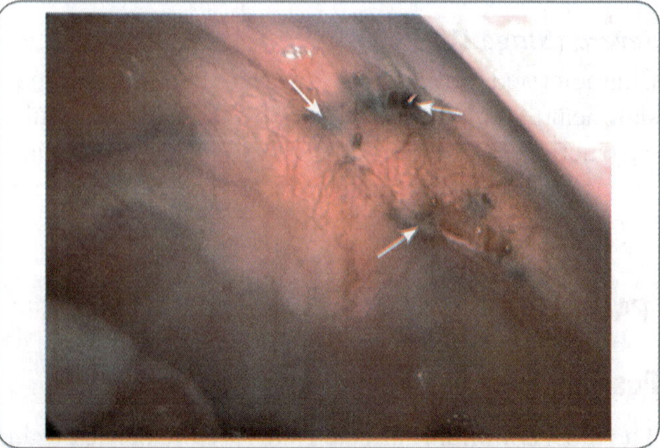

**Fig. 15.4** Peritoneal endometriosis (*Source:* Wikimedia)

protruding into the posterior fornix. These lesions may ulcerate and present with cyclical or irregular bleeding. The lesion may also infiltrate backwards into the wall of the rectum. **Similar findings may also be seen in carcinoma of the vagina.**

### Intestinal Endometriosis

Sigmoid and rectal endometriosis are the common sites of intestinal involvement. Small bowel, caecum and appendix are less commonly affected. This condition is very often diagnosed as carcinoma.

### Endometriosis in Unusual Sites

- Endometriosis can develop in the **umbilicus** due to the lymphatic and vascular connections and present as black nodule which enlarges and becomes painful during menstruation.
- Endometriosis can also occur in **laparotomy scars** (myomectomy, caesarean section, hysterotomy), **perineal wound** and in the **scar of an excised Bartholin cyst**. The affected area swells up and becomes painful during menstruation; sinus may develop discharging menstrual blood.
- **Urinary system** can also be affected with involvement of the bladder and the ureter. Bladder involvement can present with recurrent urinary infections or cyclical haematuria.
- Other areas that can be affected are **round ligament** and **labia majora.**
- Distant sites such as **lungs and pleura** can also be affected and these cases present with cyclical pleural pain, hemothorax, and haemoptysis (**vicarious menstruation**).

## DIAGNOSIS OF ENDOMETRIOSIS

There is considerable overlap of symptoms of endometriosis with other gynecological and non-gynecological conditions. Therefore, making a clinical diagnosis is a challenge.

- **Asymptomatic** Approximately 25% of patients with endometriosis are completely asymptomatic and diagnosed while investigating cases of infertility.
- **Symptomatic** When they are symptomatic, they present with congestive dysmenorrhea, deep dyspareunia, pelvic pain, infertility and other cyclical pain related to bowel and bladder.

### Symptomatology

Symptoms largely depend on the location of the endometriotic lesion, and the severity of symptoms may not correlate with the extent of the disease. Patients with very minimal disease may have severe symptoms and those with stage IV disease may not have any symptoms.

#### Pain

Pain is one of the most common symptoms of endometriosis. Patients typically present with pelvic pain, dysmenorrhea and dyspareunia. The pain in endometriosis may be due to bleeding and fibrosis in areas with rich nerve supply or due to the production of cytokines and other inflammatory cells and activation of macrophages.

##### *Pelvic pain*

The pain can be excruciating and debilitating, may be intermittent, or constant or related to menstrual cycle. The pain is often associated with dysmenorrhea, dyspareunia, lower abdominal pain and back ache. Pain can be provoked by activities such as walking or standing for too long. There are associated bowel and bladder symptoms. The patient can present with pelvic discomfort, deep-seated pelvic pain appreciated in the region of mid-pelvis referred to the sacrum, lumbar region, rectum and lower abdomen. When the chocolate cyst ruptures, there is acute pain mimicking appendicitis/ectopic gestation.

##### *Dysmenorrhea*

Patients with endometriosis usually present with progressively increasing congestive dysmenorrhea or the pain can occur before, during and after periods. Dysmenorrhea may not be seen in few cases, as some lesions may not menstruate or may be inactive for several years.

##### *Deep dyspareunia*

The pain is felt deep during sexual intercourse due to the stretching of the uterosacral ligaments, recto-vaginal septum, retroverted uterus and the ovaries and the pain can persist for up to 48 hours after sexual activity.

##### *Ovulation pain*

This results from stretching of the endometrial implants on the surface of the ovary at the time of ovulation.

##### *Low backache*

It is commonly associated with endometriosis in the POD, uterosacral ligaments and rectovaginal septum and Presario nerve endometriosis.

#### Menstrual disturbances

Heavy menstrual bleeding can occur due to pelvic congestion, and frequent periods can occur due to ovarian involvement. Endometriosis should be suspected when there is pre-menstrual spotting.

#### Other symptoms

Headache, low-grade fever, depression, anxiety, susceptibility to infection, chronic fatigue syndrome are other generalised symptoms. They can present with painful bladder syndrome, painful bowel syndrome and fibromyalgia.

#### *Bowel symptoms*

Bowel symptoms are very common with endometriosis and are caused by irritation to the bowel by endometrial implants lying in adjacent areas such as POD, back of uterus, serosa of the bowel, etc. Patients can present with nausea, vomiting, abdominal bloating, diarrhea, rectal pain, constipation, abdominal cramping, sharp gas pain and painful bowel movements; rectal bleeding can occur during periods if the endometriosis has ulcerated into the lumen.

#### *Bladder symptoms*

Endometriosis of anterior surface of the uterus or outer wall of the bladder can present with urinary symptoms such as urinary frequency, urgency, dysuria and haematuria. If the ureters are involved, patients present with flank pain radiating to groin.

#### *Respiratory symptoms*

If the lungs and pleura are involved, endometriosis can present with cyclical pleuritic pain and haemoptysis can also occur.

#### Cutaneous endometriosis

In scar endometriosis, painful nodules are seen over the skin, visible to the naked eye, may appear blue or can bleed during menstruation.

### Endometriosis and Infertility

Endometriosis is seen in nearly 30–50% of women with infertility.

#### Causes

The causes of infertility due to endometriosis are:

- Pelvic pain and dyspareunia discourage or reduce frequency of coitus.
- Distorted adnexal anatomy inhibit ovum capture after ovulation by the Fallopian tubes.
- Ovarian endometriosis may be so extensive that it destroys the normal ovarian tissue causing anovulation.
- In endometriosis, the peritoneal milieu is altered by an increased presence of macrophages, 'T' lymphocytes and their mediators. These can destroy the spermatozoa and oocytes and impair fertilisation. Moreover, the oocyte quality and early embryo development are poor in women suffering from endometriosis.
- Ovarian function can also be impaired due to anovulation, leuteal phase defect, prostaglandin-induced luteolysis and oocyte maturation defects.

## CLINICAL EXAMINATION

Pelvic examination findings may be normal in early-stage disease. However, in advanced-stage disease, the uterus is retroverted and fixed and the fornices will be tender. There may be cervical motion tenderness. Painful nodules can also be felt in the cul-de-sac, well appreciated by rectal examination. Enlarged, tender, cystic adnexal masses may suggest an endometrioma. All the above findings may suggest endometriosis but are not diagnostic.

## INVESTIGATIONS

#### *USG examination*

Transvaginal ultrasonography (TVS) may be useful in the diagnosis of endometrioma and in distinguishing endometrioma from other adnexal masses. The cyst wall appears irregular with low echoes (Fig. 15.5) and clumps of dense high-level echoes representing blood clots. On Doppler, the blood flow is scant in endometrioma.

#### *CT scan*

This is not useful in the diagnosis of endometriosis, but may be helpful in diagnosing ureteric involvement when contrast is used.

#### *MRI*

MRI is useful in diagnosing deep pelvic endometriosis, recto-sigmoid lesions and endometriosis of the bladder. But, endometriotic implants and adhesions may not be picked up.

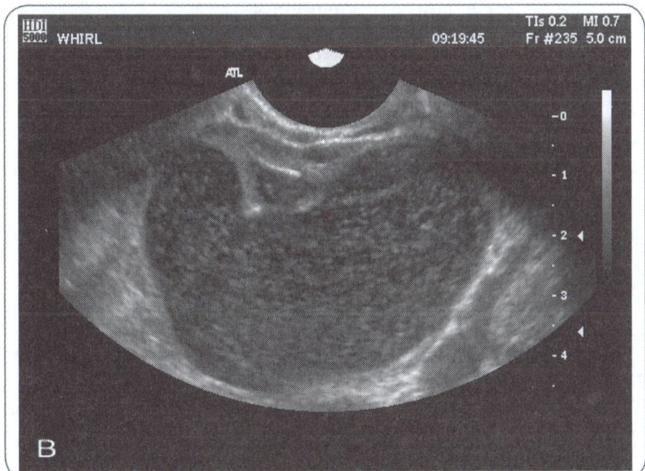

**Fig. 15.5** Image of ovarian endometrioma showing hypoehoic structure exhibiting low-amplitude uniformly distributed echotexture in the cavities of the cysts (*Source:* Chizen, D, Pierson, R, Glob. libr. women's med.)

### *Laparoscopy*

The only definitive way to diagnose endometriosis is to visualise the deposits laparoscopically and confirm by biopsy. Laparoscopy is considered **"the Gold standard"** for the diagnosis of endometriosis. Characteristic appearances associated with recent and active endometriosis are peritoneal implants, vesicles, yellow-brown peritoneal patches and red flame-like lesions. Burnt out lesions or inactive lesions appear as black deposits laden with haemosiderin. Endometriomas and deep infiltrating nodules are other common findings.

### *Serum CA 125 levels*

CA 125 levels may be elevated in women with endometriosis, but, not helpful in the initial diagnosis, but may indicate recurrence during follow-up.

### *Other investigations*

Depending on the symptoms, further investigations may be required such as cystoscopy for bladder endometriosis, sigmoidoscopy and colonoscopy for transmural bowel lesions and USG-guided fine needle aspiration for endometriosis in the recto-sigmoid, recto-vaginal septum or in the abdominal scars.

## DIFFERENTIAL DIAGNOSIS

There are some gynecological and non-gynecological conditions that mimic endometriosis.

**Differential Diagnosis of Endometriosis**

| Gynecological conditions | Non-gynecological conditions |
|---|---|
| • PID<br>• Pelvic adhesions<br>• Masses<br>• Leiomyoma<br>• Adenomyosis<br>• Ovarian malignancy<br>• Calcified tuberculous lesions | • Inflammatory bowel disease<br>• Irritable bowel syndrome (IBS)<br>• Interstitial cystitis<br>• Myofascial pain<br>• Appendicitis<br>• Bowel cancer |

## MANAGEMENT

Endometriosis is a difficult disease to treat, and there is no permanent cure for the disease. Recurrence rate is around 60%. Removal of the ovaries and the resultant fall in estrogen levels offers the most effective treatment. A multidisciplinary approach would be required in severe endometriosis, involving urologists, gastroenterologists, pain specialists and psychiatrists.

The aim of management is:

- To relieve pain
- To maintain adequate sexual function
- To promote the possibility of pregnancy in infertile women

The factors determining the treatment options are as follows:

- Age of the patient
- Desire for child bearing
- Severity of her symptoms
- Extent of the disease—superficial/nodular with or without endometrioma
- Previous treatment

Patients with endometriosis can be grouped under the following categories:

- Adolescent girls
- Young women of reproductive age group, who are desirous of pregnancy
- Women in whom childbearing is completed
- Patients with recurring symptoms

### Management of Endometriosis in Adolescent Girls

In the adolescent girls, it is difficult to make a diagnosis of endometriosis because it is difficult to distinguish endometriosis from primary dysmenorrhea. Figure 15.6 depicts a flowchart for the management of endometriosis in adolescent girls.

- **As endometriosis is a progressive disease, the diagnosis of endometriosis should not be missed.**

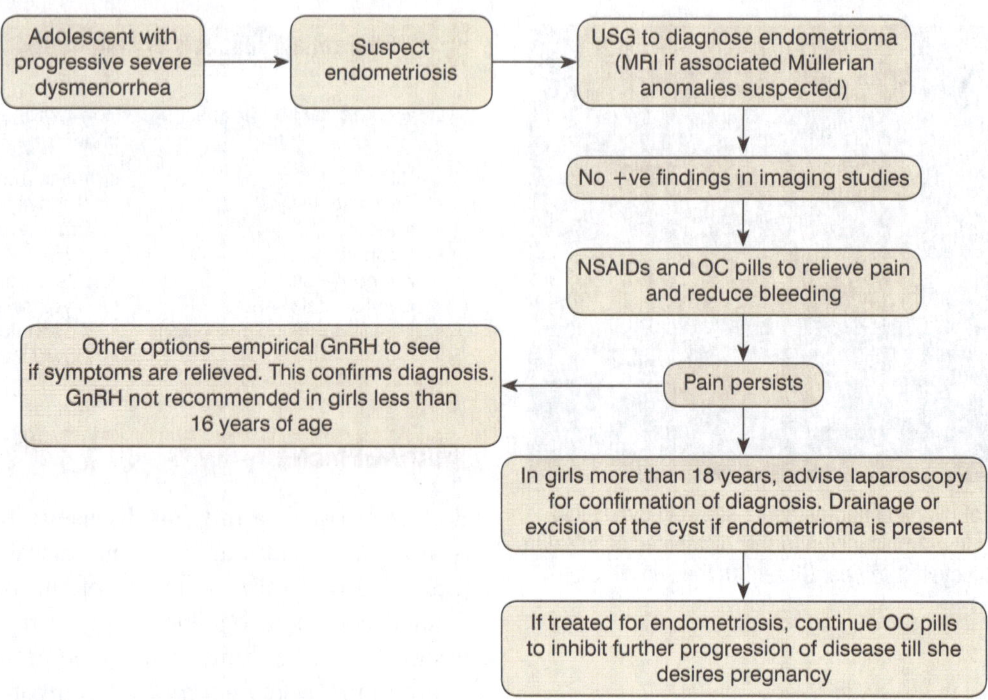


**Fig. 15.6** Flowchart for the management of endometriosis in adolescent girls

- In adolescents presenting with progressive / severe dysmenorrhea, endometriosis should be suspected and it is important to perform USG to diagnose endometriomas. If necessary, MRI is performed to diagnose Müllerian anomalies which can be associated with endometriosis.
- If there are no positive findings on imaging studies, the initial management should be with non-steroidal anti-inflammatory drugs (NSAIDS) and cyclical combined oral contraceptive (COC) pills to relieve the pain and to reduce the amount of bleeding.
- If the pain is still persistent and the girl is more than 18 years, laparoscopy is advised to confirm the diagnosis. If an endometrioma is present at the time of laparoscopy, drainage/excision of the cyst can be undertaken.
- If endometriosis was diagnosed and treated laparoscopically, OC pills are continued to inhibit further progression of the disease, until they reach the age of marriage and desire pregnancy.
- The other option is to give empirical GnRH to see whether symptoms are relieved, which will confirm the diagnosis. GnRH is not recommended in girls less than 16 years of age.

## Management of Endometriosis in Infertile Women

In infertile women with endometriosis, semen analysis, ovulatory status and tubal patency test by laparoscopy should be carried out.

#### Management of minimal or mild endometriosis in infertile women

In women with minimal or mild endometriosis, the tubes and ovaries are normal and there are no endometriotic cysts involving the ovaries. In these women, there are three options—conservative management, surgical management and assisted reproductive techniques.

### Expectant Management

When endometriosis is the only factor and all other factors are normal, expectant management (wherein no definitive treatment is given for endometriosis) can be undertaken and a significant proportion of couples will conceive spontaneously without treatment.

### Medical Management

Medical management with GnRH, OC pills, and Danazol are not advised as they inhibit ovulation and delay conception.

### Surgical Management

At the time of laparoscopy, ablation of endometriotic lesions can be undertaken.

#### Super-ovulation and IUI

In women with mild endometriosis, ovarian stimulation with gonadotropins and intrauterine insemination (IUI) increase the pregnancy rates.

### IVF

In couples with minimal or mild endometriosis, IVF may be undertaken if there is associated factor like male infertility, or when they have not conceived with expectant/superovulation and IUI/surgical treatment.

## Management of Moderate or Severe Endometriosis

- In the management of moderate or severe endometriosis with infertility, there is no place for expectant management or medical management.
- Surgical management is undertaken to excise or ablate all visible endometriosis and adhesions and correct pelvic anatomy as far as possible. If endometrioma are present, they are either ablated or excised. Laparoscopy is preferable to laparotomy.

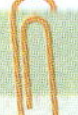

**Indications for IVF**

IVF is an early treatment option for women with moderate-to-severe disease or when surgical treatment has failed.

# EFFECT OF ENDOMETRIOSIS ON PREGNANCY

When the woman becomes pregnant after treatment for endometriosis, the following obstetric complications are likely to occur.

- Abortion
- Ectopic pregnancy
- Preterm labour

There is also increased incidence of

- Placenta previa
- PPH
- Adherent placenta

Endometriosis of recto-vaginal septum can interfere with cervical dilatation and even cause obstruction.

# EFFECT OF PREGNANCY ON ENDOMETRIOSIS

Pregnancy has a beneficial effect on endometriosis and the endometriosis can disappear. The disappearance of endometriosis during pregnancy is due to the absence of ovulation and menstruation in addition to the decidual changes in the endometrium causing necrosis and absorption.

# MEDICAL THERAPY FOR ENDOMETRIOSIS

Endometriosis is a recurring disease and medical therapy should be viewed as symptomatic control rather than curative.

## Mechanism of Action

Medical therapy aims at interrupting the cyclical ovarian hormone production and establishes a steady state. This hormonal steady state results in sub-optimal milieu for endometriotic lesions to develop.

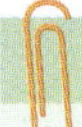

**Indications**

- When fertility is not the major issue
- In early stage disease
- Management of adolescents with endometriosis
- Recto-vaginal disease to reduce pain
- The recurrence of symptoms may be as high as 50% after discontinuing the treatment for 12–24 months.

## Drugs Used in Endometriosis

Table 15.1 lists the drugs used in endometriosis.

### Non-hormonal therapy

Non-steroidal anti-inflammatory drugs are useful in the management of endometriosis-related pain especially in adolescents and in the early-stage diseases.

### Combined oral contraceptive pills

- Combined estrogen and progesterone induces a pseudo-pregnancy state.
- This is the first line of therapy in patients in whom OC pills are not contraindicated.
- They act by reducing the menstrual flow, causing decidualisation of endometriotic implants, with decreased proliferation and increased apoptosis.
- Combined OC pills can be used in a cyclical fashion or continuous fashion for 6–9 months. But complications of uninterrupted use should be kept in mind.

### Progestogens

- Progestogens are also one of the first-line treatments. They also act by inducing pseudo-decidual endometrial response.
- Commonly used progestogens are:
  Medroxy-progesterone acetate 30 mg/day
  Depot medroxy-progesterone acetate 150 mg IM every 3 months

These drugs are used for 9–12 months.
Dienogest is newer progesterone used in the management of endometriosis.

- **Side effects** With prolonged use, weight gain, irregular bleeding, depression, osteoporosis and amenorrhea can occur. These agents are often well-tolerated with minimal side effects.

#### Levonorgestrel-releasing device (LNG intrauterine device)

Action is locally on the endometrium where the concentration of levonorgestrel is high and induces atrophy and pseudo-decidualisation of the endometrium.

#### Danocrine

- It is an isoxazol derivative of 17-alpha ethinyl testosterone.
- *Dose* 400–800 mg daily for 3–12 months
- *Mechanism of action* They act by inhibiting steroidogenesis and producing a pseudo-menopause state.
- Side effects are hot flushes, acne, reduced libido, oily hair and skin, muscle cramps, can virilise a female fetus. As the side effects are bothersome, this is not used as the first-line management.

#### Gestrinone

- It is a 19-nortestosterone derivative exhibiting androgenic, antiprogestogenic, antiestrogenic and antigonadotropic properties. It causes endometrial atrophy by a mechanism similar to danazol. The side-effects are also similar to danazol, hence it is not used.

#### GnRH analogues

- Both agonists and antagonists induce medical menopause by depleting the endogenous gonadotropins, interrupting the menstrual cycle, resulting in a hypo-estrogenic state, endometrial atrophy and amenorrhea.
- The GnRH agonists have significant side effects primarily related to hypogonadotropic state such as vasomotor symptoms, vaginal dryness, decreased libido, joint pain and loss of bone mass. GnRH may lead to bone loss up to 13% over a period of 6 months. Therefore, estrogen-progesterone add-back therapies are recommended if used longer than 6 months. However the effect on bone is partly reversible on stopping the drug.
- GnRH are not recommended for adolescents because of the effect on the bone mass.
- *Commonly used drug* Goserelin 3.6 mg injection SC every 4 weeks for 3–4 months.

## Surgical Therapy

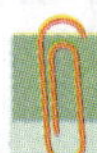

**Indications**

- Surgery should be the first choice in women who wish to conceive, and in those with endometrioma.
- Surgery can also be undertaken in women with early stage disease, who have failed to respond to medical therapy.

Surgical methods include conservative surgery and radical methods.

#### Conservative methods

- At the time of laparoscopy, if small, active endometriotic implants are found, they can be electro-coagulated and adhesions can be lysed.
- If small endometrioma are found, they can be drained.
- If the endometrioma is more than 4 cm, after draining, the cyst wall has to be removed to prevent recurrences.
- In order to relieve pain, interruption of nerve pathways by ablating the utero-sacral ligaments may be required in few cases.

#### Radical methods

In women who have completed the family, hysterectomy with bilateral salpingo-oophorectomy and removal of all endometriotic implants is undertaken.

**Table 15.1** Medical therapy for endometriosis

| Drug | Duration of use | Mechanism of action | Side-effects |
|---|---|---|---|
| Combined OC pills | Continuous/cyclic 9 months to one year | Pseudo-pregnancy state | Weight gain, depression, headache, acne, bloating, and breast tenderness |
| Progestogens | Continuous for 9 months | Pseudo-pregnancy state | Weight gain, irregular bleeding, depression, osteoporosis and amenorrhea |
| LNG-IUS | Approved for 5 years | Pseudo-pregnancy state | |
| Danazol | 9 months | Pseudo-menopause state | Hot flushes, acne, reduced libido, oily hair and skin, muscle cramps |
| GnRH-a (with or without add-back therapy) | 6 months | Pseudo-menopause state | Vasomotor symptoms, vaginal dryness, decreased libido, joint pain and loss of bone mass. |

*Case study*

*A 28-year-old lady married for 3 years, mother of a two-year-old child presents with severe deep-seated pain during coitus for the past six months. She has been on NSAIDs and oral contraceptive pills without any relief. Pelvic examination revealed the uterus to have restricted mobility and minimal forniceal tenderness.*

*a) Which condition could be responsible for her symptoms?*

*b) What investigation will confirm the diagnosis?*

*c) What are the medical management options available for this woman?*

# REVIEW QUESTIONS

### Long-Answer Question

Define endometriosis. Discuss the various probable theories for the development of endometriosis.

### Short-Answer Questions

1. What are the risk factors for developing endometriosis?
2. Describe briefly the various symptoms of endometriosis.

## MCQs

**1. Which is the most common symptom of endometriosis?**

a) Dysmenorrhea b) Dyspareunia
c) Pelvic pain d) All of the above

**2. Which investigation is the "Gold Standard" in the diagnosis of endometriosis?**

a) Laparoscopy
b) USG
c) MRI
d) CT scan

**3. Which two of the following are true with regards to endometriosis**

a) It is a malignant condition.
b) It occurs commonly in multiparous women.
c) It is estrogen-dependent.
d) It leads to infertility.

**4. The mechanism of action of LNG IUS in the management of endometriosis is:**

a) Pseudo-menopause state
b) Pseudo-pregnancy state
c) Preventing sperm penetration
d) Temporarily blocking the Fallopian tubes

# Amenorrhea

## AT A GLANCE

Etiology
Primary Amenorrhea
A. Genital Tract Anomalies
i. Absence of Vagina
ii. Transverse Septum of Vagina
iii. Agenesis of the Upper third of the Vagina
iv. Imperforate Hymen
B. Chromosomal Anomalies
i. Turner's Syndrome
ii. Androgen Insensitivity Syndrome (AIS)
C. Dysfunction of Hypothalamic-Pituitary-Ovarian Axis
Hypothalamic Amenorrhea
Pituitary Causes of Primary Amenorrhea
D. Ovarian Causes of Primary Amenorrhea
Polycystic Ovarian Syndrome (PCOS)
Ovarian Tumours
Ovarian Insensitivity Syndrome (Savage Syndrome)
E. Thyroid and Adrenal Disorders Causing Primary Amenorrhea
i. Hypothyroidism
ii. Adrenocortical Causes
F. Endometrial Causes of Primary Amenorrhea
Secondary Amenorrhea
Causes of Secondary Amenorrhea
Physiological Causes
Pathological Causes
A. Disorders Associated with a Low or Normal FSH
Hypothyroidism
B. Disorders in which the FSH is High
Primary Ovarian Failure (POF) or Premature Ovarian Insufficiency (POI)
C. Disorders with High Prolactin Levels
Hyperprolactinemia
D. Anatomic Disorders
i. Acquired Cervical Stenosis
ii. Intrauterine Adhesions (Asherman Syndrome)
E. Hyperandrogenic States
Adult-Onset Congenital Adrenal Hyperplasia (AOCAH)
Diagnosis of Secondary Amenorrhea
Investigations
Progesterone Withdrawal Test
Hormonal Evaluation
Imaging Studies
Chromosomal Analysis
Management

## INTRODUCTION

The demarcating line between delayed menarche and primary amenorrhea is an arbitrary one.

**Definition** A young girl who has not menstruated by her 16th birthday is to be considered as having primary amenorrhea rather than a delayed menarche.

> If by the age of 13 years the girl has not started menstruating with absence of secondary sexual characters like breast development, investigations for primary amenorrhea should start.

**Basic principles of menstrual function** There are five basic factors involved in the onset and continuation of normal menstruation. These are:

- normal female chromosomal pattern
- anatomical patency of the genital tract
- coordinated hypothalamo-pituitary–ovarian axis
- active support of thyroid and adrenal cortex
- a responsive endometrium

**Defect in one or more of these factors will therefore be responsible for amenorrhea, either primary or secondary.**

## ETIOLOGY

The common causes of primary amenorrhea are listed in Table 16.1.

An alternative classification of the etiology of primary amenorrhea is given in Table 16.2.

**Table 16.1** Common causes of primary amenorrhea

A. Developmental defects of genital tract:
   - Complete absence of vagina
   - Transverse septum
   - Partial absence of upper part of vagina
   - Imperforate hymen

B. Chromosomal anomalies
C. Hypothalamic, pituitary and ovarian causes
D. Dysfunction of thyroid and adrenal cortex
E. Unresponsive or absent endometrium

In a series of 217 patients with primary amenorrhea, gonadal dysgenesis was found in 13 per cent, Müllerian duct anomalies in 25 per cent, hypogonadotropic hypogonadism in 16 per cent and genital tuberculosis and testicular feminising syndrome in 2.3 per cent of the patients. In another review of 262 such patients, primary amenorrhea in 77 per cent patients was due to developmental defect of the genital tract, in 13 per cent due to chromosomal anomalies and in 3.5 per cent due to defect in hypothalamic-pituitary-ovarian axis.

## PRIMARY AMENORRHEA

The common causes for primary amenorrhea listed in Table 16.1 are discussed in detail in the following subsections.

## A. GENITAL TRACT ANOMALIES

A definite correlation almost always exists between the type of anatomic defect of the vagina and the nature of abnormalities found in the internal pelvic organs. Vaginal malformation has been classified into four grades (Table 16.3). The classification has been made on the basis of their prognosis after surgical correction.

**Table 16.2** Etiology of primary amenorrhea (Modified from: Amenorrhea, Kenneth M Bielak, MD; Chief Editor: Richard Scott Lucidi, MD, FACOG et al., Medscape)

| Gonadotrophic status | Causes | Conditions |
|---|---|---|
| Hypergonadotropic hypogonadism | Abnormal sex chromosomes | Turner syndrome (30%) |
| | Normal sex chromosomes | 46, XX (15%)<br>46, XY (3%). |
| Hypogonadotropic hypogonadism | Tumour | Unclassified malignant tumour<br>Unclassified pituitary adenoma<br>Craniopharyngioma |
| | Systemic illness | |
| | Congenital abnormalities | Congenital central nervous system (CNS) defects<br>Constitutional delay<br>Forms of hypopituitarism<br>Isolated GnRH deficiency |
| | Eating disorder | |
| | Endocrine disorders | Pseudohypoparathyroidism<br>Congenital adrenal hyperplasia (CAH)<br>Hyperprolactinemia<br>Cushing's syndrome |
| Eugonadism (pubertal delay with normal gonadotropins) | Anatomic abnormalities | Congenital absence of the uterus and vagina<br>Cervical atresia |
| | Intersex disorders | Androgen insensitivity 17-ketoreductase deficiency and inappropriate feedback |

**Table 16.3** Clinical diagnosis of primary amenorrhea associated with vaginal maldevelopment

| Grade | Type of vaginal maldevelopment | Clinical diagnosis | Co-existing abnormalities |
|---|---|---|---|
| 1 | Complete absence of vagina | True amenorrhea | Functioning uterus absent. Otherwise normal (46 XX) |
| 2 | Transverse septum of vagina | Hematocolpos and hematometra | Functioning uterus may be normal or malformed (bicornuate) |
| 3 | Partial agenesis of upper part of vagina | Hematometra only | Functioning uterus, cervix is ill-developed. |
| 4 | Annular constriction of upper part of vagina (rare) | True amenorrhea | Isthmial stenosis, uterus and adnexa normal |

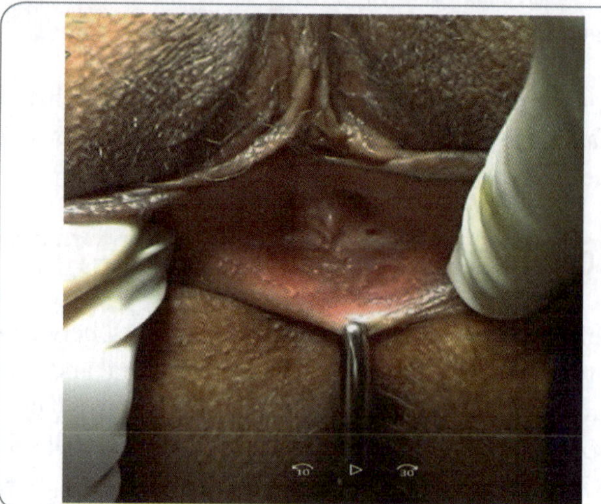

Fig. 16.1 Complete absence of the vagina (*Source:* Dr. Girija Wagh, Professor, Obstetrics & Gynecology, Bharati Vidyapeeth University Medical College)

## i. Absence of Vagina

One of the most common causes of primary amenorrhea is the absence of the vagina (Fig. 16.1) with simultaneous absence of a functioning uterus. These individuals are phenotypic females; all of them have normal gonads (ovary) and normal female karyotype. There are remnants of Müllerian tissue; the Fallopian tubes in the majority of cases are normal both anatomically and histologically. At the medial end of each Fallopian tube, there are two solid Müllerian knobs connected by a solid fibro-muscular band. The fibro-muscular band lies underneath the vesico-rectal fold of peritoneum. The solid Müllerian knobs which are embryological remnants of the adult uterus sometimes contain functionally active endometrial tissue. Behind the bladder and connected to the transverse fibro-muscular band, there is a third knob which perhaps is the lower fused portion of the Müllerian ducts. This is an embryological remnant of the adult cervix. The endocrine and ovulatory status of these individuals have been found to be normal. The pelvic findings and cytohormonal pattern are reasonably consistent and they have been grouped under a common syndrome known as **Mayer–Rokitansky–Küster–Hauser (MRKH) syndrome.** Urinary tract malformation (like pelvic kidney) is associated in about 30 per cent of cases.

### Treatment

Vaginal reconstruction is the accepted form of treatment. The principle of vaginal reconstruction is to create an avascular space between the bladder and the rectum and keep it patent by mould and graft. Various types of grafts have been used.

## ii. Transverse Septum of Vagina

There is a transverse segmental partition usually situated in the middle third of the vagina (Fig. 16.2). The uterus and cervix are normal. **Hematometra and hematocolpos are always associated with this condition.**

### Signs and symptoms

This condition can be diagnosed by periodic pain, lump in pelvis palpated by abdominal-rectal examination and occasionally, retention of urine due to the stretching of the urethra.

Sometimes the transverse septum may be confused with partial agenesis of the upper third of the vagina. In both the conditions there will be an abdomino-pelvic lump due to hematometra with or without hematocolpos.

### Treatment

The treatment is surgical incision of the obstructing partition.

## iii. Agenesis of the Upper Third of the Vagina

Agenesis of the upper third of the vagina and transverse septum may reveal the same clinical features. But from a therapeutic point of view these two conditions are entirely different.

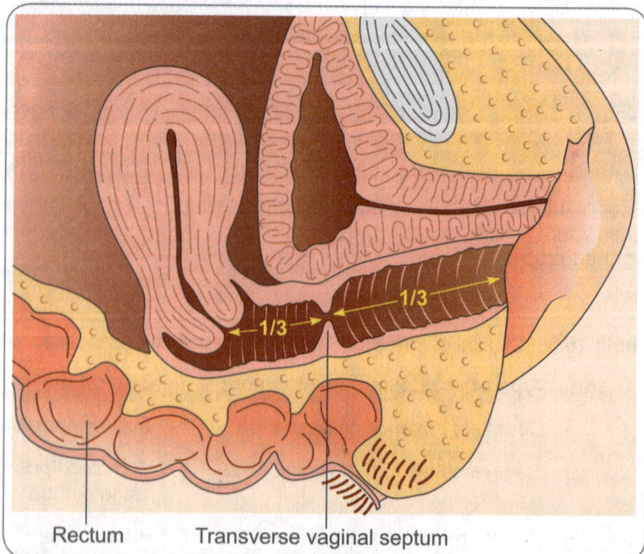


Fig. 16.2 Transverse vaginal septum (*Source:* http://www.slideshare.net/mohamedjammal9/congenital-malformations-of-genital-organs)

| Transverse septum | Partial agenesis |
|---|---|
| Upper part of vagina, cervical and uterine canal are normal and patent | In addition to vaginal agenesis, the cervix is rudimentary and non-canalised, while the uterus may be functioning |

## iv. Imperforate Hymen

In this condition there is **cryptomenorrhea** (hidden menstruation). It can easily be differentiated from the complete absence of vagina in a postpubertal or adolescent girl. The obstructing membrane or partition in both the conditions exist at the level of introitus (*see* Fig. 5.6).

### Signs and symptoms

In an adolescent girl with imperforate hymen in addition to amenorrhea there may be symptoms of periodic lower abdominal pain and occasionally retention of urine.

### Examination

On local examination, a bluish bulge on the obstructing membrane is visible at the introitus. Abdominal rectal examination will reveal a pelvic lump due to hematocolpos and hematometra.

### Treatment

Treatment is simple; cruciate incision and excision of the hymen allowing spontaneous drainage of blood collected inside the vagina and the uterus.

## B. CHROMOSOMAL ANOMALIES

The two most common conditions due to chromosomal anomalies are Turner's syndrome and testicular feminising syndrome.

## i. Turner's Syndrome

Turner (1938) described a series of female patients with sexual infantilism, webbing of neck, retardation of growth and bilateral cubitus valgus (Fig. 16.3). It was later found that such individuals had no ovaries but merely **streak gonads**. At that time, ovarian agenesis and dysgenesis and Turner's syndrome were considered synonymous.

### Clinical features

A large number of additional physical features have since been observed in pure Turner's syndrome cases, like for example, 'shield' chest, high arch palate, low-set ears, deafness, pigmented soles and coarctation

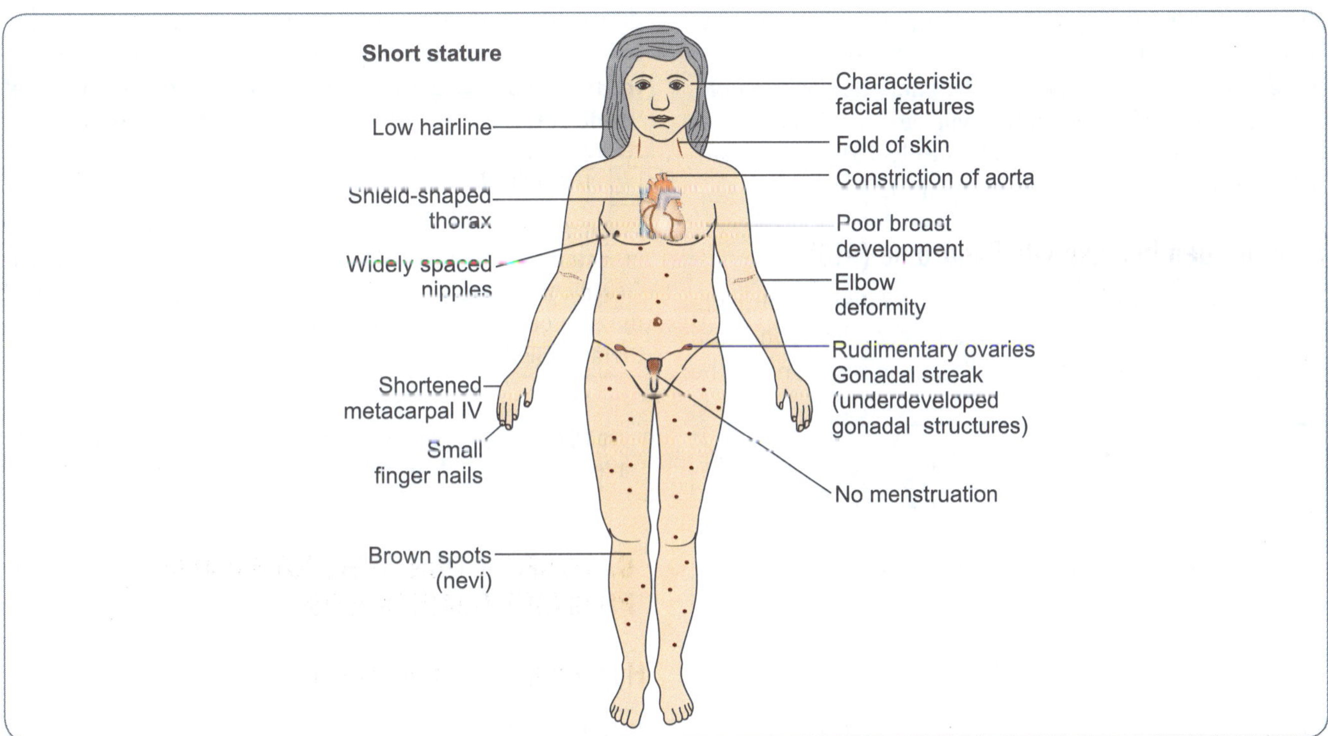


**Fig. 16.3** Turner's syndrome (note the short stature, webbing of the neck and cubitus valgus)

of aorta. These have been referred to as **Turner's stigmata.**

In Turner's syndrome, the ovarian development is normal until 20 weeks of intrauterine life and oocytes are found in the ovaries until this stage. Thereafter there is failure of the oocytes to undergo further maturation, which requires the influence of both X chromosomes. In Turner's the karyotype is 45, XO and there is only one X chromosome and the oocytes begin to undergo a process of atresia (Fig. 16.4). This probably continues beyond birth and in some cases till late puberty.

The ovary in most individuals at this stage consists mainly of stroma and is therefore unable to produce estrogen. There is normal female type organ development as the absence of the Y chromosome means the presence of uterus, tubes and vagina. The loss of one X chromosome is associated with short stature since the determining genes for height are lost. In chromosomal mosaicism (46XX/45X), the proportion of each cell line determines the manifestation of the condition. This means that individuals with a higher percentage of 45XO cells will have more features of Turner's syndrome. The presence of some normal 46XX cells indicates the possibility of ovarian differentiation and the associated development of secondary sexual characteristics. Approximately 10–15 per cent of girls exhibit some estrogenic activity.

**Even with Turner's stigmata, all women are not amenorrheic.** This will depend on the degree of deletion of genetic material in the X chromosome. The loss of the short or long arm of a chromosome may be complete or partial and the genetic material lost determines the impact of Turner's features on the patients. For example, the incidence of amenorrhea will be 35 per cent with long arm deletion while it will be only 15 per cent with deletion of short arm of the X chromosome.

### ii. Androgen Insensitivity Syndrome (AIS)

This was formerly known as testicular feminising syndrome. This is an X-linked recessive condition resulting in failure of normal masculinisation of the external genitalia in chromosomally male individuals. This could be either

- Complete androgen insensitivity syndrome (CAIS) or
- Partial androgen insensitivity syndrome (PAIS)

This differentiation depends on the amount of residual receptor function. Both complete and partial AIS individuals will have 46XY chromosome.

Those with CAIS will have normal labia, clitoris, and vaginal introitus with well-developed breasts, scanty or absent pubic and axillary hair.

The testes are hormonally competent and the plasma testosterone levels of these patients are identical to those seen in postpubertal normal males. Müllerian inhibitory factor (MIF) of testes is normal and therefore there is suppression of Müllerian tissue like uterus, fallopian tubes and upper vagina. Though the entire length of vagina has been presumed to be Müllerian in origin, the 'short blind' vagina present in testicular feminising syndrome has developed from the remnants of the urogenital sinus. Both the testes are found either in the inguinal canal, labia majora (Fig. 16.5) or rarely, in the 'ovarian fossa'. These are normal testes with normal production of testosterone and normal conversion to dihydrotestosterone (DHT). Since the condition is familial, it is not unusual to have sisters with the same defect. The main complaint is of primary amenorrhea.

Feminine development at puberty is thought to be due to normal adrenal and testicular estrogens acting on end organs which are resistant to androgens. **These individuals though categorised under the heading of 'male intersex' should be brought up as females.**

#### Treatment

Gonadectomy is indicated, because these gonads situated in ectopic sites are liable to undergo malignant change. Treatment therefore consists of removal of gonads, excision of the enlarged phallus followed by female hormone replacement therapy (HRT).

In all these cases where gonadectomy is indicated, it is performed after the age of 20 or on completion of the bone growth.

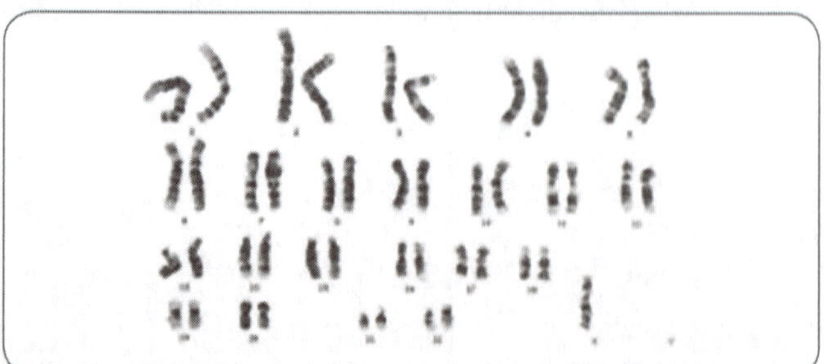

**Fig. 16.4** 45, X karyotype, showing an unpaired X at the lower right (*Source:* Wikipedia)

## C. DYSFUNCTION OF HYPOTHALAMIC-PITUITARY-OVARIAN AXIS

### Hypothalamic Amenorrhea

Primary amenorrhea may be due to functional or organic causes in the hypothalamus.

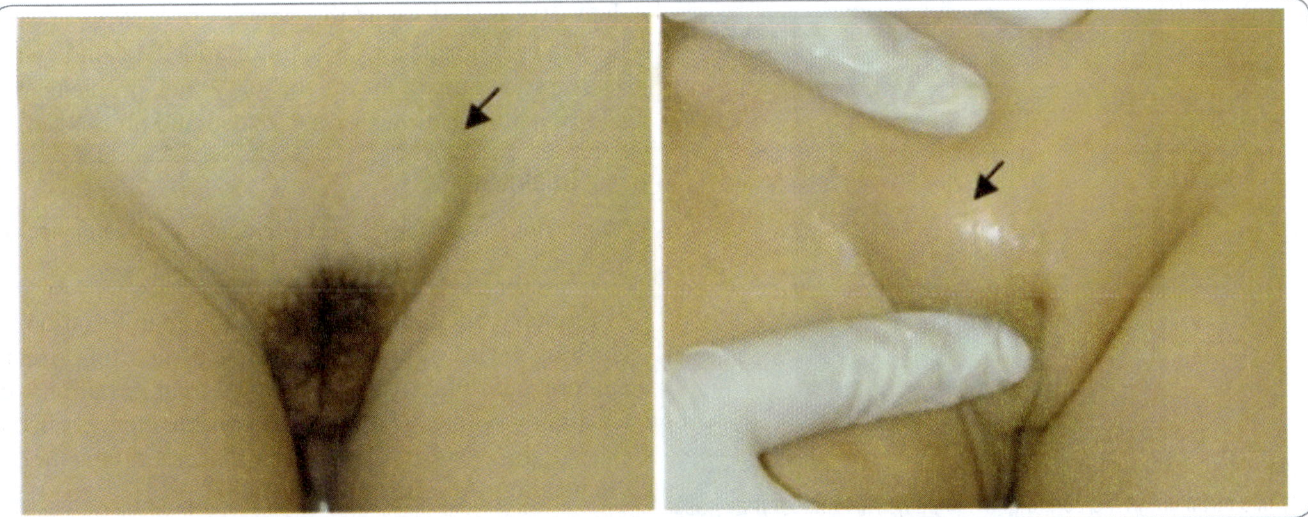

**Fig. 16.5** Labioscrotal swelling with the gonad (testes) in a case of testicular feminising syndrome (*Source:* BMC Research Notes 2011 4:173/© de Mello et al.)

#### Functional causes

##### *i. Anorexia nervosa*

This is a psychological disorder affecting children and adults equally. Growth and secondary sexual characteristics are normal but subsequently they regress. The fault lies in the pulsatile release of gonadotropins because of the effect of low body mass on the secretion of pulsatile GnRH.

##### *ii. Excessive exercise*

As in anorexia nervosa, **excessive exercise** like those undertaken by athletes may be responsible for primary amenorrhea. Reduction of body fat may lead to suppression of GnRH release leading to failure in establishing menstruation.

#### Organic causes

##### *i. Hypopituitarism*

This may be associated with short stature, obesity, peculiar distribution of fat (**adiposogenital dystrophy**).

The condition is very rare. Treatment and prognosis are unsatisfactory.

##### *ii. Olfactogenital syndrome (Kallman's syndrome)*

In this condition, the hypothalamus lacks the ability to produce GnRH and therefore there is hypogonadotropic state. The pituitary is normal and stimulation with GnRH leads to normal release of gonadotropins. The patient also suffers from anosmia. It is presumably due to a genetic defect and may occur either sporadically or in families.

## Pituitary Causes of Primary Amenorrhea

#### a. Empty sella syndrome

This syndrome is characterised by absence of sufficient pituitary tissue. Usually the endocrine function is normal but sometimes adequate amount of FSH is not produced in response to the GnRH secreted by the normally functioning hypothalamus. These patients are therefore hypogonadotropic but the problem lies at the level of pituitary rather than the hypothalamus.

#### Investigations

A CT scan of the pituitary fossa or an MRI will identify this syndrome.

#### b. Tumours

Tumours responsible for primary amenorrhea are the following.

i. **Craniopharyngioma**, also known as **Rathke's pouch tumour**, arises from embryonic squamous cell rests which persist after migration of stomodial epithelium to the anterior pituitary. These tumours are common in children and adolescents but may occur at any age.
   **Clinical presentation** of these tumours are usually with visual and neurological symptoms, with variable degree of hypopituitarism and primary amenorrhea.
   **Diagnosis** is by CT scan (Fig. 16.6) and MRI. Surgical approach is usually by craniotomy.

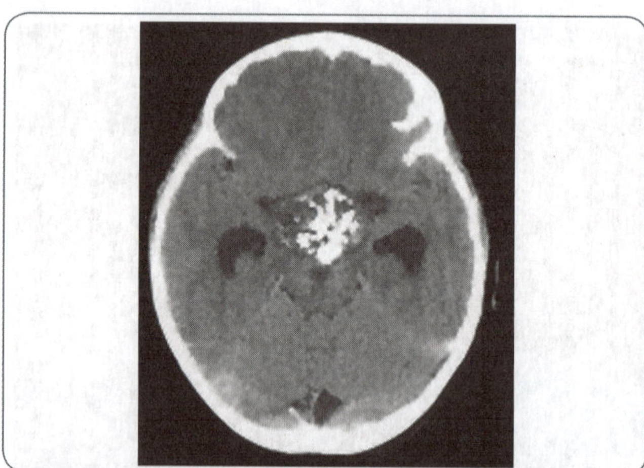

**Fig. 16.6** CT scan of the brain showing a craniopharyngioma (white structure in the centre of the image). This tumour may cause hypopituitarism and requires surgical removal. (*Source:* Orphanet Journal of Rare Diseases 2007 2:18/© Garnett et. al.)

ii. A rare type of **pituitary adenoma** is responsible for acromegaly leading to primary amenorrhea. This type of pituitary adenoma is responsible for production of excess growth hormone (GH). Over 99 per cent of cases of acromegaly are due to pituitary adenoma and less than one per cent is due to excessive production of hypothalamic growth hormone releasing hormone (GHRH) causing somatotropic hyperplasia of the pituitary. If the condition occurs before puberty, it may accelerate linear growth and culminate with gigantism. Apart from neurological manifestations, 'if the tumour is large it may produce gonadal dysfunction leading to amenorrhea. Hyperprolactinemia may be present in up to 40 per cent of patients with acromegaly, causing amenorrhea in these cases. It can be treated by surgical excision of the tumour followed by radiotherapy.

   **Treatment** Medical treatment consists of administration of bromocriptine and somatostatin analogues.

iii. The more common type of pituitary adenoma is **prolactinoma.** Prolactinoma is associated more frequently with secondary rather than primary amenorrhea. Prolactinoma may also be associated with primary amenorrhea. Apart from amenorrhea, **galactorrhea is an outstanding**, though not invariable, clinical symptom.

**Investigations** Estimation of serum prolactin will settle the diagnosis of hyperprolactinemia with or without prolactinoma. If the prolactin level is more than 100 ng/mL or if the coned down view of sella turcica is abnormal, a CT scan or an MRI is indicated. The association of headache or visual problems are additional indications for a CT scan and an MRI.

**Treatment**

Bromocriptine therapy is the standard treatment for hyperprolactinemia with or without microadenoma.

Pituitary adenoma leading to the manifestation of Cushing's syndrome may also be responsible for primary amenorrhea. Because the clinical manifestations of Cushing's syndrome are due to chronic glucocorticoid excess, this syndrome has been discussed later under the heading, Adrenocortical Defect.

## D. OVARIAN CAUSES OF PRIMARY AMENORRHEA

### Polycystic Ovarian Syndrome (PCOS)

Polycystic ovarian disease, though a common cause of secondary amenorrhea, rarely causes primary amenorrhea as well. Classic manifestations of polycystic ovarian disease are modest obesity, mild hirsutism, bilaterally enlarged ovaries, anovulation and amenorrhea. This condition is discussed in detail in Chapter 14.

### Ovarian Tumours

Apart from polycystic ovarian disease, ovarian causes of primary amenorrhea may be androgen-producing tumours of the ovary like **arrhenoblastoma (Sertoli–Leydig cell tumours)** or **hilus cell tumour of the ovary.** Defeminisation with amenorrhea is a common manifestation of these tumours. These masculinising tumours are rare.

### Ovarian Insensitivity Syndrome (Savage Syndrome)

Patients with this condition have

- normal stature
- elevated gonadotropin levels
- normal secondary sexual characteristics
- normal ovaries
- variable number of primordial follicles identified by ultrasound imaging or ovarian biopsy

Ovarian insensitivity to high level of circulating gonadotropin is attributed to a cell membrane receptor defect. Autoimmune ovarian failure may be associated with Addison's and/or Hashimoto's disease. Autoimmune ovarian failure is related to secondary rather than primary amenorrhea.

### Investigations

With the introduction of laparoscope, ultrasound and radioimmunoassay in the investigation protocol, ovarian biopsy is not indicated now for the diagnosis.

 **Treatment**

In all varieties of ovarian failure (chromosomal, genetic or autoimmune), the current approach of treatment is to achieve pregnancy, if desired, by IVF with **oocyte donation programme.**

**Estrogen hormone** treatment is indicated in young women to prevent bone loss. This could be in the form of pills, patches or vaginal ring. The treatment can be started on diagnosis and can be continued till the age of 50 the average age of menopause.

## E. THYROID AND ADRENAL DISORDERS CAUSING PRIMARY AMENORRHEA

### i. Hypothyroidism

This may be responsible for primary amenorrhea. Secondary amenorrhea is a common manifestation but primary amenorrhea is seen in cretinism. Primary hypothyroidism may be associated with primary amenorrhea. The disorders in this category include primary thyroid atrophy, post-ablative hypothyroidism and sporadic athyreotic cretinism.

Longstanding cases of primary hypothyroidism are associated with hyperprolactinemia and galactorrhea. The coexistence of hyperprolactinemia may be due to declining hypothalamic content of dopamine with ongoing hypothyroidism. This will lead to unopposed stimulatory effect of thyrotropin releasing hormone (TRH) on the pituitary cells which secrete prolactin.

 **Treatment**

Amenorrhea due to hypothyroidism is treated by replacement therapy with L-thyroxin. Hyperprolactinemia associated with hypothyroidism does not require separate treatment as control of hypothyroidism will result in correction of hyperprolactinemia.

### ii. Adrenocortical Causes

Adrenocortical causes responsible for primary amenorrhea are **congenital adrenal hyperplasia and Cushing's syndrome**.

#### Congenital adrenal hyperplasia (CAH)

Usually the non-salt-losing variety of congenital adrenal hyperplasia (CAH) lasts up to the age of puberty. Ambiguous external genitalia at birth (Fig. 16.7) without externally palpable gonads should raise the suspicion of congenital adrenal hyperplasia.

These individuals may also present at or after puberty with primary amenorrhea.

#### *Clinical presentation*

Apart from primary amenorrhea, this includes hirsutism, clitoromegaly of varying degrees (Fig. 16.7) and non-canalisation of urogenital sinus. The internal genital organs are normally feminine.

#### *Investigations*

Endocrine estimation reveals elevation of 17α-hydroxyprogesterone and testosterone. The biochemical test reveals deficiency of the adrenal enzyme 21 hydroxylase or 11β-hydroxylase. This leads to failure of normal quantity of cortisol production which in turn is responsible for elevated levels of ACTH because of defective feedback mechanism. Elevated ACTH will stimulate increased production of cortisol precursors which are converted via 17α-hydroxyprogesterone to androgens.

 **Treatment**

Treatment consists of plastic reconstruction of external genital organs and dexamethasone suppression of excess ACTH.

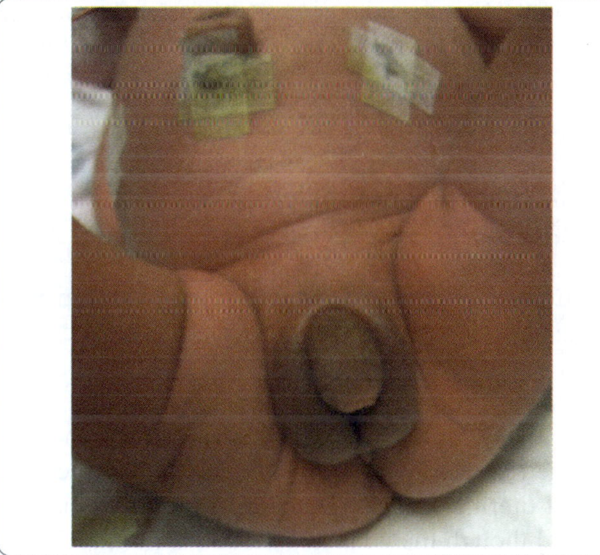

**Fig. 16.7** Ambiguous genitalia in congenital adrenal hyperplasia (*Source:* NIH)

### Cushing's syndrome

The clinical manifestations of Cushing's syndrome are the effects of chronic glucocorticoid excess. Cushing's syndrome may be due to primary pituitary dysfunction or an adrenal tumour. Pituitary dysfunction may be due to pituitary hyperplasia under the influence of excess CRH (corticosteroid releasing hormone) or due to a pituitary adenoma.

#### *Clinical features*

The classic features are

- progressive central obesity,
- typical moon faces,
- skin changes like striae,
- fragile skin with evidence of ecchymoses and
- features of hyperandrogenism like acne, mild hirsutism and occasional enlargement of clitoris (Fig. 16.8).

Moderate hypertension, glucose intolerance and hyperinsulinemia are common though true diabetes in adolescent girls is rare. Amenorrhea has been explained by negative feedback effect on gonadotropin secretion by increased levels of androgens and cortisol.

#### *Investigations*

Diagnosis is confirmed by overnight dexamethasone suppression test and estimation of 24-hour urinary free cortisol, urinary ketosteroids and 17-hydroxycorticosteroid. A CT scan of adrenal cortex and pituitary will corroborate the diagnosis of a tumour.

#### Treatment

When a tumour is detected, treatment consists of surgical removal. Postoperative radiotherapy is often essential to prevent recurrence. Other therapies include administration of centrally active drugs, adrenal enzyme inhibitors, antiglucocorticoid agents and longstanding somatostatin analogue.

## F. ENDOMETRIAL CAUSES OF PRIMARY AMENORRHEA

Intrauterine adhesions leading to primary amenorrhea are usually a sequelae of endometrial tuberculosis which is quite common in India. The size of the uterus is normal. Traumatic synechiae at this age are rare. Occasionally, in the absence of intrauterine adhesion, endometrial tissue is scanty or absent in otherwise normal uterine activity. The size of the uterus is also reduced though the gonadal function is normal. These are perhaps due to deficiency of estrogen receptors in the endometrium and myometrium.

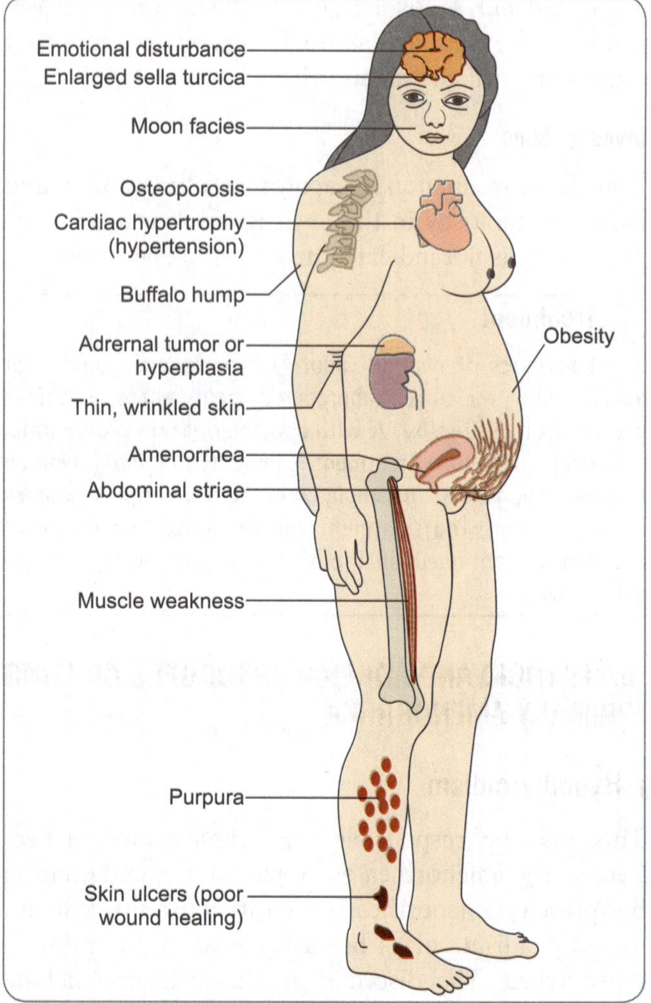


**Fig. 16.8** Symptoms of Cushing's syndrome

**Investigations** Hysteroscopy and endometrial biopsy help in the diagnosis.

## SECONDARY AMENORRHEA

Secondary amenorrhea is more common than the primary condition and about 3–5 per cent of women suffer from it.

**Definition** It is customary to use the term when there is absence of menstruation for over 3 months in a woman who has been menstruating regularly earlier.

## CAUSES OF SECONDARY AMENORRHEA

### Physiological Causes

The important physiological causes are

- pregnancy
- lactation

- menopause

**Pregnancy is the most common cause of secondary amenorrhea**. During lactational amenorrhea, ovulation and pregnancy may occur.

## Pathological Causes

The pathological causes are considered in Table 16.4.

## A. DISORDERS ASSOCIATED WITH A LOW OR NORMAL FSH

Weight loss / anorexia both anorexia nervosa and bulimia can result in amenorrhea. Weight loss is usually less severe in bulimic women whereas due to caloric restriction, self-induced vomiting and severe exercise, weight loss is more in anorexia nervosa.

### *a. Exercise-induced amenorrhea*

This is usually seen in athletes, ballet dancers and gymnasts.

### *b. Functional hypothalamic amenorrhea*

The various factors associated with functional amenorrhea may act separately or together. Exercise has been known to produce amenorrhea by increasing the level of beta endorphins.

### *c. Pituitary tumours*

Pituitary adenomas are the most common cause of acquired pituitary dysfunction. Most of them secrete prolactin. This elevated prolactin can give rise to galactorrhea and amenorrhea—the **galactorrhea–amenorrhea syndrome.**

### *d. Sheehan's syndrome*

It is a panhypopituitary condition. It usually results from severe postpartum haemorrhage with severe hypotension. The affected patient may even develop pituitary apoplexy.

### *e. Polycystic ovarian syndrome (PCOS)*

This is discussed in detail in Chapter14. Though PCOS is usually associated with oligomenorrhea, amenorrhea can also occur.

## Hypothyroidism

Thyroid disorder is a common cause of oligomenorrhea. Though the exact mechanism by which hypothyroidism causes amenorrhea is not clear, one possible explanation is as shown in the following flow diagram.

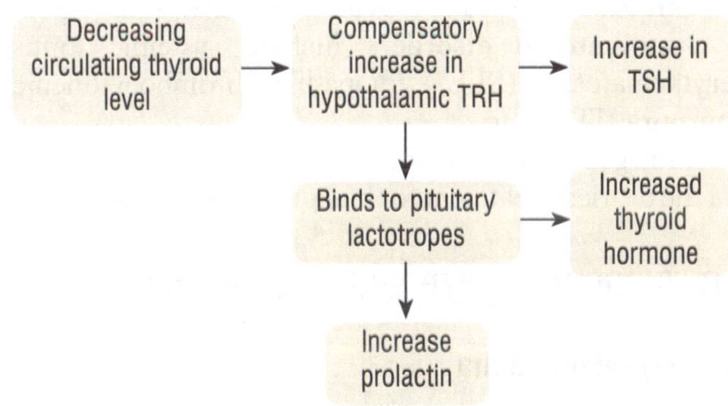


**Table 16.4** Causes of secondary amenorrhea

| | |
|---|---|
| A. Disorders associated with a low or normal FSH (66%) | • Weight loss/anorexia<br>• Non-specific hypothalamic conditions<br>• Chronic anovulation including PCOS<br>• Hypothyroidism<br>• Cushing's syndrome<br>• Pituitary tumour<br>• Empty sella syndrome<br>• Sheehan syndrome |
| B. Disorders in which the FSH is high (12%) | • 46XX spontaneous premature ovarian failure insufficiency (POI)<br>• Premature ovarian failure/insufficiency due to abnormal karyotype (45, X mosaic/ring chromosome)<br>• Pure gonadal dysgenesis |
| C. Disorders associated with a high prolactin level (13%) | • Hyperprolactinemia |
| D. Anatomic disorders (7%) | • Asherman syndrome<br>• Acquired cervical stenosis |
| E. Hyperandrogenic states as a cause of secondary amenorrhea (2%) | • Polycystic ovarian syndrome (PCOS)<br>• Ovarian tumour<br>• Non-classic congenital adrenal hyperplasia (CAH)<br>• Undiagnosed |

(Modified from: emedicine.medscape.com/article/252928-overview #a4)

## B. DISORDERS IN WHICH FSH IS HIGH

These disorders are due to hypergonadotropic hypogonadism state. In these conditions, the ovarian function is reduced or absent (hypogonadism) and the FSH and LH levels are increased (hypergonadotropic).

### Primary Ovarian Failure (POF) or Premature Ovarian Insufficiency (POI)

**Definition** POF is defined as loss of oocytes before 40 years of age. The diagnosis is confirmed by two serum FSH levels of more than 40 mIU/mL with a gap of one month between the two tests.

**Etiology** **Gonadal dysgenesis** is the most common cause of POI. Most of the affected women do not menstruate.

The other **genetic causes** are fragile X syndrome. Similarly mutations in the LH and FSH receptors have also been reported.

**Galactosemia** is a rare cause of POI.

**Infectious causes** of POI are not clearly understood.

**Autoimmune disorders** include systemic lupus erythematosus (SLE), idiopathic thrombocytopenic purpura (ITP), etc.

**Iatrogenic** ovarian failure includes surgical removal of the ovaries, treatment for malignancies, radiotherapy.

## C. DISORDERS WITH HIGH PROLACTIN LEVELS

### Hyperprolactinemia

This could be caused either by hypothalamic – pituitary stalk damage due to tumours like craniopharyngioma or suprasellar pituitary mass or due to pituitary hypersecretion in conditions like prolactinoma, acromegaly, etc. It may also result from systemic disorders like chronic renal failure or hypothyroidism or by drugs like phenothiazones, chlorpromazine, metoclopramide, etc.

Pseudocyesis is another condition with hyperprolactinemia and increased LH/FSH ratio. Pseudocyesis has endocrinological as well as psychological reasons. With the liberal use of imaging technology, delayed diagnosis of pseudocyesis has become rare.

## D. ANATOMIC DISORDERS

### i. Acquired Cervical Stenosis

Vigorous curetting (D&C), conisation, loop excision, neoplasia are some of the common causes for cervical stenosis. This may lead to amenorrhea in previously menstruating women. Postmenopausal women are initially asymptomatic until fluid (hydrometra), exudates or blood (hematometra) accumulates.

Management of cervical Stenosis requires cervical dilatation and exclusion of neoplasia.

### ii. Intrauterine Adhesions (Asherman Syndrome)

It usually follows vigorous curetting associated with postpartum hemorrhage, abortion (MTP or spontaneous) or infection. Other conditions which may give rise to intrauterine adhesions are metroplasty, myomectomy or caesarean section. As a result of these conditions the basalis layer of endometrium prevents endometrial thickening. Hence no menstruation occurs.

The diagnosis of intrauterine adhesions could be by hystereosalpingogram (HSG) (Fig. 16.9) or by hysteroscopy (Fig. 16.10).

#### *Management*

Currently the management of Asherman Syndrome is by lysis of adhesions. Where hysteroscopic facilities are not available, D&C is also effective in lysing the adhesions.

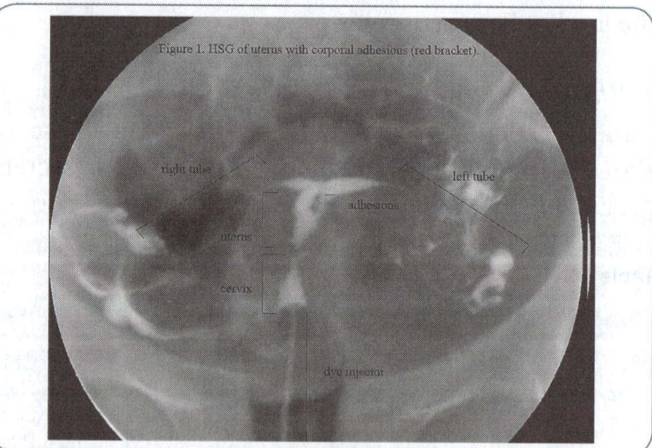


**Fig. 16.9** Hysterosalpingogram showing intrauterine adhesions (*Source:* Wikipedia)

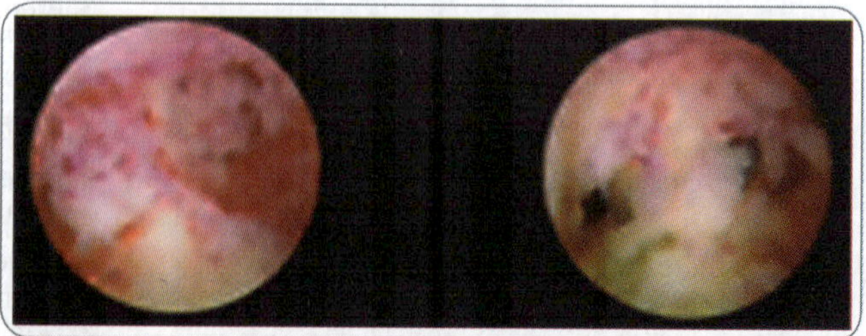

**Fig. 16.10** Hysteroscopy view of intrauterine adhesions (*Source:* Wikipedia)

Adhesiolysis by D&C is usually followed with IUCD insertion to prevent further adhesions.

## E. HYPERANDROGENIC STATES

### Adult-Onset Congenital Adrenal Hyperplasia (AOCAH)

This is also known as late-onset congenital adrenal hyperplasia (LOCAH). It is due to a mutation in the *CYP21* gene. Increased androgen levels and distorted oocyte maturation may result in anovulation and amenorrhea.

## DIAGNOSIS OF SECONDARY AMENORRHEA

The algorithm given below is a comprehensive tool for evaluating secondary amenorrhea.

- **History** The initial history should include a detailed menstrual history starting from puberty.
- **Past surgical history** Any abdominal or pelvic surgery should be carefully evaluated.
- **Physical examination** This should be followed by a thorough general physical examination with specific emphasis on height, weight, stature, visual fields, skin changes, hirsutism or acne, galactorrhea and cervical adenitis. Signs and symptoms of hypothyroidism must be carefully looked for and evaluated.
- **Genital examination** should start from examining the hair growth and its pattern. The specific points to be looked for in the genital examination are:
- Clitoromegaly
- Atrophic changes in the vaginal epithelium
- Size of the uterus
- Presence of adnexal masses
- Mobility of adnexal masses if any
- **Rectal examination** Wherever necessary rectal examination should be performed. Please refer Chapter 1 for further details

## INVESTIGATIONS

Primary investigation, like urinary pregnancy test (UPT) or ultrasound, should be done to rule out pregnancy.

### Progesterone Withdrawal Test

Progesterone withdrawal test is performed as follows:

A single injection of progesterone 50 mg IM or medroxyprogesterone acetate 10 mg daily orally for a week is given. If there is withdrawal bleeding, there is no serious disorder. The probable cause is hypothalamic dysfunction which responds to clomiphene. If there is no bleeding, ethinyl estradiol 0.05 mg daily for 20 days is given. If there is bleeding in response to this, FSH estimation helps in deciding the cause and treatment. If there is no bleeding even after the estrogens, this suggests a refractory endometrium, tuberculous endometritis or uterine synechiae.

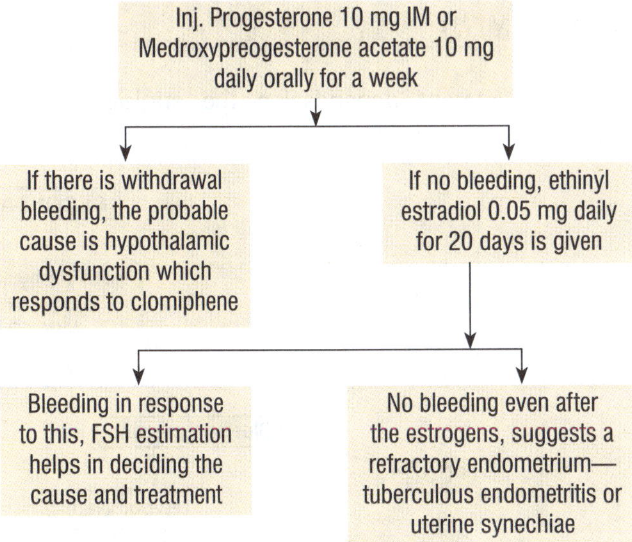


### Hormonal Evaluation

#### FSH

Normal FSH level is indicative of eugonadotropic hypogonadism like PCOS or an anatomic defect. On the other hand a low FSH suggest hypothalamic pituitary dysfunction and increased FSH is indicative of ovarian failure.

#### Prolactin and thyroid stimulating hormone

These two hormones should be tested as prolactin secreting adenoma and thyroid disease are commonly seen in secondary amenorrhea.

#### Testosterone

In women with suspected PCOS testosterone evaluation is necessary. Testosterone levels of more than 200 mg/dl is suggestive of ovarian tumour and further evaluation is necessary.

#### Dehydroepiandrosterone sulphate (DHEAS)

High normal levels are even mild elevation of DHEAS is suggestive of PCOS. Levels over 700 $\mu$g/dl is indicative of adrenal adenoma.

### Imaging Studies

Imaging techniques like ultrasonogram, CT and MRI need to be performed as necessary.

### Chromosomal Analysis

This is more important in primary amenorrhea but should also be performed in women with POI.

## MANAGEMENT

The management depends on the etiology of the condition.

- Anatomic abnormalities would require surgical correction.
- Hypothyroidism should be treated with thyroid replacement.
- Bromocriptine or cabergoline may be required in women with hyper prolactinema.
- Estrogen replacement therapy may have to be started in patients with hypogonadism to prevent osteoporosis.
- The management of PCOS is described in Chapter 14.
- Women with eating disorders will require counselling and behavioural changes.

The following flow diagram can be used for the management of secondary amenorrhea.

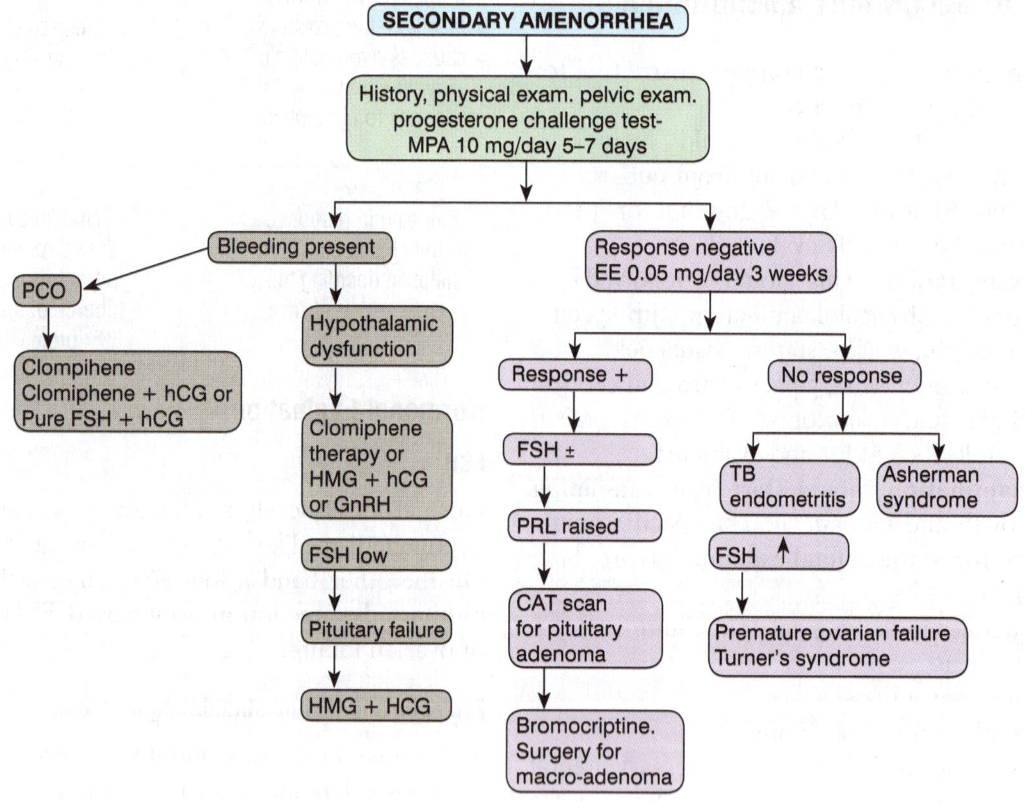


## RECAP

- A young girl who has not menstruated by her 16th birthday should be considered as having primary amenorrhea rather than a delayed menarche.
- If by the age of 13 years, the girl has not started menstruating and there is absence of secondary sexual characters like breast development, investigations for primary amenorrhea should start.
- Common causes of primary amenorrhea are developmental defects of genital tract, chromosomal anomalies, hypothalamic, pituitary and ovarian causes, dysfunction of thyroid and adrenal cortex and unresponsive or absent endometrium.
- An alternative classification based on the etiology is hypergonadotropic hypogonadism, hypogonadotropic hypogonadism and eugonadism (pubertal delay with normal gonadotropins).

- A definite correlation almost always exists between the type of anatomic defect of the vagina and the nature of abnormalities found in the internal pelvic organs.
- Absence of vagina is usually associated with urinary tract malformation (like pelvic kidney).
- Transverse septum of vagina leads to hematometra and hematocolpos.
- In partial agenesis of the upper third of the vagina, in addition to vaginal agenesis, the cervix is rudimentary and non-canalised, while the uterus may be functioning and giving rise to hematometra which requires surgical treatment.
- Imperforate hymen is associated with cryptomenorrhea.
- Chromosomal anomalies include Turner's syndrome, androgen insensitivity syndrome (AIS): (complete androgen insensitivity syndrome (CAIS) or partial androgen insensitivity syndrome (PAIS)).
- Dysfunction of hypothalamo-pituitary-ovarian axis—Functional causes of hypothalamic amenorrhea include anorexia nervosa and organic causes include hypopituitarism, olfactogenital syndrome (Kallman's syndrome).
- Pituitary causes of primary amenorrhea include empty sella syndrome.
- Tumours responsible for primary amenorrhea are craniopharyngioma and pituitary adenoma
- Ovarian causes of primary amenorrhea are Polycystic ovarian Syndrome (PCOS), ovarian tumours like arrhenoblastoma (Sertoli–Leydig cell tumours) or hilus cell tumour of the ovary.
- Patients with ovarian insensitivity syndrome (savage syndrome) are normal in stature, have elevated gonadotropin levels, normal secondary sexual characteristics with normal ovaries and variable number of primordial follicles identified by ultrasound imaging or on ovarian biopsy.
- Thyroid and adrenal disorders causing primary amenorrhea are hypothyroidism and adrenocortical causes like congenital adrenal hyperplasia, Cushing's syndrome.
- Endometrial causes of primary amenorrhea are intrauterine adhesions.
- Secondary amenorrhea is defined as the absence of menstruation for over 3 months in a woman who has been menstruating regularly earlier.
- The important physiological causes are pregnancy, lactation and menopause.
- Pathological causes are disorders associated with a low or normal FSH, disorders in which the FSH is high, disorders associated with a high prolactin level, anatomic disorders and hyperandrogenic states.
- Diagnosis of secondary amenorrhea is based on history including past surgical history, physical examination, genital examination with special emphasis on clitoromegaly, atrophic changes in the vaginal epithelium, size of the uterus, presence of adnexal masses, mobility of adnexal masses if any and rectal examination if indicated.

## REVIEW QUESTIONS

### Long-Answer Question

1. What is imperforate hymen? What complications can occur due to this condition? Discuss the management.

### Short-Answer Questions

1. Define primary amenorrhea. Enumerate the hypogonadotropic hypogonadal causes of primary amenorrhea.
2. Briefly describe the etiology, diagnosis and management of Asherman syndrome.

### MCQs

**1. The karyotype in Turner's syndrome is**
   a) 46 XY
   b) 47 XXY
   c) 47 XXX
   d) 45 XO

**2. Testicular feminising syndrome is otherwise known as**
   a) Androgen insensitivity syndrome
   b) Turner's syndrome
   c) Klinefelter's syndrome
   d) Rokitansky-Küster-Hauser syndrome

**3. Congenital adrenal hyperplasia is associated with**
   a) Increased levels of 17α-hydroxyprogesterone
   b) Reduced levels of 21-hydroxylase
   c) Reduced levels of 11β-hydroxylase
   d) Increased levels of 11β-hydroxylase

**4. Elevated levels of dehydroepiandrosterone sulphate (DHEAS) is suggestive of**
   a) Hypothyroidism
   b) Hyperthyroidism
   c) Hyperprolactinemia
   d) Polycystic ovarian syndrome

### Further Reading

Chakravarty BN. Adolescent gynecological and obstetric problems. Postgraduate obstetrics and gynecology. 4th rev. ed. Menon MKK, Devi PK, Rao KB, editors. Madras: Orient Longman; 1989.

Edmunds DK. Intersexuality. Dewhurst's Practical Paediatric and Adolescent Gyenecology. London: Butterworth; 1989. 17–20 pp.

Gun KM, Poddar DL. J Obstet Gynec India. 1978;28:1035.

Haefuer HK, Roberts JA, Schmidt RW. The University experience of clinical and pathological findings of ovarian neoplasia in children and adolescents. Adolesc Paediatr Gynaecol. 1992;5:182–187.

Rittmaster RS. Hirsutism. Lancet. 1997;349:191–195.

Saenger P. Turner's syndrome—current concepts. N Engl J Med. 1996;335:1749–1754.

# Menopause

**AT A GLANCE**


Age of Menopause
- Factors Affecting Age at Menopause
- Stages of Reproductive Aging—STRAW Report

Pathophysiology
Anatomical Changes
Hormonal Changes in Menopause
Menopausal Symptoms
Osteoporosis
Cardiovascular Disease
Individualised Plan for Management of Menopause
- Investigations

Management of Menopause


## INTRODUCTION

Menopause is a normal physiologic event. It is a retrospective diagnosis. It is a transition from the reproductive to non-reproductive phase in a woman's life.

Menopause is defined as the final menstrual period (FMP) and represents loss of ovarian follicular function.

**Spontaneous or natural menopause** is recognised to have occurred after 12 months of amenorrhea for which there are no obvious physiological or pathological causes. It is a retrospective diagnosis. It is a transition from the reproductive to non-reproductive phase in a woman's life.

**Perimenopause** is the period immediately prior to and up to 1 year after the final menstrual period. It may last for 3–5 years. The most accurate terminology for this term is menopause **transition.**

**Postmenopause** commences from the final menstrual period, regardless of whether the menopause was spontaneous or iatrogenic.

**Induced menopause** is cessation of menstruation that follows bilateral oophorectomy or iatrogenic ablation of ovarian function.

**Premature menopause** is the spontaneous menopause occurring two standard deviations (SDs) below the mean estimated age of the reference population. Traditionally menopause before 40 years of age is considered to be premature menopause.

**Delayed menopause,** though not defined, is important in terms of increased problems associated with hyperestrogenism. It is 2 SDs above the natural age of menopause in a given population.

## AGE OF MENOPAUSE

The estimated mean age of menopause is 46 years in India and is lower than Caucasians. By the year 2025, the number of postmenopausal women is expected to rise to 1.1 billion worldwide.

With women living longer than before, a majority would spend more than one-third of their life in the postmenopausal stage. The health problems cropping up during this period and related hormonal changes are now well understood. Therefore understanding and applying prophylactic measures are needed to lead a healthy and productive life.

### Factors Affecting Age at Menopause

**Age** The age at which the mother of the woman reached menopause has been found to be a important factor. This indicates a strong genetic linage in determining the age at menopause.

**Smoking** Smoking does more harm to ovaries than other lifestyle factors. Non-smokers seem to attain menopause later than smokers.

**Chemotherapy** Very often there is cessation of menstruation when the woman is on chemotherapy. Women in whom menstruation returns after chemotherapy have a higher chance of getting early menopause.

**Ovarian surgery** Repeated ovarian surgeries can damage the healthy ovarian tissue leading to early menopause.

**Ethnicity** There is ethnic difference in the age at which menopause is reached. Hispanic and African–American women reach menopause earlier than Chinese and Japanese women.

Certain factors like age at menarche, pregnancy and breastfeeding and use of hormonal contraceptives are generally believed to be associated with early menopause but these factors as such do not influence the onset of menopause.

## Stages of Reproductive Aging—STRAW Report

**The anchor for the staging system is FMP (Final menstrual period).** Five stages precede and two stages follow the FMP, as shown in Fig. 17.1. What each of these stages refer to are as follows:

- Stage –5—the early reproductive period
- Stage –4—the reproductive peak
- Stage –3—the late reproductive period
- Stage –2—the early menopausal transition and
- Stage –1—the late menopausal transition.
- Stage +1a—the first year after FMP
- Stage +1b—2–5 years postmenopause
- Stage +2—the ensuing later postmenopausal years

## PATHOPHYSIOLOGY

The menopausal transition is a progressive endocrinologic continuum that takes women from regular, cyclic, predictable menses that are characteristic of ovulatory cycles to a final menstrual period associated with ovarian senescence and menopause.

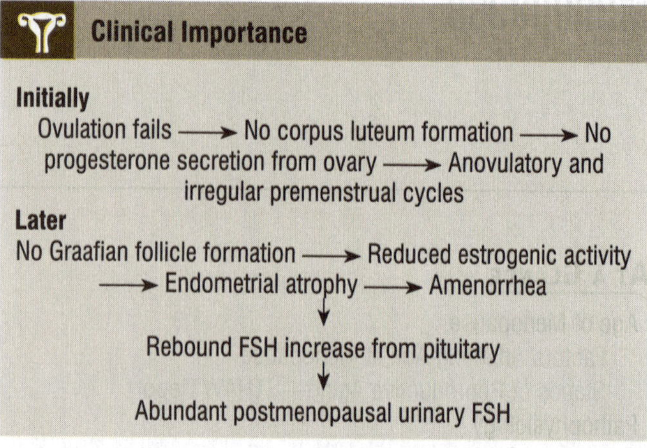

**Clinical Importance**

**Initially**

Ovulation fails ⟶ No corpus luteum formation ⟶ No progesterone secretion from ovary ⟶ Anovulatory and irregular premenstrual cycles

**Later**

No Graafian follicle formation ⟶ Reduced estrogenic activity ⟶ Endometrial atrophy ⟶ Amenorrhea

↓

Rebound FSH increase from pituitary

↓

Abundant postmenopausal urinary FSH

## ANATOMICAL CHANGES

Premenopausal ovaries have greater volume and contain follicles (Fig. 17.2a) whereas postmenopausal ovaries have smaller volume and are devoid of follicles (Fig. 17.2b).

- The uterus becomes smaller due to atrophy of its smooth muscle. During early menopausal transition, the endometrium may reflect ovulatory cycle. During the later stage, anovulation is common. So the endometrium may show estrogenic effect when unopposed by progesterone. Accordingly proliferative changes or disordered proliferative changes are the common findings on endometrial biopsy samples. After menopause, the endometrium becomes atrophic due to lack of estrogen stimulation.
- The cervix becomes smaller and the fornices disappear.

Final menstrual period (FMP) 0

| Stages | –5 | –4 | –3 | –2 | –1 | +1 | | +2 |
|---|---|---|---|---|---|---|---|---|
| Terminology | Reproductive | | | Menopausal transition | | Postmenopause | | |
| | Early | Peak | Late | Early | Late* | Early* | | Late |
| | | | | Perimenopause | | | | |
| Duration of stage | Variable | | | Variable | | (a) 1 yr. | (b) 4 yrs | Until demise |
| Menstrual cycles | Variable to regular | Regular | | Variable cycle length (> 7 days different from normal) | Intervals of amenorrhea (>42 days) | Aown × 12 noon | None | |
| Endocrine | Normal FSH | | ↑FSH | ↑FSH | | ↑FSH | | |

*Stages most likely to be characterised by vasomotor symptoms*

**Fig. 17.1** STRAW—Stages of Reproductive Ageing Workshop (*Source:* http://www.medscape.com/viewarticle/430187)

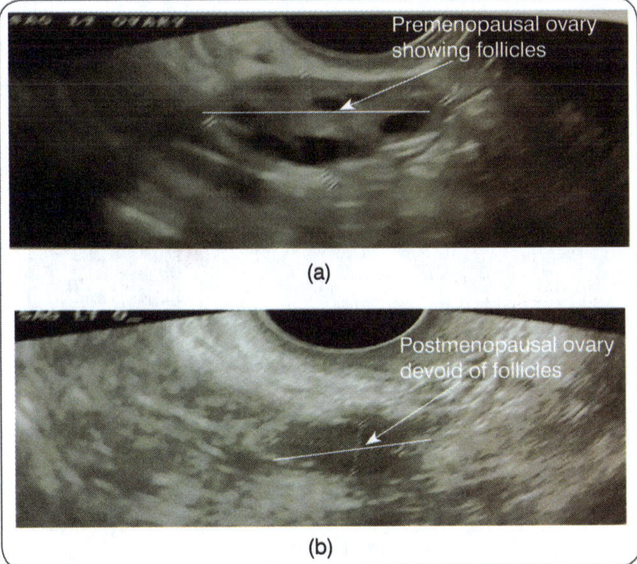


**Fig. 17.2** Transvaginal images of pre- and postmenopausal ovary (*Source:* Image from William's Gynecology 2ed by Hoffman et al. Copyright ©2012, 2008 by McGraw- Hill Companies Inc. Reproduced with permission.)

- The vulva atrophies and vagina becomes narrower, which causes dyspareunia.
- There is considerable reduction in the fat content of labia majora.
- Pubic hair is reduced and becomes grey.
- The pelvic cellular tissue becomes lax and the ligaments that support the uterus and vagina lose their tone, which predispose a woman to prolapse of genital organs.
- The vaginal epithelium becomes thin with loss of folds. Lubrication becomes less, dry and also less acidic leading to more chances of infection.
- The skin wrinkles and hair grows around chin and lips.
- Fat is deposited around breasts, hips and abdomen.

### Hormone Levels in Menopausal Women

| | |
|---|---|
| E2 | 5–25 pg/mL |
| Oestrone | 20–60 pg/mL |
| FSH | >40 mIU/mL |
| Androgen | 0.3–1.0 ng/mL |
| Testosterone | 0.1–0.5 ng/mL |
| LH | 50–100 mIU/mL |

## HORMONAL CHANGES IN MENOPAUSE

- Androgen production reduces by 50%.
- Estrogen reduces by 66%. Due to small amount of testosterone secreted by ovary, there is mild hirsutism in menopause.
- The FSH appears in high concentration in urine.
- E2/E1 ratio maintained over 1 in premenopausal period is reduced to less than 1 in postmenopausal age, causing an estrogen deficiency state. This may predispose the woman to osteoporosis and ischemic heart disease (IHD).

## MENOPAUSAL SYMPTOMS

| Type of menopausal symptom | Clinical manifestation |
|---|---|
| 1. Changes in menstrual pattern | • Shorter cycles are typical (2–7 days)<br>• Longer cycles are possible<br>• Irregular bleeding, heavy, light or spotting |
| 2. Vasomotor symptoms | • Hot flushes over face and neck due to vaso dilatation.<br>• Night sweats<br>• Sleep disturbances |
| 3. Psychological disturbances | • Depression<br>• Worsening of premenstrual syndrome(PMS)<br>• Irritability<br>• Mood swings<br>• Loss of concentration and poor memory |
| 4. Sexual dysfunction | • Vaginal dryness<br>• Decrease of libido<br>• Painful intercourse |
| 5. Somatic symptoms | • Headache<br>• Dizziness<br>• Palpitations<br>• Joint aches and back pain<br>• Breast pain |
| 6. Others | • Urinary incontinence (urge and stress), dry itchy skin, weight gain.<br>• Menopausal women, due to chronic estrogen deficiency, are liable to develop<br>– Arthritis, osteoporosis, and fracture<br>– Cardiovascular accidents, ischemic heart disease, myocardial infarction and atherosclerosis<br>– Stroke<br>– Skin changes<br>– Alzheimer's disease<br>– Ano-colonic cancer<br>– Tooth decay |

## OSTEOPOROSIS

**It needs special mention because it is a silent killer.** The modification of the bone matrix due to the effect of osteoporosis is shown in Fig. 17.3. Bone resorption follows estrogen deficiency and it affects mainly the trabecular bones of the vertebra, head of femur and the distal end of radius. This causes vertebral bone compression and **Dowager's hump** and diminishment of height (Fig. 17.4) and fracture of head of femur (Fig. 17.5).

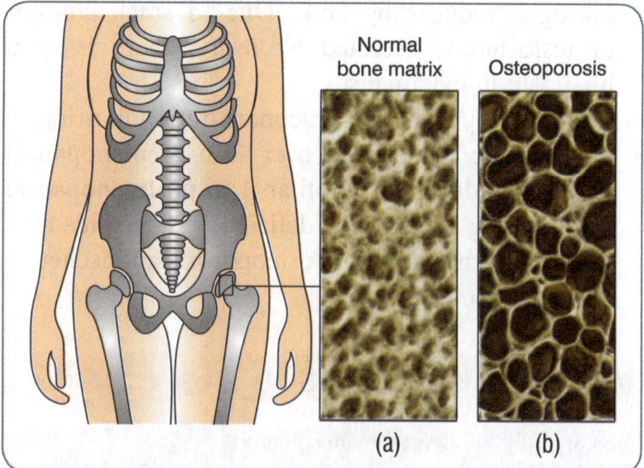


Fig. 17.3 (a) Normal bone matrix (b) Bone matrix affected by osteoporosis

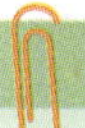

**Risk factors for Osteoporosis**

The other **high risk factors** for osteoporosis are:
- Family history
- Low calcium intake
- Low weight
- Surgical/Radiation menopause
- Thyrotoxicity
- Drugs like steroids
- Smoking, alcohol, caffeine intake
- Sedentary lifestyle

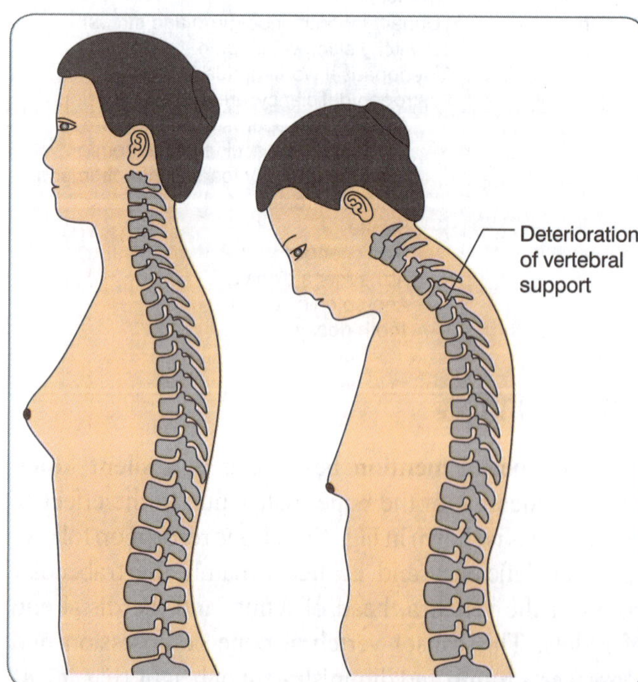


Fig. 17.4 Deterioration of vertebral support due to osteoporosis

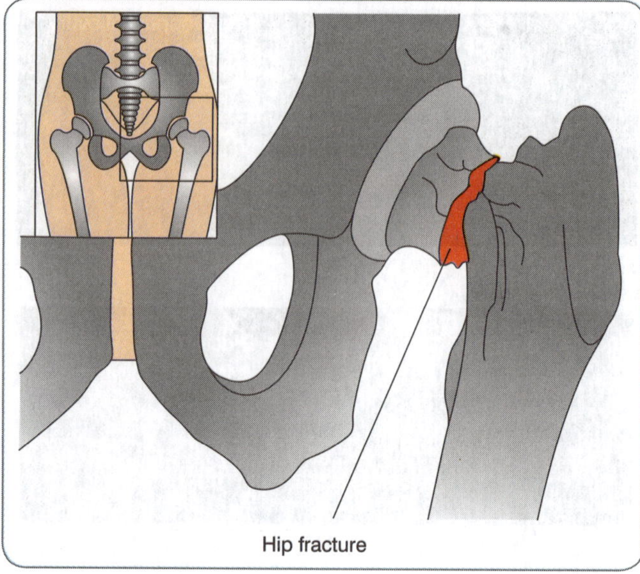


Fig. 17.5 Hip fracture

Wrist fracture is the first to occur. Hip fracture is most debilitating. Spine fracture goes unnoticed and undiagnosed.

Diminished bone mineral density (BMD) can be studied by dual energy X-ray absorptiometry (DXA).

## CARDIOVASCULAR DISEASE

Estrogen is cardioprotective by maintaining HDL and lowering LDL and triglycerides. Incidence of stroke also increases in postmenopausal women.

## INDIVIDUALISED PLAN FOR MANAGEMENT OF MENOPAUSE

Each woman needs an individualised health plan management. **It is most important to distinguish between symptomatic and asymptomatic menopausal women.** Women may present at menopausal clinic with menstrual problems, menopausal symptoms, or request for a general health check-up.

Issues in symptomatic women
- Vasomotor
- Genitourinary
- Skeletomuscular
- Sexual
- Unintended pregnancy
- Declined fertility
- Fat deposition
- Neuropsychiatric problems

## Investigations

1. History of various symptoms
2. G/E includes BP, weight, breast examination, hirsutism
3. Pelvic examination—with Pap smear
4. Blood sugar, lipid profile
5. Mammography, pelvic USG
6. Bone mineral density—by DEXA
7. Estrogen, FSH level—to decide HRT. These are particularly indicated in women with early menopause (menopause before 40 years can be thus considered), irregular menstrual pattern and following hysterectomy.
8. Serum calcium, vitamin D and phosphorus levels are indicated in those with poor calcium intake.

### DEXA scan

#### *Indications*

- DEXA scan (Figs. 17.6 and 17.7) is indicated in all women who are postmenopausal and at least 65 years of age.
- Postmenopausal and younger than 65 years who have at least one risk factor for osteoporosis (like women discontinuing estrogen or oestrogen deficiency early or premature menopause (before 40 years of age) history of amenorrhea for more than 1 year under the age of 42 years or history of maternal hip fracture after the age of 50 years) postmenopausal women with fractures.
- Bone mineral density testing may be of use in pre- and postmenopausal women with certain diseases or medical conditions like acquired immunodeficiency syndrome, chronic obstructive pulmonary disease, hyperparathyroidism, inflammatory bowel disease, rheumatoid arthritis, etc.

#### *Scoring*

The results are given as T score and the WHO standard for T score is as follows:

| Category | *T*-score |
|---|---|
| Normal | –1.0 and above |
| Low bone mass (osteopenia) | –1.0 to –2.5 |
| Osteoporosis | –2.5 and below |

T score is commonly used and it indicates the bone mineral density. Whereas a + score indicates dense bone a – score indicates less dense bones.

## MANAGEMENT OF MENOPAUSE

#### *Counselling and lifestyle changes*

Many develop pregnancyphobia and cancerphobia. It is the duty of gynaecologist to convince her after thorough examination. Advice on contraception is necessary. Contraception is very often not

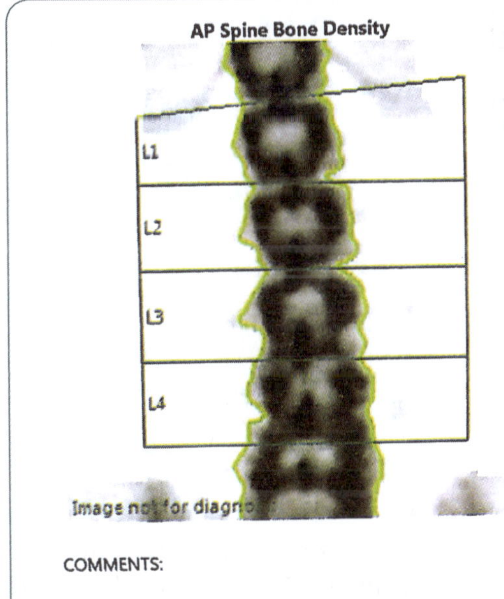


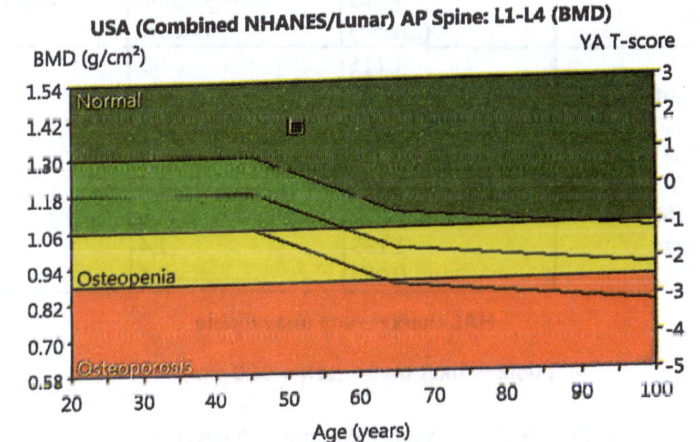


| Densitometry: USA (Combined NHANES/Lunar) | | | |
|---|---|---|---|
| Region | BMD (g/cm²) | Young-Adult T-score | Age-Matched Z-score |
| L1 | 1.309 | 1.5 | 2.0 |
| L2 | 1.363 | 1.4 | 1.9 |
| L3 | 1.405 | 1.7 | 2.2 |
| L4 | 1.469 | 2.2 | 2.7 |
| L1-L4 | 1.392 | 1.8 | 2.3 |

**Fig. 17.6** DXA report for spines

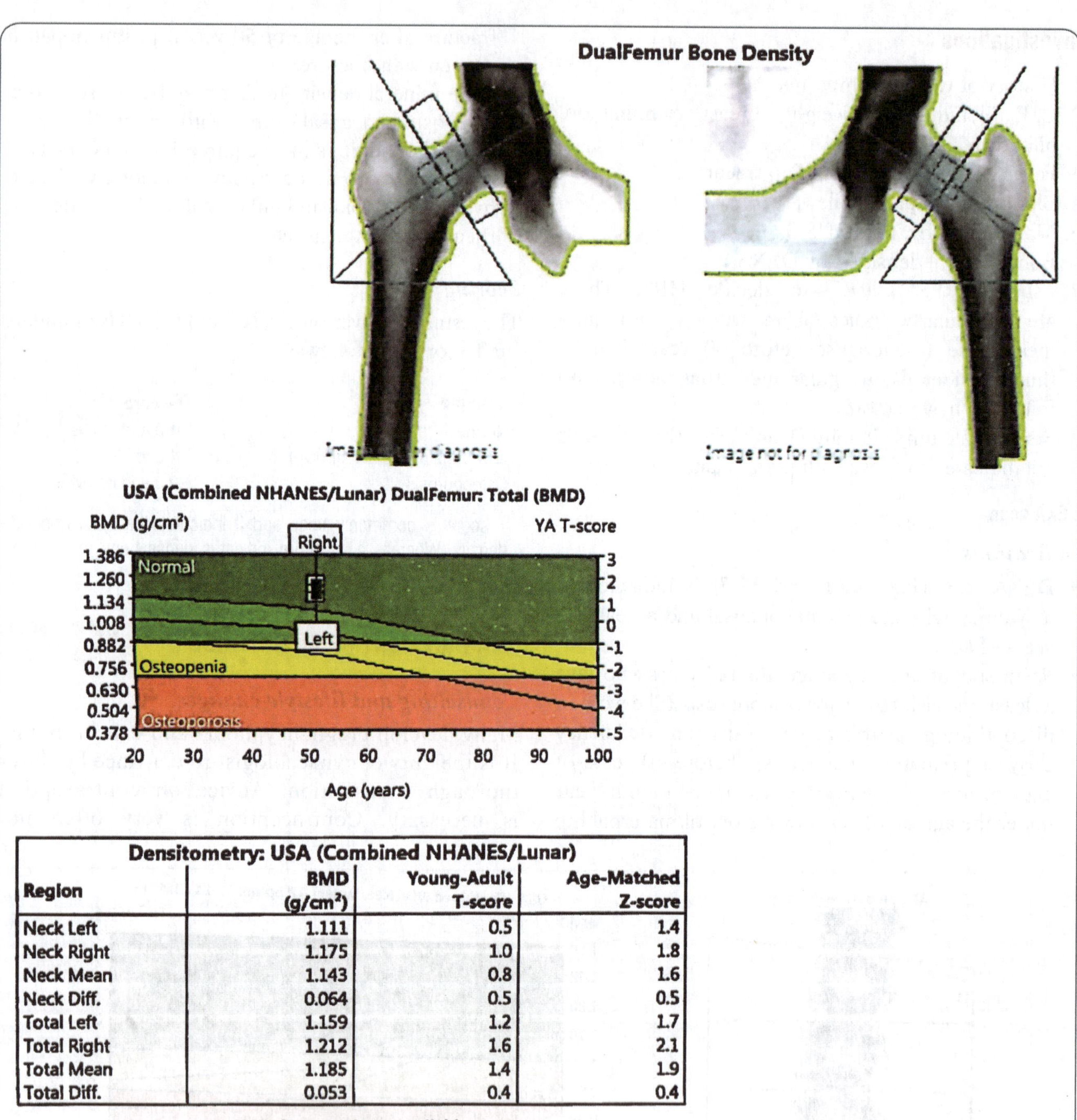


**Densitometry: USA (Combined NHANES/Lunar)**

| Region | BMD (g/cm²) | Young-Adult T-score | Age-Matched Z-score |
|---|---|---|---|
| Neck Left | 1.111 | 0.5 | 1.4 |
| Neck Right | 1.175 | 1.0 | 1.8 |
| Neck Mean | 1.143 | 0.8 | 1.6 |
| Neck Diff. | 0.064 | 0.5 | 0.5 |
| Total Left | 1.159 | 1.2 | 1.7 |
| Total Right | 1.212 | 1.6 | 2.1 |
| Total Mean | 1.185 | 1.4 | 1.9 |
| Total Diff. | 0.053 | 0.4 | 0.4 |

**Fig. 17.7** DXA report for femur

thought of in perimenopausal women. But there is a need for contraception to avoid unintended pregnancy. Those who are already on some form of contraception may continue the same if it suits them. For others barrier method, combined oral contraceptives, progesterone-only pill and intrauterine contraceptive devices can be used based on their eligibility (discussed in Chapter 33). Diet should contain at least 1.2 g of calcium, Vit D and E. Weight bearing exercises (walking and aerobics) prevent or delay osteoporosis. Yoga and meditation can reduce mental stress.

### *Menopausal transition*

Menopausal transition (MT) begins with variations in menstrual cycle length and a rise in follicle-stimulating hormone (FSH) but without any associated increase in luteinising hormone [LH], and ends with the final menstrual period. It is however confirmed only when followed by 12 months of amenorrhea.

The diagnosis is more clinical and symptomatic rather than by hormonal estimation, which are not precise. The treatment of menopausal transition is also mostly symptomatic.

### *Hormone Replacement Therapy (HRT)*

Presently this is better called as HT(Hormone Therapy).

The various drug formulations and their use have been dealt with in Chapter 18.

HT is indicated in symptomatic women who suffer from vasomotor symptoms, urinary symptoms and sexual disharmony.

The current HT recommendation is'based on short-term therapy except in the management of osteoporosis where long-term HT is recommended (see below).

**Estrogen should be given in the smallest effective dose for the shortest possible duration of 3–6 months,**

Natural equine conjugated estrogen 0.625 mg daily or

Ethinyl estradiol 0.01 mg/day are effective.

Dyspareunia, urethral syndrome and senile vaginitis respond very well to local estrogen cream.

### *Treatment of osteoporosis*

Hormone therapy is the cornerstone in prophylaxis and treatment of osteoporosis. Long-term estrogen therapy is necessary to prevent and treat osteoporosis. After menopause, women lose 3% of BMD every year. When to start HT is debatable. **HT is not recommended routinely in natural menopause unless there is definite low BMD.**

In premature menopause it is advisable as prophylaxis.

When HT is used for osteoporosis in menopause, conjugated estrogen is used in the dose of 0.625–1.3 mg.

### Other drugs used in osteoporosis management

***Tibolone*** It is a synthetic derivative of 19-nortestosterone and is considered a selective estrogen activity regulator. It has weak, estrogenic, progestrogenic and androgenic effect. It also has a selective tissue effect. Tibolone is effective in preventing bone loss and treating climacteric symptoms, without stimulating the endometrium. The effects on bone, brain and vagina can be accurately explained by the estrogenic activity of tibolone, but estrogenic activity is not expressed in the endometrium. Tibolone behaves differently from estrogen plus progestogen combinations on the breast. It is given as 2.5 mg tab daily.

***Raloxifene*** It is a selective estrogen receptor modulator (SERM). It reduces the risk of fracture by 50%. It is given in the dose of 60 mg daily. Venous thrombosis and hepatic dysfunction are contraindications. **It should not be given along with estrogen.**

***Bisphosphonates*** These reduce bone resorption through inhibition of osteoclastic activity. Also, they increase BMD by 5–10%. They are taken in the dose of 5–10 mg/day or 35–70 mg once weekly.

***Androgens*** improve libido and currently tibolone, which has a weak androgenic action can be taken (vide above).

**Contraindications for HT**

It is advisable not to use HT in the following circumstances:

- Breast cancer (particularly in estrogen and progesterone receptor positive women)
- Carcinoma endometrium
- Undiagnosed vaginal bleeding
- Active liver disease
- Hypertriglyceridemia
- Thromboembolic disorders like venous thromboembolism

Relative contraindications include

- Migraine
- Fibroid uterus
- Family history of breast cancer
- Endometriosis

### *Postmenopausal bleeding (PMB)*

**Though bleeding after one year of amenorrhea is PMB, bleeding occurring after 6 months must be investigated**. Even women without amenorrhea or irregular bleeding, if they continue to menstruate after 52 years they are to be investigated. 30–50% are attributed to malignancy. Both benign and malignant causes in the genital tract should be tested and treated. Excluding malignancy is the main aim of investigations.

***Risk factors for endometrial cancer***

- Increasing age
- Early menarche and late menopause
- Polycystic ovarian disease
- Obesity combined with diabetes
- Low parity or infertility
- Hypertension
- Unopposed oestrogen-only HRT
- Tamoxifen
- Hereditary non-polyposis colorectal carcinoma

***Etiological factors***

- The most common cause of postmenopausal bleeding (PMB) is vaginal atrophy.
- Very often the presenting symptom in a case of endometrial cancer is postmenopausal bleeding. Nearly 90% women with endometrial cancer present with postmenopausal bleeding.

The other etiological factors are

- Use of HRT
- Endometrial hyperplasia
- Endometrial or cervical polyps
- Cervical cancer
- Theca cell tumours of ovary vulval cancer
- Vaginal cancer (rarely)

The common investigations are

- Transvaginal ultrasound scan (TVS)
- Endometrial biopsy
- Hysteroscopy

***Management***

PMB should be treated as malignant unless proved otherwise. The management depends on the underlying pathology like.

## RECAP

- Normal menopause sets in around 45–51 years.
- Premature menopause occurs before 40 years.
- Late menopause is a risk factor for uterine malignancy and breast cancer.
- Proper diet, exercise, and HT when indicated.
- Not all require hormone therapy. It depends on the symptoms.
- Side effects and contraindications must be well understood.
- Proper counselling is mandatory.
- A regular follow-up is necessary for women on Hormone Therapy.
- PMB needs investigations and treatment accordingly.

## REVIEW QUESTIONS

### Long-Answer Question

1. Describe the anatomical changes in menopause.

### Short-Answer Questions

1. Describe the contraindications for hormone therapy.
2. Briefly describe the factors affecting age at menopause.

### MCQs

**1. Osteoporosis mainly affects**

a) Trabecular bones of the vertebra, head of femur and the distal end of radius
b) Skull bones
c) Only phalanges
d) Facial bones

**2. Diminished bone mineral density can be studied by**

a) Digital X-ray
b) MRI
c) Contrast CT
d) Dual energy X-ray absorptiometry (DXA)

**3. Dose of ethinyl estradiol as hormone therapy (HT) is**

a) 0.625 mg/day
b) 1.0 mg/day
c) 0.01 mg/day
d) 0.1 mg/day

**4. Raloxifene is a**

a) Selective estrogen activity regulator
b) Bisphosphonate
c) Selective estrogen receptor modulator (SERM)
d) Androgen

## Further Reading

Clinical practice guidelines on menopause. Indian menopause society. 2015.

Hoffman BL, Schorge JO, Schaffer JI et al., editors. William's Gynecology. 2nd ed. New York: McGraw-Hill; 2012.

Krishna U, Mehta RU. Osteoporosis—incidence and implications. J Ob Gyn of India. 2000;50(5):150–6.

Milsom I. Menopause-related symptoms and their treatment. Errkkola, editor. The menopause. Philadelphia: Elsevier; 2006. 16 p.

Padubidri VG, Daftary Sd. Shaw's textbook of gynecology. 16th ed. Gurgaon: Elsevier India; 2014.

# CHAPTER 18

# Hormones in Gynecology

## AT A GLANCE


Hormones at a Glance
Classification of Hormones
Hypothalamus
GnRH Analogues
- Downregulation
- Add-Back Therapy
- Commonly Used Preparations and Routes of Administration
- Indications for Usage

Pituitary
- Gonadotropins

Prolactin
Dopamine Agonists
- Bromocriptine
- Cabergoline

Adrenal
- Steroid Hormones

Selective Estrogen Receptor Modulators (SERMs)
- Clomiphene Citrate
- Tamoxifen
- Raloxifene
- Ormeloxifene

Estrogen Synthesis Inhibitors
- Aromatase Inhibitors (AI)

Progesterone
Testosterone Derivatives
- Danazol

Selective Progesterone Receptor Modulators (SPRMs) / Progesterone Antagonists
Androgens
Antiandrogens
Thyroid Hormones
Adrenal Hormones
Summary of Role of Hormones in Gynecology
- Role of Hormones in Different Conditions


## INTRODUCTION

Gynecological endocrinology is a subspecialty of gynecology. Endocrine disturbances during the different phases of female development may cause varied effects, and these are listed in Table 18.1.

**Table 18.1** Effect of endocrine disturbance in different phases of life

| Phase of life | Events due to endocrine disturbances |
|---|---|
| | Bleeding P/V<br>Hypoglycemia<br>Thyroid disturbances<br>Vulvovaginitis<br>Ambiguous genitalia |
| | Precocious puberty<br>Hormone-secreting tumours of ovary<br>Growth problems<br>CAH (Congeniital Adrenal Hyperplasia) |
| | Primary amenorrhea<br>Delayed puberty<br>PCOS (Polycystic Ovarian Syndrome)<br>Endometriosis<br>Heterosexual development<br>Puberty menorrhagia |
| 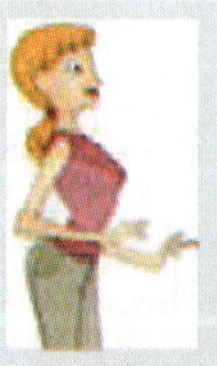 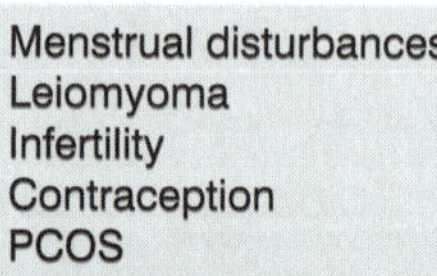 | Menstrual disturbances<br>Leiomyoma<br>Infertility<br>Contraception<br>PCOS |
| 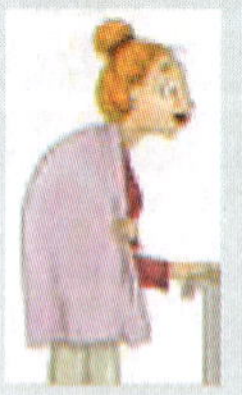 | Menopause<br>Cancers<br>Osteoporosis<br>Atrophic changes<br>Delayed menopause |

Menstruation, ovulation, reproduction, conception and contraception, sexual activity, growth, metabolism, intelligence, carcinogenesis, abnormalities of any of the events in the life of a woman—all of these require a complex interaction of the various hormones of the body.

Excess of any hormone or deficiency of many can be most often easily and effectively managed and hence a thorough knowledge of hormones used in gynecology becomes very essential.

## HORMONES AT A GLANCE

This chapter aims at briefing the student on the therapeutic role of hormones in gynecology. Table 18.2 lists the hormones and the organs that produce them.

**Table 18.2** Organs of production of various hormones

| Endocrine organ | Hormones and their analogues |
|---|---|
| Hypothalamus | GnRH analogues, clomiphene citrate |
| Pituitary | Gonadotropins, antigonadotropins (danazol and gestrinone), prolactin and its antagonists |
| Ovary | Estrogens, antiestrogens, aromatase inhibitors, SERMs (Selective Estrogen Receptor Modulators), progesterones, antiprogesterone, SPRMs (Selective Progesterone Receptor Modulators). |
| Adrenal | Androgens and antiandrogens, cortisol, DHEA (Dehydroepiandrosterone), DHEA-S (dehydroepiandrosterone sulphate) |
| Thyroid | Thyroxine and antithyroid drugs |

## CLASSIFICATION OF HORMONES

Hormones could be broadly classified as

**i) Peptide hormones** These are made up of amino acids, and their synthesis is being controlled by various enzymes. They are water-soluble; most of them thus cannot penetrate cell membrane and act through receptors and second messengers inside the cell.

**ii) Lipid hormones** These are derived from cholesterol, and are structurally similar to it. They are usually either ketones (ending with 'one') or alcohols (ending with 'ol'), e.g., sex hormones. They are only lipid-soluble, non-polar substances with no net charges and as they cannot dissolve in water they are carried by carrier proteins in the blood, but can enter into the cell easily. **Hence they have a longer half-life compared to peptide hormones.** They have their receptors on mitochondria or endoplasmic reticulum (ER). Enzymes involved in their synthesis are also located on mitochondria and ER.

**The peptide hormones of interest for a gynecologist are hypothalamic and pituitary hormones.**

It is convenient to study the hormones and their synthetic derivatives under the organ of their secretion.

## HYPOTHALAMUS

The hypothalamus secretes various hormones which control the secretions from the pituitary.

### Actions of GnRH Analogues

| Actions |
|---|
| Lowers FSH and LH levels |
| Lowers estrogen levels |
| Endometrial atrophy |
| Uterine atrophy |
| Breast atrophy |
| Medical menopause and its symptoms |
| Decreased libido |
| Osteoporosis |
| Increased risk of CVS/CNS problems |

Of these, gonadotropin releasing hormone (GnRH) is the one that is of interest to a gynecologist, which is a decapeptide with a short half-life (2–4 mins) and thus gets quickly degraded.

GnRH is secreted in a pulsatile manner, and the secretion varies in amplitude and frequency in different phases of the cycle.

## GnRH ANALOGUES

By changing one or the other amino acid in the chain, gonadotropin releasing hormone analogues (GnRH analogues) may be produced. They can be of two types:

- **Agonists** are those that bind to the pituitary gonadotropin receptors and activate them resulting in initial increase in the secretion and later suppression of gonadotropins to very low levels.
- **Antagonists,** on the other hand, have no intrinsic activity and suppress the secretion from the time they bind to the receptors.

Both result in creating a state of hypogonadism by totally suppressing the secretion of sex hormones from the gonads. As a result of this, end organs like uterus, especially endometrium, also atrophy.

**Hence GnRH analogues can be used whenever there is a need to treat hyperestrogenic state.**

### Downregulation

Agonists are known to cause a flare response due to initial stimulation, but further blockage of the receptors will cause cessation of gonadotropin secretion called **downregulation**. Hence except for this disadvantage, both agonists and antagonists can be used with the same effect. Earlier the cost factor precluded the use of antagonists but nowadays antagonists are mostly preferred of the two.

## Add-Back Therapy

Prolonged use of antagonists is not advocated for fear of osteoporosis, and other hypoestrogenic unwanted effects. If it needs to be used for more than six months, **replacement therapy** is to be initiated to combat adverse effects on bones, cardiovascular system, etc., which is called **Add back therapy**. Estrogen, progesterone, SERMs, tibolone, etc. are used for this.

## Commonly Used Preparations and Routes of Administration

**Agonists**—leuprolide, buserelin, histrelin, goserelin, deslorelin, nafarelin and triptorelin

**Antagonists**—Degarelix, Ganirelix, Cetrorelix, Abarelix, etc.

They can be used as injections (monthly, quarterly, etc.), nasal sprays or implants. The dosage of these drugs differs on the indication. However, the generally used dose is given in Table 18.3.

**Table 18.3** Routes of administration and doses of commonly used GnRH analogues

| Drug | Route of administration | Dose |
|---|---|---|
| Leuprolide | Monthly injection | 3.75 mg/monthly injection- IM/SC/Depot |
| Buserelin | Nasal spray / Injection | 200–300 μg SC/daily |
| Goserelin | Implant is injected in the SC plane in the lower abdomen—three-monthly | 3.6 mg implant<br>3.6 mg monthly depot injection |
| Triptorelin | Monthly or three-monthly injection | 3.75 mg IM/monthly<br>11.25 mg IM/three-monthly |

IM: Intramuscular; SC: Subcutaneous

## Indications for Usage

The uses of and the rationale behind using the analogues are given in the following table.

| Conditions where used | Rationale for use |
|---|---|
| Precocious puberty | To prevent early epiphyseal closure |
| Infertility | For controlled ovarian stimulation (COS) |
| Leiomyoma | To decrease the size and vascularity, and to facilitate vaginal hysterectomy |
| Endometriosis | To maintain hypoestrogenic state, for COS |
| Abnormal uterine bleeding (AUB) | Prior to endometrial ablation |
| Hormone-dependent cancers | For steroid hormone suppression, e.g., cancer prostate |
| Ovarian hyperandrogenism | For suppression, and for hirsutism |

**GnRH stimulation** GnRH is used to identify whether pituitary or the hypothalamus is at fault in certain cases of primary amenorrhea.

If the serum levels of FSH and LH increase after GnRH stimulation, it is obvious that hypothalamus is at fault, but if the GnRH stimulation has no effect on FSH and LH levels, it is clear that the pathology is at the pituitary level. This is called **GnRH stimulation** or **challenge test.**

# PITUITARY

## Gonadotropins

Gonadotropins are glycoprotein polypeptide hormones. They are secreted by the gonadotrophs of the anterior pituitary. Gonadotropins are secreted under the influence of gonadotropin releasing hormone of the hypothalamus and the secretion is controlled by feedback loops from both the pituitary and the gonads.

**FSH** and **LH** are secreted by the pituitary in varying volumes at different parts of the cycle and **human chorionic gonadotropin (hCG)** is the other hormone secreted by the trophoblastic cells of the placenta during pregnancy or in cases of gestational trophoblastic neoplasia.

### Clinical Uses

#### *Diagnostic uses*

Diagnostically, premenopausal (low levels) and postmenopausal (high levels) levels of FSH and LH are very useful. The alteration in the ratio is important in PCOS. High levels in women of reproductive age group indicate premature ovarian failure.

hCG plays an important role in the diagnosis of pregnancy, follow-up and management of ectopic pregnancy and in gestational trophoblastic neoplasia.

FSH initiates follicular growth and supports the growth of the dominant follicle. In the premenstrual phase, FSH shows slight increase which helps in recruitment of follicle for the next cycle.

LH stimulates theca cells in the ovaries, which provide androgens and hormonal precursors for estradiol production. LH surge in the midcycle triggers ovulation and helps in luteinisation of the ruptured follicle.

***Therapeutic uses***

1. Replacement therapy—in states of hypogonadotropic hypogonadism
2. Anovulatory infertility
3. Ovulation induction in assisted reproductive techniques
4. hCG for ovulation trigger and luteal support

### Preparations

It is extracted from urine—menotropins; mixture of FSH and LH available in 75–225 units.

Recombinant varieties include pure FSH and LH/hCG hCG is available as 2000–10,000 units.

| Drug | Route of administration | Dose |
|---|---|---|
| Menotropin | IM | 75 IU |
| Recombinant FSH | SC/IM | 75–150 IU |
| Recombinant LH | SC | 75 IU |
| hCG | IM | 1000–5000 IU |

IM: Intramuscular; SC: Subcutaneous

The dose is the standard available dose and the actual dose varies with the condition being treated.

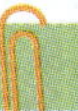

### Side Effects of Gonadotropins

- Multiple ovulation and multiple pregnancy
- Ovarian hyperstimulation syndrome (OHSS)
- Increased risk of ovarian cancer in long-term usage

## PROLACTIN

Prolactin is a single-chain peptide with 198 amino acids secreted from the lactotrophs of the pituitary gland in response to eating, mating, estrogen treatment, ovulation and nursing.

Its secretion is under the negative control of dopamine secreted by the hypothalamus and is stimulated by the hypothalamic thyroid releasing hormone.

It stimulates breast to secrete milk (oxytocin causes ejection of milk).

The following are the causes for hyperprolactinemia.

### Causes for Hyperprolactinaemia

| |
|---|
| Prolactin-secreting tumours (PRL >200) |
| Hypothyroidism |
| Dopamine-depleting drugs |
| Antidopaminergic drugs |
| Hypothalamic diseases |

Prolactin inhibitors are drugs which are used for inhibiting prolactin release. Dopamine is a prolactin inhibitor which acts on the D2 receptors and inhibits prolactin.

## DOPAMINE AGONISTS

| Drug | Route | Dose |
|---|---|---|
| Bromocriptine | Oral | 1.25, 2.5 up to 10 mg/day |
| Gabergoline | Oral | 0.25–0.5 mg |

### Bromocriptine

It is an ergot derivative and has a potent dopaminergic action. It decreases GI motility and stimulates the chemoreceptor trigger zone in the brain. Bromocriptine reduces prolactin secretion from the pituitary gland. It is used in the dose of 1.25, 2.5 to 10 mg/day.

GI side effects like nausea, vomiting and constipation make it an unpopular drug.

**Indications** It is used in hyperprolactinemia, anovulatory infertility, amenorrhea and any other situation of hyperprolactinemia, Parkinsonism (acts like levodopa) and acromegaly (reduces growth hormone secretion).

In Sheehan's syndrome, hypoprolactinemia may be the first symptom with lactation failure.

### Cabergoline

This is an ergot derivative with longer half-life which enables less frequent dose—weekly twice initially (0.25–0.5 mg) and later weekly once.

Compared to bromocriptine, the side effects are also lesser.

**Indications**

- Hyperprolactinemic states
- For lactation suppression
- Uterine leiomyoma
- Acromegaly
- Parkinson's disease

**Note** Pergolide has been withdrawn from therapeutics for fear of heart valve damage.

## ADRENAL

### Steroid Hormones

Ovaries, testis, adrenals and peripheral fat are the steroid-producing organs.

All steroid hormones are derived from cholesterol probably derived from LDL or by denovo synthesis.

The process involves different steps using multiple enzymes.

Different products (steroidogenesis) are derived by various processes like the reduction in the number of carbon atoms, deoxygenation, dehydrogenation, acetylation, etc.

The products are progesterone, adrenal steroids, androgens and estrogens.

Though the hormones of interest for a gynecologist are sex steroids, many endocrine abnormalities like precocious puberty, heterosexual development and ambiguous genitalia may involve adrenal steroid synthetic pathway abnormalities also.

**Estrogens** In 1929, Adolf Butenandt and Edward Adelbert Doisy isolated estrogen and determined its structure.

The first orally effective estrogen, Emmenin, was introduced in 1930 and it was derived from the late-pregnancy urine which was found to contain the glucuronide of estriol, which is water-soluble and becomes active in the body after hydrolysis.

Estrogens are produced in the ovary, adrenals and peripheral fat.

**The three major naturally occurring estrogens in women are estrone (E1), estradiol (E2), and estriol (E3).**

As they are not orally active, many other compounds have been synthesised for clinical use.

Estradiol is the predominant estrogen during reproductive years in terms of serum levels and potency.

Estrone is the predominant circulating estrogen during menopause.

Estriol is the predominant circulating estrogen in pregnancy.

Estriol is the weakest and estradiol the strongest with 80 times potency of estriol.

Another type of estrogen called **estetrol (E4)** is produced only during pregnancy.

All the three naturally occurring estrogens (E1, E2 and E3) are used clinically.

**Secretion of Estrogens**

| Period of life | Site of production | Quantity |
|---|---|---|
| Reproductive age group | Ovarian follicles | 10–100 mcg/day |
| Pregnancy | Placenta | 30 mg/day |
| Postmenopausal | Peripheral fat | 2-10 mcg/day |

***Classification*** Table 18.4 gives the classification of estrogens.

**Table 18.4** Classification of estrogens

| | |
|---|---|
| 1. Natural estrogens | Estradiol, estriol, estrone<br>Micronised estradiol |
| 2. Conjugated equine estrogens | Premarin |
| 3. Conjugated estrogens (prodrugs, get converted to estradiol and have longer duration of action) | Esters of estradiol<br>Estradiol cypionate<br>Estradiol acetate<br>Estradiol valerate<br>Estradiol benzoate<br>Esters of estrone and estriol<br>Estrone sulphate<br>Estriol succinate |
| 4. Non-conjugated synthetic estrogens | 17-alpha ethynyl estradiol<br>Mestranol |
| 5. Synthetic non-steroidal estrogens | Stilbesterol<br>DES |
| 6. Receptor modulators / antiestrogens | Pure agonist/antagonist:<br>Fulvestrant<br>Mixed agonist and antagonist:<br>Triphenylethylene derivatives<br>Clomiphene citrate, Tamoxifen<br>Non-steroidal sulphur-containing raloxifene |
| 7. Xenoestrogens (occurring in the environment) | Phytoestrogens (plant-derived)<br>Mycoestrogens (fungus-derived) |

**Actions of estrogen** Table 18.5 lists the various actions of estrogen.

## Preparations and uses

**Natural estrogens** Estradiol not being effective orally has no therapeutic applications. Its micronised form is orally effective and is used specially in Hormone Replacement Therapy (HRT). Conjugated varieties are used in fertility disorders.

Estrone sulphate is used for HRT, others like estriol succinate are used for early menopausal symptom management especially for urogenital symptoms. The less potent of these like estriol succinate has no effect on endometrium, and hence no risk of cancer.

**Ethinyl estradiol** This is the most commonly used drug. Addition of ethinyl group at the 17$^{th}$ alpha position enhances its potency and makes it orally active. Hence even at a very low dose its effect is maximum. It is useful for contraception in the dose of 20–50 mcg and 6–10 mcg for HRT. Depending on whether 20 mcg is used or 50 mcg is used, the oral pills are classified as low-dose or high-dose pills.

**Routes of administration** Estrogen is used as oral, transdermal, topical gels, emulsions and lotions,

Table 18.5 Actions of estrogen

| | |
|---|---|
| Structural effects | Endometrial proliferation<br>Myohyperplasia<br>Uterine growth<br>Increased tubal motility<br>Breast parenchymal proliferation and vascularity |
| Bone | Reduced resorption<br>Increased bone formation<br>Epiphyseal closure |
| Femininity and secondary sexual characters | Female body contour<br>Breast development<br>Pubic hair development vulval, vaginal growth<br>Glycogen deposition in vagina<br>Increased cervical gland activity |
| Metabolism | Fat—Increases HDL, reduces LDL, Increases triglycerides, increases fat deposition salt and water retention<br>Protein—Hepatic synthesis of binding proteins increased<br>Carbohydrate—Increased insulin sensitivity, decreased fasting insulin and increased insulin clearance. |
| Vasoprotective | May decrease the risk of atherogenesis |
| Coagulation | Factors II, VII, IX, X, antithrombin III, and plasminogen are increased along with increased adhesiveness of platelets. |
| GIT | Reduced bowel motility and increased cholesterol in bile |
| Pregnancy | Maintenance |
| Pituitary | Depresses FSH and favours LH secretion |

intravaginal creams, tablets, and vaginal rings (Table 18.6). Transdermal patch or gel utilises lower dose, ensures uniform delivery, reduces dosing frequency, has ease of termination of drug delivery. It is available as 0.05 mg/day patch, which has to be changed twice weekly.

## Therapeutic uses

1. *HRT* For postmenopausal and surgical menopausal HRT, conjugated estrogens are preferred.

   For menopausal symptoms—urogenital, atrophic symptoms and hot flashes—premarin and/or phytoestrogens may be used.
2. *Contraception* Ethinyl estradiol is used in the dose of 20–35 mcg per tablet along with various progesterone preparations. It is used as vaginal ring and injectables.
3. *Replacement* In hypogonadotropic states like Turner's syndrome.
4. *Abnormal uterine bleeding (AUB)* For control of acute bleeding episode, 25 mg IV premarin is used.
5. Carcinoma prostate
6. *Antiestrogens* For breast cancer and osteoporosis
7. *To work up a case of secondary amenorrhea* If a patient does not bleed with progesterone withdrawal and if addition of estrogen results in bleeding, the fault is in the ovarian or higher compartment. If there is no bleeding even after adding estrogen, then the fault is in the endometrium.
8. *Lactation suppression* To stop lactation by suppression of prolactin secretion by the anterior pituitary, EE 0.2 mg daily for two days and 0.1 mg daily for three more days is given. Bromocriptine/cabergoline are preferred over estrogens due to the risk of venous thromboembolism (VTE).
9. *Along with clomiphene citrate (CC)* To improve the cervical mucus and endometrium, patients on ovulation induction with CC may require addition of estrogen.
10. *Hypoplastic uterus* For achieving uterine growth.

Table 18.6 Various estrogen preparations

| Preparations | Equivalent potency | Dosage | Availability |
|---|---|---|---|
| Estriol succinate | | 2–4 mg/day | Cream 15 g/tube (Evalon), 1 mg and 2 mg tablets |
| Estriol | 12 mg | 12 mg (cream) | |
| Micronised estrogens | | 1–2 mg | |
| Estradiol | 5 mg | Not used | 1 mg and 5 mg injections |
| Estradiol valerate | | | 2–20 mg every other week |
| Ethinyl estradiol | 50 mcg | 10–50 mcg | 0.01 mg |
| Stilbesterol (DES) | 5 mg | | 5 mg tablets |
| Premarin | 3.75 mg | 0.625 mg – 1.3 mg | Tabs: 0.3, 0.625, 0.9, 1.25, 2.5 mg<br>Vaginal cream: 0.625 mg |
| Mestranol | 80 mcg | | |
| 17-beta estradiol | | 0.5–1 mg/day<br>50 mcg/day | Tabs: 0.5, 1, 1.5, 2 mg<br>Transdermal patch: 25, 37.5, 50, 75, 100 mcg/day |

### Adverse effects of estrogen

1. Oral administration causes nausea, vomiting and diarrhea.
2. Cardiovascular effects:
   - Risk of venous thromboembolism
   - Increase in plasma triglycerides
   - Hypertension, edema
3. Others:
   - Gall bladder disease
   - Risk of breast and endometrial carcinoma
   - Hyperpigmentation
   - DES: vaginal adenocarcinoma in the daughters

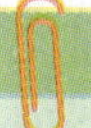

**Adverse Effects of Estrogen**

- Nausea, vomiting and diarrhea
- Risk of venous thromboembolism
- Increase in plasma triglycerides
- Hypertension, edema
- Gall bladder disease
- Risk of breast and endometrial carcinoma
- Hyperpigmentation
- DES: vaginal adenocarcinoma in the daughters

## SELECTIVE ESTROGEN RECEPTOR MODULATORS (SERMs)

Estrogen acts via two categories of receptors, alpha and beta.

- Estrogen receptor α (ERα) is found in endometrium, breast cancer cells, ovarian stromal cells, and the hypothalamus.
- ERβ has been documented in the brain, bone, heart, and endothelial cells.

Varieties of drugs have been designed which either selectively act as agonist or antagonist to the receptors or find a wide clinical application. For example, Tamoxifen, is an antagonist in breast and is, therefore, used in breast cancer treatment but it is an ER agonist in bone (thereby preventing osteoporosis and so is favourable) and a partial agonist in the endometrium (increasing the risk of uterine cancer).

### Clomiphene Citrate

This is a very commonly used SERM for inducing ovulation. It is used in oligo- or anovulation in a dose of 50–150 mg/day, once daily from the 3rd day of the cycle for 5 days. It can also be started on the 4th or 5th day of the cycle and given for five days. The starting dose is 50 mg/day, which can be increased by 50 mg every month up to a maximum of 150 mg/day and rarely to 200 mg/day.

It is also used in smaller doses of 25–50 mg/day in male hypogonadism.

It is used with an advice for the couple to have timed intercourse, or during an IUI cycle with follicular monitoring with ultrasound, or for an IVF cycle along with gonadotropins.

It acts by blocking estrogen receptors in the hypothalamus and thus preventing negative feedback of estrogen on GnRH and thus continuously stimulating follicle growth through FSH.

#### Adverse reactions

Most common is reversible ovarian enlargement.

Visual symptoms like blurred vision and double vision are reported in 1–10% of patients. Headaches, hot flashes, abnormal uterine bleeding and/or abdominal discomfort also have been reported.

Rarely ovarian hyperstimulation syndrome can occur.

Clomiphene can lead to multiple ovulation, hence increasing the chance of twins (10% of births).

**If used for more than a year it may increase the risk of ovarian cancer.**

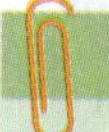

**Adverse Reactions of Clomiphene Citrate**

Reversible ovarian enlargement
Blurred vision and double vision
Headaches, hot flashes, abnormal uterine bleeding and/or abdominal discomfort
Ovarian hyperstimulation syndrome
Multiple ovulation
May increase the risk of ovarian cancer.

### Tamoxifen

This is a SERM being extensively used in both female and male breast cancers.

It belongs to triphenylethylene group and has antagonistic action on breast cancer cells, agonistic action on bone and partial agonistic action on endometrium. Thus patients on tamoxifen for breast cancer need to be monitored for endometrial hyperplasia/cancer periodically.

#### Uses

- In estrogen receptor positive male and in female breast cancer for about 5–10 years.
- As on ovulation-inducing agent in infertility, from 3rd to 7th day, once a day in the dosage of 40 mg/day.

- In the chemoprevention of breast cancer in susceptible individuals and to prevent cancer in contralateral breast.
- To prevent gynaecomastia.

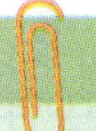

**Side Effects of Tamoxifen**

- Endometrial hyperplasia/cancer
- Beneficial effect on bone—avoids resorption
- Beneficial effect on lipid profile and thus cardioprotective

## Raloxifene

This has estrogenic actions on bone and antiestrogenic actions on the uterus and breast. It is used in

- The prevention of osteoporosis in postmenopausal women
- Postmenopausal women at high risk for invasive breast cancer.

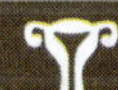

**Clinical Importance**

**Side effects**

- Menopausal symptoms
- Venous thromboembolism (VTE)

## Ormeloxifene

This is the other SERM used as a weekly-once contraceptive in the dose of 60 mg once a week **(Saheli)**. It is a non-steroidal oral contraceptive.

It is also used in cases of abnormal uterine bleeding.

# ESTROGEN SYNTHESIS INHIBITORS

## Aromatase Inhibitors (AI)

Aromatase is the enzyme that synthesises estrogen. As breast and ovarian cancers require estrogen to grow, AIs are taken to either block the production of estrogen or block the action of estrogen on receptors They inhibit conversion of androgens to estrogen and thus all estrogen-dependent breast tumours could be effectively treated by them.

The clinically used drugs are Anastrozole, Exemestane and Letrozole.

| Drug | Route of administration | Dose |
|---|---|---|
| Letrozole | Oral | 2.5 mg/day |
| Anastrozole | Oral | 1 mg/day |
| Exemestane | | 25 mg/day |

The dose has to be adjusted depending on the indication and the patient's condition.

They are used in postmenopausal women with breast cancer.

It can be used in gynaecomastia, endometriosis and non-obstructive azoospermia.

**Clinical Importance**

**Side Effects of Aromatase Inhibitors**

The more common side effects include

- Back pain
- Bone pain
- Hot flashes (sudden sweating and feeling of warmth)
- Joint pain
- Muscle pain

Other less common side effects are:

- Anxiety
- Confusion
- Constipation
- Diarrhea
- Dry mouth
- Headache
- Increased thirst
- Loss of appetite or weight loss
- Metallic taste
- Skin rash or itching

# PROGESTERONE

Natural progesterone is usually obtained from compounds derived from soybeans and Mexican yam roots. The hormone needs to be extracted or synthesised.

### Actions of Progesterone

Progesterone is a key component in the regulation of normal female reproductive function.

It acts through 2 types of receptors, **PR-A and PR-B.**

#### *In pregnancy*

Progesterone facilitates implantation, and maintenance of pregnancy, by promoting uterine growth and suppressing myometrial contractility (uterine quiescence).

#### *On the uterus*

It is totally antiestrogenic in nature. It reduces myometrial activity and tubal motility and makes the cervical mucus more viscous. Progesterone also facilitates endometrial differentiation and maturation, decidualisation thereby preparing the endometrium for implantation.

### *Breast*

Whereas progesterone facilitates lobular-alveolar development in puberty, in pregnancy it aids in preparation for milk secretion and suppression of milk protein synthesis before parturition.

### *Brain*

It mediates signals required for sexually responsive behaviour (which is well established in animal studies).

### *Bone*

Progesterone may play a role in bone remodeling.

## Classification

The classification of progesterone is as given in Table 18.7.

## Progesterone Compounds

Most of the progesterone compounds have antiestrogenic action. Some of them have androgenic and anabolic action as they are derivatives of 19-nortestosterone. The newer ones have least androgenic action and the fourth-generation progesterones have antiandrogenic action too. Their actions are shown in Table 18.8.

### *Micronised progesterone*

Micronising increases the half-life of progesterone and reduces its destruction in the GIT. By decreasing particle size, it increases the dissolution of the drug.

Serum concentrations are more rapidly achieved than with injectable preparation. Absorption is enhanced twofold when it is taken with food.

It has no adverse effects on mood, cholesterol or HDL. It has no adverse effect on pregnancy outcome. It is anxiolytic and causes sedation which may have a therapeutic advantage.

It is available as 100–400 mg tablets and can be used orally and also as vaginal tablets 2–3 times a day or as an injectable once a day.

**Table 18.7** Classification of progesterone

| Class of Progesterone | | Drug |
|---|---|---|
| Natural progesterone and micronised progesterone | | |
| | First Generation-21 carbon pregnane derivative | Dehydroretroprogesterone (Duphaston)<br>Esters of progesterone<br>17-alpha hydroxyprogesterone caproate<br>17-alpha hydroxyprogesterone acetate |
| | 17-alpha hydroxyprogesterone acetate derivatives (pregnanes) | Medroxyprogesterone acetate<br>Megestrol acetate<br>Chlormadinone acetate<br>Cyproterone acetate |
| | 17-alpha hydroxynorprogesterone caproate derivatives (norpregnanes) | Gestonorone<br>Nomegestrol acetate |
| | 19-norprogesterone derivatives (norpregnanes) | Demegestone<br>Promegestone<br>Nestorone<br>Trimegestone |
| | Alkyl derivatives of testosterone | Ethisterone, dimethisterone and Danazol |
| Derivatives of progesterone | Alkyl derivatives of 19 nor testosterone | Estrane group (First generation)<br>Nor ethisterone<br>Norethisterone acetate<br>Norethynodrel<br>Allylestranol<br>Gonane group (Second generation)<br>Norgestrel and levonorgestrel<br>Newer gonanes (Third generation)<br>Desogestrel<br>Etonogestrel<br>Gestodene<br>Norgestimate<br>Norelgestromine (Constituent of a Transdermal contraceptive) |
| | New progestins (Fourth generation) | Drospirenone<br>Dienogest<br>Trimegestone<br>Nestorone<br>Nomegestrol acetate |

**Table 18.8** Actions of progesterone

| Progesterone | Route | Actions | | | | |
|---|---|---|---|---|---|---|
| | | Estrogenic | Antiestrogenic | Androgenic | Antiandrogenic | Anabolic |
| Progesterone | IM | – | + | – | – | – |
| Hydroxyprogesterone | IM | – | – | Slight | – | – |
| Medroxyprogesterone | IM/Oral | Slight | + | + | – | – |
| Megestrol | Oral | – | – | + | + | – |
| Dydrogesterone | oral | – | + | – | – | – |
| 19-nortestosterone derivatives | | | | | | |
| Desogestrel | Oral | – | + | – | – | – |
| Norethynodrel | Oral | + | – | – | – | – |
| Lynestrenol | Oral | + | – | + | – | + |
| Norethindrone | Oral | Slight | + | + | – | + |
| Norethindrone acetate | Oral | Slight | + | + | – | + |
| Ethynodiol diacetate | Oral | Slight | + | + | – | – |
| L-Norgestrel | Oral | – | + | + | – | + |

### *Dydrogesterone*

- It is a progesterone derivative with no androgenic, estrogenic, or anabolic action.
- It has no effect on metabolism, lipid profile or on clotting factors.
- It is 10–30 times more potent than progesterone.
- It shows very good progestational activity in a dose of 10–20 mg/day.
- But it does not have a good hemostatic activity.
- It is not a good agent to control HPA axis and thus not useful for contraception.
- But it is a good agent to induce withdrawal bleeding.
- It can be considered suitable for HRT.
- It is also a good agent to manage luteal phase defect and support.

### *Medroxyprogesterone*

- Being an ester, it has longer duration of action.
- It can be used both orally and as an intramuscular injection.
- It has a very good cycle control, hence is very useful for contraception.
- It is a good agent to induce withdrawal bleeding.
- It has good progestational activity.
- Because of its prolonged action, it is a good agent for HRT.
- As it is a good endometrial protecting agent, it is useful for managing precancerous conditions of endometrium and cancer of endometrium.
- This too is a poor hemostat, hence not the preferred agent for hemostasis in heavy menstrual bleeding.
- It is used in the dose of 2.5–20 mg/day orally and for contraception as 150 mg/3 months IM injection.

### *17-alpha-hydroxyprogesterone*

This is an ester with a prolonged action.

Weekly administration in the dose of 250–500 mg IM injection is the general practice.

Historically, it was used for supporting pregnancy.

### *19-nortestosterone derivatives*

#### Estranes

- Norethisterone and norethinodrel are examples.
- Orally active in a very small dose.
- Good as haemostats.
- Useful as contraceptives in combination with estrogens.
- Have good progestational activity.
- The disadvantage is their inherent androgenic activity with adverse actions on lipid profile.

#### Gonanes

- They share all the properties of estranes.
- Levonorgestrel (LNG) is the most commonly used preparation with the advantage of lower dose but has increased androgenic effects.
- Apart from being used as a component of oral contraceptive, LNG is also used as intrauterine system (LNG IUS).

#### Newer gonanes

- Desogestrel is the most popular member of this group.

- Methylene radical at 11th position makes it lipid-friendly, decreases androgenic effects and offers excellent endometrial protection in small doses of 150 mcg/day.
- It has a prolonged duration of action.

### 4th generation progesterones

- Have antiandrogenic action
- Good progestational activity
- Used in combination with estrogen especially in situations like hyperandrogenic states

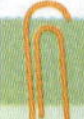

**Side Effects of Progesterone**

No major side effects are reported with the use of progesterone. Some of the minor effects are

- Fatigue
- Somnolence
- Edema
- Abdominal bloating
- Anxiety
- Irritability
- Depression
- Myalgia

### Uses

#### *In abnormal uterine bleeding*

Acute control of endometrial bleeding 10–30 mg/day of norethisterone for 3–5 days followed by tapering the dose over 3 weeks.

Endometrial protection in anovulatory cycles by using medroxyprogesterone acetate (MPA)/ Norethisterone from $5^{th}$–$25^{th}$ day of the cycle or from 15–$25^{th}$ day.

Anovulatory puberty menorrhagia not responding to antifibrinolytics.

LNG IUS for long-term protection of endometrium.

#### *In endometriosis*

Danazol 600–800 mg/day for 6–9 months.

Continuous progesterone usage—Norethindrone, Dienogest, MPA can be used.

Injectable progesterone also may be used.

#### *In contraception*

Levonorgestrel, desogestrel in combined OC pills

Levonorgestrel IUCD and in emergency contraception

MPA and norethisterone enanthate as injectable preparations

Desogestrel as progesterone only contraception

Subcutaneous implants and in dermal patches

Etonogestrel in vaginal ring contraceptive

#### *In hormone replacement therapy (HRT)*

Postmenopausal or surgical menopausal situations requiring HRT, 1.5–2.5 mg MPA, 0.1 mg norethindrone acetate, 0.5 mg drospirenone, 50 mg micronised progesterone, desogestrel, LNG IUS, dydrogesterone 10 mg/day may be used.

#### *In pregnancy*

In recurrent pregnancy loss, progesterone is used as an immune modulator.

Also used in pre-term labour and luteal phase defect (LPD).

Micronised progesterone, dydrogesterone, 17-alpha hydroxyl progesterone caproate are the preferred agents.

#### *In oncology*

MPA and megestrol have been used in endometrial cancer (including metastatic endometrial cancer), endometrial hyperplasia, breast cancer and occasionally for prostate cancer. It has also been used in uterine sarcomas.

#### *Miscellaneous uses*

Premenstrual syndrome, dysmenorrhea, progesterone challenge test in cases of secondary amenorrhea, medical curettage before initiating any long-term therapy in hyperestrogenic states.

## TESTOSTERONE DERIVATIVES

### Danazol

- It is basically ethisterone with an isoxazole moiety and is the only agent used therapeutically.
- It possesses weak progestational, androgenic, and glucocorticoid activities.
- It binds to sex hormone-binding and corticosteroid-binding globulins and is an inhibitor of p450 enzymes.
- It was primarily used in endometriosis, But subsequently, it has found its way in the management of fibrocystic disease of the breast, hematologic or allergic disorders also.
- Androgenic side effects are unwanted hair growth, acne, irreversible deepening of the voice, adverse blood lipid profiles, decrease in the breast size. Some patients may experience weight gain and fluid retention.
- Danazol should not be used in pregnancy and in liver diseases.

| Summary of use of commonly used progestogens | | | | | | | |
|---|---|---|---|---|---|---|---|
| **Drug** | **Dosage** | **Contra-ception** | **HRT** | **Haemostat** | **Endo. Protection** | **Withdrawal** | **Others** |
| Micronised progesterone | 100–400 mg | No | Yes | No | No | Yes | Luteal phase support |
| MPA | 2.5–3.0 mg<br>150 mg IM | Yes | Yes | No | Yes | Yes | Ca endometrium |
| 17-alpha OH Prog | 250–500 mg IM | No | No | No | No | No | Pregnancy support and Ca endometrium |
| Norethisterone | 5–10 mg<br>2–3 times a day<br>IM injection | Yes | Yes | Yes | Yes | Yes | |
| Danazol | 200–800 mg/day | No | No | No | No | No | Endometriosis |
| Levonorgestrel | 250 mcg<br>150 mcg<br>52 mg IUS | Yes | No | No | Yes | No | Emergency contraception<br>PMS |
| Desogestrel | 75 mcg/day | Yes | Yes | No | Yes | No | Progesterone only pill |

- Usual dosage is 400–800 mg/day for 6–9 months.

## SELECTIVE PROGESTERONE RECEPTOR MODULATORS (SPRMs) / PROGESTERONE ANTAGONISTS

Progesterone acts through 2 types of receptors. Depending on their action on the receptors **PR-A** or **PR-B,** the family is given the name progesterone receptor ligands. The activity of these compounds are spread across a spectrum, with one end of the spectrum being the **agonists** which include all progestins and the other end which are **antagonists** like mifepristone; the ones with both agonistic and antagonistic activity are known as **selective progesterone receptor modulators (SPRMs)** and they occupy intermediate positions. This is diagrammatically shown in Fig. 18.1.

They do not cause profound estrogen deficiency or decrease in bone mineral density.

## ANDROGENS

Androgens do not find any therapeutic application in gynecology, but play a major role in diagnostic workup of cases of hyperandrogenic states like hirsuitism, virilism, PCOS, etc., but a certain level of androgen activity is also needed for normal female physiology.

Androgens have some role in causing mineralisation of bones especially in postmenopausal women (probably due to aromatisation to estrogens in periphery).

### Effects

- Increased muscle mass
- Increased red blood cell production
- Maintain normal bone density

### Clinical Uses

Dehydroepiandrosterone sulphate (DHEA-S) is used to increase the ovarian reserve in the dose of 25 mg 3 times a day for a couple of months.

### Toxicity

- Masculinising actions are most noticeable in women
- Hepatic dysfunction
- Cholestatic jaundice
- Elevation of liver enzymes
- Hepatocellular carcinoma

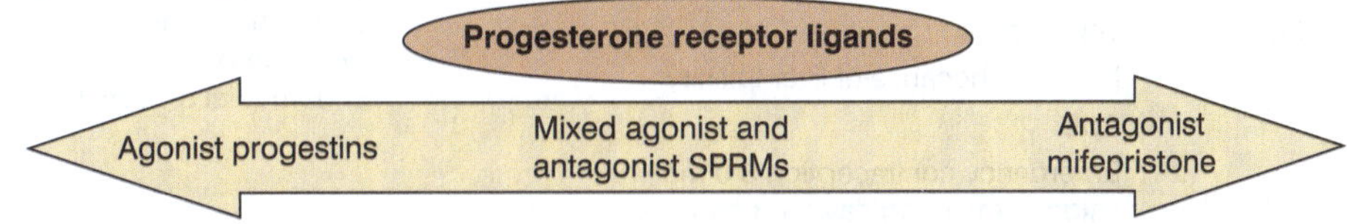


**Fig. 18.1** Diagrammatic representation of SPRMs

## ANTIANDROGENS

Antiandrogens were first discovered in the 1960s. They prevent the expression of androgens like testosterone, on the response tissues. They act either by blocking the androgen receptors or by altering the production of androgens.

Antiandrogens are used in cases of hirsuitism, virilism, PCOS (along with estrogens) and also for contraception as some of them have progestational activity (cyproterone acetate).

### Classification

- Receptor inhibitors
  - Flutamide
  - Spironolactone
- 5-α-reductase inhibitors
  - Finastride
- Gonadotropin-releasing hormone analogues
- Combined hormonal contraceptives
- Inhibitors of steroid synthesis

### Sites of Action

The following flowchart shows the sites of action of the various antiandrogens.

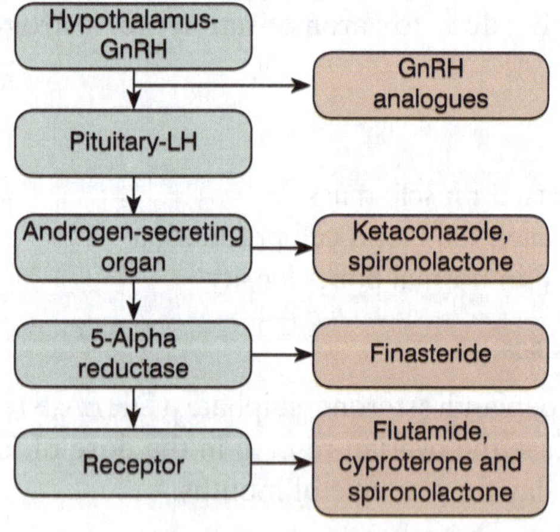


## THYROID HORMONES

T3, T4 and TSH are the hormones of interest for gynecologists.

Treating hypothyroidism and hyperthyroidism becomes crucial in infertility, anovulation, pregnancy and menstrual disturbances.

Supplementation with levothyroxine is the most effective and simple intervention in hypothyroidism. Treating subclinical hypothyroidism is becoming very common in pregnancy.

Hypothyroidism may be found in association with hyperprolactinaemia also. Thyroid levels should be stabilised prior to initiating treatment for high prolactin levels.

## ADRENAL HORMONES

They are used in working up cases of precocious puberty, ambiguous genitalia, virilism and other hyperandrogenic states, amenorrhea. Estimation of 17-alpha hydroxyl progesterone, ACTH stimulation test, dexamethasone suppression test are the applications.

## SUMMARY OF ROLE OF HORMONES IN GYNECOLOGY

The role of hormones in gynecological diagnosis is summarised in the following table.

| Hormones | Diagnostic application |
|---|---|
| GnRH and analogues | GnRH stimulation test in primary amenorrhea |
| FSH & LH | 3rd day FSH for ovarian reserve<br>FSH & LH for diagnosing menopause<br>In PCOS-Reversal of ratio<br>To diagnose premature ovarian insufficiency<br>Low FSH and LH in hypothalamic or |

| Summary of SPRMs | | |
|---|---|---|
| **Compounds** | **Uses** | **Rationale** |
| Mifepristone (RU486) | Medical termination of pregnancy 200–600 mg<br>Intrauterine fetal demise termination<br>Leiomyoma 25–50 mg/day for 3 months<br>Endometriosis<br>Emergency contraception<br>Cushing's syndrome | Direct antiproliferative effects on the endometrium<br>Antiproliferative effect on smooth muscle cells of myometrium<br>Antiglucocorticoid action<br>Suppression of late follicular development<br>Ovulation suppression<br>LH surge block<br>Endometrial receptivity alteration |
| Telapristone (CDB-4124) | Leiomyoma | |
| Onapristone | Not used because of liver toxicity | |
| Asoprisnil (J867) | AUB | |
| Ulipristal (CDB-2914) | Emergency contraception 3 0 mg<br>Leiomyoma 5 mg/day for 3 months<br>Preoperative in leiomyoma | |

| | |
|---|---|
| | hypophyseal disorders in primary and secondary amenorrhea<br>LH surge to identify ovulation |
| hCG | Diagnosis of pregnancy<br>Follow-up in ectopic pregnancy on medical or conservative management<br>Follow-up of gestational trophoblastic diseases |
| Prolactin | Hyperprolactinemia |
| Ethinyl estradiol | Estrogen challenge in secondary amenorrhea<br>Levels to correlate with follicular activity in ART cycles |
| Progesterone | Progesterone challenge test<br>Grey zone of beta hCG in ectopic pregnancy (Progesterone of >24 ng/mL is diagnostic of intrauterine pregnancy and <5 ng/mL of unsuccessful pregnancy) |
| 17-alpha OH progesterone | In congenital adrenal hyperplasia diagnosis |
| Free testosterone, DHEA-S | Hyperandrogenism—to diagnose androgen-secreting tumours |
| Fasting insulin and insulin resistance | PCOS |

Therapeutic applications have already been discussed under each hormone.

## Role of Hormones in Different Conditions

### Amenorrhea

Primary amenorrhea without secondary sexual characters—FSH and LH levels are used to differentiate ovarian from hypothalamo-hypophyseal causes.

Hypogonadotropic hypogonadism is successfully managed with gonadotropins.

Gonadal agenesis or dysgenesis requires hormone replacement to develop secondary sexual characters.

Hypoplastic uterus can be managed by high doses of estrogen and progesterone.

Amenorrhea—Primary and secondary (Asherman's syndrome, premature ovarian failure, Sheehan's syndrome, Simmond's disease, thyroid disorders, hyperprolactinemia) can be differentiated by gonadotropin levels.

Estrogen and progesterone supplementation is useful in Asherman's syndrome post adhesiolysis. Premature ovarian failure too requires hormone replacement therapy.

Adrenal and gonadal pathology should be looked for in heterosexual development in a female. Surgical correction or hormone antagonists may have to be used.

Precocious puberty—adrenal hormone and sex hormone work up and if found to be constitutional, needs to be managed with GnRH analogues to prevent premature epiphyseal closure.

### Menstrual disturbances

Progesterone, SERMs, combined OC pills, LNG IUS may be used in cases of heavy menstrual bleeding and endometrial hyperplasia.

For dysmenorrhea and premenstrual syndrome, combined OC pill therapy may be useful in spasmodic variety.

### Endometriosis

Progesterones are the mainstay of treatment: GnRH analogues, danazol may have to be considered in some cases. LNG IUS may be useful in adenomyosis.

### Leiomyoma

Medical management has seen a great deal of development with GnRH analogues, progesterone, progesterone antagonists, aromatase inhibitors, SPRMs, cabergoline, etc.

### Infertility

For infertility evaluation, ovulation induction, luteal support and ART, gonadotropins, SERMs, progesterone, GnRH analogues, hCG and aromatase inhibitors are extensively used.

DHEA-S is used with an intention of improving ovarian reserve (patients with low AMH).

Hirsuitism—Hormones are used for both diagnostic workup with adrenal and gonadal androgens to localise the pathology and subsequently antiandrogens are used in the management.

### Pregnancy events

Abortions / recurrent pregnancy loss (RPL)—Role of progesterone and hCG in supporting pregnancy is a debatable issue, but one of the extensively used indication.

In ectopic pregnancy, hCG and progesterone are useful mainly for diagnosis and follow-up.

### Contraception

Probably the maximum use of hormones happens in this sector in various forms.

### Menopausal problems

Urogenital problems, vulvovaginitis (even in prepubertal girls), preoperative estrogen in postmenopausal long-standing genital prolapse and osteoporosis are conditions which require estrogens or SERMs in various forms. With the outcomes of the Woman's Health Initiative (WHI) and The Million Women Study, postmenopausal hormone replacement has become a controversial issue.

### Oncology

Progesterone and SERMs are used in endometrial carcinoma and cancer breast respectively in certain cases.

Benign ovarian tumours—many of the suspected functional cysts of the ovary are treated with combined OC pill though the evidence do not support it.

### Miscellaneous

Ambiguous genitals, Turner's syndrome, adrenogenital syndrome, gonadal dysgenesis, androgen insensitivity syndrome, Klinefelter's syndrome are some of the conditions which may need hormone estimation at some stage of evaluation and some of them might require hormonal therapy for various reasons.

## RECAP

- Hypothalamus and pituitary are the masters of the endocrine orchestra in our body.
- Gonadotropin releasing hormones and their analogues have a wide application in present-day gynecological practice.
- Gonadotropins are extensively used in anovulatory infertility.
- Thyroid and adrenal glands and their hormones play an important role in regulation of menstrual cycle and in the reproductive function of a woman.
- All sex steroids are derived from cholesterol.
- Enzyme defects can cause problems in sexual development, menstruation and reproduction.
- Estrogens and progesterones and their derivatives are used for many of the gynecological disorders like AUB, leiomyoma, endometriosis, cancer, etc.
- Receptor modulators and antagonists of the ovarian steroids also find important application.
- Hormones are extensively used in contraception, infertility and menstrual disturbances.
- Androgens have no therapeutic role, but antiandrogens are used in hyperandrogenic states.

## REVIEW QUESTIONS

### Long-Answer Questions

a. What are the actions of progesterone in a woman? Discuss the medical management of endometrial hyperplasia in a 30-year-old woman with one living child.

b. Discuss the various progesterone preparations used in clinical practice and the different routes of administration.

c. What are the uses of estrogens in gynecology?

### Short Notes

a. Clomiphene citrate

b. Gonadotropins

c. GnRH analogues in gynecology

d. Hirsutism

e. Medical management of uterine leiomyoma

f. Human chorionic gonadotropin

g. Danazol

### MCQs

**1. Which of these progesterones has an anabolic action?**

a) Desogestrel b) Dydrogesterone
c) Medroxyprogesterone d) Lynestrenol

**2. The predominant circulating estrogen in pregnancy is**

a) Estriol b) Estrone
c) Estradiol d) All of the above

**3. Which of these is not a GnRH analogue?**

a) Buserelin b) Ganirelix
c) Triptorelin d) Deslorelin

**4. Phytoestrogens are derived from**

a) Antiestrogens b) Fungus
c) Plant
d) Non-conjugated synthetic estrogens

# Chapter 19

# Malignant Diseases of the Vulva, Vagina and Fallopian Tube

**At a Glance**

Premalignant Lesions of the Vulva
Classification of VIN (ISSVD 2004)
Carcinoma of the Vulva
Melanoma of the Vulva
Pre-Malignant Epithelial Changes of the Vagina (VaIN)
**Malignant Tumours of the Vagina**
Carcinoma of the Vagina
Clear Cell Adenocarcinoma
Sarcoma of the Vagina
Verrucous Carcinoma
Adenocarcinoma
Embryonal Rhabdomyosarcoma (Sarcoma Botryoides)
Primary Carcinoma of the Fallopian Tube

## PREMALIGNANT LESIONS OF THE VULVA

Though vulvar cancer is rare, 90% of vulvar cancer develops through precancerous lesions known as **vulvar intraepithelial neoplasia (VIN)** (Fig. 19.1).

### Classification of VIN (ISSVD 2004)

| VIN Type | |
|---|---|
| VIN, usual type<br>• Warty<br>• Basaloid<br>• Mixed | This includes former VIN 2,3 and vulvar carcinoma in situ |
| VIN, differentiated type | Includes about 10% of former VIN3 lesions |
| VIN, unclassified type | Rare paget lesions |

**Etiology** In the etiology of this condition, viruses, especially the **human papilloma virus (HPV),** are incriminated, though the **herpes simplex virus (HSV-2)** infections cannot be ruled out in a few cases.

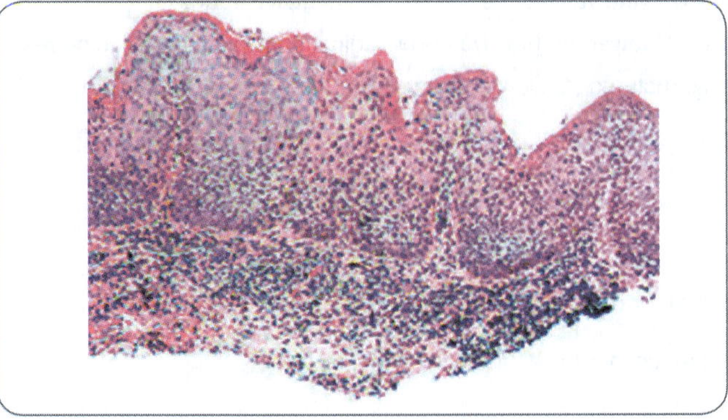

**Fig. 19.1** Vulvar intraepithelial neoplasia (*Source:* Wikimedia / © 2011 Michael Bonert)

**Incidence** The VIN is being diagnosed with increasing frequency especially among women less than 40 years of age; this may be either due to a true increase in the incidence or because of the increasing recognition of the disease.

**Symptoms** The most common symptoms are

1. Pruritus
2. Vulvar pain
3. Soreness and dyspareunia
4. Warty lesions

**Diagnosis** Confirmation of diagnosis is by **biopsy** and histopathological examination. The best area for biopsy is detected by colposcopic examination of the vulva and perianal area. This is known as **vulvoscopy.**

Biopsy can be taken using a **Keyes punch biopsy forceps.**

**Management**

***VIN1*** Though 2004 ISSVD has removed VIN1 category, those diagnosed with this lesion earlier need not be treated, but reassessed for progression. Reassessment includes gross inspection or vulvoscopy and biopsy as clinically indicated.

***VIN 2 and 3*** All high-grade VIN lesions should be treated by either excision or ablation.

## CARCINOMA OF THE VULVA

Carcinoma of the vulva is relatively rare and accounts for about 5 per cent of all malignant tumours of the female genital tract.

**Incidence** Its incidence is more in the white than in the coloured races. It is mostly found in women over 60 years.

**Etiology** The cause is not clear. In older patients, it is more common in single, nulliparous women. It is also common in younger women with a history of STD, including HPV infection. Though a vulvar carcinoma may develop in an apparently normal skin, in 30–40 per cent of patients, there is a past history of dysplasia as early as 10 years. Leukoplakia, especially of the hyperkeratotic type, is known to lead to the development of invasive cancer.

**Risk factors**

- Obesity
- Hypertension (in 30–50%)
- Diabetes (in 10%)
- Smoking
- HIV infection by producing immunosuppression and increasing chances of HIV infection

**Symptoms**

- It may start as an ulcer in a leukoplakic patch.
- The ulceration may spread progressively with the patient complaining of pain, pruritus and bleeding.
- The patient usually reports late for treatment because she feels shy discussing her symptoms. Although a carcinoma arises on a body surface and is hence easily detectable, a delay of 6–12 months in seeking medical attention is common.

**Sites**

- In older women The lesion begins more anteriorly on the vulva, and the clitoral or preputial site is common.
- In younger women, the fourchette is the most common site. The labia majora are involved in about 40 per cent of these cases, the labia minora or clitoris in about 20 per cent and the perineum much more rarely.

**Pathology**

Approximately 90 per cent of tumours are squamous cell cancers. They may be intraepithelial or invasive. Most of them are well differentiated with **keratinisation** and **epithelial pearl formation**. They may arise from the skin, and the subcutaneous tissue of the vulva, often from the labia, and rarely from the urethra or the glandular elements. A slow-growing, locally invasive, rarely metastatic wart-like variant of squamous cell carcinoma is called **verrucous carcinoma**. When a carcinoma arises from the Bartholin's gland, it is an adenocarcinoma.

**Spread**

- **Direct spread** The growth may involve the rest of the vulva, urethra, perineum and in advanced cases the rectum and the vagina, or may get fixed to the pubic bone.
- **Lymphatic spread** It also metastasises to the regional lymph nodes.
- **Hematogenous spread** It spreads to distant sites like the lungs via the bloodstream.

**Staging** The staging of vulvar carcinoma as recommended by the International Federation of Gynecology and Obstetrics (FIGO) is given in Table 19.1 and Fig. 19.2. The staging helps in the management, prognostication and international comparison of the results of the therapy.

**Table 19.1** Staging of vulvar carcinoma (FIGO, 2009)

| Stage | Characteristics |
|---|---|
| I | Tumour confined to the vulva |
| IA | Lesions ≤2 cm in size, confined to the vulva or perineum and with stromal invasion ≤1.0 mma, no nodal metastasis |
| IB | Lesions >2 cm in size or with stromal invasion >1.0 mma, confined to the vulva or perineum, with negative nodes |
| II | Tumour of any size with extension to adjacent perineal structures (1/3 lower urethra, 1/3 lower vagina, anus) with negative nodes |
| III | Tumour of any size with or without extension to adjacent perineal structures (1/3 lower urethra, 1/3 lower vagina, anus) with positive inguinofemoral lymph nodes |
| IIIA | i) With 1 lymph node metastasis (≥5 mm), or<br>ii) 1–2 lymph node metastasis(es) (<5 mm) |
| IIIB | i) With 2 or more lymph node metastases (≥5 mm), or<br>ii) 3 or more lymph node metastases (<5 mm) |
| III C | With positive nodes with extracapsular spread |
| IV | Tumour invades other regional (2/3 upper urethra, 2/3 upper vagina), or distant structures<br>Tumour invades any of the following: |
| IVA | i) upper urethral and/or vaginal mucosa, bladder mucosa, rectal mucosa, or fixed to pelvic bone, or<br>ii) fixed or ulcerated inguinofemoral lymph nodes |
| IVB | Any distant metastasis including pelvic lymph nodes |

FIGO = International Federation of Gynecology and Obstetrics.

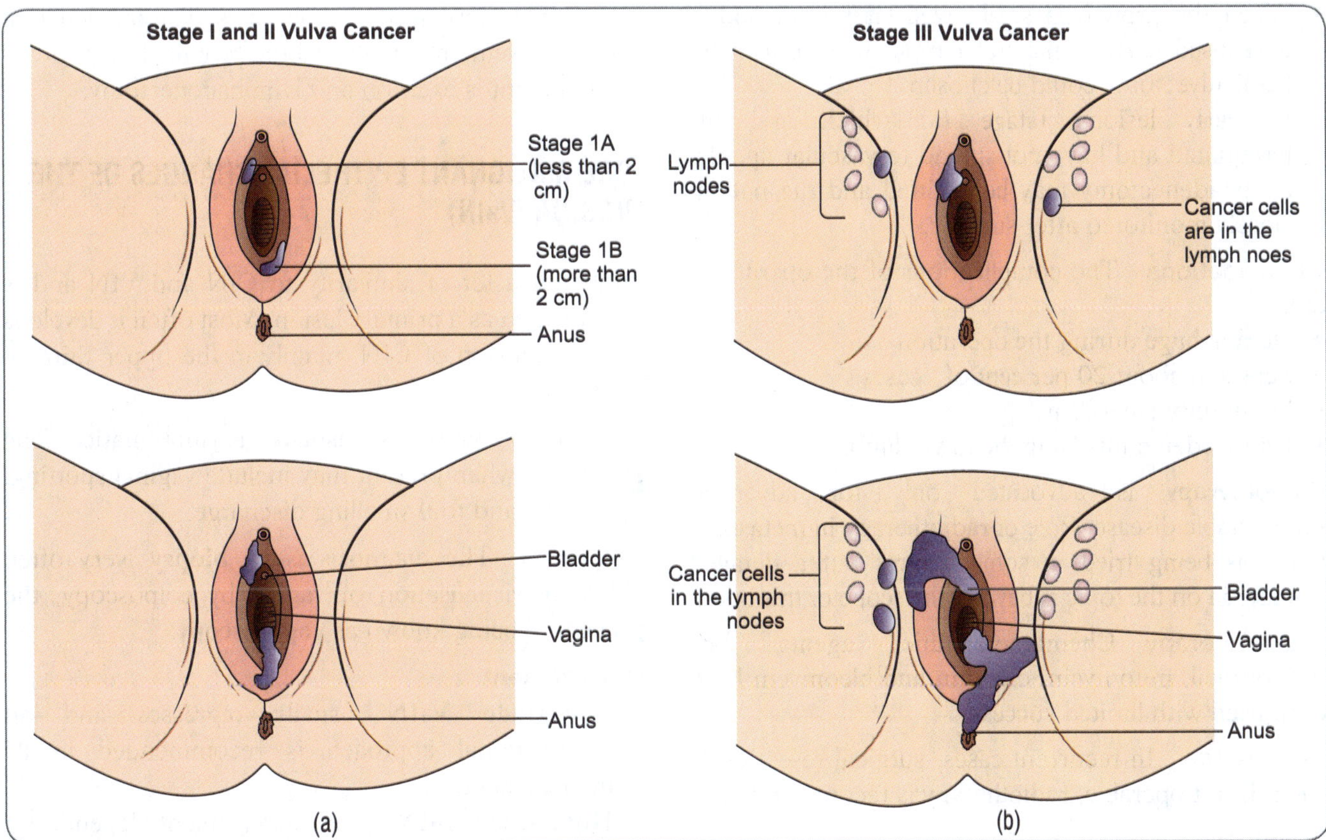


**Fig. 19.2** Stages of vulvar cancer. (a) Stage I and II (b) Stage III

## Diagnosis

- **Physical examination** In a typical case, the diagnosis can be made by inspection, palpation of the lesion and by observing its edges. If a thorough physical examination is not possible due to patient's discomfort. Examination under anesthesia will be helpful.

**Biopsy** from the ulcer is diagnostic.

- CT, MRI and PET scans are useful in women with large tumours and extensive invasion to adjacent areas. MRI scan helps in the identification of involved lymph node and also the fixity of the tumour.

**Differential diagnosis** The following conditions may simulate vulvar cancer

- Syphilis
- Tuberculosis
- Rodent ulcer
- Condylomata of the vulva

***Lymphatics of the vulva*** The lymphatics of the vulva have been discussed in detail in chapter 3. In about 50 per cent of cases, the lymph nodes may be involved. The lymph nodes draining the vulva are mainly the superficial inguinal group and the external iliac group. The superficial inguinal group consists of the horizontal nodes along the inguinal ligament and the vertical nodes around the saphenous opening and the great saphenous vein. These latter nodes drain into the deep femoral especially into the gland of Cloquet or Rosenmuller (which is located at the upper end of the femoral canal and underneath the inguinal ligament). The external iliac group is located along the external iliac artery and at the bifurcation of the common iliac artery. **The lymphatics of the vulva freely anastomose across the midline** and hence bilateral block dissection of the lymph nodes along with radical vulvectomy is necessary in case of vulvar cancer.

**Treatment** **Surgery** is the treatment of choice and the operation which gives the best results is **radical vulvectomy along with dissection of the regional, superficial and deep nodes** (as devised by Taussig and modified by Way).

**Two-stage procedure** There is no doubt that radical vulvectomy and regional node dissection performed in one stage give the best five-year survival results. However, when the patient's general condition is poor on account of age or concomitant disease, it may be desirable to perform a two-stage operation instead.

- When the growth is small, well lateralised and is diagnosed early, unilateral lymphadenectomy with hemivulvectomy could be chosen.
- In early lesions (stage Ia) which are differentiated and have not spread to vascular spaces, lymphadenectomy may be omitted and the patient closely monitored after surgery.

**Complications** The complications of the operations are:

- Hemorrhage during the operation
- Sepsis in about 20 per cent of cases
- Pulmonary embolism
- Lymphedema involving the lower limbs

**Radiotherapy** is advocated only for advanced unresectable disease. Role of radiotherapy in metastatic nodes is being tried in some centres but a detailed discussion on the topic is beyond the scope of this book.

**Chemotherapy** Chemotherapeutic agents like fluorouracil, mitomycin, cisplatin and bleomycin have been tried with limited success.

**Recurrence** In recurrent cases, surgical resection is tried. If not operable, radiotherapy is recommended.

### Prognosis

- The important prognostic factors in cancer of the vulva are
  - the stage of the disease
  - involvement of the urethra, vagina or anal canal
  - the histological type
  - its operability
  - the involvement of regional nodes
- A complete excision of the primary tumour yields a five-year survival rate of 80 per cent in the absence of lymph node metastases.
- In tumours less than 2 cm in diameter, the lymph node involvement is 10–15 per cent, but when it increases in size, the risk of metastases is higher.
- The five-year survival with lymph node involvement varies from 15–30 per cent.
- In general, about 40 per cent of patients undergoing surgery will have positive lymph nodes. Involvement of the bladder or rectum worsens the prognosis.

## MELANOMA OF THE VULVA

This is a rare tumour but is exceedingly fatal. The histological appearance does not differ from that of malignant melanomas in other parts of the body. These frequently tend to be very large on the vulva, much larger than those seen at other sites. The incidence of node involvement is high and the prognosis is poor.

Treatment is excision and lymphadenectomy.

## PRE-MALIGNANT EPITHELIAL CHANGES OF THE VAGINA (VaIN)

VaIN has a lot of similarity to CIN and VIN and is rarely found as a primary lesion. Most often it develops as an extension of CIN, mainly in the upper third of the vagina.

**Symptoms** VaIN is usually asymptomatic. The symptoms when present may include vaginal spotting, discharge, and foul smelling discharge.

**Diagnosis** The diagnosis is by **biopsy**, very often aided by visualisation of vagina by colposcopy, the procedure being known as **vaginoscopy**.

### Management

- **Low-grade VaIN** usually regresses and an observational approach is recommended in its management.
- **High-grade VaIN** The management depends on the location and number of lesions, sexual activity of the individual, length of the vagina, prior radiation therapy if any, in those with previous VaIN, prior treatment modalities and the expertise of the clinician.

  Management options include:

1. Excision
2. Carbon dioxide laser ablation
3. Radiation therapy and
4. Off-label use of 5FU as a medical ablation.

## MALIGNANT TUMOURS OF THE VAGINA

## CARCINOMA OF THE VAGINA

Primary carcinoma of the vagina forms 1 per cent of genital malignancy in women and is mostly seen in postmenopausal women. It may present as an ulcer or a cauliflower-like, easily bleeding growth in the middle or upper part of the vagina (Figs. 19.3 and 19.4). In over 95 per cent of cases it is an epidermoid carcinoma. Adenocarcinoma occasionally arises from mesonephric remnants or from vaginal endometriosis. The patient usually complains of irregular vaginal bleeding or foul-smelling discharge.

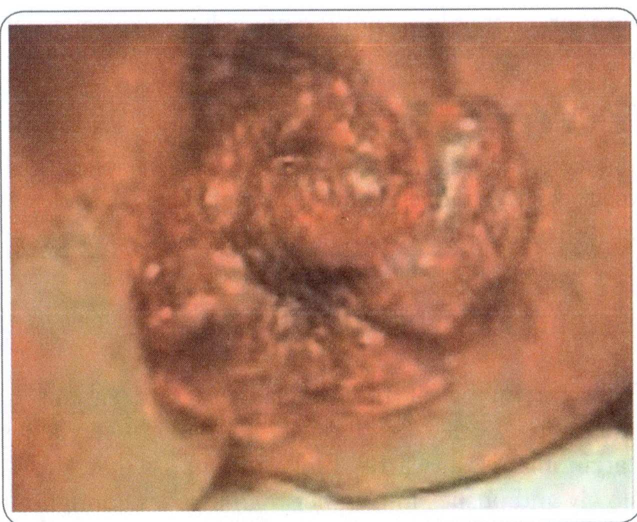

**Fig. 19.3** Carcinoma vagina (*Source:* Image from William's Gynecology 2ed by Hoffman et al. Copyright ©2012, 2008 by McGraw- Hill Companies Inc. Reproduced with permission.)

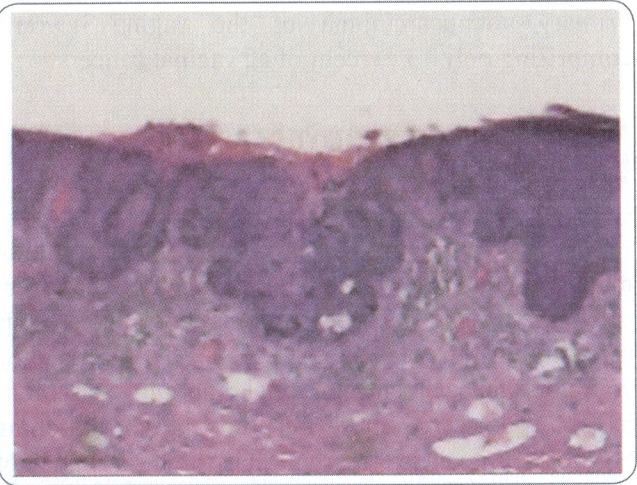

**Fig. 19.4** Histopathological picture of carcinoma vagina (*Source.* Image from William's Gynecology 2ed by Hoffman et al. Copyright ©2012, 2008 by McGraw-Hill Companies Inc. Reproduced with permission.)

**Table 19.2** FIGO staging of carcinoma of the vagina

| Stage | Characteristics |
|---|---|
| I | The carcinoma is limited to the vaginal wall. |
| II | The carcinoma has involved the subvaginal tissue but has not extended to the pelvic wall. |
| III | The carcinoma has extended to the pelvic wall. |
| IV | The carcinoma has extended beyond the true pelvis or has involved the mucosa of the bladder or rectum; |
| IVA | bullous edema as such does not permit a case to be allotted to stage IV. |
| IVB | Tumour invades bladder and/or rectal mucosa and/or direct extension beyond the true pelvis. Spread to distant organs. |

FIGO = International Federation of Gynecology and Obstetrics.

Primary carcinoma of the vagina is rare. Mostly the vaginal malignancy is secondary to primary growth arising from the cervix or the vulva. In the primary vaginal lesion, the cervix is healthy.

If the cervix is also involved, it is most likely to be a primary cervical cancer.

The staging of vaginal carcinoma as recommended by FIGO is given in Table 19.2.

## Symptoms

- Most vaginal cancers develop in the upper third of the vagina.
- Vaginal bleeding is the most common complaint associated with vaginal cancer.
- Pelvic pain and vaginal discharge may also be noted.
- Less frequently, lesions involving the anterior vaginal wall may lead to dysuria, hematuria, retention, or urgency.
- Alternatively, constipation may be the presenting symptom in those with lesions of the posterior wall. Most vaginal cancers develop in the upper third of the vagina.

## Diagnosis

- In all women, during pelvic evaluation, the vagina should be inspected as the speculum is being inserted or removed.
- If a gross lesion is found, vaginal cancer should be considered and confirmed by punch biopsy. Biopsy may be obtained with a Tischler biopsy forceps.
- Computed tomographic (CT) scanning can delineate the size and extent of many tumours.
- However, if the extent of cancer expansion is unclear, magnetic resonance (MR) imaging helps to visualise the extent of involvement.
- As in cervical cancer, an examination under anesthesia may be helpful to clinically stage the patient and further guide treatment.
- Proctosigmoidoscopy to a depth of at least 15 cm can detect local bowel invasion.
- In the presence of anterior tumours, cystourethroscopy helps to identify bladder or urethral involvement.

**Prognosis** Since the vagina is a thin-walled tube richly supplied with lymphatics and is intimately related to the bladder in front and the rectum behind, the prognosis in vaginal carcinoma is poor. The five-year survival rate is about 20–30 per cent. The growth spreads rapidly to the surrounding paravaginal tissues and neighbouring viscera. The proximity of the bladder and rectum also pose problems during therapy.

### Treatment

***Stage I*** Both surgery and radiotherapy are options for stage I disease. However, surgery is preferred for most if negative surgical margins can be achieved.

Surgery includes radical vaginectomy and pelvic lymphadenectomy for most tumours located in the upper third of the vaginal vault.

***Stage II*** Both surgery and radiation are options for stage II cancers.

***Stage III and IVA*** For advanced disease, external beam radiation alone or combined with brachytherapy is usually administered (Frank, 2005). Concurrent chemotherapy with cisplatin as a radiation adjunct is also generally recommended.

***Stage IVB*** The most common sites of distant spread include liver, lungs and bones. Metastatic vaginal cancer is not curable, and treatment may include systemic chemotherapy or supportive hospice care.

## CLEAR CELL ADENOCARCINOMA

This is a rare type of vaginal cancer seen in adolescent girls who have been exposed prenatally to Diethyl Stilboestrol (DBS) administered to the mother in the first trimester of pregnancy. Some of these patients earlier show evidence of vaginal adenosis. This type of cancer is mostly seen in the upper third of the anterior vaginal wall as a nodular or polypoidal, friable, easily bleeding mass.

### Treatment

In early cases, radical surgery (radical hysterectomy with vaginectomy and pelvic lymphadenectomy) is the treatment of choice. In advanced cases, radiation therapy is advised.

## SARCOMA OF THE VAGINA

This is rare and is seen mostly in children. An interesting variety of sarcoma is the grape-like sarcoma of the vagina, also called **sarcoma botryoides**, first described over a hundred years ago. It is a polypoidal tumour consisting of grape-like, pinkish, polyp-like masses filling the vagina and protruding through the vulva. In advanced stages it infiltrates into the surrounding tissues and into the abdomen. It is a mixed mesodermal tumour containing undifferentiated mesodermal and striped muscle fibres.

### Treatment

The radical surgical removal (radical hysterectomy and total vaginectomy) is the best line of treatment though the five-year survival rate is quite low.

## VERRUCOUS CARCINOMA

This carcinoma of the vagina is a rare variant of squamous cell carcinoma. Grossly, verrucous carcinoma is a warty, fungating mass that grows slowly and pushes into rather than invades contiguous structures.

## ADENOCARCINOMA

Primary adenocarcinoma of the vagina is rare, comprising only 13 percent of all vaginal cancers.

## EMBRYONAL RHABDOMYOSARCOMA (SARCOMA BOTRYOIDES)

Embryonal rhabdomyosarcoma is the most common malignancy of the vagina in infants and children. Most are of the subtype sarcoma botryoides. This rare tumour develops almost exclusively in girls aged younger than 5 years. Embryonal rhabdomyosarcomas have a poor prognosis, but the subtype sarcoma botryoides is easy to treat and has the best chance of cure.

## PRIMARY CARCINOMA OF THE FALLOPIAN TUBE

This carcinoma was considered a rare entity till recently. However, the fimbria of the Fallopian tube has recently been identified as an origin for many high-grade pelvic serous carcinomas. Hence there is a renewed interest in Fallopian tube carcinoma.

The following criteria have to be satisfied if the tumour is to be considered a primary Fallopian tube carcinoma.

1. The tumour must be located macroscopically within the tube or its fimbriated end.
2. Additionally, the uterus and ovary must not contain carcinoma, or if they do, it must be clearly different from the Fallopian tube lesion.

**Table 19.3** FIGO staging of carcinoma of the Fallopian tube

| Stage | Characteristics |
|---|---|
| I | Growth limited to the Fallopian tubes |
| IA | Growth is limited to one tube, with extension into the submucosa and/or muscularis, but not penetrating the serosal surface; no ascites |
| IB | Growth is limited to both tubes, with extension into the submucosa and/or muscularis, but not penetrating the serosal surface; no ascites |
| IC | Tumour either stage IA or IB, but with tumour extension through or onto the tubal serosa, or with ascites present containing malignant cells, or with positive peritoneal washings |
| II | Growth involving one or both Fallopian tubes with pelvic extension |
| IIA | Extension and/or metastasis to the uterus and/or ovaries |
| IIB | Extension to other pelvic tissues |
| IIC | Tumour either stage IIA or IIB and with ascites present containing malignant cells or with positive peritoneal washings |
| III | Tumour involves one or both Fallopian tubes, with peritoneal implants outside the pelvis and/or positive regional lymph nodes. Superficial liver metastasis equals stage III. Tumour appears limited to the true pelvis, but with histologically proven malignant extension to the small bowel or omentum |
| IIIA | Tumour is grossly limited to the true pelvis, with negative nodes, but with histologically confirmed microscopic seeding of abdominal peritoneal surfaces |
| IIIB | Tumour involving one or both tubes, with histologically confirmed implants of abdominal peritoneal surfaces, none exceeding 2 cm in diameter. Lymph nodes are negative |
| IIIC | Abdominal implants >2 cm in diameter and/or positive retroperitoneal or inguinal nodes |
| IV | Growth involving one or both Fallopian tubes with distant metastases. If pleural effusion is present, there must be positive cytology to be stage IV. Parenchymal liver metastases equals stage IV. |

Primary Fallopian tube carcinoma (PFTC) is one of the rare female genital cancers. It is usually seen in the 4th and 5th decade of life with an average age of 55–60 years. The exact etiology is unknown.

**Clinical features** Vaginal bleeding and abdominal pain are the two most common presenting symptoms. The other symptoms include ascites and abdominal mass. ***Latzko's triad* of symptoms,** consists of intermittent profuse serosanguinous vaginal discharge, colicky pain relieved by discharge, and abdominal or pelvic mass . The other feature of PFTC is ***Hydrops tubae profluens***, whih is considered to be a pathognomonic feature. It is intermittent vaginal discharge of clear or blood-tinged fluid spontaneously or on pressure followed by shrinkage of an adnexal mass; but it is now found that this feature is elicitable in less than 10% of PFTC patients. The staging of carcinoma of the Fallopian tube as recommended by FIGO is given in Table 19.3.

**Diagnosis** The diagnosis is usually by imaging technique. Ultrasound, CT and MRI all have been used. Transvaginal ultrasound is found to be better than abdominal ultrasound but the image is not pathognomonic of Fallopian tube cancer (Fig. 19.5). CT and MRI can contribute to the diagnosis.

The primary treatment modality is surgery, irrespective of the staging. However most of the patients even in early stage cancer of the Fallopian tube receive adjuvant chemotherapy to prevent spillage into the abdominal cavity. The aim of the surgery is both staging and debulking. Along with the tubes, the ovaries, uterus, cervix, infracolic omentectomy, retroperitoneal lymphadenectomy and peritoneal washing/biopsy are taken during surgery.

**Recurrences** are associated with a poor prognosis. The overall survival rate varies from 55–60% in early stages to less than 10% in late stage cancer of the Fallopian tube.

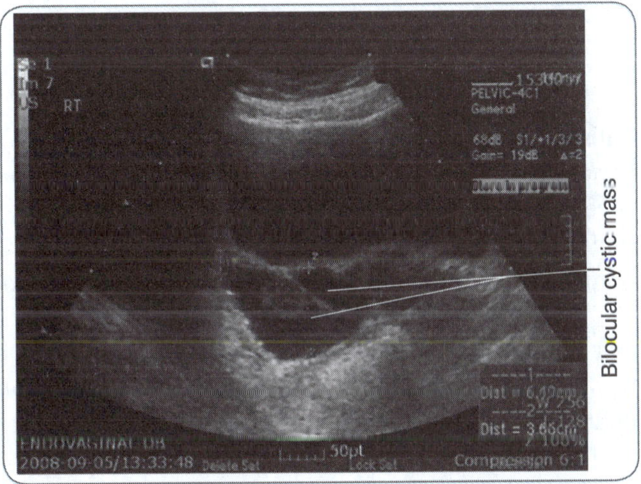


**Fig. 19.5** Ultrasonogram of ca FT showing a bilocular cystic mass with intramural nodule (*Source:* Copyright © 2012. Korean Society of Obstetrics and Gynecology. Reproduced with permission)

> ***Case study***
>
> *A 65-year-old lady comes with complaints of ulcer over the vulva. She also complains of itching in the vulva. Both complaints are of six months duration. Local examination reveals a 3 × 3 × 2 cm ulceration over the upper part of the right vulva.*
>
> *a) How will you confirm the diagnosis?*
> *b) Can this lesion spread to the opposite side also, if so trace the pathway of spread?*
> *c) Discuss the management?*

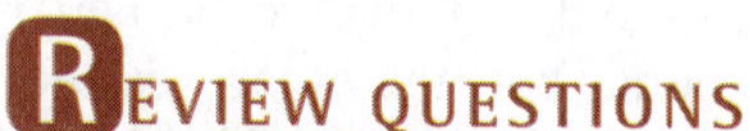

## REVIEW QUESTIONS

### Long-Answer Question

Discuss the lymphatics of the vulva. Classify vulvar cancer.

### Short-Answer Questions

1. What are the criteria to be satisfied for a tumour to be considered a primary Fallopian tube carcinoma? What are the clinical features of primary Fallopian tube carcinoma?
2. What is vaginal intraepithelial neoplasia (VaIN)? Discuss the diagnosis and management of the same.

### MCQs

1. **Embryonal rhabdomyosarcoma is the most common malignancy of**
   a) The vagina in infants and children
   b) The vulva in infants and children
   c) The vagina in women over 70 years of age
   d) The vulva in women 45–60 years of age.
2. **Vaginal carcinoma in over 95% of patients is**
   a) Squamous cell carcinoma
   b) Epidermoid carcinoma
   c) Adenocarcinoma
   d) Mucinous carcinoma
3. **Epithelial pearl formation is characteristic of**
   a) Fallopian tube carcinoma
   b) Vaginal carcinoma
   c) Cervical carcinoma
   d) Carcinoma of the vulva
4. **What percentage of vulvar carcinoma develops through vulvar intraepithelial neoplasia (VIN)?**
   a) Nearly 90%
   b) Nearly 10%
   c) Nearly 50%
   d) Do not develop from VIN

### Further Reading

Cavanagh D. Vulde val carcinoma: controversies in management. Br J Obstet Gynecol. 1996;103:293–300.

Green TH. 1977. Gynecology. 3rd edn. Boston: Little Brown; 1977.

Hoffman BL, Schorge JO, Schaffer JI et al., editors. William's Gynecology. 2nd ed. New York: McGraw-Hill; 2012.

Hoffmann MS, Cavanagh D. Malignancies of the vulva. ***Te Linde's Operative Gynecology.*** Rock JA and Thompson JD, editors. New York: Lippincott-Raven; 1996. 1331–82 pp.

Mac Dermott RIJ. 1995. Bacterial vaginosis—A review. Br J Obstet Gynecol. 1995;102:92–4.

Novak ER. Novak's text book of gynecology 10th ed. Baltimore: Williams and Wilkins; 1981.

Reichman RC, Badger GJ, Mertz GJ, et al. Treatment of recurrent genital herpes simplex infections with oral acyclovir. A controlled trial. JAMA. 1984 Apr 27;251(16):2103–2107.

Shepherd JH. Cervical and vulva cancer changes in FIGO definitions of staging. Br J Obstet Gynecol. 1996;

Society of Gynecologic Oncologists 1998. Practice guidelines: vaginal cancer. Oncology. 1998;12:449–52.

Sowmini CN. STD in Gynecology. Postgraduate obstetrics gynecology. 4th ed. Menon MKK, Devi PK, Rao KB, editors. Madras: Orient Longman; 1989.

WHO Technical Report Series 73. Expert Committee on Venereal Diseases. Geneva: WHO; 1986.

# Malignant Lesions of the Cervix

## At a Glance

Incidence of Cervical Cancer
Etiopathogenesis of Cervical Cancer
Risk Factors
Signs and Symptoms
Diagnosis
Modes of Spread
Specific Investigations
Colposcopy
Histological Types of Cervical Cancer
Differential Diagnosis
Staging
Treatment
Radical Trachelectomy
Types of Hysterectomy
Cancer Cervix in Other Situations
Cervical Cancer During Pregnancy
Stump Carcinoma
Recurrent Carcinoma Cervix
Management

**Cervical cancer is a preventable cancer because it has a long preinvasive state that lasts for about 10–15 years.** In spite of this fact, worldwide it is the 4th most common cancer among women, after breast, colorectal, and lung cancers with an estimated 527,624 new cases and 265,672 deaths in 2012 (GLOBOCAN).

Almost 70% of the global disease burden is seen in lower-middle-income countries and more than one-fifth of all new cases are diagnosed in India. In high-income countries, reduction of cancer cervix is a success story by effective screening and appropriate treatment for precancerous lesions. But in India, screening is limited. Opportunistic screening is patchy and not ideal.

## INCIDENCE OF CERVICAL CANCER

About 122,844 new cervical cancer cases are diagnosed annually in India (estimations for 2012). Cervical cancer ranks as the 2nd leading cause of female cancers in India and it is also the second most common female cancer in women aged 15 to 44 years in India. It is therefore a matter of public health, as it affects women within the reproductive age group. About 67,477 cervical cancer deaths occur annually in India (estimations for 2012).

The majority of cases are squamous cell carcinoma followed by adenocarcinoma. Of late the incidence of adenocarcinomas is increasing.

Screening and prevention has been dealt with in detail in the chapter on benign lesions of cervix. (Chapter 9).

Cervical cancer screening has decreased the incidence of and mortality from this condition. Methods for screening include evaluation with the Papanicolaou (Pap) test (cytology) and testing for high-risk types of human papilloma virus (HPV). Cervical cancer screening detects pre-invasive neoplasia, thereby making treatment possible before the disease becomes invasive; invasive disease may also be detected.

## ETIOPATHOGENESIS OF CERVICAL CANCER

The link between genital HPV infections and cervical cancer was first demonstrated in the early 1980s by Harold zur Hausen, a German virologist. Since then, the link between high-risk HPV types and cervical squamous cell carcinoma has become well known. In 1996, the World Health Organisation recognised HPV as an important cause of cervical cancer. Worldwide HPV has been implicated in 99.7% of cervical squamous cell carcinomas. The magnitude of the association between HPV and cervical carcinoma is higher than that for the association between smoking and lung cancer.

The HPV genome consists of a single molecule of double-stranded, circular DNA containing approximately 7900 base pairs. The genome is functionally divided into three regions which control

DNA replication, viral replication and encode the structural proteins for viral capsid.

Of the 15 oncogenic types of HPV, HPV 16 and 18 account for 70% of cervical cancer.

## RISK FACTORS

**1. Low socioeconomic status and low education status**

- Low priority for women's health issues
- Lack of knowledge among women about the relevance of symptoms
- Belief that there is no cure for cancer
- Improper utilisation of the available health care facilities.

**2. Sexual activity at an early age** This increases the risk of HPV infection. Having multiple sexual partners at any time as well as having sex with a person who has or had multiple sexual partners increase the risk of cervical cancer. Age is an important determinant of risk of HPV infection. The HPV prevalence reaches its peak in young adults (18 to 30 years of age) and declines at older ages.

**3. Age at first full-term pregnancy** Cervical cancer risk among parous women is 77% higher in those who were under 17 years at their first full term pregnancy, compared to those aged 25 or older; the risk decreases with older age at first full-term pregnancy. The association with age at first full-term pregnancy is limited to squamous cell carcinoma, with no association for adenocarcinoma.

**4. Cigarette smoking** The incidence of both high-grade squamous lesions and cervical cancer is 2 to 3 times high in HPV-infected women and present and past smokers. The probable mechanism is direct exposure of the DNA in cervical epithelial cells to tobacco end products like nicotine and aromatic hydrocarbons, which leads to reduction of Langerhans cells (these cells are responsible for the clearance of the HPV infection) in the cervix of smokers.

**5. Disease and drugs** The primary immune response to HPV infection is cell-mediated; therefore in women with conditions that impair cell mediated immunity such as end-stage renal disease or HIV, the risk of developing cervical cancer is 6 times more than women in general population. Cervical cancer risk among women with HIV may be reduced by treatment with appropriate antiretroviral therapy, which improves immune function and helps to clear HPV infection.

Cervical dysplasia risk is higher in women who are on long-term use of steroids, immunosuppressants for connective tissue disorders like systemic lupus erythematosus, rheumatoid arthritis, inflammatory bowel disease, autoimmune disorders and following organ transplantation. These drugs increase the risk of acquisition, persistence and progression of HPV disease.

**6. Reproductive history** High parity increases the risk of cervical cancer.

Cervical cancer risk is 15% higher in women who have had 1 full-term pregnancy compared with those who have had none; the risk increases with number of full-term pregnancies.

There is a 65% higher chance of development of cervical cancer in women with 7+ full-term pregnancies.

**7. Sexually transmitted disease** When a HPV-positive woman gets infected with sexually transmitted infections (STI), the risk of developing cervical cancer is increased. This may reflect her reduced ability to clear HPV infection due to immune suppression by other STIs. HPV-positive women with *Chlamydia trachomatis* (CT) infection have a higher risk of developing cervical cancer than those without CT infection.

But recent meta-analysis shows that cervical cancer risk is not associated with herpes simplex virus 2 infection, as previously thought.

Similarly there is no association between cervical adenocarcinoma and CT infection.

**8. Environmental factors** Based on limited evidence, tetrachloroethylene is classified by the International Agency for Research on Cancer (IARC) as a cause of cervical cancer.

**9. Genetic predisposition** Genetic predisposition has been found to be a contributing factor in cervical cancer. Heredity could affect many factors contributing to the development of cervical cancer, including susceptibility to HPV infection, ability to clear HPV infection, and time taken for development of the disease.

## SIGNS AND SYMPTOMS

The symptoms associated with cervical cancer are common and non-specific but may indicate significant pathology and should be investigated appropriately.

**Early cervical cancer** patients usually have normal general health.

**Late stage cervical cancer** symptoms may be profuse bleeding from the friable growth that causes anaemia and cachexia, frequency of micturition, dysuria, haematuria and incontinence due to fistula (indicating bladder involvement). Similarly diarrhea, rectal pain, bleeding PR and fecal incontinence due to fistula indicate bowel involvement. Extensive parametrial involvement results in unilateral/bilateral hydronephrosis, ureteral obstruction and pyelonephritis. Whereas compression of venous and lymphatic channels results in pedal edema, involvement of nerve plexus in the uterosacral ligaments produce pelvic pain.

**Symptoms and Signs**

- Inter-menstrual bleeding (IMB)
- Postcoital bleeding (PCB)
- Postmenopausal bleeding (PMB)
- Abnormal appearance of the cervix (suspicion of malignancy)
- Watery vaginal discharge (blood-stained)
- Pelvic pain
- Pedal edema
- Urinary symptoms
- Gastrointestinal disturbances

## DIAGNOSIS

Patients who present with any of the above bleeding symptoms should be thoroughly investigated with history, per speculum examination, pelvic, bimanual and rectal examination.

**Speculum examination** This reveals the nature of the growth–Ulcerative/nodular/exophytic growth, necrotic fungating growth with foul-smelling profuse watery, purulent, blood-tinged discharge (Fig. 20.1).

**Bimanual examination** This reveals (Fig. 20.2)

- Induration
- Extent of the growth
- Size of the uterus and mobility

Enlarged uterus may be due to the tumour growth invading the endometrial cavity or due to endocervical growth that occludes the internal os causing pyometra/haematometra.

**Rectal examination** This reveals,

- Extension of the disease, cervical size and shape when the fornices are obliterated,
- Parametrial involvement

**Rectovaginal examination** Vaginal extension may reveal thickened, firm, irregular rectovaginal septum (Fig. 20.3).

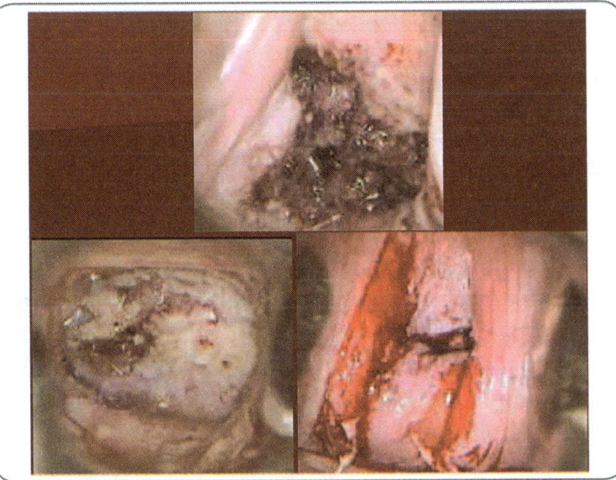

**Fig. 20.1** Speculum examination showing cancer cervix tissue and bleeding

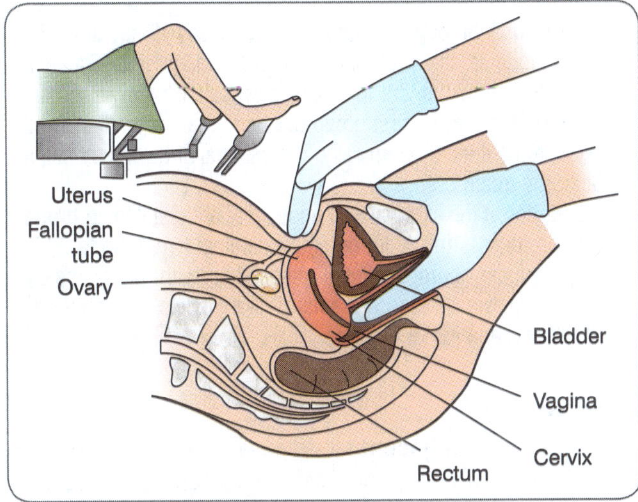


**Fig. 20.2** Bimanual palpation of the uterus

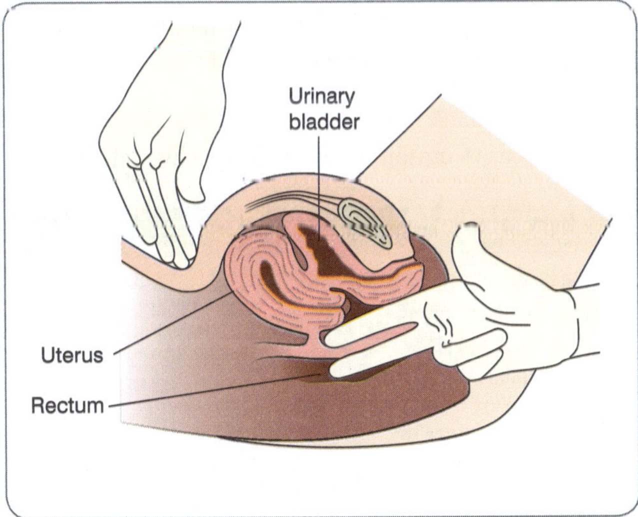


**Fig. 20.3** Bidigital (rectovaginal) examination

Parametrial extension involvement extending up the lateral pelvic walls and uterosacral ligaments is well appreciated by this examination.

## MODES OF SPREAD

### *Lymphatic spread*

Here the spread is through the extensive lymphatic plexus that accompanies the uterine veins. They drain into the paracervical, parametrial, obturator, internal, external, common iliac lymph nodes and finally para-aortic lymph nodes. Involvement of pelvic or para-aortic lymph nodes in most histological types of cervical cancer is the greatest single predictor of long-term survival.

#### Sentinel Node Biopsy

**Sentinel node biopsy is being used for early diagnosis.** The sentinal node is the first node/group of nodes that drains a primary tumour. After the injection of isosulfan/methylene blue around the tumour the first group of nodes that are blue-stained is dissected out laparoscopically. The sentinal node biopsy helps to tailor the treatment.

The nodes at the external iliac nodes that are distal to common iliac bifurcation is the most common sentinel lymph node. This biopsy reduces complications associated with unnecessary extensive pelvic node dissection like pelvic lymphocele, lymphedema and nerve damage.

### *Local spread*

Through the adjacent nodes it spreads to the parametrium up to pelvic side walls causing ureteral stenosis.

Cancer cervix can also spread superiorly into the endometruim, anteriorly into the bladder through vesicouterine ligaments and posteriorly into the rectum through rectal and uterosacral ligaments.

### *Blood spread*

Metastasis are frequently seen in lungs, liver and bones.

#### General Investigations

- Urinalysis
- Complete hemogram
- Blood sugar levels
- Renal function test
- Liver function test
- Serum electrolytes
- Blood grouping and typing
- Chest X-ray
- ECG

An elevated creatinine level suggests urinary tract involvement. Elevated liver function tests suggest liver involvement, and an elevated serum calcium level suggests bone involvement.

## SPECIFIC INVESTIGATIONS

### Colposcopy

The main objectives of colposcopy are the following:

- To study the cervix when Pap smear detects abnormalities
- To locate the abnormal areas and take biopsy
- To study the extent of the lesion
- Conservative surgery under colposcopic guidance
- Follow-up

#### Colposcopic findings of invasive cancer

1. Irregular surface contour with loss of surface epithelium
2. Abnormal blood vessels
3. Colour tone change—When acetic acid is applied to the cervix, a dense intense aceto-white area appears fast and it remains visible for for some time before disappearing.
4. The diagnosis is confirmed by colposcopy-directed biopsy using Tischler's forceps combined with endocervical curettings. Histopathology Examination Report (HPE) confirms the type of lesion. **When Cervical Intraepithelial Neoplasia Stage 3 (CIN3) is reported on HPE, ideally it has to be followed by conisation (either in the form of electrosurgical excision / cold knife) to rule out micro-invasion.**

## HISTOLOGICAL TYPES OF CERVICAL CANCER

The invasive squamous cell carcinoma arises from the squamous component of the cervix in the transformation zone and adenocarcinoma arises from the glandular component of the cervix. Squamous cell carcinoma accounts for 70% of the tumours arising from the cervix.

#### Types of Cervical Cancers

**Types of Squamous Cell Carcinoma**

- Keratinising
- Non-keratinising
- Basaloid
- Verrucous
- Warty
- Papillary

- Lymphoepithelioma-like
- Squamotransitional cell

**Types of Adenocarcinoma**

*Mucinous adenocarcinoma*

- Endocervical
- Intestinal
- Signet-ring cell
- Villoglandular
- Minimal deviation

*Endometrioid adenocarcinoma*

*Clear cell adenocarcinoma*

*Serous adenocarcinoma*

*Mesonephric adenocarcinoma.*

Adenocarcinoma accounts for 25% of the cervical cancers. Since the the signs and symptoms of adenocarcinoma are mostly hidden, they are detected in late stage.

**Types of Mixed Cervical Carcinoma**

- Adenosquamous carcinoma
- Glassy cell variant
- Adenoid cystic carcinoma
- Adenoid basal carcinoma

**Neuroendocrine Tumours of the Cervix**

- Large cell neuroendocrine tumours
- Small cell carcinoma
- Carcinoid
- Atypical carcinoid tumours

**Other Malignant Tumours**

- Sarcoma of the cervix
- Malignant lymphomas
- Metastatic Cancers

## DIFFERENTIAL DIAGNOSIS

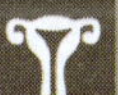

### Clinical Importance

**Differential diagnosis**

- Cervical tuberculosis
- Syphilitic ulcer
- Cervical ectopy
- Fibroid polyp
- Products of conception in incomplete abortion

### *Cervical tuberculosis*

The diagnosis of cervical TB is difficult clinically as the symptoms and physical examination usually do not give clues to the disease. Pelvic organs are infected from a primary focus, usually the chest, by hematogenous spread. Often the primary lesion would be healed at presentation. The macroscopic findings of cervical TB can vary. There may be a hypertrophy of the cervix or a friable papillary or vegetative growth simulating cervical cancer. The diagnosis of cervical TB is usually made by histological examination of a cervical punch biopsy specimen.

### *Syphilitic ulcer*

It is a single, firm, painless ulceration with a clean base and sharp borders. The diagnosis is confirmed by VDRL, Fluorescent Treponemal Antibody Absorption Test (FTA-Abs) and cervix biopsy.

### *Cervical ectopy*

The cervix looks red and angry when there is a large ectopy. On colposcopy, ectocervix is seen to be covered by a single layer of columnar cells with typical grape-like villi with blood vessel at the central core.

### *Fibroid polyp*

Here a thick broad fleshy mass is seen protruding through the os. When it is ulcerated and infected, it resembles a growth. The diagnosis is confirmed by biopsy.

### *Products of conception*

When products of conception protrude through the cervix it looks like soft vascular friable growth with foul-smelling discharge. However on colposcopy this is neither aceto-white nor Schiller test-positive. Ultrasound of the pelvis, suction evacuation and histopathology confirms retained products.

## STAGING

**Unlike other gynecological cancers, cancer cervix is clinically staged** (Figs. 20.4–20.10). The stage of the disease is an important criterion for long-term survival. In the developing countries it has been emphasised that only clinical staging should be continued as more elaborate investigations are needed for lymph node assessment which constitutes a part of surgical staging. Table 20.1 shows the staging of carcinoma of the cervix uteri as per the FIGO classification.

### Surgical Procedures for Cervical Cancer Staging

FIGO allows the following procedures for staging colposcopy—endocervical curettings, conisation, hysteroscopy, cystoscopy, proctoscopy, intravenous pyelogram, chest X-ray, skeletal X-ray. If proctoscopy or cystoscopy (bullous edema) is abnormal, a biopsy must be done and if positive to place the patient in a stage IVA category.

Additional modalities like computerised tomography (CT), magnetic resonance imaging (MRI) and positive emission tomography (PET) can be used when available.

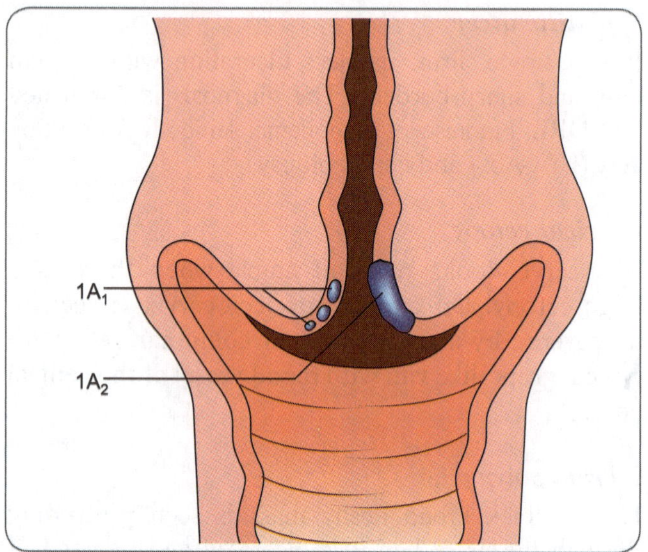


Fig. 20.4 Cervical carcinoma: Stage IA

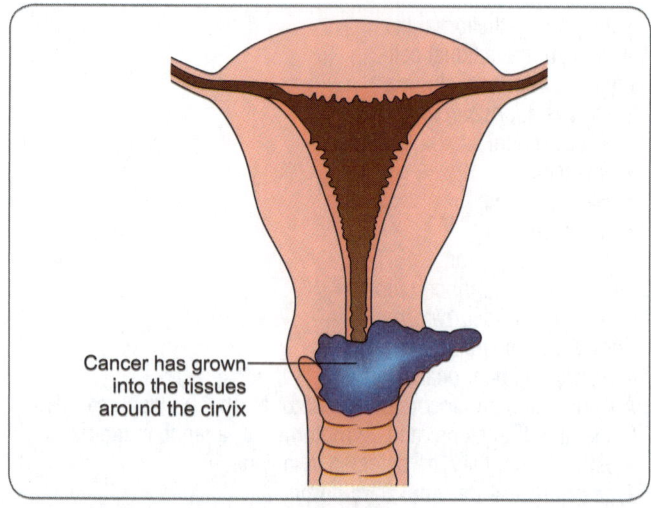


Fig. 20.7 Cervical carcinoma: Stage 2B

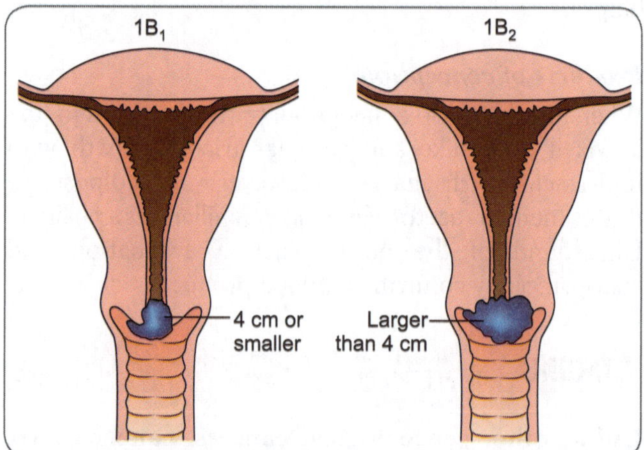


Fig. 20.5 Cervical carcinoma: Stage 1B

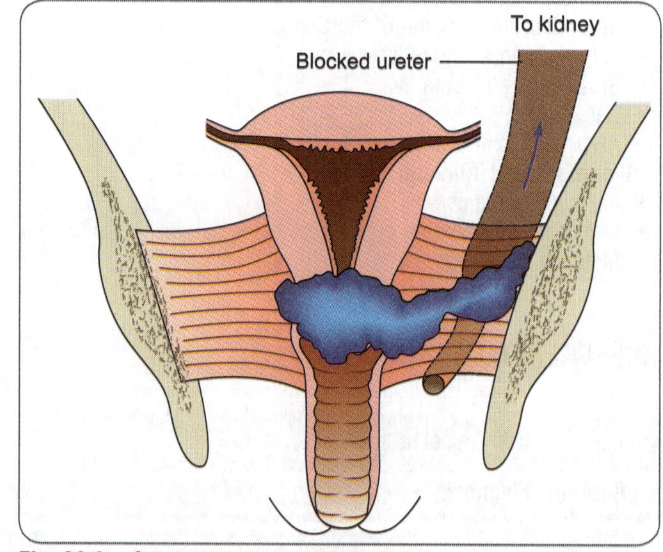


Fig. 20.8 Cervical carcinoma: Stage 3B

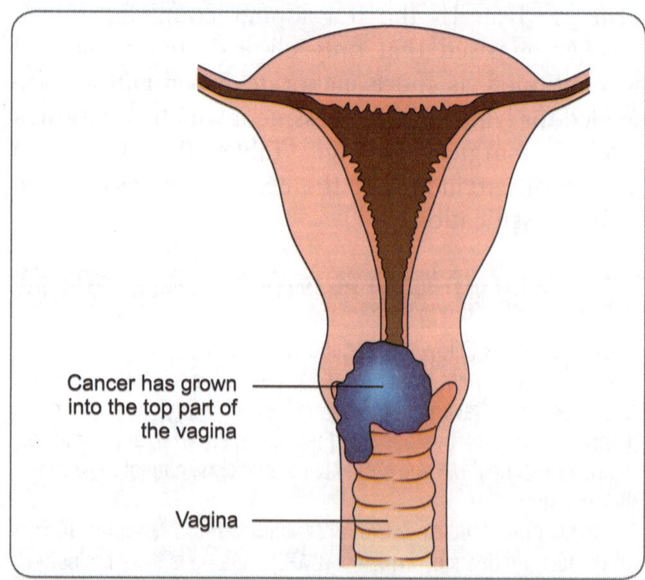


Fig. 20.6 Cervical carcinoma: Stage 2A

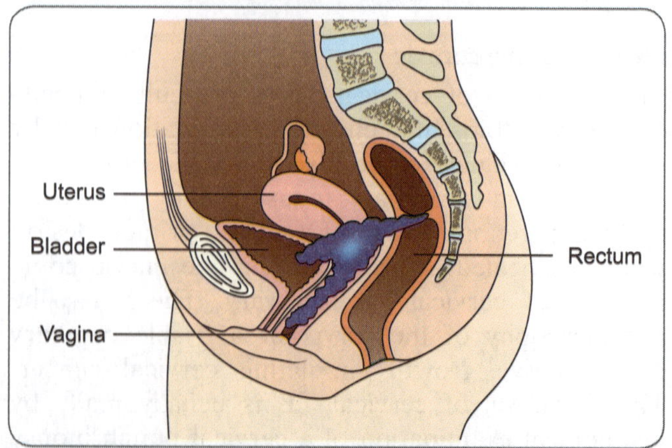


Fig. 20.9 Cervical carcinoma: Stage 4A

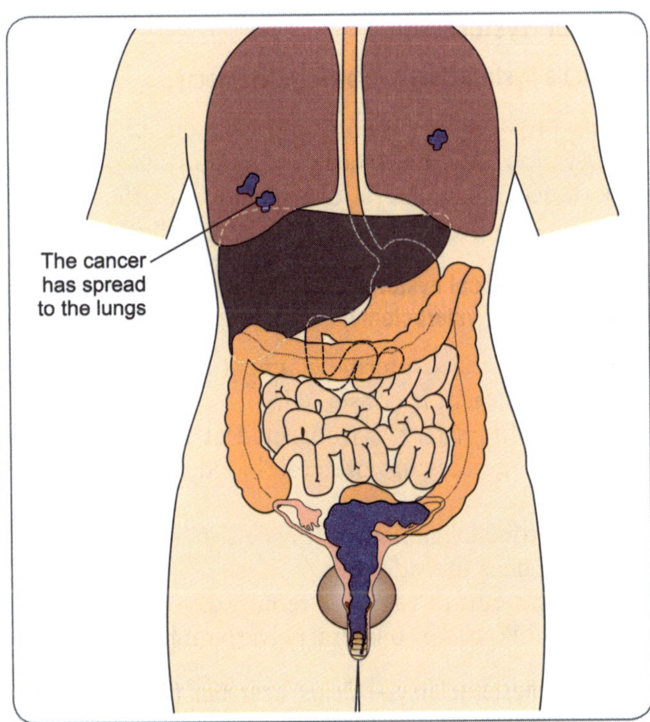


**Fig. 20.10** Cervical carcinoma: Stage 4B

- **Chest X-ray** has identified metastases in 4% of women with clinical stage IIB or greater disease. In patients with FIGO stage IB disease there is a very low likelihood of pulmonary metastases.
- **CT scan,** compared to X-ray chest, is more accurate in identifying pleural effusion, thoracic nodes and parenchymal metastases.
- **Ultrasound** is used in assessment of
- Primary tumour size
- Nodal status
- Confirm pyometra.
- **IV urogram** is used for diagnosing hydroureter and hydronephrosis.
- **Examination under anaesthesia (EUA):** EUA allows a more thorough visual inspection of the upper vagina and a better bimanual examination of the parametria. **Patients who have a large-volume tumour and require cystoscopy or proctoscopy may benefit from simultaneous EUA.**

EUA, particularly when performed by a gynecologic oncologist and a radiation oncologist at the same time, may increase the accuracy of clinical staging by 25%.

- **CT scan** helps in assessing size, extent of disease, hydroureter and hydronephrosis and in determining the lymph node status.
- **MRI** is more accurate than CT for radiological staging of cancer cervix.
- **MRI scores over CT in diagnosis of early-stage cervical cancer.**
- **PET-CT** can assess the primary tumour as well as detect metastatic spread better than other modalities.

**PET has the potential for more accurately selecting patients for different treatment modalities.**

**Table 20.1** Staging of carcinoma of the cervix uteri (FIGO classification)

| Stage | Characteristics |
|---|---|
| Stage I | The carcinoma is strictly confined to the cervix (extension to the corpus would be disregarded) |
| IA | Invasive carcinoma which can be diagnosed only by microscopy, with deepest invasion ≤5 mm and largest extension ≤ 7 mm |
| IA1 | Measured stromal invasion of ≤3.0 mm in depth and extension of ≤7.0 mm |
| IA2 | Measured stromal invasion of >3.0 mm and ≤5.0 mm with an extension ≤7.0 mm |
| IB | Clinically visible lesions limited to the cervix uteri or pre-clinical cancers greater than stage IA2 * |
| IB1 | Clinically visible lesion ≤4.0 cm in greatest dimension |
| IB2 | Clinically visible lesion not > 4.0 cm in greatest dimension |
| Stage II | Cervical carcinoma invades beyond the uterus, but not to the pelvic wall or to the lower third of the vagina |
| IIA | Without parametrial invasion |
| IIA1 | Clinically visible lesion ≤4.0 cm in greatest dimension |
| IIA2 | Clinically visible lesion > 4 cm in greatest dimension |
| IIB | With obvious parametrial invasion |
| Stage III | The tumour extends to the pelvic wall and/or involves lower third of the vagina and/or causes hydronephrosis or non-functioning kidney** |
| IIIA | Tumour involves lower third of the vagina, with no extension to the pelvic wall |
| IIIB | Extension to the pelvic wall and/or hydronephrosis or non-functioning kidney |
| Stage IV | The carcinoma has extended beyond the true pelvis or has involved the mucosa of the bladder or rectum. A bullous edema, as such, does not permit a case to be allotted to Stage IV |
| IVA | Spread of the growth to adjacent organs |
| IVB | Spread to distant organs |

*All macroscopically visible lesions—even with superficial invasion—are allotted to stage IB carcinomas. Invasion is limited to a measured stromal invasion with a maximal depth of 5.00 mm and a horizontal extension of not >7.00 mm. Depth of invasion should not be >5.00 mm taken from the base of the epithelium of the original tissue—superficial or glandular. The depth of invasion should always be reported in mm, even in those cases with "early (minimal) stromal invasion" (~1 mm). The involvement of vascular/lymphatic spaces should not change the stage allotment.

**On rectal examination, there is no cancer-free space between the tumour and the pelvic wall. All cases with hydronephrosis or non-functioning kidney are included, unless they are known to be due to another cause.

## TREATMENT

| Stage | Description | Treatment |
|---|---|---|
| Stage IA1 | ≤3 mm invasion, no lymphovascular space involvement (LVSI). | Conisation or type I hysterectomy |
| Stage IA1 | ≤3 mm invasion with LVSI | Radical trachelectomy or type II radical hysterectomy with pelvic lymph node dissection |
| IA2 | Lesion has stromal invasion between 3 and 5 mm | Radical trachelectomy or type II radical hysterectomy with pelvic lymph node dissection |
| IB1 | | Radical trachelectomy or type III radical hysterectomy with pelvic lymphadenectomy |
| IB2 | | Type III radical hysterectomy with pelvic and para-aortic lymphadenectomy or primary chemoradiation |
| IIa | | Type III radical hysterectomy with pelvic and para-aortic lymphadenectomy or primary chemoradiation |
| IIb, IIIa, IIIb | | Primary chemoradiation |
| IVa | | Primary chemoradiation or primary exenteration |
| IVb | | Primary chemotherapy ± radiation |

## Radical Trachelectomy

**Indication** This is the choice of surgery in young women in whom fertility preservation is desired. Pre-operative MRI is mandatory.

**Contraindication** Trachelectomy is contraindicated when the tumour extends beyond internal os.

**Procedure** Abdominal radical trachelectomy can be done by open method, laparoscopic and robotic modalities.

With midline incision, a thorough evaluation of abdomen and pelvis is done. If the para-aortic nodes are involved and they are found to be positive on frozen section, procedure is abandoned and a radical hysterectomy is proceeded.

In a radical hysterectomy, the cervix, proximal vagina, parametrial and paracervical tissues are removed.

Ureters are deroofed, retracted laterally to enable the removal of the parametrial and paracervical tissue.

## Types of Hysterectomy

### 1. Simple hysterectomy (Type I hysterectomy)

In case of young patients who are anxious to conceive, preservation of the ovarian function is of prime importance. Here lateral transposition of the ovaries are done to protect the ovaries during radiotherapy.

### 2. Modified radical hysterectomy—Wertheim's operation (Type 2 radical hysterectomy)

The anterior vesico-uterine ligament is divided but the posterior ligament is conserved.

The uterine artery is transected at the level of the ureter but preserving ureteral blood supply to the ureter.

The cardinal ligament is divided in its midportion instead of near the sidewalls.

A smaller cuff of vagina is removed.

This is followed by bilateral pelvic lymphadenectomy.

### 3. Radical hysterectomy— Meigs' operation (Type 3 radical hysterectomy)

Hysterectomy is performed with resection of the parametrium up to the side walls.

Ureters are completely dissected from their bed and bladder and rectum mobilised.

Most of the uterosacral and cardinal ligaments are removed. Upper one-third of the vagina is also removed. This is followed by bilateral pelvic lymph node dissection.

**Nerve-sparing radical hysterectomy** (NSRH) is a technique in which the neural part of the cardinal ligament which encloses the inferior hypogastric plexus, as well as the bladder branch is preserved. By this method the bladder's innervation is safe and its functional recovery is more rapid with drastic improvement in the quality of life.

### 4. Ultra-radical surgery—Brunschwig operation (pelvic exenteration)

**Indications**

- Stage IVA disease,
- Central pelvic recurrent carcinoma without any metastasis
- Completely resectable tumour mass
- Absence of ureteral obstruction, sciatic pain or unilateral leg edema,
- Women should be psychologically and physically adjusted to cope with urinary and fecal stoma.

**Contraindication** Cancer cervix that has spread with distant metastasis.

**Types**
1. Anterior exenteration
2. Posterior exenteration

### Prognosis of Cervical Cancer

| Stage of cervical cancer | 5-yr survival rate% |
|---|---|
| IA | 100 |
| IB | 85 |
| IIA | 65 |
| IIB | 45 |
| III | 20–40 |
| IVA | 18–35 |

## CANCER CERVIX IN OTHER SITUATIONS

### Cervical Cancer During Pregnancy

Incidence of invasive cancer is 1.2 in 10,000.

**Conisation is contraindicated in first trimester.** Management depends on
- period of gestation
- survival of the fetus
- wish of the patient.

Microinvasive cancer can be followed up to term.

In all other advanced stages of cancer cervix in pregnancy, treatment modality is same as in the non-pregnant state.

### Stump Carcinoma

This develops in the cervical stump left behind after subtotal hysterectomy, the incidence being 1%.

True stump carcinoma develops after 2 years of primary surgery and has the following features.
- Difficulty in treatment due to adhesion.
- Radiation is technically difficult.
- 5-year survival 30–60%.

### Recurrent Carcinoma Cervix

Risk factors
- Size of tumour
- Lymph-vascular space invasion
- Positive lymph node
- Advanced stage of the primary tumour

Most common site of recurrence is pelvic side wall.

Occurs mostly in the first 2 years following primary treatment.

Recurrence is confirmed by FNAC or trucut needle biopsy.

The extent of the disease is confirmed by cystoscopy, proctoscopy, CT, MRI, and PET.

## MANAGEMENT

Recurrent growth following radiotherapy can be treated by hysterectomy or exenteration.

Lateral recurrence is managed by radiotherapy in a previously operated woman.

To conclude, cancer cervix is the second most common cancer affecting women in the developing nations. It is essentially a clinically staged disease.

The stage at the time of diagnosis determines the treatment and long time prognosis. Effective screening and HPV vaccination holds a great promise in reducing the disease burden.

Though various surgical options are detailed, as mentioned above, in most of the centres, cancer cervix from Stage IIB onwards is treated either by radiotherapy or by chemotherapy or a combination of both—chemoradiation.

Chemotherapy is either with cisplatin singly or in combination with other drugs like Topotecan or Gemcitabine, or Paclitaxel. The details of chemotherapy are given in Chapter 24 and of Radiotherapy in Chapter 25.

## RECAP

- Cervical cancer is a preventable cancer because it has a long preinvasive state that lasts for about 10–15 years.
- About 122,844 new cervical cancer cases are diagnosed annually in India. About 67,477 cervical cancer deaths occur annually in India.
- The majority of cases are squamous cell carcinoma followed by adenocarcinoma.
- Risk factors: Low socioeconomic status, sexual activity at an early age has an increased risk of HPV infection, age at first full-term pregnancy, cigarette smoking, disease and drugs, reproductive history, sexually transmitted disease, environmental factors, genetic predisposition.

- Symptoms and signs—inter-menstrual bleeding (IMB), postcoital bleeding (PCB), postmenopausal bleeding (PMB), abnormal appearance of the cervix (suspicion of malignancy), watery vaginal discharge (blood-stained), pelvic pain
- Differential diagnosis—Cervical tuberculosis, syphilitic ulcer, cervical ectopy, fibroid polyp, products of conception in incomplete abortion.
- Treatment—Stage IA1—Conisation or type I hysterectomy
- Stage IA1 with LVSI—Radical trachelectomy or type II radical hysterectomy with pelvic lymph node dissection.
- Stage IA2—Radical trachelectomy or type II radical hysterectomy with pelvic lymph node dissection.
- Stage IB1—Radical trachelectomy or type III radical hysterectomy with pelvic lymphadenectomy.
- Stage IB2—Type III radical hysterectomy with pelvic and para-aortic lymphadenectomy or primary chemoradiation.
- Stage IIa—Type III radical hysterectomy with pelvic and para-aortic lymphadenectomy or primary chemoradiation.
- Stage IIb, IIIa, IIIb—Primary chemoradiation.
- Stage IVa—Primary chemoradiation or primary exenteration
- Stage IVb—Primary chemotherapy ± radiation.
- However, in practice, chemoradiation or radiation is the treatment of choice from Stage IIB onwards.

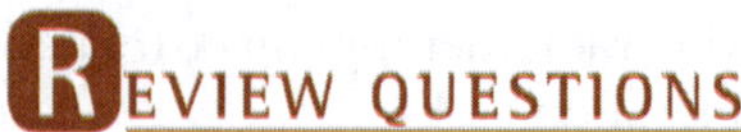

## REVIEW QUESTIONS

### Long-Answer Question

Discuss the risk factors for carcinoma cervix. What are the indications for Type I hysterectomy (simple hysterectomy) in the management of cervical cancer?

### MCQs

**1. Treatment of Stage IA1 cancer cervix with lymphovascular space involvement (LVSI) is**

a) Conisation
b) Type I hysterectomy
c) Radical trachelectomy or type II radical hysterectomy with pelvic lymph node dissection
d) Type III radical hysterectomy with pelvic and para-aortic lymphadenectomy

**2. Stage IIIA cancer cervix is**

a) Clinically visible lesion > 4 cm in greatest dimension
b) Tumour involving lower third of the vagina, with no extension to the pelvic wall
c) The carcinoma extended beyond the true pelvis or involving the mucosa of the bladder or rectum
d) Spread of the growth to adjacent organs

**3. Sentinal node is**

a) First node/group of nodes that drains a primary tumour
b) A lateral node in the pelvic wall
c) Farthest node from the cervix
d) Any node which shows malignant involvement

**4. Parametrial extension involvement extending up to lateral pelvic walls and uterosacral ligaments are appreciated best by**

a) Speculum examination
b) Rectal examination
c) Bimanual pelvic examination
d) Rectovaginal examination

### Further Reading

Borruto F, De Ridder M, editors. HPV and cervical cancer: achievements in prevention and future prospects. New York: Springer Verlag Inc; 2012.

Coppleson M. editor. Gynecologic oncology: fundamental principles and clinical practice. London: Churchill Livingstone; 1991, 1 & 2 vol.

IARC-WHO. IARC handbook of cancer prevention. IARC Press; 2005, 10 vol.

Rajaram S, Chitrathara K, Maheswari A. Cervical cancer: contemporary management. New Delhi: Jaypee Brothers; 2012. Ahuja M, Basu P, Banerjee D. Precancerous lesions of the cervix: prevention, early diagnosis and management. London: JP Medical Publishers; 2014.

Singer A, Monaghan JM, Swee Chong Quek. Lower genital tract precancer: colposcopy, pathology and treatment. Hoboken: Wiley-Blackwell; 2008.

# CHAPTER 21

# Malignant Neoplasm of the Uterus

## AT A GLANCE


- Incidence
- Classification
  - International Federation of Gynecology and Obstetrics (FIGO) Histological Grading
  - TNM Classification for Endometrial Cancer
- Etiological Risk Factors
- Pathophysiology
- Histological Types
- Metastasis
- Clinical Features
  - Symptoms
  - Signs
- Investigations and Diagnosis
- Staging
- Management
  - Surgery
  - Add-On Therapy
  - Chemotherapy
  - Radiotherapy
  - Hormonal Therapy
  - Monitoring
- Prognosis
  - Survival Rates
  - Recurrence
- Uterine Sarcomas
  - Pathology
  - Signs and Symptoms
  - Management


## INTRODUCTION

**Endometrial cancer (EC)** is a cancer of the endometrium. **Endometrial carcinoma is sometimes loosely referred to as "uterine cancer", although it is distinct from other forms of uterine cancer such as cervical cancer, uterine sarcoma, and trophoblastic disease**. The most frequent type of endometrial cancer is endometrioid carcinoma, which accounts for more than 80% of cases. Occasionally some cases of uterine cancer may be in the form of sarcomas or squamous cell carcinoma.

Endometrial cancer is the result of the abnormal growth of the epithelial cells that have the ability to invade or spread to other parts of the body. It occurs most commonly after menopause, more common during the 6th and 7th decades of life, with the mean age of patients being 65 years.

> **Corpus Cancer Syndrome**
>
> It is a triad of obesity, high blood pressure and diabetes with endometrial carcinoma. 40% of cases are related to obesity and others associated with excessive estrogen exposure, high blood pressure and diabetes.

Endometrial cancer is commonly diagnosed by endometrial biopsy or by taking samples during dilation and curettage. A Pap smear is not typically sufficient to show endometrial cancer. The leading treatment option for endometrial cancer is abdominal hysterectomy with bilateral salpingo-oophorectomy. In more advanced cases, radiation therapy, chemotherapy or hormone therapy may also be recommended. If the disease is diagnosed at an early stage, the outcome is favourable.

## INCIDENCE

Endometrial carcinoma is the third most common cause of death in cancers after ovarian and cervical cancer. In 2012, endometrial cancers occurred in 320,000 women and caused 76,000 deaths. It is more common in the developed world and is the most common cancer of the female reproductive tract in developed countries. It is the most common gynecologic malignancy and the fourth most common cancer in women in the United States. The rates of endometrial cancer have risen in a number of countries between the 1980s and 2010. This is believed to be due to the increasing number of elderly people and increasing rates of obesity. Incidence of endometrial cancer in all four parts of India as per the National Registry is somewhere between 5–8% of all genital tract cancers.

## CLASSIFICATION

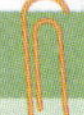

### WHO Classification

**A. Epithelial cell tumours**

1. **Endometrioid carcinoma** It is the most common type and is found in up to 90% of cases, with histology showing recognisable malignant glands and glandular cells in the better-differentiated (low-grade) forms
   a. Variant with squamous differentiation (adenoacanthoma)
   b. Villoglandular variant
   c. Secretory variant
2. Serous endometrial intra-epithelial carcinoma
3. Serous carcinoma
4. Mucinous carcinoma
5. Clear cell carcinoma (1–6% of cases)

**B. Neuroendocrine tumours**

1. Low-grade (carcinoid tumour)
2. High-grade (small cell neuroendocrine carcinoma; large cell neuroendocrine carcinoma)
3. Mixed cell adenocarcinoma
4. Undifferentiated carcinoma
5. De-differentiated carcinoma

**C. Mesenchymal tumours**

1. Leiomyoma
2. Smooth muscle tumour of uncertain malignant potential
3. Leiomyosarcoma
4. Endometrial stromal and related tumours
5. Miscellaneous mesenchymal tumours

**D. Mixed epithelial and mesenchymal tumours**

1. Adenomyoma
2. Adenosarcoma
3. Carcinosarcoma (malignant Müllerian mixed tumour [MMMT])
4. Atypical polypoid adenomyoma (Fig. 21.1)
5. Adenofibroma

**E. Miscellaneous tumours**

1. Neuroectodermal tumours
2. Adenomatoid tumour
3. Germ cell tumours

**F. Lymphoid and myeloid tumours**

1. Lymphomas
2. Myeloid neoplasms

**G. Secondary tumours**

### International Federation of Gynecology and Obstetrics (FIGO) Histological Grading

Endometrial carcinoma is graded as low-grade (well differentiated) or high-grade (poorly differentiated), based on histopathology and evaluation of the tumour cell morphology and growth pattern. Some clinicians will also use 3 levels of grading based on histological tumour pattern:

1. G1: non-squamous or non-morular solid growth pattern of 5% or less
2. G2: non-squamous or non-morular solid growth pattern of 6% to 50%
3. G3: non-squamous or non-morular solid growth pattern of more than 50%

### TNM Classification for Endometrial Cancer

| Primary tumour (T) | FIGO stages | Surgico-pathologic findings |
|---|---|---|
| TX | | Primary tumour cannot be assessed |
| T0 | | No evidence of primary tumour |
| Tis* | | Carcinoma in situ (preinvasive carcinoma) |
| T1 | I | Tumour confined to corpus uteri |
| T1a | IA | Tumour limited to endometrium or invades less than one half of the myometrium |
| T1b | IB | Tumour invades one half or more of the myometrium |
| T2 | II | Tumour invades stromal connective tissue of the cervix but does not extend beyond uterus** |
| T3a | IIIA | Tumour involves serosa and/or adnexa (direct extension or metastasis) |
| T3b | IIIB | Vaginal involvement (direct extension or metastasis) or parametrial involvement |
| | IIIC | Metastases to pelvic and/or para-aortic lymph nodes |
| | IV | Tumour invades bladder mucosa and/or bowel mucosa, and/or distant metastases |
| T4 | IVA | Tumour invades bladder mucosa and/ or bowel mucosa (bullous edema is not sufficient to classify a tumour as T4) |

* FIGO no longer includes stage 0 (Tis)
**Endocervical glandular involvement should only be considered as stage I and no longer as stage II

## ETIOLOGICAL RISK FACTORS

Risk factors for endometrial cancer include:

1. Obesity
2. Diabetes mellitus
3. Use of tamoxifen in breast cancer—Tamoxifen, has been associated with endometrial cancer in approximately 0.1% of users, particularly older women, but the benefits for survival from tamoxifen generally outweigh the risk of endometrial cancer.
4. Nulliparity and elderly age
5. Early menarche and late menopause
6. High levels of estrogen—an estimated 40% of cases of high estrogen are thought to be related

to obesity. The excess of adipose tissue increases conversion of androstenedione into estrone. Higher levels of estrone in the blood cause less or no ovulation and exposes the endometrium to continuously high levels of estrogens. Polycystic ovary syndrome (PCOS), which also causes irregular or no ovulation, is associated with higher rates of endometrial cancer for the same reasons as obesity. Specifically, obesity, type II diabetes, and insulin resistance are risk factors for Type I[1] endometrial cancer.

7. Whereas taking estrogen alone increases the risk of endometrial cancer, taking both estrogen and progesterone in combination, as in most oral contraceptive, pills, decreases the risk.
8. Unopposed estrogen replacement therapy during menopause is another risk factor. Higher doses or longer periods of estrogen therapy have higher risk of endometrial cancer. Women of lower weight are at greater risk from unopposed estrogen. A longer period of fertility—either from an early first menstrual period or late menopause—is also a risk factor. Unopposed estrogen raises an individual's risk of endometrial cancer by 2–10 folds, depending on the weight of the woman and the length of the therapy.
9. Genetic predisposition—Overall, genetic causes contribute to 2–10% of endometrial cancer. Lynch syndrome, an autosomal dominant genetic disorder that mainly causes colorectal cancer, has a 40–60% risk of developing endometrial cancer especially before menopause.
10. Family history—the inherited genetic condition **Cowden syndrome** can cause endometrial cancer. Women with this disorder have a 5–10% lifetime risk of developing endometrial cancer, compared to the 2–3% risk for unaffected women.
11. Endometrial hyperplasia is a significant risk factor because hyperplasia can and often will develop into adenocarcinoma, though cancer can develop without the presence of a hyperplasia. Within ten years, 8–30% of atypical endometrial hyperplasias develop into cancer, whereas 1–3% of non-atypical hyperplasias do so.
12. Smoking, breast feeding and the use of progestin are protective against endometrial cancer. Smoking provides protection by altering the metabolism of estrogen and promoting weight loss and early menopause. This protective effect lasts long after smoking is stopped.

[1]Type 1 cancers are the most common type. They are usually endometrioid adenocarcinomas, and are linked to excess estrogen in the body. They are generally slow growing and less likely to spread.

## PATHOPHYSIOLOGY

In 10–20% of endometrial cancers, mostly Grade 3, mutations are found in a tumour suppressor gene, commonly *p53* or *PTEN*.

*PTEN* and *p27* loss of function mutations are associated with endometrial cancer with good prognosis, particularly in obese women.

The *Her2/neu* oncogene, which indicates a poor prognosis, is seen in 20% of endometrioid and serous carcinomas.

*CTNNB1* (beta-catenin; a transcription gene) mutations are found in 14–44% of endometrial cancers and may indicate a good prognosis. Beta-catenin mutations are commonly found in endometrial cancers with squamous cells.

*ERID1A* gene mutations also lead to endometrial cancers.

## HISTOLOGICAL TYPES

Histologically, endometrial carcinoma can be divided into two subtypes.

**I. Endometrioid adenocarcinoma (type I)** that accounts for 90% of the tumours. They are associated with estrogen excess and obesity. The characteristic features of these tumours are as follows:
- They often arise in a background of endometrial hyperplasia.
- They occur in the early postmenopausal period.
- They generally are low-grade.
- They have a good prognosis.

**Grades of Endometrioid Adenocarcinoma**

Based on the degree of differentiation, endometrioid adenocarcinomas are subdivided into three grades:
Grade 1: Well differentiated tumours
Grade 2: Moderately differentiated tumours
Grade 3: Poorly differentiated tumours.

**II. Type II endometrial carcinomas include the clear-cell, serous papillary subtypes and carcinosarcomas.** Type II cancers have no association with estrogen excess or atypical hyperplasia, generally occur in older women, carry a worse prognosis, and spread like ovarian cancer. All type II cancers and grade 3 endometrioid tumours are classified as high-grade tumours and are associated with a poor prognosis. Recent studies suggest mutations may be present in individual genes such as *p53*, *HER2/neu*, and phosphatase and tensin homolog (PTEN) in patients with high-grade endometrial tumours. Mutant tumour suppressor *p53* overexpression has been associated with poor histological grade, non-endometrioid histology, advanced stage, and poor survival rates.

Polypoid adenocarcinoma (Fig. 21.1) are rare and usually mistaken for endometrial polyps. The woman generally presents with irregular vaginal bleeding.

## METASTASIS

Usually the cancer first spreads into the myometrium (Figs. 21.2 and 21.3) and the serosa, then into other reproductive and pelvic structures.

- **Lymphatic spread** When the lymphatic system is involved, the pelvic and para-aortic nodes are usually the first to become involved, but in no specific pattern, unlike cervical cancer.
- **Direct spread** Endometrial carcinoma frequently metastasises to the ovaries and Fallopian tubes when it is located in the upper part of the uterus, and to the cervix when the cancer is in the lower part of the uterus.
- **Hematogenous spread** More distant metastases are spread by the blood and often occur in the lungs, as well as the liver, brain, and bone. Endometrial cancer metastasises to the lungs (Fig. 21.4) 20–25% of the time, more than any other gynecologic cancer.

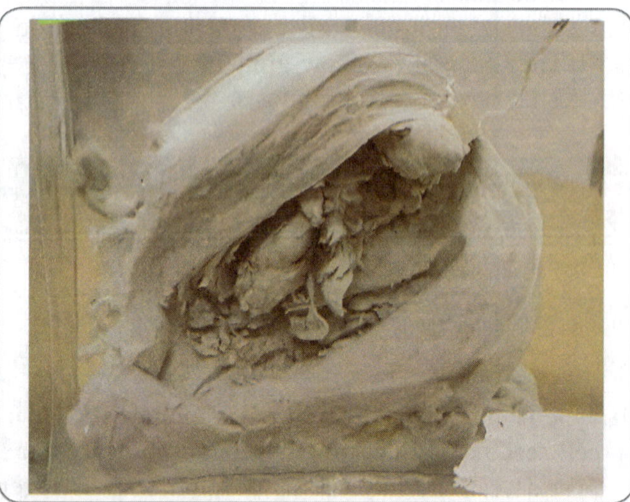

**Fig. 21.1** Polypoidal endometrial carcinoma (*Source:* Wikimedia/ © Ala'a)

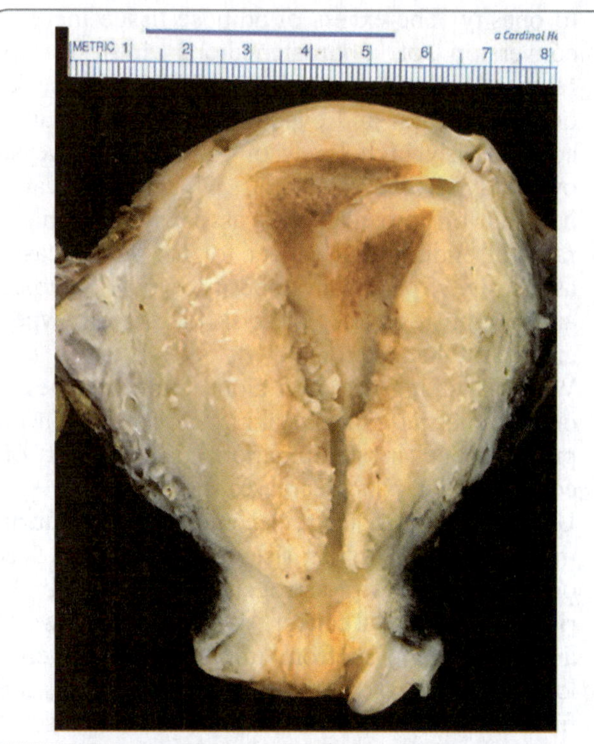



**Fig. 21.2** A stage III endometrioid adenocarcinoma that has invaded the myometrium (*Source:* Wikimedia/ © Ed Uthman)

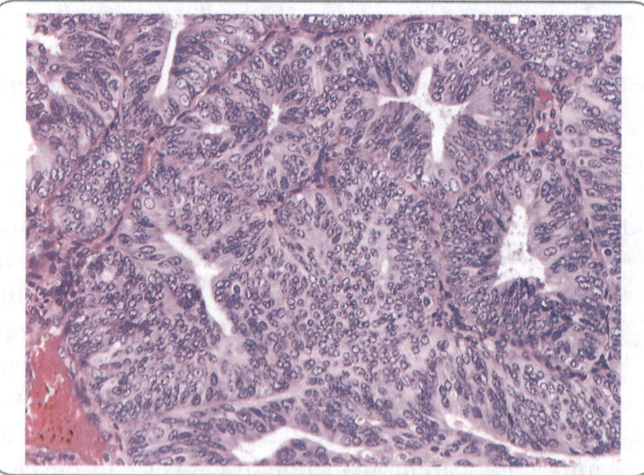

**Fig. 21.3** Endometrial adenocarcinoma showing many abnormal nuclei (*Source:* Wikimedia/ © KGH)

## CLINICAL FEATURES

### Symptoms

1. **Postmenopausal vaginal bleeding** or spotting occurs in 90% of endometrial cancer. In two-thirds

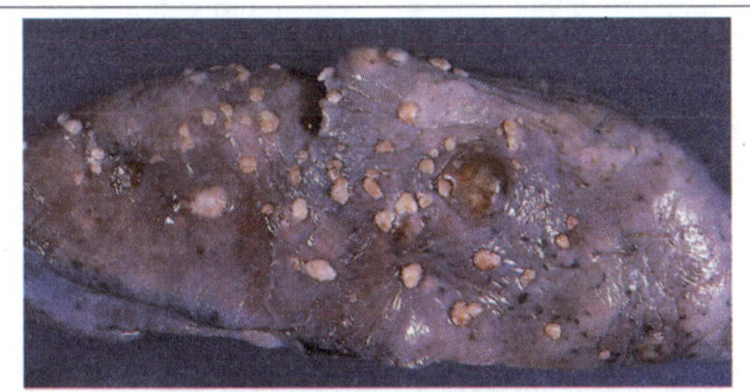

**Fig. 21.4** Metastatic endometrial cancer seen in a removed lung (*Source:* Source: Wikimedia/ © Yale Rosen)

of all cases of adenocarcinoma bleeding is especially common.

2. **Perimenopausal abnormal menstrual cycles** or extremely long, heavy, or frequent episodes of bleeding in women may also point to endometrial cancer.
3. Other symptoms include thin white or clear **vaginal discharge** in postmenopausal women and lower **abdominal pain**.
4. Other symptoms may be dependent on the spread of the disease to various organs.
5. **Spread of the disease to the bladder would result in urinary symptoms** in the form of frequency, dysuria, hematuria and spread to the bowel could result in bowel symptoms like diarrhea and dyschezia.
6. Painful sexual intercourse and pyometra are less common symptoms.

## Signs

**General physical examination**. Woman may have high BMI, may have pallor of variable degree, icteric if metastasis to liver has occurred, blood pressure may be high and pedal edema may be present.

**Systemic examination** may not reveal significant findings.

**Abdominal examination** may reveal enlarged uterus, in some cases it can be palpated abdominally or may appear as a soft, uniformly enlarged pelvic lump.

**Speculum examination** may reveal normal cervix unless cervix is involved, occasionally malignant polyp protrudes out of cervical os, blood or pus discharge may be seen trickling through the external os of cervix.

**Pelvic examination** may reveal a uniformly enlarged uterus with soft consistency, in early stages it is mobile freely with regular contour while in later stages it becomes immobile and has no regular outline.

## INVESTIGATIONS AND DIAGNOSIS

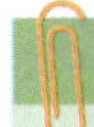

### Purpose of Investigation

The investigations are done
1. To confirm the diagnosis
2. To see the extent of disease and
3. To plan the treatment

1. **Vaginal ultrasonography** in a postmenopausal woman revealing a uterine cavity with endometrial fluid (Fig. 21.5) should arouse the suspicion of endometrial carcinoma.

   However routine screening of asymptomatic people is not recommended.
2. **Cervical screening test** A Pap smear can detect disease that has spread to the cervix so another screening method (for example endometrial biopsy or dilatation and curettage) must be used in conjunction.
3. **Endometrial aspiration cytology** (EAC) is also a method of confirming the diagnosis. However in almost 50% of cases, it may be negative and in some cases may reveal dysplasia and not malignancy. Pipelle's aspiration has been found to give better results as compared to other techniques of aspiration.
4. **Endometrial biopsy (EB)** is the less invasive option, but it may not give conclusive results every time.
5. **Dilatation and curettage** (D and C) or more correctively **fractional curettage** is used to obtain a tissue sample for histological examination. In fractional curettage, endocervix is the first sample, isthmus the second, anterior wall of the uterus the third sample, left lateral wall the fourth sample, right lateral wall the fifth sample and the sixth sample is from the fundus.

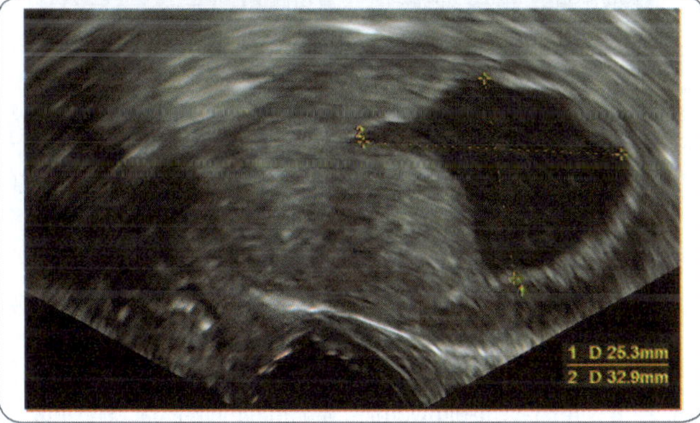


**Fig. 21.5** Vaginal ultrasonography with an endometrial fluid accumulation (darker area) in a postmenopausal uterus (*Source:* Häggström, Mikael (2014)/WikiJournal of Medicine 1 (2))

6. **CT** scans (Fig. 21.6) are used for preoperative imaging of tumours that appear advanced on physical examination or have a high-risk subtype (at high risk of metastasis). They can also be used to investigate extrapelvic disease.
7. **MRI** can be of some use in determining if the cancer has spread to the cervix or if it is an endocervical adenocarcinoma. MRI is also useful for examining the nearby lymph nodes (Fig. 21.7).
8. Hysteroscopy can help in studying the gross anatomy of the endometrium. However it may not be useful unless done in conjunction with a biopsy.
9. Positron emission tomography (PET), PET/CT, and PET/MRI have also been used in staging these patients. PET/CT is highly sensitive and specific for detecting positive pelvic and/or para-aortic lymphadenopathy as well as distant metastases in selected high-risk patients with endometrial cancer
10. **Other Tests** These include CBC, blood group and type, blood sugar, ECG, chest X-ray, liver function tests, kidney function tests and others as required according to treatment protocols.
11. **Markers** CA 125, a tumour marker that can be elevated in endometrial cancer and estrogen and progesterone receptor (ER & PR) study can be done to assess the prognosis and need for hormonal therapy. Progesterone receptor has a significant prognostic factor after clinical staging. Estrogen receptor has no significant prognostic relevance. When ER and PR and combined ER/PR status were analysed separately, patients with receptor-positive lesions had significantly better disease-free survival than those with receptor-negative lesions.

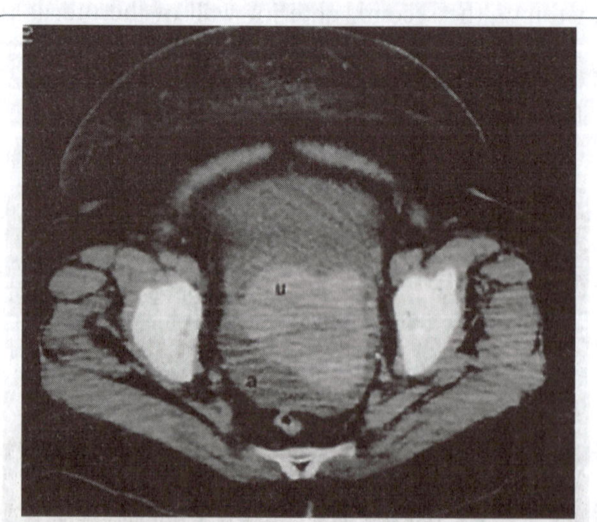


**Fig. 21.6** A 61-year-old woman with endometrial cancer. Note enlargement of the uterus (u) with a central area of hypodensity and the surrounding ascites (a) (*Source:* Abu-Yousef, M, Pelsang, R, et al, Glob. libr. women'smed).

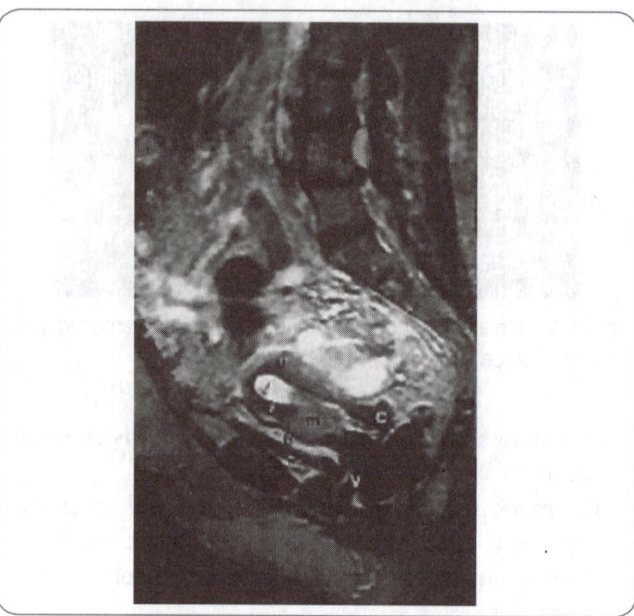


**Fig. 21.7** Sagittal T2-weighted MRI in a patient with a stage IA endometrial carcinoma shows replacement of the lower two-thirds of the hyperintense endometrium by an inhomogeneous, medium-intensity irregular mass (m) that invades the deeper layer of the myometrium anteriorly. (u, uterus; c, cervix; v, vagina; b, bladder; black arrow, endometrium; white arrow, uterine junctional zone.) (*Source:* Abu-Yousef, M, Pelsang, R, et al, Glob. libr. women'smed.)

## STAGING

Endometrial carcinoma is surgically staged (Figs. 21.8–21.11) using the FIGO cancer staging system. The 2009 FIGO staging system is as follows:

**Endometrial Carcinoma—FIGO Staging**

| Stage | Description |
|---|---|
| IA | Tumour is confined to the uterus with less than half myometrial invasion |
| IB | Tumour is confined to the uterus with more than half myometrial invasion |
| II | Tumour involves the uterus and the cervical stroma |
| IIIA | Tumour invades serosa or adnexa |
| IIIB | Vaginal and/or parametrial involvement |
| IIIC1 | Pelvic lymph node involvement |
| IIIC2 | Para-aortic lymph node involvement, with or without pelvic node involvement |
| IVA | Tumour invades bladder mucosa and/or bowel mucosa |
| IVB | Distant metastases including abdominal metastases and/or inguinal lymph nodes |

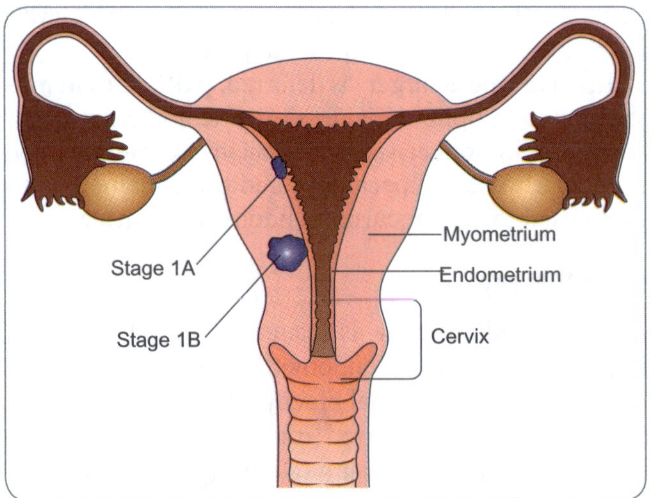


**Fig. 21.8** Diagrammatic representation of Stage 1A and 1B endometrial cancer

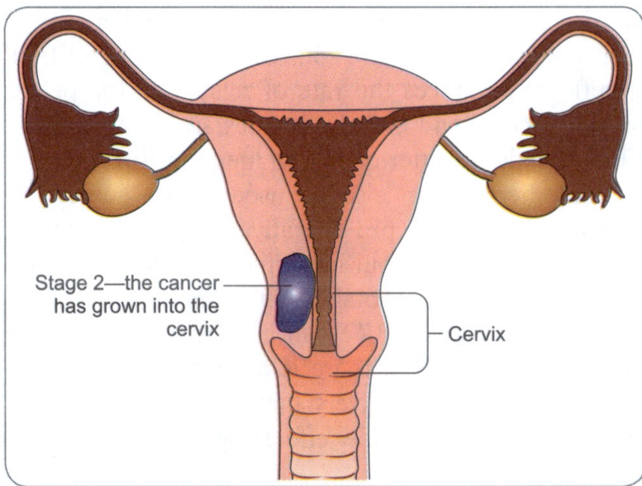


**Fig. 21.9** Diagrammatic representation of Stage 2 endometrial cancer

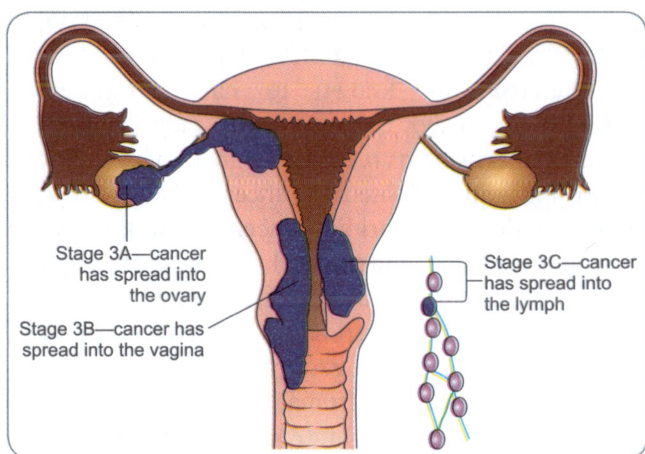


**Fig. 21.10** Diagrammatic representation of Stage 3A and 3B endometrial cancer

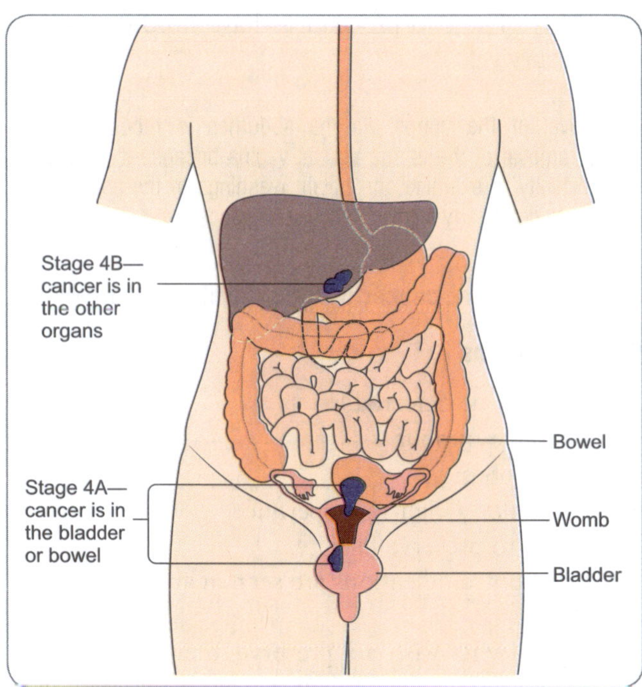


**Fig. 21.11** Diagrammatic representation of Stage 4A and 4B endometrial cancer

## MANAGEMENT

The modalities of management are primarily surgery; chemotherapy and hormonal therapy are either adjuvant options or are given in later stages. Radiotherapy is also given as an adjuvant but not primarily.

### Surgery

Almost 90% of women with endometrial cancer are treated with some form of surgery. Surgical treatment typically consists of hysterectomy including a bilateral salpingo-oophorectomy.

- Lymphadenectomy of pelvic and para-aortic lymph nodes is performed for tumours of histologic grade II or above.
- The topic of lymphadenectomy and what survival benefit it offers in stage I disease is still being debated.
- In stage III and IV cancers, cytoreductive surgery is the norm and a biopsy of the omentum may also be included.
- In stage IV disease, where there are distant metastases, surgery can be used as part of palliative therapy.

Laparotomy is the traditional surgical procedure; however, laparoscopy is associated with lower operative morbidity. The two procedures have no difference in overall survival.

Removal of the uterus via the abdomen is recommended over removal of the uterus via the vagina because it gives the opportunity to examine and obtain washings of the abdominal cavity to detect any further evidence of cancer.

Staging of the cancer is done during the surgery.

### Contraindications

Surgery may be deferred in

- inoperable tumour,
- massive obesity,
- a particularly high-risk operation,
- a desire to preserve fertility.

These contraindications are seen in about 5–10% of cases.

Women who wish to preserve their fertility and have low-grade stage I cancer can be treated with progestins, with or without concurrent tamoxifen therapy. This therapy can be continued until the cancer does not respond to treatment or until childbearing. Uterine perforation may occur during a D&C or an endometrial biopsy.

**Side effects** of surgery to remove endometrial cancer can specifically include sexual dysfunction, temporary incontinence, and lymphedema, along with more common side effects of any surgery.

## Add-On Therapy

There are a number of possible additional therapies. Surgery can be followed by radiation therapy and/or chemotherapy in cases of high-risk or high-grade cancers. This is called adjuvant therapy.

## Chemotherapy

**Adjuvant chemotherapy** is a recent innovation consisting of combination of paclitaxel (or other taxanes like docetaxel), doxorubicin (and other anthracyclines), and platins (particularly cisplatin and carboplatin). Adjuvant chemotherapy has been found to increase survival in stage III and IV cancer more than added radiotherapy. Mutations in mismatch repair genes, like those found in Lynch syndrome, can lead to resistance against platins, meaning that chemotherapy with platins is ineffective in people with these mutations. Side effects of chemotherapy are common. These include hair loss, low neutrophil levels in the blood, and gastrointestinal problems.

In cases where surgery is deferred, **palliative chemotherapy** is an option; higher-dose chemotherapy is associated with longer survival. Palliative chemotherapy, particularly using capecitabine and gemcitabine, is also often used to treat recurrent endometrial cancer.

## Radiotherapy

Adjuvant radiotherapy is commonly used in early-stage (stage I or II) endometrial cancer. It can be delivered through vaginal brachytherapy (VBT), which is becoming the preferred route due to its reduced toxicity, or external beam radiotherapy (EBRT). In the case of endometrial cancer, the radiation source is placed directly in the vagina. VBT is used to treat any remaining cancer solely in the vagina, whereas EBRT can be used to treat remaining cancer elsewhere in the pelvis following surgery. However, the benefits of adjuvant radiotherapy are controversial. Though EBRT significantly reduces the rate of relapse in the pelvis, overall survival and metastasis rates are not improved. VBT provides a better quality of life than EBRT.

Radiotherapy can also be used before surgery in certain cases. When pre-operative imaging or clinical evaluation shows tumour invading the cervix, radiation can be given before a total hysterectomy is performed. Brachytherapy and EBRT can also be used, singly or in combination, when there is a contraindication for hysterectomy. Both delivery methods of radiotherapy are associated with side effects, particularly in the gastrointestinal tract.

## Hormonal Therapy

Hormonal therapy is only beneficial in certain types of endometrial cancer. It was once thought to be beneficial in most cases. If a tumour is well-differentiated and known to have progesterone and estrogen receptors, **progestins** may be used in treatment. Progestin receptors function as tumour suppressors in endometrial cancer cells. About 25% of metastatic endometrioid cancers show a response to progestins. Also, endometrial stromal sarcomas can be treated with **hormonal agents,** including tamoxifen, hydroxyprogesterone caproate, letrozole, megestrol acetate, and medroxyprogesterone. This treatment is effective in endometrial stromal sarcomas because they typically have estrogen and/or progestin receptors. Progestin receptors function as tumour suppressors in endometrial cancer cells. Preliminary research and clinical trials have shown these treatments to have a high rate of response even in metastatic disease.

### Monitoring

The tumour marker **CA 125** is frequently elevated in endometrial cancer and can be used to monitor response to treatment, particularly in serous cell cancer or advanced disease. Periodic **MRIs or CT scans** may be recommended in advanced disease and women with a history of endometrial cancer should receive more frequent pelvic examinations for the five years following treatment.

#### Follow-up

Examinations conducted every three to four months are recommended for the first two years following treatment, and every six months for the next three years.

Women with endometrial cancer should not have routine surveillance imaging to monitor the cancer unless new symptoms appear or tumour markers begin rising. Imaging without these indications is discouraged because it is unlikely to detect a recurrence or improve survival, and because it has its own costs and side effects. If a recurrence is suspected, **PET/CT scanning** is recommended.

## PROGNOSIS

### Survival Rates

5-year relative survival rates in the US by FIGO stage

| Stage | 5-year survival rate |
|---|---|
| I-A | 88% |
| I-B | 75% |
| II | 69% |
| III-A | 58% |
| III-B | 50% |
| III-C | 47% |
| IV-A | 17% |
| IV-B | 15% |

The five-year survival rate for endometrial adenocarcinoma following appropriate treatment is 80%. Most women, over 70%, have FIGO stage I cancer, which has the best prognosis. Stage III and especially Stage IV cancers have poor prognosis, but these are relatively rare, occurring in only 13% of cases. The median survival time for stage III–IV endometrial cancer is nine to ten months. Older age indicates a worse prognosis. In the United States, white women have a higher survival rate than black women, who tend to develop more aggressive forms of the disease by the time of their diagnosis. Tumours with high progesterone receptor expression have a good prognosis compared to tumours with low progesterone receptor expression; 93% of women with high progesterone receptor disease survived to three years, compared with 36% of women with low progesterone receptor disease. Heart disease is the most common cause of death among those who survive endometrial cancer, with other obesity-related health problems also being common.

### Recurrence

**Rates** Recurrence of early-stage endometrial cancer ranges from 3 to 17%, depending on primary and adjuvant treatment. Most recurrences (75–80%) occur outside of the pelvis, and most occur two to three years after treatment, 64% after two years and 87% after three years.

**Factors influencing recurrence** Higher-staged cancers are more likely to recur, as are those that have invaded the myometrium or cervix, or that have metastasised into the lymphatic system. Papillary serous carcinoma, clear cell carcinoma, and endometrioid carcinoma are the subtypes at the highest risk of recurrence. High-grade histological subtypes are also at a higher risk for recurrence.

**Sites of recurrence** The most common site of recurrence is in the vagina; vaginal relapses of endometrial cancer have the best prognosis. If relapse occurs from a cancer that has not been treated with radiation, EBRT is the first-line treatment and is often successful.

Other common recurrence sites are the pelvic lymph nodes, para-aortic lymph nodes, peritoneum (28% of recurrences), and lungs, though recurrences can also occur in the brain (<1%), liver (7%), adrenal glands (1%), bones (4–7%; typically the axial skeleton), lymph nodes outside the abdomen (0.4–1%), spleen, and muscle/soft tissue (2–6%).

#### Treatment

If a cancer treated with radiation recurs, pelvic exenteration is the only option for curative treatment. Palliative chemotherapy, cytoreductive surgery, and radiation are also performed. Radiation therapy (VBT and EBRT) for a local vaginal recurrence has a 50% five-year survival rate. Pelvic recurrences are treated with surgery and radiation, and abdominal recurrences are treated with radiation and, if possible, chemotherapy.

## UTERINE SARCOMAS

Sarcoma of the uterus is a rare but highly malignant tumour and account for <1% of all gynecological malignancies and 2–5% of uterine malignancies.

### Pathology

The three main pathological groups are:

- Endometrial stromal sarcoma
- Uterine leiomyosarcoma and
- Carcinosarcomas

Of these, leiomyosarcoma is more common followed by carcinosarcoma and endometrial stromal carcinoma.

### Signs and Symptoms

The common signs and symptoms include unusual or postmenopausal bleeding which should be investigated to rule out sarcoma also. The other symptoms include pelvic pain, pressure symptoms and unusual vaginal discharge. Similarly a non-pregnant uterus that enlarges quickly should be viewed with suspicion and investigated further. However, none of the signs are specific.

### Management

Total abdominal hysterectomy with bilateral salpingo-oophorectomy is the standard treatment. The role of lymphadenectomy is controversial and depends on the tumour histology. Similarly adjuvant chemo- and radiotherapy are also of limited benefit.

### Treatment

Treatment at a Glance

| Stage of the disease | Treatment |
|---|---|
| Stage 1 A Grade 1 and 2 | Hysterectomy with bilateral salpingo-oophorectomy |
| Stage 1A G3 | Hysterectomy with bilateral salpingo-oophorectomy (BSO) with or without pelvic and para-aortic lymphadenectomy |
| Stage 1B G1–3 | Hysterectomy with bilateral salpingo-oophorectomy with or without pelvic and para-aortic lymphadenectomy |
| Stage II | Radical hysterectomy with BSO with pelvic and para-aortic lymphadenectomy |
| Stage III and IV A | Maximal cytoreductive surgery with omental biopsy |
| Stage IV B | Palliative surgery |
| **Chemotherapy** | |
| Stage III and IV | Adjuvant chemotherapy with paclitaxel, doxorubicin and platins |
| **Radiotherapy** | |
| Stage I or II | Adjuvant radiotherapy is commonly used in early-stage by vaginal brachytherapy (VBT), or external beam radiotherapy (EBRT). |
| Special circumstances | When the cervix is invaded by the tumour, radiation can be given before a total hysterectomy is performed.<br>Brachytherapy and EBRT can also be used, singly or in combination, when there is a contraindication for hysterectomy. |
| **Hormonal therapy** | |
| Well-differentiated tumour with progesterone and estrogen receptors, | Progestins |
| Endometrial stromal sarcoma | Hormonal agents, including tamoxifen, hydroxyprogesterone caproate, letrozole, megestrol acetate, and medroxyprogesterone. |

**Case study**

*A 45-year-old lady who had attained menopause two years back and with diabetes and hypertension for the past 10 years reports with profuse bleeding per vaginum on and off for the past 6 months. Non-specific managements were of no effect. She says she is losing weight and also gives history of loss of appetite. She is also anemic.*

*a) What is the probable diagnosis?*

*b) How would you confirm the diagnosis?*

*c) How would you manage her?*

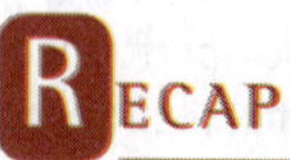
ECAP

- The most frequent type of endometrial cancer is endometrioid carcinoma, which accounts for more than 80% of cases.
- It occurs most commonly after menopause, more common during the 6th and 7th decades of life.

- A triad of obesity, high blood pressure and diabetes with endometrial carcinoma is called **corpus cancer syndrome**.
- Whereas taking estrogen alone increases the risk of endometrial cancer, taking both estrogen and progesterone in combination, as in most oral contraceptive pills decreases the risk.
- Between two and five percent of cases are related to genes inherited from the parents.
- Endometrial carcinoma is the third most common cause of death in cancers behind ovarian and cervical cancer.
- Incidence of endometrial cancer in all four parts of India as per National Registry is somewhere between 5–8 % of all genital tract cancers.
- Risk factors are obesity, diabetes mellitus, use of tamoxifen, nulliparity and elderly age, early menarche and late menopause, high levels of estrogen, unopposed estrogen replacement therapy during menopause, genetic predisposition, family history, endometrial hyperplasia.
- Smoking, breast feeding and the use of progestin are protective against endometrial cancer.
- Histologically, endometrial carcinoma can be divided into two subtypes—endometrioid adenocarcinoma (type I) and type II endometrial carcinoma includes the clear-cell, serous papillary subtypes and carcinosarcomas.
- Usually the cancer first spreads into the myometrium and the serosa, then into other reproductive and pelvic structures. More distant metastases are spread by the blood and often occur in the lungs, as well as the liver, brain, and bone. Endometrial cancer metastasises to the lungs 20–25% of the time, more than any other gynecologic cancer.
- Symptoms include postmenopausal vaginal bleeding or spotting, perimenopausal abnormal menstrual cycles, white or clear vaginal discharge in postmenopausal women and lower abdominal pain. spread of the disease to the bladder would result in urinary symptoms and to the bowel to bowel symptoms like diarrhea and dyschezia.
- Signs: General physical examination, systemic examination, abdominal examination may reveal enlarged uterus; in some cases it can be palpated abdominally or may appear as a soft, uniformly enlarged pelvic lump; speculum examination, pelvic examination may reveal a uniformly enlarged uterus with soft consistency; in early stages it is mobile freely with regular contour while in later stages it becomes immobile and has no regular outline.
- Investigations: Vaginal ultrasonograpy, cervical screening test, endometrial aspiration cytology, endometrial biopsy, dilatation and curettage, CT scans, MRI, hysteroscopy, positron emission tomography.
- Other tests: CBC, blood group and type, blood sugar, ECG, chest X-ray, liver function tests, kidney function tests.
- Markers: CA-125 can be elevated in endometrial cancer and estrogen and progesterone receptor (ER & PR) study.
- The modalities of management are primarily surgery; chemotherapy and hormonal therapy are either adjuvant options or are given in later stages. Radiotherapy is also given as an adjuvant and not primarily.
- The five-year survival rate for endometrial adenocarcinoma following appropriate treatment is 80%. Stage III and especially Stage IV cancers have poor prognosis, but these are relatively rare.
- Tumours with high progesterone receptor expression have a good prognosis compared to tumours with low progesterone receptor expression.
- Heart disease is the most common cause of death among those who survive endometrial cancer, with other obesity-related health problems also being common.
- Recurrence of early-stage endometrial cancer ranges from 3 to 17%.

## REVIEW QUESTIONS

### Long-Answer Question

Discuss the clinical signs, symptoms and investigations in a case of endometrial carcinoma.

### Short-Answer Questions:

1. Describe the staging of endometrial cancer.
2. Write briefly on hormonal therapy in endometrial cancer.

### MCQs

1. **The most frequent type of endometrial cancer is**
   a) Endometrioid carcinoma
   b) Serous endometrial intra-epithelial carcinoma
   c) Serous carcinoma
   d) Mucinous carcinoma
2. **Risk factors for endometrial cancer include all except**
   a) Diabetes mellitus

b) Obesity
c) Use of tamoxifen
d) Younger age and multiparity

**3. Significant prognostic factor after clinical staging is**
a) CA-125
b) Progesterone receptor
c) Estrogen receptor
d) Carcinoembryonic antigen (CEA)

**4. Adjuvant chemotherapy has been found to increase survival in**
a) Recurrent endometrial cancer
b) Mutations in mismatch repair genes
c) Stage III and IV cancer
d) Lynch syndrome

**Further Reading**

Ahluwalia M, Light AM, Surampudi K, Finn CB. Transitional cell carcinoma of the endometrium: a case report and review of the literature. International Journal of Gynecological Pathology. 2006;25(4):378–82.

Biswas A, Oh PI, Faulkner GE, Bajaj RR, Silver MA, Mitchell MS, Alter DA. Sedentary time and its association with risk for disease incidence, mortality, and hospitalization in adults: a systematic review and meta-analysis. Annals of Internal Medicine. 2015;162(2):123–32.

Burke WM, Orr J, Leitao M, Salom E, Gehrig P, Olawaiye AB, Brewer M, Boruta D, Villella J, Herzog T, Abu Shahin F. Endometrial cancer: A review and current management strategies: Part I. Gynecologic Oncology. 2014;134(2):385–92.

Coleman RL, Ramirez PT, Gershenson DM. Neoplastic diseases of the ovary. In Lentz GM, Lobo RA, Gershenson DM, Katz VL, editors. Comprehensive Gynecology. 6th ed. St. Louis: Mosby; 2013.

Colombo N, Preti E, Landoni F, Carinelli S, Colombo A, Marini C, Sessa C. Endometrial cancer: ESMO clinical practice guidelines for diagnosis, treatment and follow-up. Annals of Oncology. 2011;22 (Supplement 6): vi35–vi39.

Goodrich S, Kebria-Moslemi M, Broshears J, Sutton GP, Rose P. Primary squamous cell carcinoma of the endometrium: two cases and a review of the literature. Diagnostic Cytopathology. 2013;41(9):817–20.

Hoffman BL, Schorge JO, Schaffer JI, Halvorson LM, Bradshaw KD, Cunningham FG, editors. Endometrial cancer. Williams gynecology. 2nd ed. New York: McGraw-Hill; 2012. 819 p.

Johnson N, Bryant A, Miles T, Hogberg T, Cornes P. Adjuvant chemotherapy for endometrial cancer after hysterectomy. The Cochrane Database of Systematic Reviews. 2011;(10):CD003175.

Luo L, Luo B, Zheng Y, Zhang H, Li J, Sidell N. Levonorgestrel-releasing intrauterine system for atypical endometrial hyperplasia. The Cochrane database of systematic reviews. 2013;6:CD009458.

Mani RS. The emerging role of speckle-type POZ protein (SPOP) in cancer development. Drug Discovery Today. 2014;19(9):1498–502.

Mariño-Enríquez A, González-Rocha T, Burgos E et al. Transitional cell carcinoma of the endometrium and endometrial carcinoma with transitional cell differentiation: a clinicopathologic study of 5 cases and review of the literature. Human Pathology. 2008;39(11):1606–13.

PDQ. NIH. 28 February 2014.

Staley H, McCallum I, Bruce J. Postoperative tamoxifen for ductal carcinoma in situ. The Cochrane database of systematic reviews. 2012;10:CD007847.

Suh DH, Kim JW, Kang S, Kim HJ, Lee KH. Major clinical research advances in gynecologic cancer in 2013. Journal of Gynecologic Oncology. 2014;25(3):236–48.

Thaker PH, Sood AK. Molecular Oncology in Gynecologic Cancer. In Lentz GM, Lobo RA, Gershenson DM, Katz VL, editors. Comprehensive gynecology, 6th ed. St. Louis: Mosby; 2014.

CHAPTER 22

# Malignant Ovarian Tumours

## AT A GLANCE


Incidence
Epidemiology
Pathogenesis
- Fathalla's Incessant Ovulation Theory
- Gonadotropin Theory
- Ascending Carcinogens
- Modern Theory

Classification
Pathology
- Germ Cell Tumours

Tumour Spread
Clinical Features
Signs
Diagnosis
- General Investigations
- Tumour Markers
- Imaging Modalities
- Genetic Studies
- Multimodal Evaluation

Screening for Ovarian Cancer
Staging of Ovarian Cancer
Management
- Staging Laparotomy
- Chemotherapy
- Radiotherapy

Important Non-epithelial Tumours
- Dysgerminoma
- Granulosa Cell Tumour


Christmas day of 1809 saw a revolution in the history of ovarian tumour management when Dr Ephraim McDowell operated upon a patient with benign ovarian tumour successfully without anaesthesia! Malignancies are known from time immemorial in this organ and a journey along the time line shows the evolution of management options from simple surgery, radical surgery, radiotherapy evolution and chemotherapeutic interventions. Today, tumour markers, imaging modalities, fertility-sparing procedures, and risk-reducing strategies have made an ocean of difference in their management.

Ovaries are made up of varieties of cells some of which are totipotent; they have potential for uncontrolled proliferation and hence varieties of tumours are known to occur in the ovaries. It could be from the surface epithelium, germ cells, sex cord stromal cells, connective tissue cells, etc., which can be appreciated in the WHO classification of ovarian tumours. These are the most lethal of all gynecological cancers as the diagnosis is made most often in stage 3 or 4, putting the overall 5-year survival at 45%.

## INCIDENCE

- Across the globe, ovarian cancer is the seventh most common cancer in women, responsible for 1.4 lakh deaths annually.
- Fiji has the highest rate of ovarian cancer, followed by Latvia and Bulgaria.
- About 58% of ovarian cancer cases occur in less developed countries.
- The highest incidence of ovarian cancer is in Europe and Northern America; and the lowest incidence in Africa and Asia.
- In India it is third only to cancer cervix and cancer breast, seeing a whooping increase in incidence and death, by 153% and 122% respectively from 1990 to 2013.

## EPIDEMIOLOGY

**Age** 1$^{st}$ and 2$^{nd}$ decade tumours are more likely to be germ cell tumours or sex cord – stromal tumours. In the 5$^{th}$ decade, it is low malignant potential (LMP) tumours and in the 6th decade it is often epithelial ovarian cancers.

**Race** Caucasians are affected more than Asians.

**Genetic** *BRCA1* and *2* mutation, *p53* suppression, *KRAS* activation are some of the genetic causes.

**Geographic area** Found more in Europe compared to USA, but least in Japan.

**Diet** High calorie and fatty diet increase the incidence of ovarian cancer.

**Familial nature** This is genetically determined.

**Habits** Women using talc over undergarments have a higher predilection for developing ovarian tumors. Smoking may increase the risk for of mucinous tumours.

**Menstrual issues** Early menarche and late menopause predispose the woman to cancer ovary. Women with lesser number of ovulations are more protected from cancer ovary.

**Reproductory aspects** Pregnancy and lactation decrease the risk. More the number of pregnancies more is the protection.

**Contraception** OC pills offer a great protection. Tubectomy offers some protection.

**Other diseases** Hysterectomy for any other reason decreases the risk. Cancer breast, gastro-intestinal cancers may increase the risk. Type 1 tumour may arise in an endometrioma. In 20% of cases, cancer endometrium may be associated with endometrioid carcinoma of ovary.

## PATHOGENESIS

Many theories have been proposed to explain the pathogenesis of the ovarian cancer with supportive and contradictory evidences for them, thus none being conclusive.

Genetic predisposition with *KRAS* activation, *p53* suppression and *BRCA 1, 2* mutations can predispose a woman to an early onset of cancer ovary.

### Fathalla's Incessant Ovulation Theory

Any situation that causes repeated ovulation or multiple ovulation, continuously damages the ovarian surface epithelium; repeated attempts of the epithelium at regeneration may result in DNA damage, mutations and uncontrolled proliferation. On the other hand, factors that cause decreased ovulation like multiparity, breastfeeding and OC pill usage protect the woman from cancer ovary. More ovulation by induction with gonadotropins, early menarche, late menopause and nulliparity predisposes a woman to cancer ovary. But the fact that PCOS women with no ovulation are more predisposed to cancer ovary contradicts this theory.

### Gonadotropin Theory

Excessive gonadotropins either exogenous (administered for ovulation induction) or endogenous (PCOS, menopause), may continuously stimulate the ovary with their high levels and may be responsible for ovarian cancer.

### Ascending Carcinogens

There could be environmental carcinogens which might ascend up the genital tract through cervix and cause cancer in the ovary. Particles of talc used on the undergarments or napkins are thought to be responsible for the carcinogenesis. Protection offered by tubal ligation and hysterectomy may support this theory.

### Modern Theory

It was thought that ovarian carcinomas are derived from the ovarian surface epithelium and that subsequent metaplasia leads to the development of the various cell types. But now the ovarian tumours at large are studied as Types 1 and 2.

- **Type 1** Evolve from surface epithelium from a precursor lesion, are more indolent, start as benign, evolve to borderline variety and then to invasive variety. They are mostly confined to the ovary, have a stable genome and no *p53* mutations. They include endometrioid, clear cell, mucinous, low-grade serous, and transitional cell carcinomas.
- **Type 2** Arise de novo from ovarian/fimbrial epithelium or from the tubo-ovarian junction cells. They are more aggressive, diagnosed at an advanced stage, have *p53*/*BRCA 1* or *2* mutations. They include high-grade serous carcinomas, undifferentiated carcinomas, and carcinosarcomas.

The ovarian surface epithelium is histologically similar to the epithelium that lines the peritoneum. This probably explains the shared origin of the ovarian epithelial tumour and the primary peritoneal tumours.

## CLASSIFICATION

The latest classification of ovarian tumours into type 1 and type 2 is based on the histogenesis of the tumours and their progression. It also indicates their prognosis (Fig. 22.1).

But the histological classification of the tumours as given by WHO comprises the entire gamut of the ovarian tumours—benign, borderline and malignant. It separates ovarian neoplasms according to the most probable tissue of origin: surface epithelial (65%),

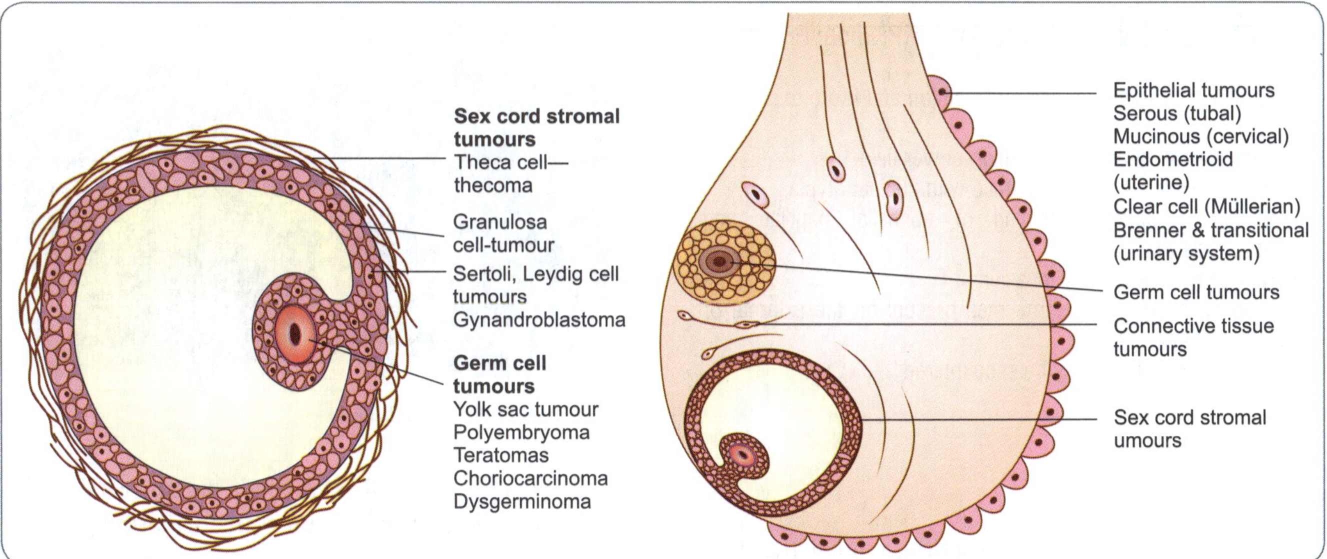


**Fig. 22.1** Origin of ovarian tumour from different cell lines

germ cell (15%), sex cord – stromal (10%), metastases (5%), miscellaneous.

Surface epithelial tumours are further classified by cell type (serous, mucinous, endometrioid, etc.) and atypia (benign, borderline or malignant; malignant may be invasive or non-invasive). 90% malignant tumours are surface epithelial.

Epithelial tumours are related to one or the other cells of origin from the urogenital system. Serous (Fallopian tube), mucinous (endocervical), endometrioid (endometrium), transitional (urinary system), clear cell (Müllerian).

Germ cell tumours arise from any of the developing part of the embryo—totally undifferentiated (dysgerminoma), yolk sac origin (yolk sac tumour), trophoblast origin (choriocarcinoma), embryonal origin (polyembryoma), development towards any of the germ layers (teratoma). They help to find the tumour marker with each tumour variety also.

### Classification of Ovarian Tumours

1. **Surface epithelial-stromal tumours** Each divided as benign, borderline and malignant.
   - Serous tumours
   - Mucinous tumours, endocervical-like and intestinal type
   - Endometrioid tumours
   - Clear cell tumours
   - Transitional cell tumours
     - Brenner tumour (3 varieties)
     - Transitional cell carcinoma (non-Brenner type)
   - Epithelial-stromal
     - Adenosarcoma
     - Carcinosarcoma (formerly mixed Müllerian tumours)
2. **Sex cord-stromal tumours**
   - Granulosa tumors
   - Fibromas
   - Fibrothecomas
   - Thecomas
   - Sertoli cell tumours
   - Leydig cell tumours
   - Sex cord tumour with annular tubules
   - Gynandroblastoma
   - Steroid (lipid) cell tumours
3. **Germ cell tumours**
   - Teratoma Immature, mature, solid, cystic (dermoid cyst)
   - Monodermal (e.g., struma ovarii, carcinoid)
   - Dysgerminoma
   - Yolk sac tumour (endodermal sinus tumour)
   - Choriocarcinoma
   - Mixed germ cell tumours
4. **Malignant, not otherwise specified metastatic cancer from non-ovarian primary**
   Colonic, appendiceal, gastric, breast

## PATHOLOGY

**80% epithelial, 10% sex cord stromal, 5% germ cell and 5% others.**

The benign variety of some of the tumours may be the precursors of their malignant counterparts. LMP (low malignant potential) or borderline tumours are specifically found with epithelial ovarian tumours which are diagnosable on the basis of only histopathology, and the malignant tumours with some special characters need to be clearly delineated by pathological examination.

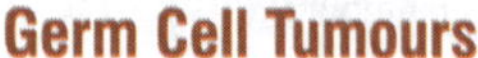

**Characteristics of Borderline/LMP Tumours**

- Epithelial hyperplasia with stratification and more than 4 cell layers
- Less than 4 mitoses per 10 high-power field
- Altered nucleo-cytoplasmic ratio with nuclear atypia
- Slight-to-complex branching of epithelial papillae and pseudopapillae
- No destructive stromal invasion
- Grossly, papillae are sometimes present on the external or internal surfaces
- Occasional spread may be encountered

## Germ Cell Tumours

### Dysgerminoma

This may develop in a dysgenetic gonad if there is a Y chromosome.10–30% are bilateral. Solid tumours are of moderate size (5–15 cm). Histopathology reveals large cells arranged in an alveolar pattern and mimics gonadal structure. It may show areas of choriocarcinoma, sertoli/Leydig cell tumours also. Germ cell tumours could be associated with pregnancy.

### Teratoma

Teratomas are classified as immature and mature. When the immature component is more, they are more likely to be malignant. Immature teratomas (Figs. 22.2, 22.3 and 22.4) are undifferentiated masses of solid tumour with poor prognosis and a disease of childhood. Neural element differentiation is considered for grading. Benign variety may contain hairs, teeth, bones, formed organs, etc., all arising from a projection from the inner wall of the cyst called Rokitansky's protuberance. This is a common site of malignant transformation

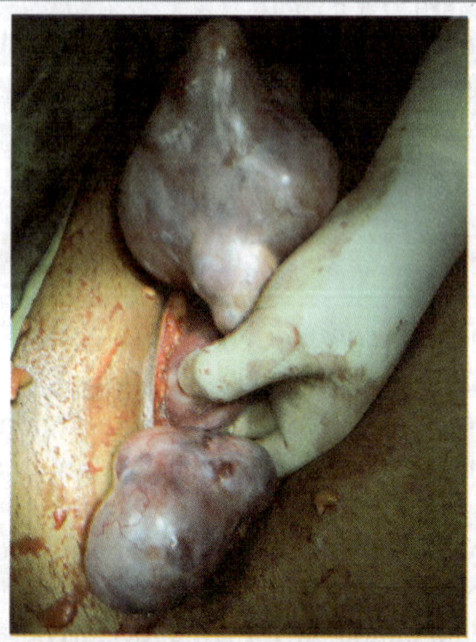

**Fig. 22.2** Immature teratoma in a 16-year-old girl

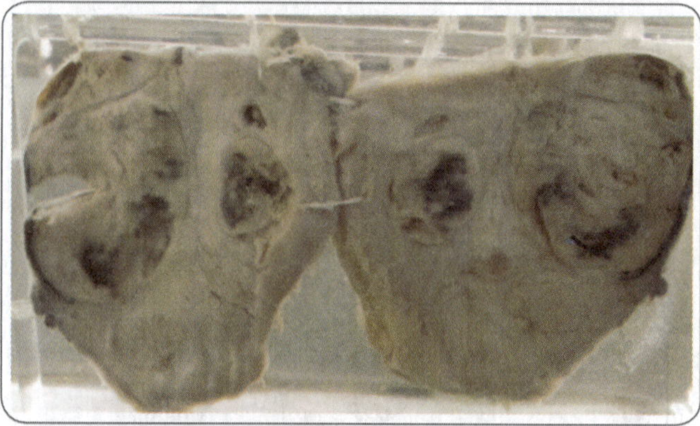

**Fig. 22.3** Immature teratoma

### Endodermal sinus tumours (yolk sac tumours)

These are rapidly growing encapsulated solid tumours with areas of cystic degeneration and are 100% unilateral. They show cystic areas with projecting vascular core containing glomerulus-like structure called **Schiller-Duval body.** They secrete alpha-fetoprotein.

### Embryonal carcinoma

These are large, and 65% of them are unilateral and secrete hCG and AFP. They may secrete estrogen also. These are common in younger age.

### Primary choriocarcinoma

These occur in young patients. They are hCG-secreting and very rare. Sheets of syncytiotrophoblasts are seen in histopathology. The prognosis is poor.

### Polyembryoma

Early embryonic differentiation structures may be found.

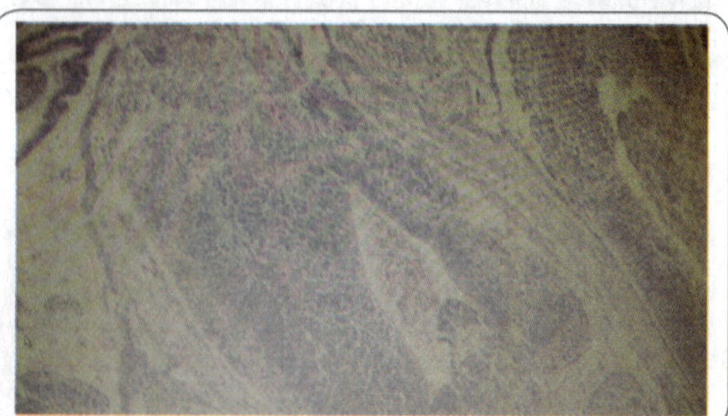

**Fig. 22.4** Immature cells

### Extragonadal germ cell tumours

These can form when the germ cells go astray during their migration from yolk sac to gonads.

### Mixed germ cell tumours

Such tumours also can occur. Most common among them is dysgerminoma with endodermal sinus tumour.

### Sex cord – stromal tumours

#### *Granulosa cell tumours*

They grow to a moderate size (2–20 cm), are rarely bilateral and occur in the 2nd or 6th decade commonly (Fig. 22.5). They are estrogen-secreting. The granulosa cell tumours are smooth, lobulated solid tumours with histopathology showing sheets of cells arranged as undifferentiated cells, in trabecular form or follicular pattern. **Call–Exner bodies** (Fig. 22.6) which are small cell clusters around a central cavity are seen. Coffee bean nuclei are characteristic of this tumour. Inhibin is the marker.

#### *Sertoli–Leydig cell tumour*

This is usually seen in the 3rd or 4th decade of life. They form 0.2% of ovarian cancers. Tubule formation, androgen secretion and heterosexual development are the hallmarks.

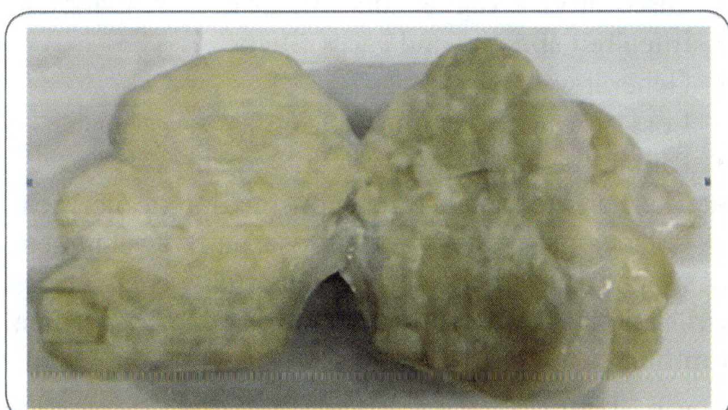

**Fig. 22.5** Granulosa cell tumour

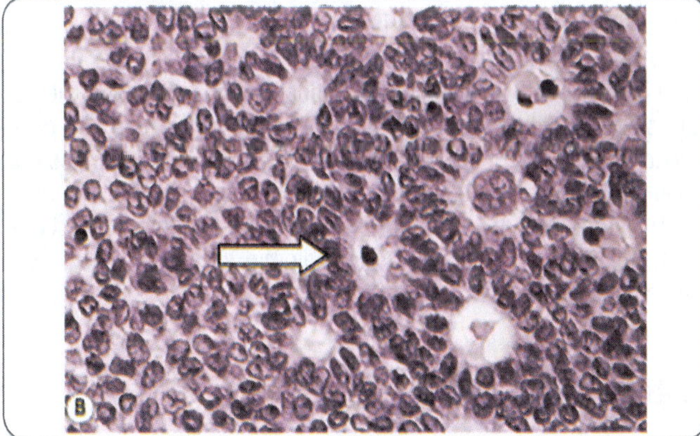

**Fig. 22.6** Granulosa cell tumour showing Call–Exner bodies (arrow)

### Kruckenberg tumours

These tumours are bilateral, soft, solid with smooth surface and slight bosselations. They are freely mobile, mostly associated with ascites, neither infiltrating through the capsule nor adhering to the surrounding structures. The shape of the ovary is maintained. Microscopy reveals cellular and myxomatous stroma with signet ring cells. They usually occur as secondaries from stomach, breast or colon. Their spread is through retrograde lymphatic spread. Treatment consists of treating the primary and removing the ovaries. Characteristics of some of the malignant tumours of the ovary are given in Table 22.1.

## TUMOUR SPREAD

**Spread to contiguous structures** This is the most common mode of spread. Surface breach causes tumour cells to exfoliate to peritoneal cavity, spread to pelvic organs like uterus, tubes, other ovary, bladder surface, colonic surface, pouch of Douglas, peritoneum, uterosacral ligaments, peritoneal surface (initially microscopic and later macroscopic) and to the omentum which forms an indurated mass many a times adherent to the tumour and classically known as **omental cake.**

**Lymphatic spread** Ovarian cancer can spread to any of the pelvic nodes—internal iliac, external iliac, common iliac, obturator nodes. It can directly spread to para-aortic nodes as it is supplied by ovarian vessels which is a direct branch of aorta. Left ovarian tumour

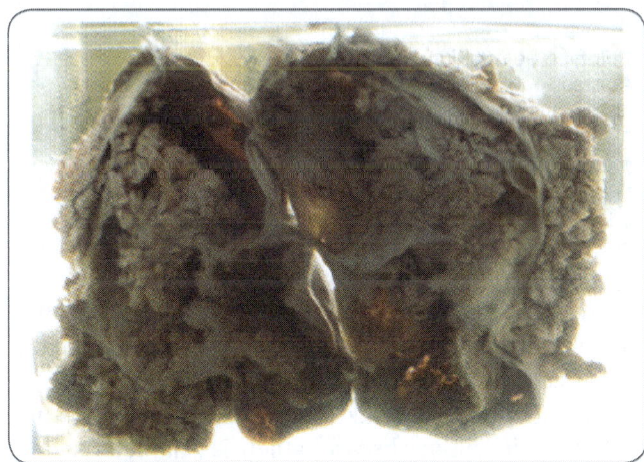

**Fig. 22.7** Serous cystadenocarcinoma (Gross)

**Table 22.1** Characteristics of some malignant ovarian tumours

| Tumour | Gross appearance | Microscopy | Special feature |
|---|---|---|---|
| Serous Cysadenocarcinoma (75%) (Fig. 22.7) | 50% bilateral<br>Fairly large<br>Cystic Semisolid (2/3) or solid<br>Adhesions, excrescences, deposits are common | Papillary, glandular with papillae, or sheets of cells in high grade. Cells with features of malignancy—Hyperchromatic nucleus, altered nucleo-cytoplasmic ratio, multiple nucleoli, etc. | Psammoma bodies |
| Mucinous cystadenocarcinoma (20%) | 10% bilateral, very large, multiloculated. At one site tuft of lobules suggesting the growing end is seen. Occasionally adhesions seen | Locules with polysaccharide-rich mucinous fluid. Lined by columnar cells. | Pseudomyxoma peritonei, Association with mucocele of appendix and teratoma of ovary |
| Endometrioid carcinoma (2%) | Large with smooth surface with excrescences sometimes | Solid, cystic, filled with blood or fluid. Glandular cells resembling endometrium with scanty stroma. Squamous metaplasia, areas of serous or mucinous features may be seen | |
| Clear cell carcinoma (1%) | | Tubulocystic, reticular, papillary and solid varieties | Tumour not graded<br>Hobnail cells |
| Malignant Brenner tumour (1%) | Very small, diagnosed many a times on histology, occasional estrogenic activity | Central core lined by columnar epithelium with sheets of squamous or transitional cells suggesting Brenner tumour with malignant transitional epithelium | Can cause postmenopausal bleeding |

can spread to left supraclavicular nodes, which is an important sign to be looked for.

**Transcoelomic spread** This type of spread may result in pleural effusion associated with a few ovarian tumours.

**Vascular spread** Parenchymal deposits to liver, lungs and even to skeletal system and brain may occur rarely with ovarian tumours.

## CLINICAL FEATURES

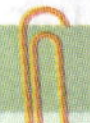

**3 Ds of Ovarian Cancer**

Distension
Discomfort
Dyspepsia

**Points to be noted in history**
Age, socioeconomic status, past history of breast Ca, family history of ovarian, colon or breast Ca, parity, contraceptive practice, breast feeding, ovulation induction, IVF

**Points in examination**
Pallor, cachexia, Supraclavicular lymph node, Unilateral pedal edema, Bilaterality of tumour, ascitis, consistency, surface, fixity, irregularity, tenderness in the tumour

Ovarian cancer is typically a postmenopausal disease affecting women in their 5$^{th}$ and 6$^{th}$ decade. Germ cell and sex cord – stromal tumours can occur in childhood, adolescence and reproductive age group.

It is a deceptive disease which is characterised by being asymptomatic in the early stages and associated with vague non-specific symptoms in advanced stages; both of this is the reason for delay in the diagnosis and adverse outcome.

- Abdominal distension—Tumour and fluid
- Discomfort—Vague pain or heaviness in abdomen
- Impaired appetite and early satiety
- General weakness
- Loss of weight (significant loss)
- Pain in the later stages
- Mass per abdomen-rarely constipation or diarrhea

Precocious puberty, heterosexual development, postmenopausal bleeding, menstrual irregularities, virilisation, etc. are the symptoms of **sex cord – stromal tumours.**

**Acute features** Pain could be due to torsion and haemorrhage or nerve involvement, intestinal obstruction or urinary retention. Chest symptoms like cough, breathlessness, haemoptysis can occur.

Ovarian fibroma associated with ascites and right-sided pleural effusion constitute the features of **Meig's syndrome.** In case pleural effusion and ascites are associated with other varieties of ovarian tumours, it is called **pseudomeig's syndrome**.

The mechanism of ascites is due to peritoneal implants and pleural effusion due to transcoelomic spread or rarely lung metastasis.

## SIGNS

- Features of anaemia
- Cachexic look

- Wasted muscles with distended abdomen
- Pedal edema—pelvic adhesions with lymphatic involvement usually causing unilateral lower limb edema
- Lymphadenopathy—Palpable left supraclavicular node is a significant finding
- Hirsutism, signs of precocious puberty, change in voice, trunkal obesity may be noticed in hormone-secreting tumours.

**Characteristics of Ovarian Mass**

Growth : Rapidly growing
Size : Medium to large
Surface : Irregular
Bilaterality
Consistency : Solid, cystic and variable
Mobility : Restricted
Tenderness : May be present
Ascites : Usually present
Organomegaly : If involved

Respiratory system examination may reveal pleural effusion more on the right side.

- Abdominal examination may reveal ovarian mass

Most of the features described help to differentiate the malignant mass from its benign counterpart.

Uterus which is normal sized in a postmenopausal woman with adnexal mass, estrogenic features in the external genitals and vagina may be encountered in estrogen-secreting tumours, and virilisation features may be seen in androgen-secreting tumours.

## DIAGNOSIS

Whenever a patient with mass per abdomen presents in whom there is a suspicion of malignant ovarian tumour, the following algorithm helps in arriving at the diagnosis.

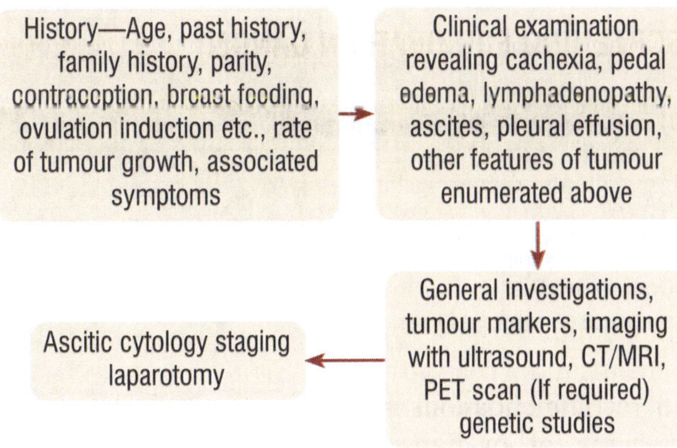


### General Investigations

Complete blood count, blood sugar, blood urea nitrogen, serum creatinine, and if planning for surgery, VDRL, HIV 1 & 2, HBsAg, HCV, blood grouping and Rh typing, ECG, echocardiogram if required, chest X-ray needs to be done. The pre-operative workup may be followed as per the hospital protocol.

### Tumour Markers

They are also called biomarkers. They may be secreted by cancer cells or may be secreted by other tissues of the body in the presence of cancer elsewhere. They may be important for diagnosis, follow-up and prognostication of a tumour (Table 22.2). Some ovarian tumours are known to have specific tumour markers which could be glycoproteins or hormones.

**Table 22.2** Some tumour markers

| Tumour marker | Tumour | Importance |
|---|---|---|
| CA -125<br>CA-199<br>HE-49 (human epidermal factor) | Epithelial cancers<br><br>More sensitive mainly for serous tumours | Diagnosis, follow-up and prognostication |
| Alpha fetoprotein | Yolk sac tumour, embryonal cell carcinoma | Diagnosis, follow-up, staging |
| Carcino-embryonic antigen | Mucinous tumours | Diagnosis & follow-up |
| LDH 1 & 2 | Dysgerminoma | Diagnosis & follow-up |
| Beta hCG | Choriocarcinoma,embryonal cell carcinoma | Diagnosis & follow-up |
| Inhibin | Granulosa cell tumour | Diagnosis & follow-up |

### Imaging Modalities

#### Ultrasound scan

Transabdominal and transvaginal USG (Fig. 22.8) which complement each other may give valuable information. Bilaterality, multiloculations, thick capsule and/or septae, solid components, surface or septal excrescences, ascites, liver metastasis, etc. are the strong morphological features of malignancy on ultrasound examination. This is further strengthened if the Doppler flow study shows a Pulsatility Index $<1.0$ and Resistive Index of $<0.4$, indicating low impedance flow.

#### CT/MRI

This can show the exact nature, spread, lymph node involvement and other organ metastasis (Figs. 22.9 and

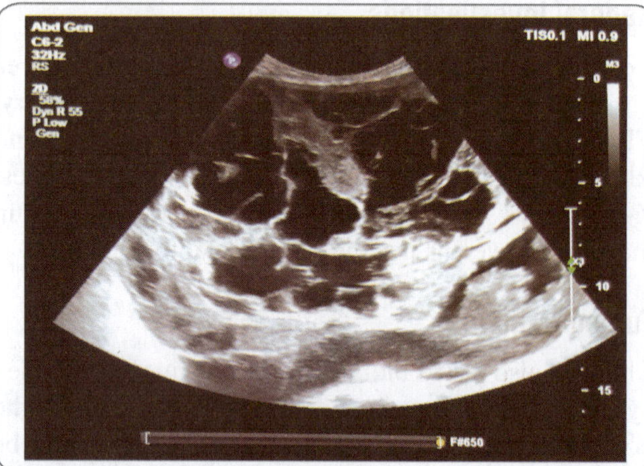

Fig. 22.8 USG—multiloculations, thick septae, excrescences

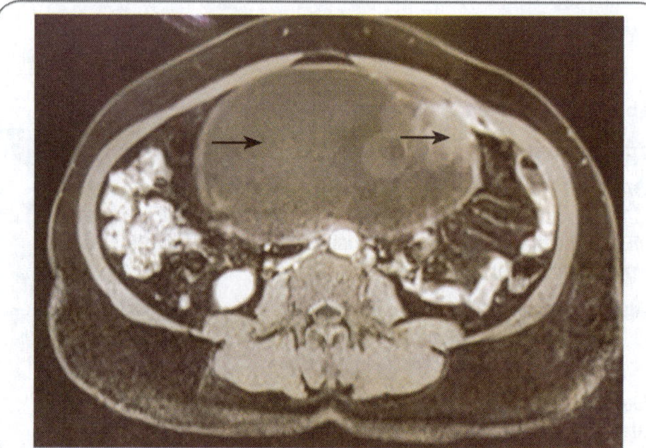

Fig. 22.9 CT scan—arrow marks showing the masses

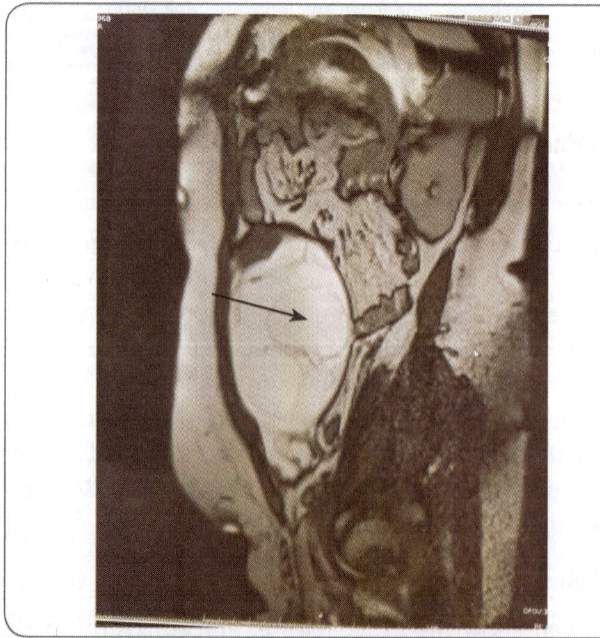

Fig. 22.10 MRI—huge mass with solid components

22.10), and may suggest about immediate operability of the tumour.

### PET scan

This shows the areas of high metabolic rate and thus can pick up small secondaries, but because of the cost, it is not routinely used.

### Chest X-Ray

Confirms effusion and can pick up lung secondaries.

## Genetic Studies

BRCA 1 and BRCA 2 mutations can be looked into in cases of familial occurrence.

## Multimodal Evaluation

Clinically it is very important to evaluate an adnexal mass regarding its malignant potential. Many multimodal evaluation systems have been used to calculate the risk and to diagnose malignancy Table 22.3.

Table 22.3 Multimodal evaluation systems

| Morphology Index (MI) of the tumour by transvaginal ultrasound | 0–10 scale <5 is benign, > 5 is malignant |
|---|---|
| Risk Of Malignancy Index (ROMI) | Age<br>Menopausal status (pre/ postmenopausal)<br>CA 125 level<br>>35 IU/L postmenopausal and >200 IU/L premenopausal<br>USG findings |
| OVA 1 (FDA-Approved) | Combine the 5 serum markers—CA 125, transthyretin (prealbumin), apolipoprotein A1, transferrin and β2 microglobulin, and menopausal status—into a numerical score. |
| Risk of Malignancy Algorithm (ROMA) (FDA Approved) | A quantitative serum test that combines HE4, CA 125 and menopausal status into a numerical score. |

## SCREENING FOR OVARIAN CANCER

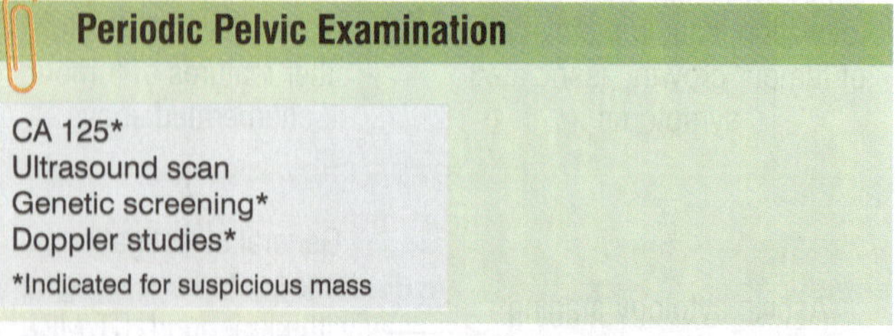

### Periodic Pelvic Examination

CA 125*
Ultrasound scan
Genetic screening*
Doppler studies*
*Indicated for suspicious mass

No recommendations have been made for universal screening of ovarian cancer as the modalities are neither very sensitive or specific nor very cost-effective. But a **selective screening** strategy may be adopted in cases with history of breast cancer, family history of breast, ovarian or colon cancer. **Women with known mutation of BRCA 1 or 2 also need to be screened.**

Screening modalities that could be adopted are shown in the Table 22.3.

## STAGING OF OVARIAN CANCER

Table 22.4 shows the staging of ovarian cancer.

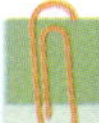

**Preventive Strategy**

- High-risk women may undergo prophylactic oophorectomy (does not prevent peritoneal cancer)
- OC pill usage
- Limiting number of ovulation induction cycles
- Screening selected population
- Effective evaluation of adnexal mass

## MANAGEMENT

A suspected case of ovarian malignancy requires near-accurate diagnosis by the various investigatory modalities and it is better to proceed with a procedure called ***staging laparotomy***.

### Staging Laparotomy

Surgical procedure involves a midline or paramedian incision.

If ascites is present, fluid is collected; otherwise 50–100 mL saline is instilled into the peritoneal cavity and washings collected for cytological examination.

A systematic examination of all visceral surface is done in an anticlockwise direction through right paracolic gutter, liver, undersurface of diaphragm, spleen, lieno and renal ligaments, left paracolic gutter, omentum, pouch of Douglas, bladder surface, and sigmoid colon.

Pan hysterectomy is done (uterus with both adnexae).

Biopsy is taken from all suspicious areas.

Otherwise biopsy is taken from the peritoneal surfaces, scrapings from the diaphragm.

Lymph nodes are examined and lymphadenectomy done if necessary.

Omentectomy, is routinely done (Fig. 22.11).

In addition, adequate **debulking or cytoreduction** may require excision of bowel segments, spleen, surface

**Table 22.4** FIGO ovarian cancer staging, effective January 1, 2014

| **STAGE I:** | **Confined to ovaries** | |
|---|---|---|
| Stage IA | Tumour limited to one ovary, capsule intact, no tumor on surface, negative washings. | |
| Stage IB | Tumour involves both ovaries otherwise like IA. | |
| Stage IC | Tumour limited to one or both ovaries | |
| IC1 | Surgical spill | |
| IC2 | Capsule rupture before surgery or tumour on ovarian surface. | |
| IC3 | Malignant cells in the ascites or peritoneal washings | |
| **STAGE II:** | **Tumour involves one or both ovaries with pelvic extension (below the pelvic brim) or primary peritoneal cancer** | |
| II A | Extension and/or implant on uterus and/or Fallopian tubes | |
| II B | Extension to other pelvic intraperitoneal tissues | |
| **STAGE III:** | **Tumour involves one or both ovaries with cytologically or histologically confirmed spread to the peritoneum outside the pelvis and/or metastasis to the retroperitoneal lymph nodes** | |
| IIIA | Positive retroperitoneal lymph nodes and/or microscopic metastasis beyond the pelvis | |
| III A1 | Positive retroperitoneal lymph nodes only | |
| | IIIA1 (i) | Metastasis ≤ 10 mm |
| | IIIA1 (ii) | Metastasis > 10 mm |
| III A2 | Microscopic, extrapelvic (above the brim) peritoneal involvement ±, positive retroperitoneal lymph nodes | |
| III B | Macroscopic, extrapelvic, peritoneal metastasis ≤ 2 cm ±, positive retroperitoneal lymph nodes. Includes extension to capsule of liver/spleen. | |
| III C | Macroscopic, extrapelvic, peritoneal metastasis > 2 cm ±, positive retroperitoneal lymph nodes. Includes extension to capsule of liver/spleen. | |
| **STAGE IV:** | **Distant metastasis excluding peritoneal metastasis** | |
| IV A | Pleural effusion with positive cytology | |
| IV B | Hepatic and/or splenic parenchymal metastasis, metastasis to extra-abdominal organs (including inguinal lymph nodes and lymph nodes outside of the abdominal cavity) | |

Histologic type including grading should be designated at staging.

- Primary site (ovary, Fallopian tube or peritoneum) should be designated where possible.
- Tumours that may otherwise qualify for stage I but involved with dense adhesions justify upgrading to stage II if tumour cells are histologically proven to be present in the adhesions.

lesion, lymphadenectomy, all aiming at excising the tumour load as much as possible leaving behind lesions <1 cm or microscopic in size.

In young patients with non-epithelial tumours and unilateral tumour without any other involvement, fertility-sparing surgery in the form of unilateral oophorectomy may be considered.

In LMP tumours also, unilateral tumour excision, confirmation by frozen section may be adequate. But follow-up is necessary.

## Chemotherapy

Management of ovarian cancer is revolutionised because of the chemotherapeutic interventions. Taxanes and platinum-based chemotherapy are the preferred modes.

Drugs used are **Paclitaxel and Carboplatin**—paclitaxel 175 mg/M$^2$, carboplatin AUC5-6 3–6 cycles are used, once in 3 weeks.

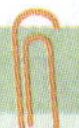

**Paclitaxel**

It is a taxane. Acts on microtubule formation and prevents spindle formation during metaphase. Can cause hair loss, arthralgia, myalgia, etc. **Dose is 80–175 mg/M$^2$. Docitaxel** is another member of the family with lesser incidence of neurological side effects, arthralgia, myalgia.

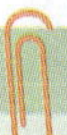

**Carboplatin**

Platinum-based chemotherapeutic agent used in Ovarian carcinoma. Interferes with DNA repair. Preferred over Cisplatin for lesser nephrotoxicity, nausea and vomiting. It has more of myelosuppressive effect. Dose is calculated looking at creatinine clearance and area under the curve (AUC). **Usual dose is AUC 5-7**

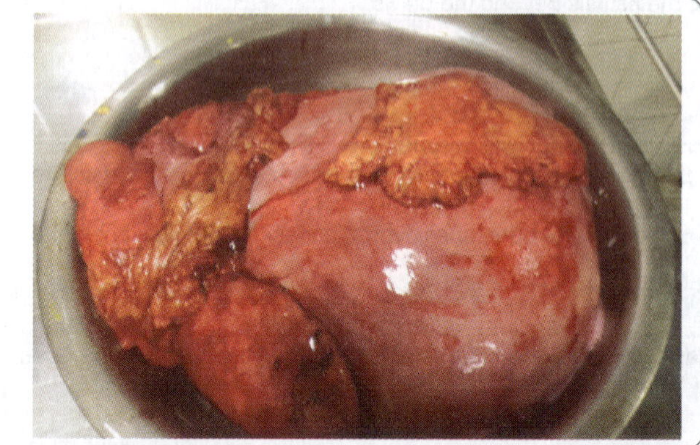

**Fig. 22.11** Surgical specimen of ovarian tumour with uterus and omentum

### Neoadjuvant chemotherapy

In advanced ovarian cancer, 2–3 cycles of chemotherapy before surgery (Fig. 22.12) would make the surgery more feasible and decreases the surgical morbidity and improves the patient's symptoms.

### Intraperitoneal chemotherapy

Cisplatin and paclitaxel have been used in stage 3 ovarian carcinoma intraperitoneally with the same results as with intravenous therapy. Patient compliance is less with this mode.

### Dose-dense chemotherapy

Paclitaxel used weekly instead of once in 3 weeks along with carboplatin once in 3 weeks is called dose-dense chemotherapy which might give better results.

When patient relapses in spite of chemotherapy, it could be **platinum-sensitive** cases when relapse occurs 6 months after chemotherapy. In **platinum-resistant** cases, relapse occurs within 6 months. **Platinum refractory** patients show advances during treatment. In sensitive cases, repeat chemotherapy with platinum drugs may be used. Carboplatin alone also can be used if they are sensitive to paclitaxel.

Otherwise second-line drugs like Topotecan, Gemcitabine, liposomal doxorubicin may be used.

A new drug called Bevacizumab which prevents neovascularisation may be used with any regime.

| Primary debulking surgery | Neoadjuvant chemotherapy |
|---|---|
| Reduces tumour bulk<br>Removes chemoresistant resting cells<br>Improves quality of life<br>Reduces bowel symptoms<br>Ascites is reduced<br>Early satiety reduced<br>Chemotherapy becomes more effective<br>Lesser dose of drugs would suffice | Ascites reduced<br>Tumour bulk reduced<br>Quality of life improves<br>General condition improves<br>Cytoreduction better<br>Surgical morbidity reduced<br>Per operative bleeding reduced |

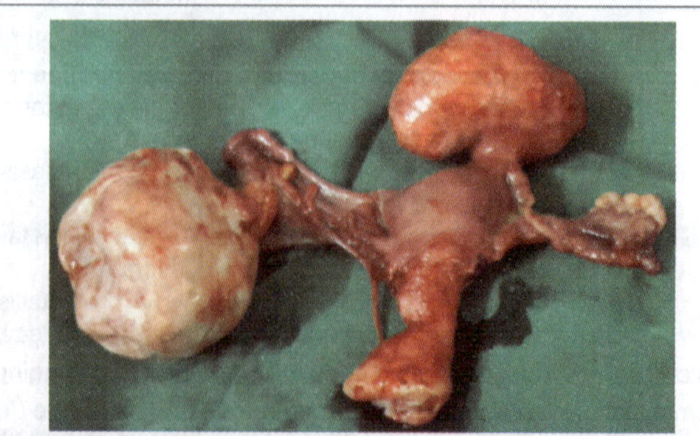

**Fig. 22.12** Postchemotherapy surgical specimen

### Treatment

| Stage | Treatment | 5-year survival |
|---|---|---|
| Stage 1 low risk | Staging laparotomy and fertility-sparing surgery may be considered | 94% |
| Stage 1 high risk* | TAH+BSO and omentectomy, staging procedure | |
| Stage 2 | Cytoreduction or neoadjuvant chemo followed by surgery | 73% |
| Stage 3 | Neoadjuvant chemotherapy followed by cytoreduction Intraperitoneal chemotherapy may be considered | 25–30% |
| Stage 4 | Palliative, neoadjuvant chemo, rarely surgery | 15% |

*Surface excrescences, pre-surgery rupture, ascites, positive peritoneal cytology, adhesions

## Radiotherapy

This has no major role in the management of ovarian cancer as it involves whole abdominal radiation which causes more of morbidity.

**Second look laparotomy** is not resorted to now adays, but secondary cytoreductive surgery is done following neoadjuvant chemotherapy and in recurrent cases.

**Complications and palliation** Intestinal obstruction is the most common terminal event which requires symptomatic management. Surgical correction is associated with greater risk of mortality.

## IMPORTANT NON-EPITHELIAL TUMOURS

Most of them are fast growing and can cause pain due to capsular stretch, haemorrhage and necrosis, occasionally torsion. Most of them are unilateral except dysgerminoma. In those presenting in early stage, surgery with chemotherapy is the preferred treatment option. Though they are radiosensitive (germ cell tumours) radiation can compromise with fertility and hence not used.

### Dysgerminoma

This is the most common germ cell tumour. It is a disease of 1$^{st}$ or 2$^{nd}$ decade. 10–15% are **bilateral**. LDH 1 and 2 could be the markers for undifferentiated germ cell tumour. Malignant tumours are usually diagnosed in stage1. Staging is similar to the staging of any ovarian cancer. Unilateral oophorectomy usually suffices. Inspection of the other ovary, or staging procedures needs to be done. Adjuvant BEP (Bleomycin, Etoposide and Cisplatin) is the combination chemotherapy preferred in this tumour. Dysgenetic gonads are likely to develop it. Thus karyotyping may be indicated in dysgerminoma. Presence of calcifications suggests association with gonadoblastoma. 5-year survival for Stage 1 is >95%.

### Granulosa Cell Tumour

It is a sex cord – stromal tumour secreting estrogen. It is usually **unilateral**. It can be found in children or in the postmenopausal women and is of bimodal occurrence. Early-stage diagnosis and indolent behaviour make the prognosis good.

- Pre-pubertal—can cause precocious puberty
- Reproductive age group—can present with AUB
- Postmenopausal women—postmenopausal bleeding, 25–50% show endometrial hyperplasia and some of them may have endometrial carcinoma. Biopsy is usually required. They secrete inhibin.

Granulosa cell tumour should be considered in a premenopausal woman with amenorrhea, infertility and raised inhibin.

Earlyl-stage disease can be treated with surgery alone but the later stage disease requires adjuvant chemotherapy with BEP regime.

The other solid tumours which secrete estrogen, like thecoma and fibroma, are usually benign.

## RECAP

- Common cancer in women with bad prognosis because of late diagnosis.
- Varieties of tumour can occur in the ovary
- Childhood tumours are most likely to be malignant and non-epithelial.

- Infertility, ovulation induction and familial disposition cause ovarian cancer while OC pills, breast feeding and tubectomy decrease the risk of ovarian cancer.
- Multimodal diagnosis combining clinical features, tumour markers and imaging modalities will aid in near-accurate diagnosis.
- Surgicopathological staging is the procedure of choice.
- Cytoreductive surgery followed by chemotherapy is the preferred mode of treatment.
- Screening and preventive strategy may be adopted in high-risk population.
- Non-epithelial tumours usually carry a better prognosis and are diagnosed early.

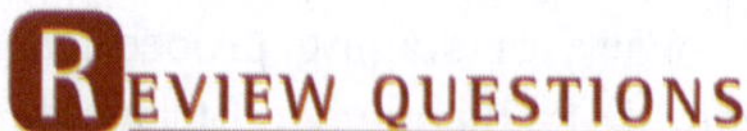

## REVIEW QUESTIONS

### Long-answer questions

Discuss the management of ovarian carcinoma in a 60-year-old woman.

### Short-Answer questions

Write short notes on

i. Kruckenberg tumours
ii. Dysgerminoma
iii. Chemotherapy for ovarian cancer
iv. Staging of ovarian carcinoma

### MCQs

**1. Which of these is not a sex cord – stromal tumour**

a) Sertoli cell tumours
b) Leydig cell tumours
c) Gynandroblastoma
d) Brenner tumour

**2. Call–Exner bodies are seen in**

a) Granulosa cell
b) Kruckenberg tumours
c) Serous cystadenocarcinoma
d) Endometrioid carcinoma

**3. Neoadjuvant chemotherapy is used in**

a) Early-stage ovarian cancer
b) Advanced ovarian cancer
c) Dose-dense chemotherapy
d) Intraperitoneal chemotherapy

### Further Reading

Ayhan A, Reed N, Gultekin M, Dursun P, editors. Text book of gynaeological oncology. Ankara: Gunes Publishing; 2016.

Barakat RR, Berchuck A, Markman M, Randall ME. Principles and practice of gynaecological oncology. 6th ed. Philadelphia: Wolters Kluver; 2013.

Berek JS , Hacker NF, editors. Berek & Hacker's gynecologic oncology. 6th ed. Philadelphia: Wolters Kluver; 2015.

Hoffman B, Schorge J, Schoffer J, Halvorson L, Bradshaw K, Cunningham F. William's gynecology. 2nd ed. New York: McGraw-Hill; 2012.

# CHAPTER 23

# Gestational Trophoblastic Disease

## AT A GLANCE


Molar Pregnancy
- Pathogenesis
- Clinical Findings
- Diagnosis
- Management

Gestational Trophoblastic Neoplasia (GTN)
- Clinical Findings
- Diagnosis
- Investigations
- Metastatic GTN
- Chemotherapy

Placental Site Trophoblastic Tumour (PSTT)
Epithelioid Trophoblastic Tumour (ETT)
Subsequent Pregnancy After Chemotherapy


## INTRODUCTION

*Trophoblastic Tumour is God's first cancer and Man's first Cure!*

— Hertig

Gestational trophoblastic diseases (GTDs) are pregnancy-related trophoblastic proliferative abnormalities. They refer to a spectrum of diseases. The malignant forms of Gestational trophoblastic disease are termed Gestational Trophoblastic Neoplasia (GTN). These malignancies develop weeks or years following any type of pregnancy, but frequently occur after hydatidiform mole.

**Incidence** Molar pregnancy is common in Oriental countries — Philippines, China, Indonesia, Japan and India. The incidence in India is one in 400, and 80% of the cases are uncomplicated. Based on a thorough pathologic review the incidence of complete and partial mole was 1 : 1945 and 1 : 695 respectively.

### Risk Factors

1. **Age** Both extremes of reproductive ages are vulnerable.
   - Less than 15 years—double the risk
   - more than 40 years—7.5 times risk

   The probable reason may be that oocytes are undergoing abnormal fertilisation during this period.

   Paternal age of more than 45 also carries 4-fold increased risk.
2. **History of previous mole** After one mole, risk of recurrence is 1.5–2% (Garret 2008). After two molar pregnancies, risk is 23% (Berkowitz et al).
3. **Ethnicity** Asians, Hispanics, American Indians are more predisposed (Drake 2006, Lee2011).

## MOLAR PREGNANCY

In molar pregnancy, there is villous stromal edema and trophoblastic proliferation.

Based on the degree of histological changes, karyotype difference, and presence or absence of embryonic elements, it is classified as **complete** (Fig. 23.1) or **partial mole** (Fig. 23.2). Table 23.1 lists the features of a complete and partial mole.

### Pathogenesis

With rare exceptions, molar pregnancies arise from chromosomally abnormal fertilisations as shown in Fig. 23.3.

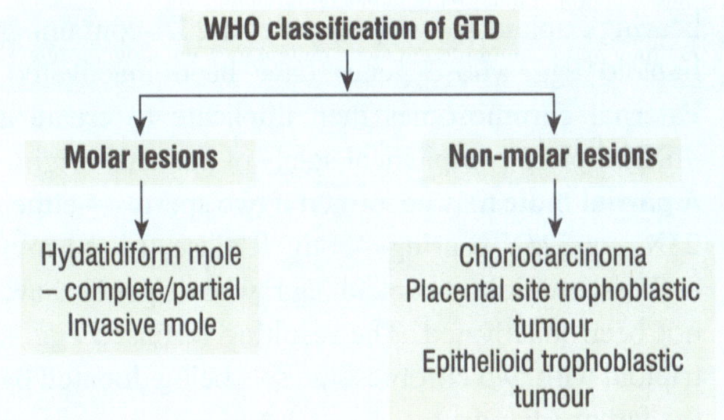

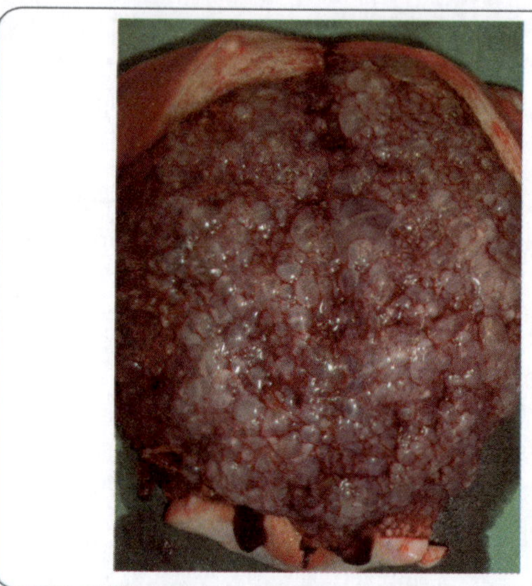

**Fig. 23.1** Complete mole (*Source:* © Prof Jonathan Carter/ Sydney Local Health District. Reproduced with permission)

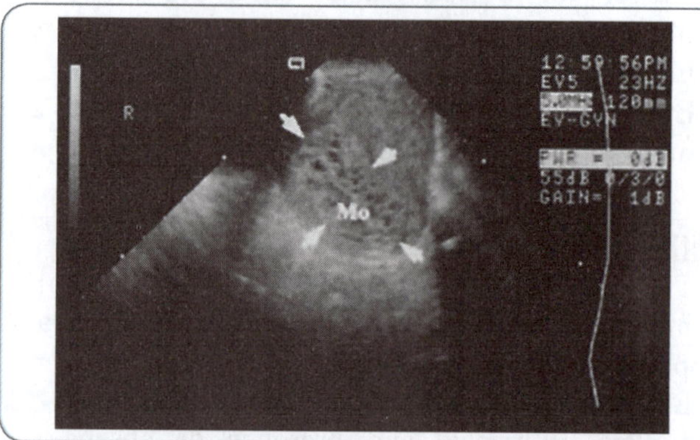


**Fig. 23.2** Partial mole: Endovaginal scanning provides superior resolution of the non-pregnant or very early pregnant pelvic organs. This is a midline endovaginal view of an anteflexed uterus filled with clusters of tiny anechoic areas and is the image of a hydatidiform mole (Mo). The outline of the mole is indicated (arrowheads). The transducer in the vaginal fornix is at the top of the image, the maternal abdominal wall is to the left, and the cul-de-sac would be to the right. (*Source:* Watson, W, Seeds, J, Glob. libr. women's med.)

A. 46XX **complete mole** may be formed if a 23X bearing haploid sperm penetrates a 23X-containing haploid egg whose genes have been inactivated. Paternal chromosomes then duplicate to create a 46XX diploid complement solely of paternal origin.

B. A **partial mole** may be formed if two sperms—either 23X- or 23Y-bearing—both fertilise (dispermy) a 23X-containing haploid egg whose genes have not been inactivated. The resulting fertilised egg is triploid with two chromosome sets being donated by the father (diandry).

**Table 23.1** Features of partial and complete moles

| Feature | Partial Mole | Complete Mole |
|---|---|---|
| Karyotype | 69, XXX or 69, XXY | 46,XX |
| **Clinical presentation** | | |
| Diagnosis | Missed abortion | Molar gestation |
| Uterine size | Small for dates | Large for dates |
| Theca lutein cysts | Rare | 25–30% of cases |
| Initial hCG levels | <100,000 mIU/mL | >100,000 mIU/mL |
| Medical complications | Rare | Uncommon |
| Rate of subsequent GTN | 1–5% of cases | 15–20% of cases |
| **Pathology** | | |
| Embryo-fetus | Often present | Absent |
| Amnion, fetal erythrocytes | Often present | Absent |
| Villous edema | Focal | Widespread |
| Trophoblastic proliferation | Focal | Slight to severe |
| Trophoblastic atypia | Mild | Marked |
| P57 immunostaining | Positive | Negative |

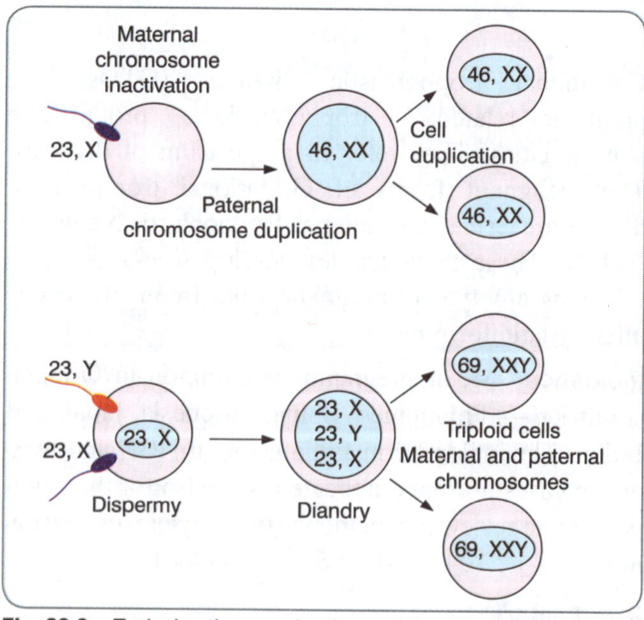


**Fig. 23.3** Typical pathogenesis of complete and partial mole

## Clinical Findings

Molar pregnancies present to the clinicians as follows:

Amenorrhea, vaginal bleeding (95%)

Uterus enlarged to more than the period of amenorrhea (50%)

Hyperemesis (25%)

Theca lutein cysts (50%)

Pre-eclampsia (25%)
and
Hyperthyroidism (5%)

But the clinical presentation has changed remarkably now because prenatal care is sought earlier and sonography is virtually universal. So it is possible to diagnose molar pregnancy even before any of these symptoms arise.

## Diagnosis

Period of amenorrhea followed by bleeding or occasionally passage of vesicles.

Serum beta hCG – raised.

Ultrasound is the mainstay of diagnosis. The appearance is described as typical **snowstorm.**

## Management

Regardless of uterine size, suction evacuation is the preferred treatment.

Preoperative cervical dilatation with an osmotic agent is recommended if the cervix is minimally dilated. Adequate anaesthesia, sufficient IV access, and blood banking support is imperative.

### Precautions to be taken during suction curettage

- It is preferable to evacuate the mole with oxytocin infusion.
- Heavy bleeding should not deter from cervical dilatation. With suction curettage, uterus usually dramatically reduces in size and bleeding will get controlled.
- When needed, uterotonic agents like methyl ergonovine (0.2 mg IM), Carboprost (250 µg IM) and Misoprostol (220 µg rectally) can be used. After completion, all tissues collected should be sent for histological evaluation.

> Anti-D **must** be given to the Rh-negative mother after evacuation of the mole.

Hysterectomy with mole in situ with ovarian preservation may be preferred in women aged 40 years and older, since approximately a third will develop GTN, and hysterectomy may reduce this likelihood (Hanna 2010). But even in them, follow-up is essential. Theca lutein cysts at the time of hysterectomy, even if large, do not require removal because they spontaneously regress after molar evacuation.

### Follow-up after molar evacuation

During every follow-up visit, clinical, biochemical and sonographic evaluation must be done.

**β-hCG levels** should be assessed every week ***until*** it is normal for 3 consecutive weeks (Fig. 23.4). Following this, β-hCG should be monitored every month till it is normal for 6 months. It can take 12–14 weeks to become normal. Because most of the malignant sequel happen at that time, follow-up till then is necessary.

Pelvic examinations are performed while hCG values are elevated to monitor the involution of pelvic structures and to aid in the early identification of vaginal metastases. New pregnancy should be ruled out by clinical examination and sonographic evaluation. This is more relevant in women with irregular follow-up and in those not following contraceptive advice properly.

### Contraceptive advice after molar evacuation

> To avoid confusion caused by rising beta hCG levels from new pregnancy, contraception is essential.

Barrier method, oral contraceptive pills (OCP) and DMPA injection can all be used.

It has been found that there is no increased incidence of persistent disease with OCP use and regression time is also not influenced by OCP.

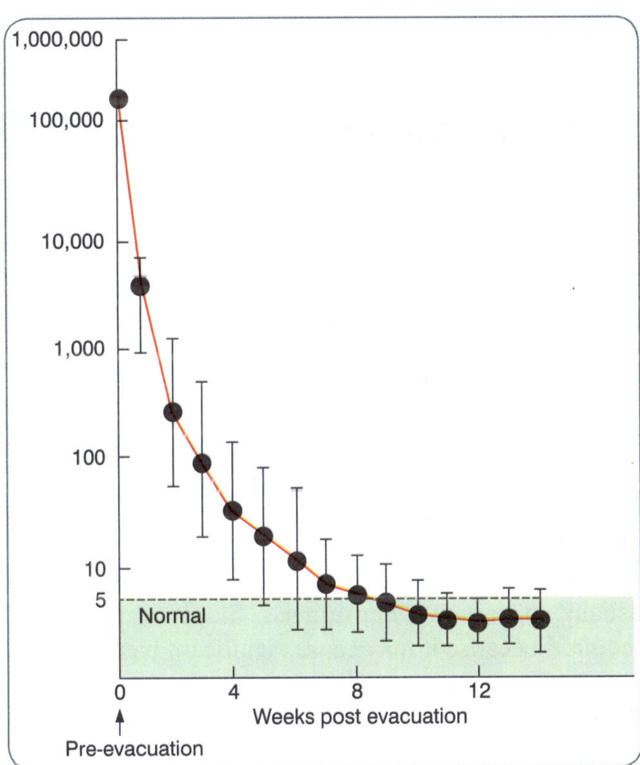


**Fig. 23.4** Normal regression of β-hCG after molar evacuation

Because of the risk of perforation, IUCD is avoided until hCG becomes undetectable.

Prophylactic chemotherapy after molar evacuation is not routinely given because of risk of drug resistance, toxicity and need for follow-up.

### *Phantom hCG*

False +ve elevation of hCG due to heterophilic antibodies that are detected during hCG assays is known as Phantom hCG. It can be confirmed by finding of 5-fold difference with alternative immunoassays, finding that a heterophilic antibody blocking agent prevented/limited false detection and negative urine test.

## GESTATIONAL TROPHOBLASTIC NEOPLASIA (GTN)

This group includes

- Invasive mole,
- Choriocarcinoma,
- Placental site trophoblastic tumour and
- Epithelioid trophoblastic tumour.

Half follow molar pregnancy, a fourth follow miscarriage or ectopic, and another fourth after a preterm or term pregnancy.

### Clinical Findings

They are characterised clinically by their aggressive invasion into the myometrium and propensity to metastasise. The most common finding with GTN is irregular bleeding associated with uterine sub-involution.

**Criteria for Diagnosing GTN**

1. Plateau of serum β-hCG for four measurements during a period of 3 weeks or longer
2. Rise of serum β-hCG level of >10%
3. Serum β-hCG levels detectable for 6 months or more.
4. Histological criteria for choriocarcinoma.

### Diagnosis

Consideration of the possibility of GTN is the most important factor in its recognition. Unusually persistent bleeding after any type of pregnancy should prompt serum β-hCG estimation and consideration for diagnostic curettage. Lower genital tract metastasis usually appears as a bluish mass. Biopsy of this is not required because it may cause significant bleeding.

### Investigations

1. Baseline serum beta hCG
2. Complete hemogram
3. TVS
4. Search for metastasis—LFT, RFT, chest X-ray, brain and abdominopelvic imaging.

#### FIGO staging of GTN

**Stage I**—Patients have persistently elevated hCG levels and tumour confined to the uterine corpus

**Stage II**—Patients have metastases to the vagina and pelvis or both

**Stage III**—Patients have pulmonary metastases with or without uterine, vaginal or pelvic involvement

**Stage IV**—Patients have advanced diseases and involvement of the brain, liver, kidneys or gastrointestinal tract

### Metastatic GTN

Metastatic GTN occurs in about 4% of patients after evacuation of complete mole but it is seen more often when GTN develops after non-molar pregnancies. Symptoms of metastasis may result from spontaneous bleeding at metastatic foci. The most common sites of metastasis are lung (80%), vagina (30%), pelvis (20%), liver (10%) and brain (10%).

**Pulmonary metastasis** (Fig. 23.5) may present as chest pain, cough, hemoptysis, dyspnea or asymptomatic lesion visible in chest radiography. The four principal pulmonary patterns are the following.

1. Snowstorm pattern
2. Discrete rounded densities
3. Pleural effusion
4. Pulmonary artery occlusion by emboli

**Vaginal metastasis** occurs in 30% of cases, which may present as suburethral nodule or nodules in the

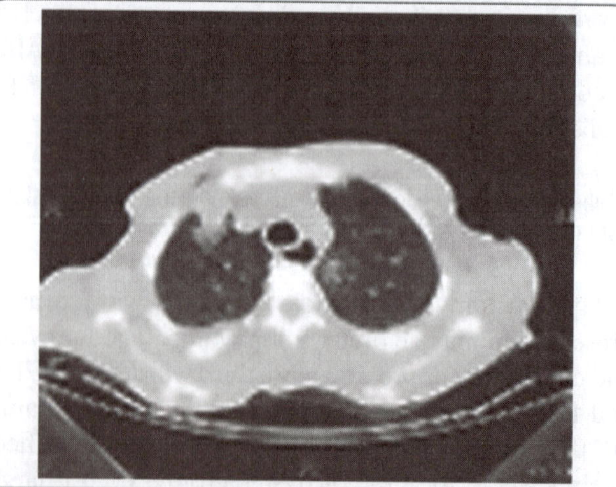

**Fig. 23.5** CT scan showing pulmonary nodules suggestive of metastases (*Source:* Wikimedia)

fornices. These are highly vascular and may bleed vigorously when biopsied.

**Hepatic and CNS metastases** occur in advanced cases.

### WHO Prognostic Scoring

| World Health Organization risk scoring system based on prognostic factors | | | | |
|---|---|---|---|---|
| | Score | | | |
| **Prognostic factors** | **0** | **1** | **2** | **4** |
| Age (Y) | <40 | >39 | — | — |
| Antecedent pregnancy | Mole | Abortion | Term | — |
| Interval (mo)* | <4 | >3, <7 | >6, <13 | >12 |
| Pretreatment serum hCG (mIU/mL) | $<10^3$ | $10^3$ to $<10^4$ | $10^4$ to $<10^5$ | $>10^5$ |
| Largest tumour, including uterine (cm) | — | 3 to <5 | >4 | — |
| Site of metastases | Lung | Spleen, kidney | Gastrointestinal tract | Brain, liver |
| Number of metastases | — | 1–4 | 5–8 | >8 |
| Prior failed chemotherapy | — | — | Single drug | Two drugs |

1. Plateau of serum β-hCG for four measurements during a period of 3 weeks or longer
2. Rise of serum β-hCG level of >10%
3. Serum β-hCG levels detectable for 6 months or more.
4. Histological criteria for choriocarcinoma.

### Chemotherapy

A detailed account of chemotherapy is given in Chapter 24.

## PLACENTAL SITE TROPHOBLASTIC TUMOUR (PSTT)

Placental site trophoblastic tumour is an uncommon but important variant of choriocarcinoma, which consists predominantly of intermediate trophoblast. They tend to remain confined to the uterus, metastasising late in their course. Relative to their mass, these tumours produce small amount of hCG and human placental lactogen (hPL). In contrast to other trophoblastic tumours, placental site tumours are relatively insensitive to chemotherapy. So treatment is hysterectomy.

## EPITHELIOID TROPHOBLASTIC TUMOUR (ETT)

This is a rare tumour different from choriocarcinoma and PSTT. The patient might give history of remote pregnancy or prior pregnancy is not established. There is proliferation of intermediate trophoblasts. Since ETT does not respond well to chemotherapy, hysterectomy is the treatment of choice. There is a 20–25% chance of metastasis.

## SUBSEQUENT PREGNANCY AFTER CHEMOTHERAPY

Patients treated successfully using chemotherapy can expect normal reproduction in the future.The logic of waiting for 6 months after last course of chemo before allowing to attempt pregnancy is that all oocytes that are in different phases of maturation and that are exposed to chemotherapy, would have undergone natural atresia by that time.

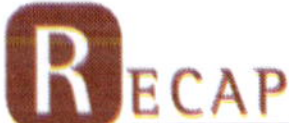

## RECAP

- Complete molar pregnancies are generally diploid and all chromosomes have paternal origin.
- Partial moles are triploid and the extra set of chromosomes are paternal.
- Complete moles are nowadays diagnosed earlier in pregnancy and there is lesser frequency in patients presenting with classic symptoms and signs.
- USG is the mainstay in diagnosis.
- Suction curettage is the treatment option for molar pregnancy.
- GTN responds very well to chemotherapy.
- Single agent chemotherapy achieves a high remission rate in non-metastatic, low-risk and low-risk metastatic GTN.
- Normal reproductive future is possible after remission with chemotherapy.
- Regular follow-up is essential in gestational trophoblastic disease.

## REVIEW QUESTIONS

### Long-answer Question

1. Discuss the risk factors for molar pregnancy. How do you differentiate complete mole from partial mole?

### Short-Answer questions

1. Briefly describe gestational metastatic neoplasia (GTN)
2. Write briefly on:
   a) Contraception after evacuation of molar pregnancy
   b) Phantom hCG

### MCQs

**1. Which is not a presentation of molar pregnancy?**
   a) Amenorrhea
   b) Hyperemesis
   c) Polycystic ovaries
   d) Theca lutein cysts

**2. According to WHO prognostic scoring, which score is low risk?**
   a) 5–7
   b) 8 and above
   c) 0
   d) 4 and below

**3. Stage II of FIGO staging of GTN is**
   a) Patients have persistently elevated hCG levels and tumour confined to the uterine corpus.
   b) Patients have pulmonary metastases with or without uterine, vaginal or pelvic involvement.
   c) Patients have advanced diseases and involvement of the brain, liver, kidneys or gastrointestinal tract.
   d) Patients have metastases to the vagina and pelvis or both.

### Further Reading

Berek J, editor. Berek & Novak's Gynecology. 15th ed. New York: Wolters Kluwer; 2012.

Cunningham FG. Williams Obstetrics. 24th edition. New York: McGraw-Hill Education. 2014.

Dutta DC. Haemorrhage in early pregnancy. In: Konar H, editor. Textbook of Obstetrics. 6th ed. Kolkata: New Central Book Agency; 2004. 159–202 pp.

Hoffman BL, Schorge JO, Bradshaw KD, Halvorson LM, Schaffer JI, Corton MM, editors. William's Gynecology. 3rd ed. New York: McGraw-Hill Education; 2016.

Padubidri VG, Daftary Sd. Shaw's textbook of gynecology. 13th ed. Gurgaon: Elsevier India; 2004.

# Chapter 24

# Chemotherapy in Gynecology

**At a Glance**


Incidence
Principles of Chemotherapy
Assessment
Calculation of Dose
Role of Chemotherapy in Treatment of Gynecological Cancers
Classification of Antineoplastic Drugs
Common Side Effects of Chemotherapy
Targeted Therapy
Immunotherapy
CT Treatment for Various Types of Gynecological Malignancies
Cancer Ovary
Germ Cell Tumours
Sex Cord – Stromal Tumours
Fallopian Tube Carcinoma
Primary Peritoneal Carcinoma
Cancer Cervix
Vulvar Cancer
Vaginal Cancer
Gestational Trophoblastic Disease (GTD)
Cancer Endometrium
Uterine Sarcoma


According to WHO (2011) cancer causes more deaths than coronary artery disease or stroke. It is predicted that there will be 20 million cancer cases by early 2025 especially in low and middle income countries. **GLOBOCAN** project is a comprehensive cancer surveillance database managed by the International Association of Cancer Registries (IARC), whose aim is to calculate the incidence, prevalence and mortality worldwide due to major types of cancers in 184 countries of the world. Globocan 2012 says more than one-fifth of new cases are diagnosed in India. In India 8,00,000 new cases are registered every year and lung and oral cancers are most common among men and breast and cervical cancers are common among women.

## INCIDENCE

In women 50 60% of cases occur in cervix, breast, ovary and uterus and nearly two-thirds present only in the advanced stage. Annually 1,22,844 cervical cancer cases are diagnosed in India and 67,477 die, roughly 1 out of 2 die due to the disease. The crude incidence rate of endometrial cancer has increased from 1.6/1 lakh population in 1982–1987 to 2.1/1 lakh population in 2006–2008. Most of these changes are due to environmental pollution, smoking and life style changes.

The treatment of cancer requires surgery, radiotherapy and chemotherapy but the recent advances in cancer therapy also include molecularly targeted therapy and immunotherapy.

The outcome of gynecological cancers have improved due to advances in radical surgery, radiation and chemotherapy. Surgery is the mainstay of treatment but there will be microscopic or macroscopic disease left behind even after complete surgery which results in recurrences later.

## PRINCIPLES OF CHEMOTHERAPY

The growth characteristics of normal and tumour tissues are different, and modern chemotherapy exploits this differential feature of normal and tumour tissues. Normal cell replication proceeds through a number of phases (Fig. 24.1) which are regulated by internal and external factors. Different chemotherapeutic drugs act in different phases of the cell cycle.

The **$G_0$ phase** (gap 0 or the resting phase) of the cell cycle is programmed for specialised functions and enters active cycling when triggered by growth factors or signals. **Glucocorticoids act in this phase.**

The **$G_1$ phase (gap 1 or interphase)** can be of variable length and associated with protein and RNA synthesis, DNA repair and cell growth. **L-asparaginase acts in this phase.**

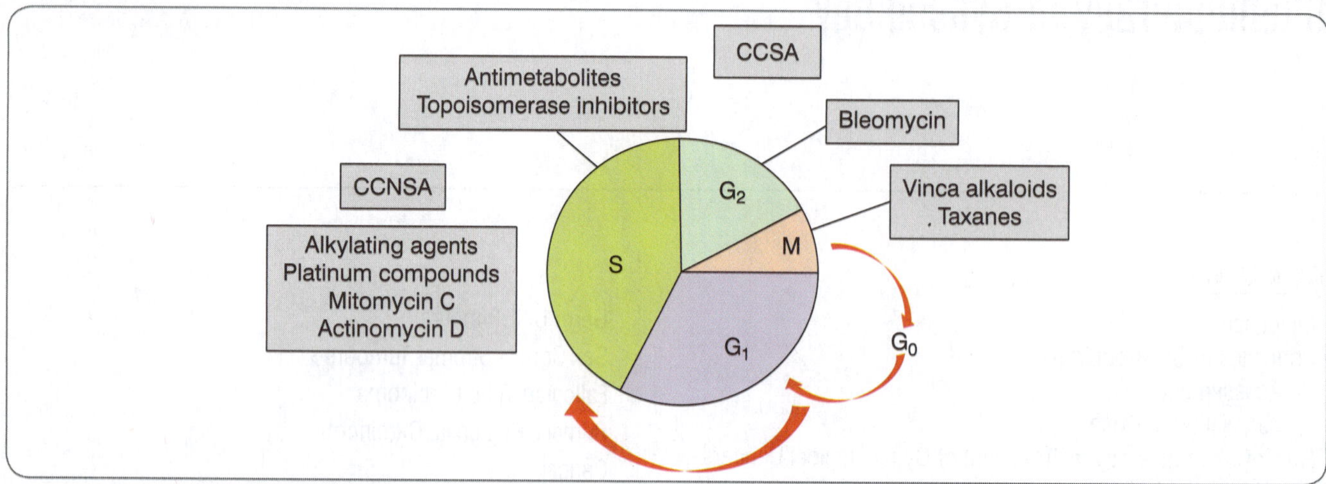


**Fig. 24.1** Phases of cell cycle

The **S phase (DNA synthesis)** is the phase where the DNA doubles. **Most alkylating agents and antimetabolites act in this phase.**

The **$G_2$ phase (gap 2)** is the phase where protein and RNA synthesis continue and precursors of mitotic spindle are produced. **Plant alkaloids and bleomycin act in this phase.**

**During the M phase (mitosis)**, the cell divides into two with the segregation of genetic material and the new cells enter either into $G_0$ or $G_2$ phase and initiate another cell cycle. **Plant alkaloids act in this phase.**

The **cell cycle checkpoints** are where the dividing cells are stopped before DNA synthesis and mitosis to ensure that the cell has the correct and non-defective DNA.

Most chemotherapeutic agents affect DNA, RNA or protein synthesis in the cell and when interference in synthesis or function in neoplastic cell population is sufficiently great, a proportion of cells die. Some cells die due to direct effect of chemotherapy and some due to chemotherapy-induced apoptosis. Often cell death occurs after several divisions of the cell.

**Clinical Importance**

Only a proportion of cells die with one cycle of chemotherapy, hence repeated doses must be given at specific intervals to eradicate all cancer cells.

Rapidly dividing cells are sensitive to chemotherapy and cells in $G_0$ phase are less sensitive. Hence not only cancer cells but also the rapidly proliferating cells of bone marrow, hair follicles and gastrointestinal mucosa are affected by chemotherapeutic agents. This results in side effects like neutropenia, anaemia, thrombocytopenia due to marrow suppression, alopecia due to loss of hair follicles and mucositis due to loss of gastrointestinal lining cells. But the normal cells in the gut and bone marrow regenerate and the patient recovers from side effects and also hair regrows once chemotherapy is completed.

**Combination chemotherapy** is preferred over single agents because of superior therapeutic benefit and prevention of development of resistance to drugs. **Drugs with different mechanism of action may produce additive or synergistic benefit and hence total or near-total eradication of cancer cells can occur.** Drugs with non-overlapping toxicity should be combined like one drug with myelotoxicity and another with gastrointestinal or dose-limiting renal or hepatic toxicity. Dose intensity and schedule should be maintained during treatment.

Chemotherapy agents affect DNA,RNA or protein synthesis in the cells and cause death. Rapidly dividing Cells are sensitive to chemotherapy. Not only cancer cells but rapidly proliferating cells of the bone marrow, gastrointestinal mucosa and hair follicles are affected.

Targeted agents target molecules that are uniquely or abnormally expressed within the cancer cells while sparing the normal cells.

In immunotherapy, a patient's own immune system is stimulated to eliminate cancer cells.

## Assessment

Before chemotherapy, one should assess the patient's performance status, nutrition, age, comorbidities like diabetes and renal, hepatic or cardiac illness.

**Patients with poor performance, who are frail and elderly with extensive metastatic disease and poor general condition should not be offered chemotherapy.**

## Calculation of Dose

Chemotherapy drugs are calculated according to the body surface area and most of them are given intravenously in a diluted form.

Since neutropenia can occur between 7–14 days, total WBC count should be checked on the 14th day after chemotherapy.

## ROLE OF CHEMOTHERAPY IN TREATMENT OF GYNECOLOGICAL CANCERS

1. Chemotherapy is **curative** in certain malignancies, e.g., **choriocarcinoma and germ cell tumours of the ovary.**

2. **Adjuvant chemotherapy** This is given to patients after definitive surgery, who have no evidence of residual disease but are at high risk for relapse. Adjuvant chemotherapy has proven benefit in breast cancer, osteogenic sarcoma and colon cancer and early-stage epithelial ovarian cancer.

### Adjuvant Systemic Chemotherapy

Adjuvant systemic chemotherapy is given
- To eradicate the microscopic disease and to prevent or delay recurrences.
- As a curative in some cancers like choriocarcinoma and germ cell tumours of the ovary.
- As a palliative in advanced and disseminated disease to improve quality of life.

3. **Neoadjuvant chemotherapy** In patients with **advanced ovarian cancer** where the disease is not amenable for initial surgery, chemotherapy can be given to reduce the tumour volume and after 3–4 cycles, surgery can be done. Neoadjuvant chemotherapy not only reduces the tumour burden but also reduces the tumour vascularity, improves appetite of the patient and quality of life, reduces intra- and postoperative complications. Neoadjuvant chemotherapy can also be given in cancer **cervix Stage IB2 prior to surgery**.

4. **To prolong disease-free and median overall survival** Primary chemotherapy in patients with **advanced epithelial ovarian cancer** shows high response rates to chemotherapy. In tumours with intermediate and lower response rates like advanced cervical and endometrial cancer, and uterine mixed Müllerian tumours, chemotherapy produces limited improvement in median overall survival.

5. **Palliative chemotherapy** is given in advanced and recurrent disease after prior chemotherapy to control symptoms and improve quality of life.

### Role of Chemotherapy in Gynecological Cancer

1. **Curative:** In choriocarcinoma and germ cell tumours
2. **Adjuvant:** In early-stage ovarian cancer
3. **Neoadjuvant:** In advanced ovarian cancer, cancer cervix IB2
4. **To prolong disease-free and overall survival** In advanced epithelial ovarian cancer
5. **Palliative** In all advanced and recurrent ovarian, endometrial and cervical cancers

## CLASSIFICATION OF ANTINEOPLASTIC DRUGS

Based on their action on the phase of cell cycle they can be divided into:

1. **Cell cycle non-specific agents** (phase non-specific, CCNSA): Acts in all phases of cell cycle, even in $G_0$, e.g., alkylating agents.
2. **Cell cycle specific agents** (phase specific, CCSA): Acts in specific phases of cell cycle, e.g., vinca alkaloids, antimetabolites.

**The commonly used chemotherapeutic agents and other class of drugs in treating gynecological cancers are listed in** Table 24.1.

**Table 24.1** Some chemotherapeutic agents and other drugs used in gynecological cancers

| Class | Drugs |
|---|---|
| 1. Alkylating agents | Cisplatin, carboplatin, cyclophosphamide, chlorambucil |
| 2. Antimetabolites | Methotrexate, 5-fluorouracil, gemcitabine, leucovorin, capecitabine |
| 3. Antitumour antibiotics | Actinomycin D, doxorubicin, bleomycin, liposomal doxorubicin, epirubicin |
| 4. Mitotic spindle agents | Paclitaxel, docetaxel, albumin-bound paclitaxel, vincrine, vinblastine |
| 5. Topoisomerase inhibitor | Etoposide, topotecan, irinotecan |
| 6. Monoclonal antibody | Bevacizumab (anti-VEGF antibody) |
| 7. Hormonal agents | Tamoxifen, medroxyprogesterone acetate, megestrol, aromatase inhibitor, LHRH agonists |
| 8. m-TOR inhibitor | Temsirolimus |
| 9. PARP-1 inhibitor | Olaparib |
| 10. Immunotherapy | Anti-PD-1 (Pembrolizumab) and Anti PD-L1 (Nivolumab) antibodies. CAR T cell therapy |
| 11. Cancer vaccines | Prophylactic vaccine: HPV vaccine, Therapeutic: dendritic cell vaccine. |

## COMMON SIDE EFFECTS OF CHEMOTHERAPY

***1. Hypersensitivity*** Anaphylactic reactions can occur with paclitaxel, carboplatin and etoposide. Premedication should be given to prevent them.

***2. Gastrointestinal toxicity*** Nausea, vomiting, stomatitis and diarrhea are the gastrointestinal side effects. Antiemetic agents are given for all chemotherapeutic agents.

Highly emetogenic drugs like cisplatin and cyclophosphamide should receive adequate antiemetic drugs. 5-hydroxytryptamine (5-HT3) receptor antagonist Ondansetron or Granisetron or neurokin-1 inhibitor Aprepitant can be given with steroids (dexamethasone) and lorazepam.

***3. Bone marrow toxicity*** Neutropenia is the most common toxicity due to chemotherapeutic agents, and typically occurs 7–14 days after chemotherapy. Alkylating agents, paclitaxel, docetaxel, topotecan and carboplatin are known to cause myelosuppression. Moderate anaemia can occur with repeated chemotherapy. Thrombocytopenia can occur with carboplatin. Bone marrow toxicity is dose-limiting and more myelosuppression is seen with intense and high-dose chemotherapy. Cumulative toxicity is seen with alkylating agents.

***4. Genitourinary toxicity*** Cisplatin causes renal toxicity and it can be prevented with adequate hydration. Hemorrhagic cystitis is produced by cyclophosphamide, ifosfamide which can be prevented by simultaneous use of mesna.

***5. Alopecia*** Loss of hair can be partial or total. Drugs like doxorubicin, paclitaxel, docetaxel and etoposide produce total alopecia. Carboplatin, cisplatin, cyclophosphamide and ifosfamide produce partial hair loss. Alopecia is temporary, and hair growth resumes when chemotherapy is discontinued.

***6. Neurotoxicity*** Peripheral neuropathy is a common side effect of cisplatin, paclitaxel, docetaxel and vincristine. The grade of neuropathy ranges from grade I to IV which can be paraesthesia, numbness to severe motor and sensory deficits that incapacitate the patient.

***7. Other toxicities*** Skin toxicity, nail discoloration, sexual dysfunction due to chemo and radiation, premature menopause in patients who get prolonged treatment for high-risk gestational trophoblastic disease, hepatic dysfunction and ototoxicity are some of the other side effects.

***8. Long-term toxicity*** Second malignancy, either leukemias (e.g., due to etoposide within 5 years) or solid tumours (due to alkylating agents after 5–10 years) can occur.

## TARGETED THERAPY

Targeted therapy blocks proliferation of cancer cells by interfering with specific molecules required for tumour development and growth. Some of these molecules are present in normal tissues but are overexpressed or mutated in tumours. **Unlike cytotoxic drugs which affect all proliferating cells, targeted therapy affects cells with specific abnormality.**

### Common Toxicity of Chemotherapy

1. Hypersensitivity reactions: Paclitaxel, Etoposide
2. Bone marrow toxicity: Neutropenia, anaemia, thrombocytopenia
3. Alopecia
4. GI toxicity: Nausea,vomiting,diarrhea
5. Genitourinary toxicity: Cisplatin—neprotoxicity, Cyclophosphamide—hemorrhagic cystitis
6. Neurotoxicity: cisplatin and paclitaxel—peripheral neuropathy
7. Others: Skin hyperpigmentation (cyclophosphamide, bleomycin), gonadal toxicity-premature menopause (high-risk GTD), sexual dysfunction after chemotherapy and radiation

**Molecular targets** play an important role in signal transduction pathways that control tumour cell growth, proliferation, migration, angiogenesis and apoptosis. These targets are often present inside the cell.

Targeted therapy includes **tyrosine kinase inhibitors and monoclonal antibodies.** Tyrosine kinase inhibitors are also called '**small molecules**' because of their small size and hence they enter the cell. Monoclonal antibodies are larger in size, cannot enter the cell and act on cell-surface receptors.

**Tyrosine kinase** is an enzyme which plays a critical role in modulation of growth factor signalling inside the cell (Fig. 24.2). Activation of these kinases occurs in cancer resulting in increased proliferation of cells and metastasis.

Tyrosine kinase inhibitors (Fig. 24.3) play an important role in blocking the signalling cascade within the cell. They are divided into receptor tyrosine kinases and non-receptor tyrosine kinases.

**Receptor tyrosine kinases** have an extracelluar ligand, a transmembrane domain and an intracellular catalytic domain.

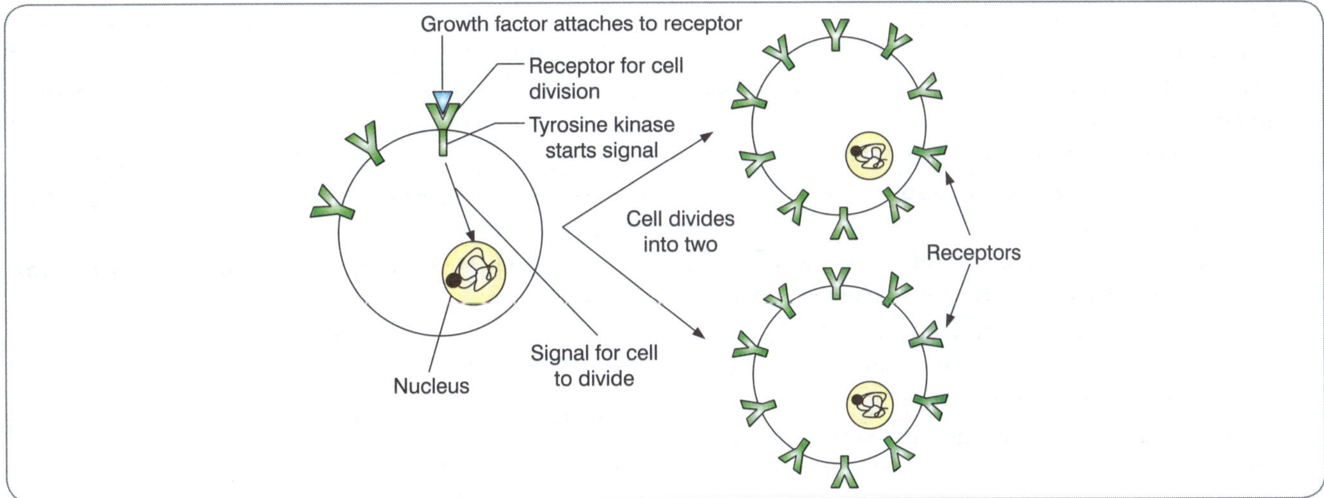


**Fig. 24.2** Activity of tyrosine kinase in cell division

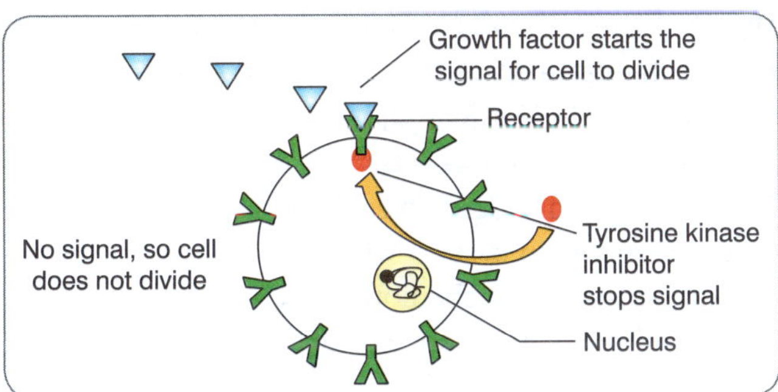


**Fig. 24.3** Inhibition of cell division by tyrosine kinase inhibitor

Ligand-binding results in dimerisation of tyrosine kinase leading to autophosphorylation of intracellular domain and subsequent signalling results in cell proliferation, migration, angiogenesis and apoptosis.

Examples are **epidermal growth factor receptor** (EGFR) family members, **vascular endothelial growth factor receptor** (VEGFR) and **platelet-derived growth factor receptors** (PDGFR $\alpha$ and $\beta$).

**Non-receptor tyrosine kinases** relay or transmit intracellular signals to the cytoplasm, inner surface of the cell and nucleus. After stimulation, they also activate cellular signalling pathways, e.g., BCR-ABL, c-KIT and c-Src.

Dysregulation of tyrosine kinases in cancer cells where proteins get fused to tyrosine kinases leads to constant autophosphorylation and activation. This occurs as a result of chromosomal translocations like t(9;22) which results in formation of BCR-ABL protein in chronic myeloid leukemia (CML). The drug used for treatment of CML is Imatinib, tyrosine kinase inhibitor (TKI). Other TKIs are dasatinib, nilotinib, ponatinib and crizotinib.

**EGFR targeting agents** Erlotinib, Geftinib, Afatinib

**Multikinase inhibitors** Pazopanib, sunitinib, sorafenib, regorafenib

**Monoclonal antibodies (MAbs)** These monoclonal antibodies act at the cell surface level where they bind to proteins or receptors and directly affect ligand-receptor reactions. They can also mediate antibody-dependent cell-mediated cytotoxicity or complement-mediated lysis. They are classified into unconjugated, conjugated and radioimmunoconjugates, e.g., unconjugated MAbs—rituximab, trastuzumab, obinutuzumab, cetuximab, bevacizumab, panitumumab.

**Conjugated MAbs** Brentuximab vedotin, ado-trastuzumab emtansine

**Radioimmunoconjugates** Ibritumomab tiuxetan

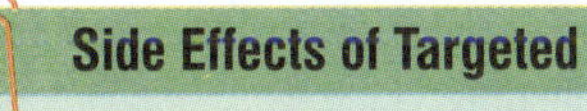

### Side Effects of Targeted Therapies

Fatigue, skin rashes, diarrhea, mucositis, fluid retention, hypertension, proteinuria, deep vein thrombosis, hypo- or hyperpigmentation of skin

## IMMUNOTHERAPY

Immunotherapy is where the patient's own immune system is stimulated to eliminate cancer cells.

1. It can be **non-specific** stimulation of immune response by one of the following.
   a) cytokines like IL-2 in melanoma or
   b) Inhibition of regulatory factors with anti-CTLA-4 antibodies like ipilimumab in melanoma,

c) Anti-PD-1 antibodies (Pembrolizumab and Nivolumab) in lung cancer and melanoma.

2. **Active immunisation** using cancer vaccines, which can be
   a) Prophylactic vaccines like HPV vaccine against cancer cervix and HBV vaccine against hepatocellular carcinoma.
   b) Therapeutic vaccines like Sipleucel-T in castration-resistant prostate cancer (which contains autologous antigen presenting cells, prostate acid phosphatise and granulocyte macrophage colony-stimulating agent)
3. Passive or adoptive cell therapy which includes donor lymphocyte infusion (DLI), tumour infiltrating lymphocytes (TIL), chimeric antigen receptor (CAR) T cells, natural killer (NK) cells therapy.

## CT TREATMENT FOR VARIOUS TYPES OF GYNECOLOGICAL MALIGNANCIES

### Cancer Ovary

The types of ovarian tumours, etiological factors, signs and symptoms and diagnosis are described in Chapter 22. Once diagnosed, they should be subjected for staging laparatomy. Complete removal of the tumour is the goal. **Optimal surgery is defined as residual tumour of <1 cm size (GOG criteria) at the end of surgery**. Surgery includes removal of all tumours and ovaries, total hysterectomy, pelvic lymphadenectomy and infracolic omentectomy.

> **Chemotherapy in Ovarian Cancer**
>
> **Early-stage ovarian cancer**
> Stage IA, IB, Gr I & II: No Chemotherapy
> Stage IA, IB, Gr III & IC all grades: chemotherapy 6 cycles (carboplatin and paclitaxel)
>
> **Advanced stage**
> Stage II, III—after surgery: 6 cycles (carboplatin and paclitaxel)
> Stage III & IV—Inoperable: 3–4 cycles of neoadjuvant chemotherapy followed by surgery and chemo to complete 6 cycles (carboplatin and paclitaxel)
>
> **Intraperitoneal chemotherapy**
> In optimally debulked, stage III ovarian cancer with residual disease < 0.5 cm in centres with expertise only

**Neoadjuvant chemotherapy** can be given for patients with large tumours with gross ascites, or with extensive upper abdominal disease or pleural effusion, supraclavicular nodes, liver metastases or in patients with significant co-morbidity, or elderly with poor performance status. After 3–4 cycles of chemotherapy, interval debulking can be done.

Stage grouping is as per FIGO 2014 staging.

**All stages will require chemotherapy except stage IA, Gr I & II.**

**All histological types are treated with the same regimen.**

#### Early-stage ovarian cancer

**Stage IA, IB, Gr I & II**: no postoperative chemotherapy

**Stage IA, B, Gr III, Stage IC, all grades**: require chemotherapy (6 cycles)

**Stage II, stage III & IV**: chemotherapy (6 cycles)

**Inj. Paclitaxel** 175 mg/m$^2$, 3-hr infusion, D1

**Inj. Carboplatin** AUC 5–6, q3 wks × 6 cycles

Other chemotherapy options as first-line therapy:

1. Carboplatin and docetaxel
2. Paclitaxel (dose-dense weekly 80 mg/m$^2$) D1, 8, 15 and carboplatin every 3 wks
3. Intraperitoneal chemotherapy after optimal cytoreduction in advanced stage: IP and IV Cisplatin and paclitaxel =
   Paclitaxel 135 mg/m$^2$ IV 24 hrs D1 &
   Cisplatin 75 mg/m$^2$ IV D2,
   Paclitaxel 60 mg/m$^2$ IP on D8, Rpt q3 wk × 6 cycles
4. Cisplatin and cyclophosphamide
5. Pegylated liposomal doxorubicin with carboplatin (for patients who are not able to tolerate paclitaxel)
6. Paclitaxel, carboplatin and bevacizumab q3 wks × 6 cycles

Intraperitoneal chemotherapy regimens have also an intravenous component so that systemic disease can also be treated.

#### Recurrent ovarian cancer—platinum-sensitive (recurrence after 12 months of last chemotherapy)

This can be treated with any of the following drugs:

- Carboplatin
- Carboplatin and paclitaxel
- Pegylated liposomal doxorubicin
- Carboplatin and gemcitabine

**Dose-dense chemotherapy** Paclitaxel used weekly instead of once in 3 weeks along with carboplatin once in 3 weeks is called dose-dense chemotherapy which might give better results.

#### Recurrent ovarian cancer—platinum-resistant (relapse <6 months after last chemotherapy)

Single agents preferred over combinations to avoid toxicity.

- Docetaxel
- Liposomal doxorubicin
- Gemcitabine
- Oral etoposide
- Weekly paclitaxel
- Weekly paclitaxel with bevacizumab
- Chlorambucil
- Cyclophosphamide
- Albumin-bound paclitaxel

A new drug called bevacizumab which prevents neovascularisation may be used with any regime.

## Germ Cell Tumours

The types of germ cell tumours, etiological factors, signs and symptoms and diagnosis are described in Chapter 22.

**Chemotherapy: PEB regimen**
Cisplatin: 20 mg/m$^2$/day × 5 days
Etoposide: 100 mg/m$^2$/day × 5 days
Bleomycin: 20 mg/m$^2$ weekly × 6 doses
Repeated q3 wks × 4 cycles

## Sex Cord – Stromal Tumours

The types of sex cord – stromal tumours, etiological factors, signs and symptoms and diagnosis are described in Chapter 22.

**Chemotherapy**
PEB regimen × 4 cycles
Or
Paclitaxel + carboplatin × 6 cycles

## Fallopian Tube Carcinoma

Rare, behaves biologically like serous carcinoma of ovary and hence staged and treated like ovarian cancer.
**Chemotherapy** The same regimens mentioned for epithelial ovarian cancer.

## Primary Peritoneal Carcinoma

The peritoneum may transform into malignant Müllerian epithelial pattern similar to epithelial tumours of the ovary. Patients will present with extensive peritoneal disease and ascites without any ovarian mass. They are treated like epithelial ovarian tumours.

**Chemotherapy** The same regimens as mentioned for epithelial ovarian cancer.

## Cancer Cervix

The types of cervical cancers, etiological factors, signs and symptoms and diagnosis are described in Chapter 20.

**Early-stage cervical cancer** can be treated with surgery or radiotherapy. Younger women may be subjected to surgery as it can preserve hormonal and sexual function. Elderly women with comorbidities and medically unfit for surgery can be treated with radiotherapy. 5-year survival for early stage is 80–90% when treated by either modality. Stage IB2, with tumours >4 cm in size can be treated with combined chemotherapy and radiation or neoadjuvant chemotherapy followed by surgery.

**Advanced stage disease, Stage IIB, III, IVA** should be treated with concurrent chemotherapy and radiation. Five-year survival rates of patients with IIB, IIIB and IV treated with only radiotherapy are 65–75%, 35–50% and 15–20% respectively. Results of 5 major clinical trials published in the end of the 1990s demonstrated that addition of chemotherapy to definitive radiation therapy reduced the risk of recurrence by 50%. Cisplatin was used in most of the trials of chemoradiation. Stage IVB disease with distant metastasis is not curable and palliative treatment is given in the form of local radiation, radiotherapy to painful areas, and chemotherapy to patients with good performance status and normal renal parameters. Chemotherapy may be with either single agents like cisplatin, carboplatin, ifosfamide or paclitaxel or with a combination of cisplatin with topotecan, gemcitabine, paclitaxel, vinorelbine or 5-fluorouracil.

In metastatic and recurrent cervical cancer, targeted therapy with bevacizumab, an anti-VGEF (vascular endothelial growth factor) antibody has shown a longer overall survival along with cisplatin and paclitaxel or with cisplatin and topotecan.

Pazopanib, an oral anti-VEGF, and platelet-derived growth factor receptor has shown activity in recurrent and metastatic cervical cancer.

#### Chemotherapy in Cancer Cervix

**Neoadjuvant chemotherapy, prior to surgery**
Stage IB2
Cisplatin + 5-fluorouracil
**Adjuvant chemotherapy**
Postoperative cases with > 4 nodes positive, margins positive, presence of lymphovascular invasion

**Concurrent chemoradiation**
Stage IIB, III, IVA
Cisplatin 40 mg/m2, weekly x 6 doses along with radiation or
Cisplatin (70 mg/m2 ) with 5-Fluorouracil(750 d1-3) q3weeks x 3 cycles, along with radiation
**Palliative chemotherapy**
Cisplatin + topotecan
Cisplatin + paclitaxel
Cisplatin + 5-fluorouracil
Cisplatin, paclitaxel and bevacizumab
Single agents—paclitaxel
Vinorelbine
Gemcitabine

## Vulvar Cancer

The types of vulvar cancer, etiological factors, signs and symptoms and diagnosis are described in Chapter 19.

**Early-stage disease** (Stages I & II) is treated with radical vulvectomy and bilateral inguinal nodal dissection. Two or more positive nodes should be treated with pelvic and inguinal radiation after surgery.

**Advanced stage disease** (Stages III & IV) can be treated with chemoradiation. Cisplatin and 5-fluorouracil or weekly cisplatin can be used along with radiation.

## Vaginal Cancer

Rare gynecological cancer. Same etiological factors like for cervical cancer play an important role in vaginal cancer especially HPV 16 which is detected in two-thirds of vaginal cancers. It presents as vaginal bleeding, discharge, pain, dyspareunia and bladder symptoms.

**VAIN III lesions** (vaginal intra-epithelial neoplasia) can be treated with simple surgical excision and/or ablation. Topical treatment with Imiquimod and topical 5 fluorouracil can be used.

All **invasive lesions, stage I–IV** should be treated with some form of radiation. Cisplatin can be used along with radiation.

## Gestational Trophoblastic Disease (GTD)

The etiological factors, signs and symptoms and diagnosis of gestational trophoblastic disease are described in Chapter 23.

**Chemotherapy in GTD**

**Low-Risk (Score 0–6)**
1. Methotrexate (Mtx) 50 mg/wk or
2. Methotrexate 1 mg/kg, D1, 3, 5, 7
   Tab.Calcium leucovorin 0.1 mg/kg, D2, 4, 6, 8 –q2 wks
3. Actinomycin-D 1.25 mg/m$^2$, q2 wks (in mtx failure)

**High-Risk (>6)**
1. EMA-CO Regimen, q2 wks
2. EMA-EP –q2 wks
3. PVB Regimen (salvage)

### Low-risk GTD (score 0–6)

Single agents:
1. Inj. Methotrexate 50 mg/weekly, IM till β-hCG becomes normal or
2. Inj. Methotrexate 1 mg/kg on D 1, 3, 5, 7
   Tab. Calcium Leucovorin 0.1 mg/kg on D2, 4, 6, 8
   Repeat cycles q2 wks till β-hCG becomes normal and 1 cycle after the remission.
3. Inj. Actinomycin-D 1.25 mg/m$^2$ IV q2 wks, till β-hCG becomes normal. This is used in patients who fail to achieve remission with methotrexate.

### High-risk GTD (score > 6)

1. EMA-CO Regimen:
   Inj. Etoposide 100 mg/m$^2$, D1 and D2
   Inj. Methotrexate 100 mg/m$^2$ IV bolus & 200 mg/m$^2$ IV infusion for 12 hrs, D1
   Inj. Actinomycin-D, 350 μg/m$^2$ IV bolus on D1 and D2
   Tab. Calcium Leucovorin 15 mg, q12 hours × 4 doses, oral, starting 24 hours from the time of methotrexate bolus.
   Inj. Vincristine 1.4 mg/m$^2$, IV bolus on D8
   Inj. Cyclophosphamide 800 mg/m$^2$, IV infusion on D8
   Cycle is repeated on D15 ie q2 wks till β-hCG becomes normal and 2 cycles should be given after remission.
2. Salvage regimens
1. EMA-EP: Etoposide, methotrexate, actinomycin-D, on D8 and etoposide and cisplatin on D1
2. PVB: Cisplatin, vinblastine, bleomycin

## Cancer Endometrium

The types of endometrial cancers, etiological factors, signs and symptoms and diagnosis are described in Chapter 21.

**Chemotherapy**

*Early-stage, low-risk:* **Stages I A & IB, Gr I & II, Endometrioid type**: Only observation.

*Early-stage, high-risk endometrial cancer*: Stages I & II, Grade III, Stage IC all grades: Radiotherapy to pelvis and vault with or without chemotherapy.

Presence of lymphovascular invasion, more than 4 nodes positive, surgical margins positive, grade III, more than 50% myometrial invasion of tumour, high-risk histologic type (papillary serous, adenosquamous, clear cell) can be given chemotherapy with radiotherapy either concurrently or sequentially.

Randomised trials show that combined modality treatment resulted in 36% reduction in risk of relapse or death.

Inj. Carboplatin AUC 5–6 + Inj. paclitaxel 175 mg/m$^2$ q3 weeks × 6 cycles

*Advanced stage (stage IIIA, IIIB, IIIC, IV) endometrial cancer* Patients with extrauterine disease by surgical staging have been known to develop recurrence without adjuvant chemotherapy. Radiation therapy can control pelvic disease, however most recurrences are extrapelvic and distant metastases in the liver, lungs and peritoneum. Hence systemic therapy is important in prevention of distant metastases. Adjuvant chemotherapy improves both progression-free and overall survival compared with radiation alone.

GOG 122 study established the role of adjuvant chemotherapy (cisplatin and doxorubicin) in patients with extrauterine disease. GOG 184 using 3 drugs (cisplatin, doxorubicin, paclitaxel) with or without radiotherapy showed there was no survival benefit with three drugs compared with use of two drugs but resulted in more toxicity.

### Chemotherapy in Cancer Endometrium

I. **High-risk early-stage:** Stage IA, IB Gr III and stage IC all grades, clear cell, uterine papillary serous carcinoma (UPSC) and squamous histologies:
   1. Carboplatin and Paclitaxel, q3 wks × 6 cycles or
   2. Cisplatin and Doxorubicin or
   3. Carboplatin and Docetaxel

II. **Stage II, III, IV endometrioid ca and clear cell, UPSC, squamous histologies:**
   1. Carboplatin and Paclitaxel, q3 wks × 6 cycles or
   2. Cisplatin and Doxorubicin, or
   3. Carboplatin and Docetaxel

III. **Recurrent and Metastatic disease:**

Carboplatin and Paclitaxel, q3 wks × 6 cycles
Cisplatin and Doxorubicin
Pegylated Liposomal Doxorubicin
Paclitaxel
Docetaxel
Topotecan
Ifosfamide

**Recommended chemotherapy regimens**

1. Inj. carboplatin AUC 5–6 + paclitaxel 175 mg/m$^2$, q3 weeks = 6 cycles is the preferred regimen.
2. Inj. cisplatin 75 mg/m$^2$ + Inj. doxorubicin 50 mg/m$^2$, q3 weeks = 6 cycles
3. Inj. Carboplatin AUC 5 + Inj. docetaxel 75 mg/m$^2$, q3 weeks = 6 cycles

### Recurrent and metastatic endometrial cancer

Generally not curable, palliative chemotherapy can be planned according to the age and co-morbidity as most of them are elderly.

Current combination chemotherapy gives a response rate of 50–60% and median overall survival of 12–15 months.

Single agents produce a response rate of 20–30%.

**Single agents** Inj. cisplatin, Inj. carboplatin, Inj. doxorubicin, Inj. liposomal doxorubicin, Inj. paclitaxel, temsirolimus, topotecan, bevacizumab, docetaxel, ifosfamide.

**Hormonal therapy** No role for adjuvant hormonal therapy.

Hormonal therapy is another option for recurrent and metastatic endometrial cancer with response rates between 20% and 30%.

Progestins, antiestrogens, gonadotropin-releasing hormone analogues, aromatase inhibitors are used.

Well-differentiated tumours, grade 1 or 2,estrogen and progestin receptor-positive tumours show better response than poorly differentiated tumour.

**Targeted agents** have also shown some activity in the management of recurrent and metastatic endometrial cancer with response rates between 5 and 15% and progression-free survival between 2–6 months. The approved targeted agents are

Antiangiogenic agent—Bevacizumab

Phosphatidylinositol 3-kinase/mTOR inhibitor—Temsirolimus

### Recurrent and Metastatic Endometrial Cancer

I. **Hormonal Therapy**
   1. **Progestins**
      A. Medroxyprogesterone acetate (MPA): Inj. MPA 1 g/wk × 6 followed by monthly till progression or oral MPA 200 mg/day
      B. Hydroxyprogesterone caproate 1 g/wk × 6, foll. by monthly till progression
      C. Megesterol acetate 160 mg/day, till progression
   2. **Antiestrogens**
      Tab.Tamoxifen 20–40 mg/day
   3. **Gonadotropin-releasing analogues**
      Inj. Leuprolide
   4. **Selective estrogen-receptor modulator**
      Anastrazole 1 mg/day
      Arzoxifene 20 mg/day

II. **Targeted agents**
1. Bevacizumab
2. Temsirolimus

## Uterine Sarcoma

The types of uterine sarcomas, etiological factors, signs and symptoms and diagnosis are described in Chapter 21.

### Chemotherapy

**Leiomyosarcoma**

1. Doxorubicin 60 mg/$m^2$
   Ifosfamide 1.2 g/$m^2$ D 1–3, rpt q3 weeks × 6 cycles
2. Gemcitabine 900 mg/$m^2$ D1 and 8
   Docetaxel 75 mg/$m^2$ q3 weeks × 6 cycles

**Carcinosarcoma**

1. Ifosfamide 1.2 g/$m^2$, D 1–3
   Cisplatin 75 mg/$m^2$, Repeat q3 weeks × 6 cycles
2. Paclitaxel 175 mg/$m^2$ D1
   Carboplatin AUC 5 D1, Repeat q3 weeks × 6 cycles

**Endometrial stromal sarcoma**

Megesterol acetate 160–360 mg/day

## RECAP

- Cancer has become the leading cause of death in the world since 2011.
- Breast and cervical cancer are the most common cancers among women in India.
- Treatment of cancer includes surgery, radiotherapy, chemotherapy, targeted therapy and immunotherapy.
- Chemotherapy interferes with cellular DNA, RNA and protein synthesis and prevents cell growth or causes apoptosis.
- In targeted therapy, drugs target molecules that are uniquely or abnormally expressed within the cancer cells while sparing the normal cells.
- In immunotherapy, the patient's own immune system is stimulated to eliminate cancer cells.
- Chemotherapy can be curative, adjuvant, neoadjuvant and palliative. The most commonly used chemotherapeutic agents in the treatment of gynecological cancers are cisplatin, carboplatin, cyclophosphamide, paclitaxel, methotrexate, 5-fluorouracil, bleomycin, etoposide, actinomycin-D.
- Targeted agents include bevacizumab, temsirolimus.
- Immunotherapy includes pembrolizumab, CAR-T cell therapy.

## REVIEW QUESTIONS

### Long-Answer Questions

1. Discuss the various chemotherapeutic regimens for treatment of cancer cervix.

### Short-Answer Questions

1. Write a note on neoadjuvant chemotherapy.
2. What are the different phases of cell cycle in which the chemotherapeutic drugs act?

### MCQs

**1. Which is not a hormonal agent?**
   a) Medroxyprogesterone acetate
   b) Aromatase inhibitor
   c) Etoposide
   d) Megesterol

**2. Which drug is not part of the PEB regimen in the treatment of germ cell tumour?**
   a) Cisplatin
   b) Etoposide
   c) Pegylated liposomal doxorubicin
   d) Bleomycin

**Further Reading**

Aswathy S, Javed R, Dinesh A. Epidemiology of cervical cancer with special focus on India. Int J Wom Health. 2015;7:405–14.

Barakat RR, Berchuck A, Markman M, Randall ME. Editors. Principles and practice of gynecologic oncology, 6th ed. Philadelphia: Lippincott Williams and Wilkins; 2013.

DeVita VT, Lawrence TS, Rosenberg SA. Cancer: Principles and Practice of Oncology. 10th ed. Philadelphia: Wolters Kluwer; 2015.

Gerber DE. Targeted therapies: a new generation of cancer treatments. American Family Physician. 2008;77(3):311–19.

Skeel RT, Khlief SN. Handbook of Cancer Chemotherapy, 8th ed. Philadelphia: Lippincott Williams & Wilkins; 2011.

Gerber DETargeted therapiesnew generationca Https://www.mycancergenome.org/content/molecular-mediciline/overview-of-targeted-therapies-for-cancer treatmentsAmerican Family Physician.2008773): 311–319Overview of Targeted Therapies in Cancer;My Cancer Genome.

Cancer growth blokers/Cancer Research UK http://www.cancerresearchuk.org/about-cancer/cancers-in-general/treatment/biological/types/cancer-growth-blockers

Chapter 25

# Radiotherapy in Gynecological Cancer

**At a Glance**


Radiation Effects
Radiation Energy
- Radiation Dose
- Tumour Clearance

Radiobiology
Tissue Tolerance
Principles of Radiation Therapy
- Process

Radiotherapy in Gynecological Malignancy
- Cervical Cancer
- Carcinoma of the Cervical Stump
- Adenocarcinoma of the Cervix
- Endometrial Cancer
- Vulvar Cancer
- Vaginal Cancer
- Ovarian Cancer

Side Effects of Radiation Therapy
- Management of Radiation Reactions

Recent Advances
- External Beam Therapy
- Brachytherapy
- Imaging
- Biological Radiotherapy Planning

Translational Research in Radiation Oncology


## INTRODUCTION

The optimal management of gynecological cancers is best provided by a multidisciplinary team consisting of gyne-oncology surgeon, radiation oncologist, medical oncologist, radiologist, pathologist, palliative care team and social worker. More than 50% of such patients need radiation therapy and in malignancy, like early cervical cancer, radiation therapy plays a curative role. This multidisciplinary approach in the management of malignant diseases has paid high dividends in recent years. Radiation therapy especially precision techniques and advanced imaging have played a vital role in improving the therapeutic benefit by maximising tumour control and minimising side effects.

**Radiation Physics** Radiation is a form of emission and propagation of electromagnetic waves in the form of rays or particles. Radiation can be non-ionising or ionising depending upon the ejection of an excited electron from an atom or a molecule. This ionising form of radiation is used in therapeutic management.

## RADIATION EFFECTS

Ionising radiation (that is, alpha, beta, gamma, X-rays and heavy particles) produce **cell damage in all living cells**. The effect depends on the energy range of the radiation, the sensitivity of the tissue and other host factors. **Radiation injury is greater in actively multiplying tissues such as the gonads, hemopoietic tissue, lymphoid tissue, intestinal mucosa and epiphyses.**

The effect of radiation is brought about both by direct and indirect means resulting in chromosomal, nuclear and cytoplasmic damage. This molecular, cellular and tissue damage ultimately results in cell death. The normal tissue in the vicinity of the tumour also suffers damage but recovers, while the damage is pronounced in the tumour because of the high degree of mitotic division of its cells.

> The main objective in radiation oncology is to minimise the radiation damage and protect the normal tissue near the tumour, while producing an intense tumour-lethal effect in the tumour volume.

## RADIATION ENERGY

Radiation oncologists now have a wide range of radiation equipment and radionuclides at their disposal. We have moved from the era of deep X-ray (200–500 kV), to **megavoltage radiation** (over one million electron volt) which has ushered in a new era in radiotherapy for gynecological malignancy.

**Advantages** The advantages of megavoltage radiation are:

- better penetration
- increased percentage depth dose
- sparing of the skin at the treatment portal
- no increased bone absorption of radiation
- a diminished bone-shielding effect and simple radiation field set-up

The telecobalt unit and linear accelerator are the widely used megavoltage equipment in most radiation therapy centres.

Recently, particle therapy with fast neutrons, protons, electrons and carbon ions with greater clinical potential have revolutionised radiation therapy. In **particle therapy,** the lethal effect of radiation does not depend largely on the degree of oxygenation of the tumour, and the central anoxic zone in the tumour also gets equally damaged. Moreover, the radiation injury is produced at a precise depth of the volume of tissue irradiated thus sparing the normal tissue in the vicinity of the tumour. **Electron therapy** is ideally suited in the treatment of vulval carcinoma.

### Radiation Dose

The required dose of radiation is determined by

- the inherent sensitivity of the tumour
- the volume of the tissue to be irradiated
- the dose constraints of surrounding normal tissues

### Tumour Clearance

A **minimal clearance** of the tumour in squamous cell carcinoma, which is a moderately sensitive tumour is needed.

A **wide clearance** in sensitive tumours like lymphoma and dysgerminoma are essential.

Local as well as systemic tolerances depend on the radiation dose and the volume of the tumour to be treated. Hence in squamous cell cancer of the cervix, a dose of 7000 8000 rads to point A, and pelvic radiation of 5000–6000 rads is delivered over a period of 5–6 weeks (based on the SI unit system, Gy representing Gray is equivalent to 100 rads and 1 cGy is 1 rad).

## RADIOBIOLOGY

The effect of radiation depends on the 4Rs of radiobiology—repair of DNA damage, repopulation, redistribution and reoxygenation of hypoxic tumour cells.

Radiosensitivity is directly proportional to the degree of mitotic activity and inversely proportional to the degree of differentiation. This means that rapidly multiplying cells and anaplastic tumours are more sensitive to radiation. Germ cell tumours such as seminomas and dysgerminomas are highly sensitive; squamous cell carcinoma is moderately sensitive and osteogenic sarcoma is radio-resistant.

## TISSUE TOLERANCE

The tissue tolerance of radiation is variable and is an important factor in radiotherapy. The tissues are classified as **serial organs** and **parallel organs** to understand and predict the potential toxicity of radiation. A damage even on a short segment of a serial organ like spinal cord can cause significant toxicity whereas a similar damage in a parallel organ like the kidneys will not cause that profound morbidity due to the parallel alignment of its functional units. The tolerance of the skin, mucosa, hemopoietic tissue, kidney, liver, brain, spinal cord, lungs, gonads, eyes and epiphyses, if exceeded, will lead to disastrous sequelae. While delivering the lethal dose to the tumour, the dose to the normal tissue and the vital organs in the neighbourhood must be kept at a minimum.

The cell culture technique helps us to study cancer cell kinetics. The premitotic (G1) and mitotic (M) phases are the phases of the cell cycle most sensitive to radiation injury. If tumour cells are made to accumulate in this sensitive phase and irradiated, maximum tumour cell death can be achieved. This process of synchronisation can be produced by certain chemical agents.

Normally a large malignant tumour has poorly oxygenised central cells (anoxic cells) which are resistant to radiation injury, and can be overcome by increasing the concentration of oxygen in the blood circulating in the tumour volume. In hyperbaric oxygen therapy, the patient is put in a chamber and the oxygen concentration is raised to about 3 atmospheric pressures which increases the radiosensitivity of normal as well as tumour tissue. Similarly the sensitivity of the tumour can be increased by certain chemicals like vitamin K, actinomycin D, methotrexate, bleomycin and metronidazole. Hyperthermia is also found to increase the sensitivity of the tumour. The time-dose fraction system is based on the repair of sub-lethal damage, reoxygenation, repopulation and redistribution of cells at the treatment site.

## PRINCIPLES OF RADIATION THERAPY

Gynecological radiation therapy can be delivered by using teletherapy (given from a distance or externally) or by brachytherapy (given from very close or within the tumour/internally).

### Process

The process of radiation therapy involves
1. Clinical evaluation to assess the extent of disease
2. Radiotherapy planning
3. Plan evaluation
4. Plan approval
5. Treatment delivery
6. Quality assurance
7. Weekly monitoring

#### Clinical evaluation

Before delivering radiation, the target is defined during the planning process (Fig. 25.1). The visible tumour as seen or felt clinically and visualised on imaging is known as Gross Tumour Volume (GTV). The subclinical component of tumour along with the GTV is known as Clinical Target Volume (CTV). Planning target volume (PTV) is a geometrical concept which is a margin given around the CTV to account for the errors during patient setup and treatment delivery.

Teletherapy can be delivered using a radioactive source like cobalt-60 or high-energy photons using linear accelerator.

#### Radiation treatment planning

***i. Conventional planning***

The first step in treatment planning is to determine the exact location of the tumour, the precise definition of tumour depth and volume (Fig. 25.2). Then the cross-section of the body contour in the tumour plane is drawn and the location of the volume of the tumour marked. In collaboration with the physicist, the appropriate field size, number and angulation are decided. While directing the radiation beam, the treatment volume and the dose that would be received by the vulnerable structures in the vicinity of the tumour are plotted. Dosimetry helps to predetermine the dose at any point in the treatment volume and to avoid over- or underdosage. Simulator Unit, a technique in which the exact treatment condition is simulated, is often used for field verification and definition. While drawing a prescription for radiation treatment, the total tumour dose, the daily dose, the number of fractions, the overall time and the ancillary devices are mentioned.

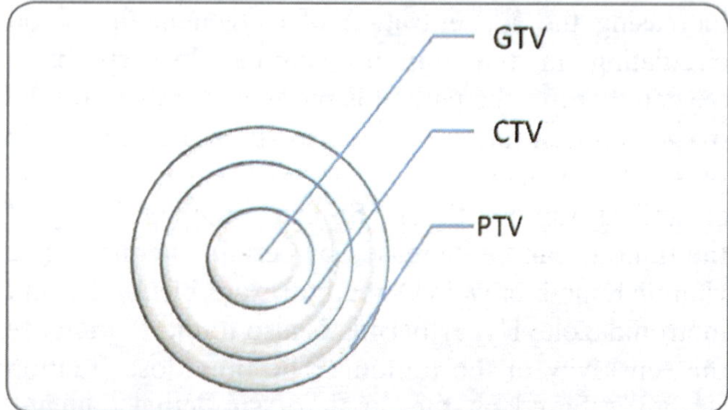


**Fig. 25.1** Defining planning process; GTV: gross tumour volume, CTV: clinical target volume, PTV: planning target volume

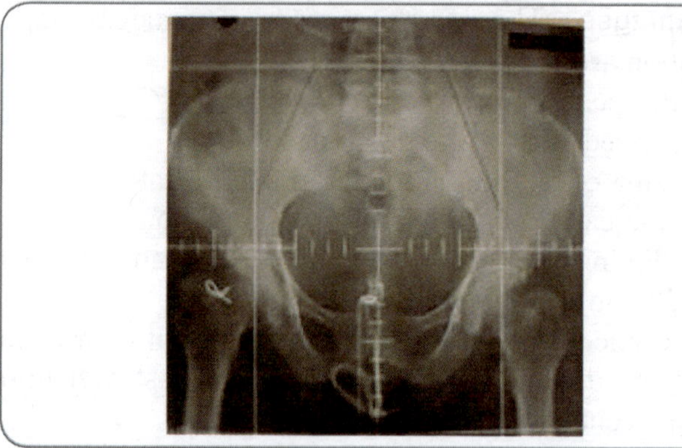

**Fig. 25.2** Conventional treatment planning

Simulation can be done by conventional method which involves acquiring a 2D orthogonal X-ray image of the area of interest with the desired treatment fields delineated on the patient body.

***ii. 3D CT planning***

A more technologically advanced method uses a CT-scan-based simulation where the patient's tumour region and the surrounding organs at risk are delineated and a 3D volume is rendered. Radiotherapy planning is then done conforming to the tumour volume as shown in Fig. 25.3.

This allows the oncologist to physically see the dose distribution to the target as well as the dose delivered to the organs at risk with the help of Dose Volume Histograms (DVHs).

***iii Intensity-modulated radiation therapy (IMRT) planning***

While 3D conformal planning optimises by defining the shape of radiation fields and optimising by modulating weightages of each beam and the use of tissue compensators, a more technologically advanced way of planning is by IMRT. During IMRT planning,

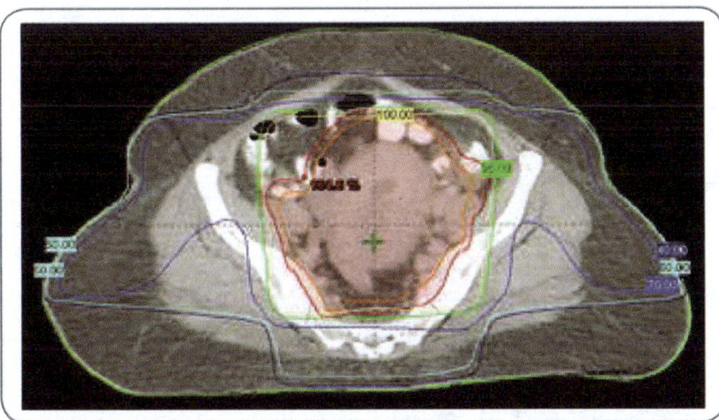

Fig. 25.3 CT-based planning

the target dose and dose constraints are predefined in the planning software and through a complex algorithm by intensity modulation, the dose is sculpted around the target while respecting the dose constraints of the surrounding organs at risk. The plan evaluation is again done using DVHs and a stringent quality assurance is necessary before starting the treatment on the patient.

### Quality assurance and treatment delivery

Once the patient's treatment plan is approved in the planning system, the calculated dose needs to be verified with the actual dose delivered on the treatment unit. This involves a complex process of physics dosimetry which often uses a phantom water bath to verify the calculated versus delivered dose.

Once the patient is positioned on the treatment couch to initiate treatment, the position is verified by a variety of systems ranging from simple skin surface markings to more advanced image-guided methods which use on-board CT scan on the therapy unit to verify the patient's anatomy rather than the skin marks alone. In precision techniques, this patient position verification is frequently repeated during the entire treatment schedule.

# RADIOTHERAPY IN GYNECOLOGICAL MALIGNANCY

## Cervical Cancer

Cervical cancer is one of the most radiosensitive tumour and has a high chance for cure with radiation. It continues to be the one of the most prevalent cancer in Indian women. **Radiation therapy plays a curative role in almost all the stages of Cervical Cancer.** The treatment for each case must be decided jointly by the radiotherapist, the gynecologist and the pathologist, and their close collaboration ensures the best outcome.

For early-stage IA, IB for medically inoperable patients and those who refuse surgery, radiation therapy is equally effective compared to surgery. For locally advanced cervical cancer IB2, IIB, III, IVA concurrent chemoradiation therapy with weekly Cisplatinum 40 $mg/m^2$ is considered the standard of care.

External radiation therapy is delivered by using a 4 field box technique to the pelvis in a dose of **50 Gy in 25 fractions, 5 fractions per week over a period of 5 weeks.** The treatment volume is planned to include the external iliac, internal iliac, obturator group of nodes. For stage IIIB tumours, the presacral nodes are also included in the radiation field to include the entire sacral hollow.

### Intracavitary brachytherapy

Once the central disease has shown good response, brachytherapy is delivered either by interdigitating with external radiation therapy or at the end of external radiotherapy. Cervical Intracavitary Brachytherapy is given by either **Low Dose Rate (LDR)** or **High Dose Rate (HDR).** Intracavitary therapy plays an important role in the treatment plan, delivering intense radiation to the cervical region with a rapid 'fall-off' of the dose to the paracervical tissue. The resultant radiation zone is pear-shaped, and the deficiency in the dose to the lateral parametria and the pelvic node is adequately supplemented and balanced by external beam therapy where parametrial radiation is needed Fig. 25.4. For Stage II, the desired total dose delivered by external radiation therapy and brachytherapy to point A is in the range of 80–85 Gy whereas for Stage III it is in the range of 85–90 Gy or equivalent.

### Interstitial brachytherapy

When at the end of external radiotherapy there is no significant reduction in the parametrium disease, intracavitary radiation therapy may not be sufficient to provide adequate dose to the parametrial disease. In such a situation interstitial brachytherapy (Fig. 25.5) is useful which uses the insertion of perineal needles in the parametrium while the patient is under anaesthesia in a lithotomy position. These needles when loaded with an Iridium-192 source along with the central uterine tandem ensure an adequate radiation dose to the residual disease. The treatment is currently delivered using a remote after loading HDR brachytherapy unit.

## Carcinoma of the Cervical Stump

In this case cancer occurs in the cervical stump following a subtotal hysterectomy. True stump cancer cases are assessed as for non-operated cases of cancer

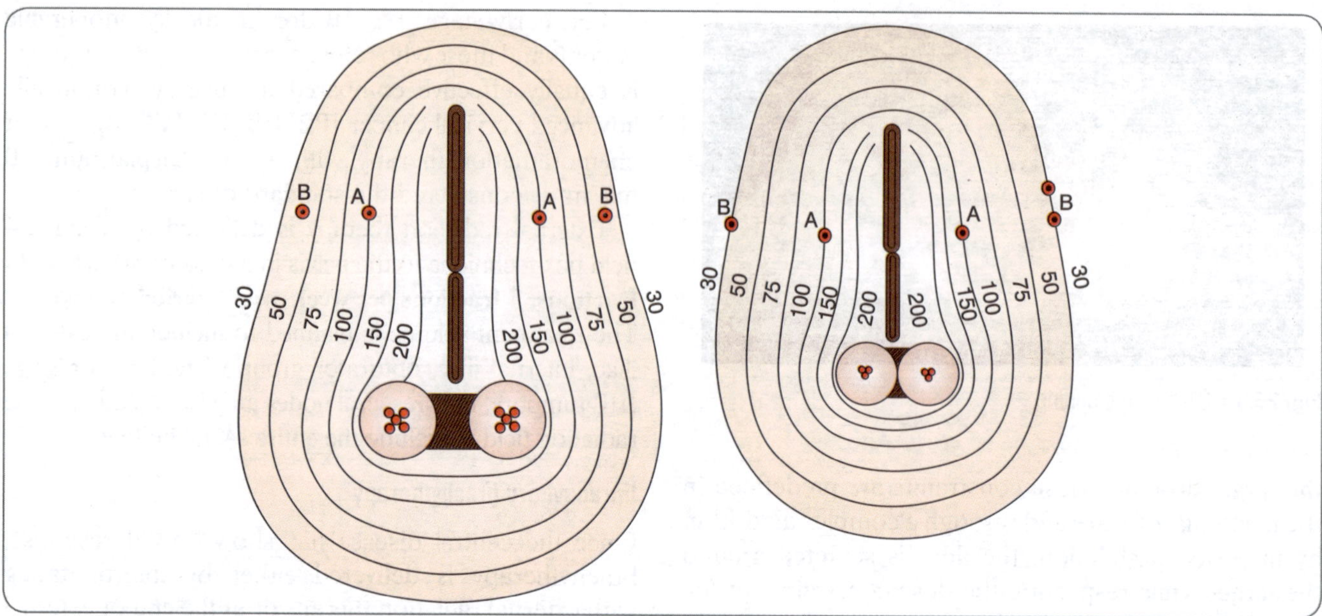


Fig. 25.4 Isodose curves of radiation for carcinoma of the cervix

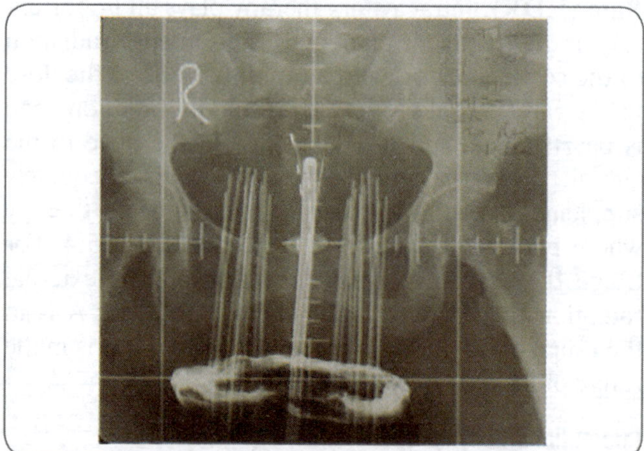


Fig. 25.5 Interstitial brachytherapy

of the cervix and intracavitary and external radiation are given. In these cases, however, the intracavitary application needs to be modified to suit the local altered anatomy. The prognosis is guarded in such cases.

## Adenocarcinoma of the Cervix

Adenocarcinoma of the cervix is generally of endocervical origin but a distinction must be made between a lesion of primarily endocervical origin and an extension of corpus cancer. The radiotherapeutic management is the same as for squamous cell carcinoma of the cervix, and a maximum tolerable cancericidal dose is planned. Because of the lower incidence of pelvic wall lymph node metastases, there is a greater emphasis on intracavitary radiation than on parametrial radiation. In radioresistant cases, radical surgery is advised.

**Pregnancy and carcinoma of the cervix** The stage of pregnancy has a great deal of influence on the line of treatment. In early pregnancy, Wertheim's hysterectomy is done for early cancer; for late cancer, radiation is given, ignoring the pregnancy. The pregnancy may terminate or spontaneous abortion may occur during therapy. For late pregnancy and early cancer, cesarean section followed by Wertheim's hysterectomy is advised; for late cancer, cesarean section followed by radiotherapy is indicated.

## Endometrial Cancer

Corpus cancer, mostly adenocarcinoma, is a disease of the postmenopausal age group and is not as sensitive to radiation as squamous cell carcinoma. The disease spreads by direct infiltration into the uterine muscle, via the lymphatics into the regional nodes and occasionally through the bloodstream to metastasise to the lungs, bones and liver. The prognosis depends on the grade of malignancy, the extent of myometrial invasion, the involvement of the internal os and the hormonal profile of the patient. In cases where the growth has infiltrated deep into the myometrium or where the nodes are positive, adjuvant radiotherapy is needed. Primary radiotherapy is indicated in elderly women with medical complications or in those where the growth has involved the cervix. In Heymann's packing technique, the uterine cavity is packed to its capacity with radioactive source capsules, delivering 6000 rads in two applications. In view of the risks and radiation hazards associated with this technique, it is not in vogue now. Usually, the conventional Manchester technique with the longest intrauterine tube is used, delivering a total of 8000 rads at 2 cm in two applications of 72 hours each, at an interval of one week. For inoperable corpus cancer, intracavitary radiotherapy is followed by external beam therapy (3000–3500 rads/four weeks). In addition to surgery and radiation, high-dose progesterone therapy is indicated in all cases showing involvement of the myometrium and internal os. Modern radiation techniques like intensity-modulated radiation therapy (IMRT) have made the delivery of postoperative radiation to patients safer and better tolerable.

### Vulvar Cancer

The most common malignant lesion of the vulva is squamous cell carcinoma. **The response to radiation is poor** due to the intolerance of the moist region to radiation and poor vascularity. Radical vulvectomy with bilateral block dissection of the nodes is preferred to radiation. In cases where surgery is not feasible, electron beam therapy is superior to other forms of radiation.

### Vaginal Cancer

**Vaginal carcinoma** is mostly of the squamous cell type. If an adenocarcinoma is encountered, a thorough search must be made for the primary in the uterus or other pelvic and abdominal organs. Direct and lymphatic spreads are common as there is a rich lymphatic anastamosis.

- Cancer in the upper third of the vagina is treated in the same way as cancer of the cervix with intrauterine and vaginal sources followed by external radiation.
- Cancer of the middle third is best treated by the megavoltage beam-directed technique. Growths arising in the lower third, if small and superficial, are treated with interstitial implantation or they are managed by external radiation. During the implantation of needles, extreme care must be taken to cover the tumour volume correctly and to avoid transfixing the bladder or the rectal mucosa. On most occasions, radiotherapy is preferred to extensive radical surgery.
- When it involves the lower third of the vagina, besides radiation to the primary growth, block dissection of the inguinal lymph nodes is also recommended.

### Ovarian Cancer

The standard of care for ovarian cancer is optimal cytoreduction with removal of uterus, ovaries, pelvic and para-aortic nodes and other tumour deposits. Treatment of advanced ovarian cancer necessitates adjuvant or neoadjuvant chemotherapy.

Due to the availability of effective chemotherapeutic agents for treating ovarian cancer, the role of radiation therapy is very limited. However earlier in adjuvant settings a historical technique "Moving Strip" technique was often practised. Recently there has been a renewed interest in assessing the feasibility of advanced radiotherapy techniques like intensity modulated radiation therapy (IMRT) with tomotherapy in ovarian cancer.There is also an emerging option of stereotactic ablative radiation (SABR) for isolated relapses in ovarian cancer.

## SIDE EFFECTS OF RADIATION THERAPY

While the aim of radiation therapy is to deliver minimal dose to the surrounding normal structures and high dose to the tumour, there is always a potential for side effects to surrounding normal structures. The radiation side effects can be

**Acute**—observed while the radiation is ongoing

**Subacute**—observed since the completion of radiation to up to 3 months

**Late**—manifest after 3 months since completing radiation and can surface even after a period of 2 years or more.

### Management of Radiation Reactions

The systemic and local radiation reactions depend on the volume of the area treated, the dose delivered and the tolerance of the tissues.

The **systemic reactions** include nausea, vomiting, anorexia, lassitude, sometimes fever and, in severe cases, convulsions. These symptoms are easily controlled with antiemetics and antihistamines.

- In case of nausea and vomiting associated with diarrhea, the electrolyte imbalance may have to be corrected, if necessary, with intravenous fluids.
- The associated leucopenia and thrombocytopenia (caused by bone marrow depression) may be transient, needing hematinics or fresh blood transfusion.
- The local radiation reactions are mainly due to mucosal intolerance. Mild degrees of enteritis, proctitis, proctosigmoiditis, colitis and cystitis may

be encountered late during therapy. Intestinal reactions are easily treated with antispasmodics, analgesics, antidiarrheal substances and a low-residue bland diet.

- The bladder symptoms are treated with a liberal fluid intake, potassium citrate mixture and urinary analgesics.
- The skin reactions are often of a mild degree and are usually not seen in megavoltage radiotherapy. The moist regions like the groin and the vulva are likely to show minimal moist peeling of the skin, for which 1% aqueous gentian violet solution is ideal. The region subjected to treatment should be kept clean and dry with talcum powder. In some cases, a late subcutaneous fibrosis may result.
- Deep pelvic fibrosis and pathological fractures are rare in clinical practice.
- Severe intestinal reactions such as gangrene of the bowel, stricture of the intestines, intestinal obstruction and fistula formation are likely when there are pre-existing adhesions in the abdominal cavity.
- The intracavitary radiation is likely to produce mild proctitis and cystitis which usually passes off with symptomatic treatment. The faulty position of the radium and the resultant high-dose effect in the paracervical tissue or the rectovaginal septum may lead to severe extrinsic rectal reaction. Severe bladder reaction may produce hematuria of varying degrees. Rectal and vaginal ulcerations are caused by a high dose of radiation.

**Late sequelae** such as vault stenosis and vaginal fibrosis are easily preventable by simple measures.

## RECENT ADVANCES

### External Beam Therapy

#### 3D Conformal Radiation Therapy (3DCRT)

With rapid improvements in technology, it is now possible to shape the area of radiation field by using a multileaf collimator which are in-built in the linear accelerator gantry head. This technique is known as 3D conformal radiation therapy which requires a "**Planning CT scan**" of the patient in the desired immobilisation position. This CT scan is then transferred onto an advanced treatment planning system where the anatomy of the tumour region and the organs at risk are reconstructed and a 3D-rendered structure set is available for "3D Planning".

#### Intensity-Modulated Radiation Therapy (IMRT)

With the introduction of multileaf collimator and complex planning algorithms, it is now possible to actually modulate the intensity of radiation so that the dose can be easily shaped even in the concavities of a treatment volume which otherwise is not possible with conventional and 3D conformal techniques (Fig. 25.6).

#### Image-Guided Radiation Therapy (IGRT)

During conventional and 3D conformal radiation, the patient is positioned daily by matching the tattoo marks on the skin surface. This is often not a true match with the patient's internal anatomy which is the actual area of treatment. This can sometimes lead to a mismatch of the planned fields and the delivered field of radiation. With the availability of on-board KV imaging and cone beam CT (CBCT) on the treatment unit, it is now possible to accurately match the patient's anatomy to achieve a highly reproducible daily treatment set-up of patients. Thus IGRT provides a technologically and biologically more accurate method of verifying and delivering radiation therapy.

#### MR-Linac

MR-Linac is one of the latest innovative ways of image-guided radiation therapy which incorporate an in-built MRI along with the linear accelerator. This option of onboard MRI will significantly enhance the quality of treatment verification by providing a superior anatomical registration.

### Brachytherapy

#### Intracavitary brachytherapy

Intracavitary brachytherapy has been the standard of care especially for locally advanced cervical cancer

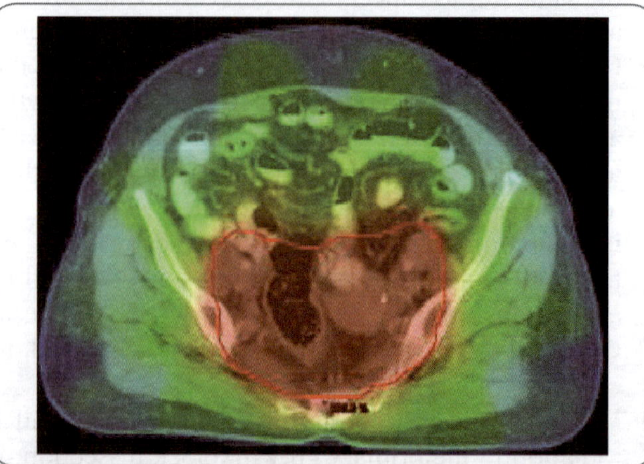

**Fig. 25.6** Intensity-modulated radiation therapy

during or at the completion of external radiation therapy. Conventionally the brachytherapy planning and dose calculation was done extrapolating the point A, rectal and bladder points using orthogonal X-ray films. This method had been successfully used for many years with reasonably good outcomes. With the availability of CT/MRI-based planning, it is now known that by using conventional method as mentioned above there is often a high probability of under-dosing the brachytherapy target volume. Several studies have shown that image-guided brachytherapy not only facilitates optimal dose delivery to the target volume but also minimises the dose to the organs at risk, which are actually visualised in a CT/MRI. Various investigators have also evaluated the role of ultrasound-guided brachytherapy for better optimisation.

## Imaging

### PET-CT

With the prompt availability of radioisotope tracers like 18 FDG (fludeoxyglucose), a functional PET-CT scan is increasingly being incorporated in the evaluation, radiotherapy planning and assessment of disease status after completing radiation therapy.

Several non-FDG-based tracers are also being studied. Among them, as markers of hypoxia within large neoplastic lesions include, 18F-MISO, 64Cu-ATSM, 18F-EF5, which highlight the presence of hypoxic areas. This imaging of hypoxic areas can be particularly useful for patients who must be treated with radiotherapy.

### Functional MRI

While MRI is known to provide a high-quality morphological imaging, another emerging role is the qualitative analysis of the water molecules diffusion in the tissues by the interpretation of the signal intensity in the area of interest by a functional MRI. The quantitative analysis can also be performed calculating the apparent diffusion coefficient (ADC) attributing absolute values in $mm^2/s$ for the signal intensity of the area of interest.

### PET/MRI

Hybrid imaging using CT scan and PET has been extensively used combining the morphological and functional data. Recently with the technological adanvces in computer software and hardware it has become possible to combine the superior morphological imaging of MRI and the functional data obtained in PET by using PET/MRI.

## Biological Radiotherapy Planning

This advanced technique incorporates acquiring the biological data from a functional scan like a PET-CT scan.The functional scan can help in identifying within the tumour volume, heterogeneous regions of variable tumour activity, which can then be selectively and differentially delivered varying the dose of radiation therapy.

## TRANSLATIONAL RESEARCH IN RADIATION ONCOLOGY

With the rapid advances in molecular biology techniques and understanding of the underlying biology of various interactions of radiation therapy, there are various biomarkers/genes under investigation which can predict the radiation response and probability of normal tissue toxicity. This area of translational research in the near future will play a major role in the practice of Personalised Radiation Oncology and also improve therapeutic benefits and ultimately the survival of cancer patients.

While it is important to be up-to-date with the modern technologically advanced radiation facilities and evidence-based medicine, it is equally important to be pragmatic especially in a resource-constrained scenario to practise what is relevant and ethically appropriate.

## RECAP

- Radiation therapy plays a significant role in the management of gynecological cancers.
- Teletherapy or external beam radiation is delivered using a radioactive cobalt-60 source or using high-energy photons with linear accelerator.
- There has been a renewed interest in the use of particle beam radiation therapy with protons and carbon ion.
- Radiotherapy is often used with a curative intent in highly radiosensitive tumours like cervical cancers.

- It also plays an important role in adjuvant settings in endometrial, vulval and vaginal cancers.
- For incurable conditions, radiation continues to offer an effective option for palliation.
- With technological advancements, precision radiation therapy techniques like IMRT and IGRT significantly improve the therapeutic benefit of radiation therapy.
- Brachytherapy plays an important role in delivering high dose from within the tumour and can be delivered by manual or remote afterloading techniques using cesium-137 or iridium-192 radioactive sources.
- Image-guided brachytherapy is an emerging modality for volume-based brachytherapy.
- Translational research in radiation oncology is investigating novel biomarkers for radiation response and toxicity so as to enable personalised radiation therapy delivery which will be the future.

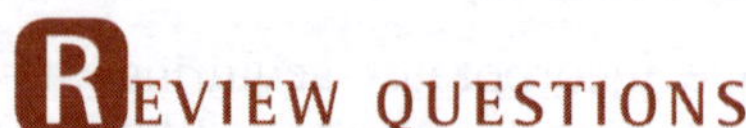

## REVIEW QUESTIONS

### Long-Answer Questions

1. Describe the role of radiation therapy in gynecological cancer.

2 What is radiation? Explain in brief the various modalities of radiation therapy used in gynecological cancers.

### Short-Answer Questions

1. What are the recent advances in external beam therapy?
2. Describe the management of radiation reaction.

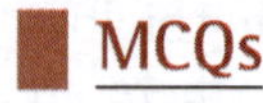

### MCQs

**1. MR Linac**

a) incorporates an in-built MRI along with the linear accelerator
b) is a form of brachytherapy
c) is the other name for PET-CT
d) is a functional MRI

**2. Cancer of the middle third of the vagina is best treated by**

a) Electron beam therapy
b) Interstitial implantation
c) Megavoltage beam-directed technique
d) Intrauterine and vaginal sources

**3 Interstitial brachytherapy is used**

a) in carcinoma of the cervical stump
b) in adenocarcinoma of the cervix
c) when cancer cervix is associated with pregnancy
d) when there is no significant reduction in the parametrium disease

**4. Intensity-Modulated Radiation Therapy (IMRT) Planning is**

a) Used in the treatment of cancer cervix
b) A radiation treatment planning method
c) Used in the treatment of endometrial cancer
d) Used in the treatment of cervical stump carcinoma

**Further Reading**

Casciato DA. Manual of clinical oncology. 7th ed. Philadelphia: Wolters Kluwer; 2015.

Hansen E, Roach III,M, editors. Handbook of evidence based radiation oncology. 2nd ed. New York: Springer; 2010.

Seshadri L. Essentials of gynaecology. 2nd ed. Gurgaon: Wolters Kluwer; 2017.

# Uterovaginal Prolapse

## At a Glance

Definition
Incidence
Supports of the Uterus
Pelvic Musculature
Etiology
Classification Systems
I. Shaw's System
II. Jeffcoate's System
III. Baden-Walker System
IV. POPQ Classification
Clinical Evaluation
Examination
Examination Components
Equipment
Patient Positioning
Documentation
Visual Inspection
Speculum and Bimanual Examination
Using the POPQ system
POPQ Measurements
Additional Examination Techniques
Simulated Apical Support
Inspection for Paravaginal Defects
Rectovaginal Examination
Neuromuscular examination
Differential Diagnosis
Management
Medical Therapy
Surgical Management

The gradual increase in life expectancy in developed countries over the past century has produced an increased demand on the health care system for geriatric population. Pelvic organ prolapse (POP) and urinary incontinence (UI) are common conditions affecting many adult women today.

## DEFINITION

Pelvic organ prolapse is the abnormal descent or herniation of the pelvic organs from their normal attachment sites or their normal position in the pelvis.

Uterovaginal prolapse is a type of displacement of the uterus and vaginal walls and is also called pelvic organ prolapse. Normally the external os of the cervix is at the level of ischial spines; if the external os moves below the level of ischial spine, it is considered as pelvic organ prolapse.

## INCIDENCE

The exact prevalence of POP is difficult to determine. However, it is estimated that the lifetime risk of requiring at least 1 operation to correct incontinence or prolapse is approximately 11%. Over 50% of asymptomatic women presenting for annual gynecological examination have at least stage 2 prolapse on examination. **Nearly 5–8% of gynecological admissions are due to symptomatic uterovaginal prolapse.**

## SUPPORTS OF THE UTERUS

A detailed account of the pelvic musculature and the uterine support is given in Chapter 3. However the relevant portions related to prolapse of the uterus will be discussed here.

### Pelvic Musculature

The uterus is maintained in its normal position by the following:

1. The **inherent muscle tone** of the uterus keeps it in the anteflexed position. In asthenic conditions and in the postpartum period, the myometrium becomes lax and the body of the uterus falls back on the cervix to lie in the line of the vagina, facilitating the descent of the uterus through the vagina on straining.

2. The **two levator ani muscles** covered by a dense layer of pelvic fascia constitute the pelvic floor (Fig. 26.1). This is pierced in the midline by the urethra, the vagina and the rectum. The levator ani muscles consist of three parts, the pubococcygeus, the iliococcygeus and the ischiococcygeus. The iliococcygeus and ischiococcygeus form the lateral part of the pelvic floor and do not directly support the pelvic viscera. The pubococcygeus is the most important part. It arises from the back of the pubic rami and passes backwards to be inserted into the coccyx and anococcygeal raphe. The innermost fibres (the puborectalis) decussate behind the rectum at the level at which it turns backward to form the anal canal. Some fibres decussate between the vagina and rectum and divide the opening in the pelvic floor into two parts, the urogenital hiatus anteriorly and the rectal hiatus posteriorly. When these fibres are stretched or torn during childbirth, the urogenital hiatus becomes patulous allowing the uterus and the vagina to prolapse through the pelvic floor. In addition to the innermost fibres of the puborectalis which decussate between the vagina and the rectum, the muscles of the perineum consisting of the bulbocavernosus, the superficial and deep transverse perineii and the sphincter ani converge on and are inserted into the perineal body. This pyramid-shaped structure lies between the lower third of the vagina and the anus and forms the central point of the perineum.
3. **Ligaments supporting the uterus** The pelvic cellular tissue is condensed to form ligaments supporting the uterus and other pelvic structures and fixing them to the side of the pelvis (Figs. 26.2 and 26.3).
   - The uterosacral ligaments pass from the supravaginal portion of the cervix and the vagina backwards lateral to the rectum to be inserted to the second and third sacral vertebrae.

     The **transverse cervical ligaments Mackenrodt's ligaments** (also called **cardinal ligaments**) extend from the cervix and from the upper part of the vagina, or to the side wall of the pelvis.
   - Anteriorly, the pubo-vesico-cervical ligament plays an important role in supporting the cervix and the bladder.

   Whereas the uterosacral ligaments keep the uterus anteverted by pulling the cervix behind, the transverse cervical ligaments help prevent the descent of the uterus whenever there is increased intra-abdominal pressure.

### Risk Factors

- Pregnancy
- Childbirth
- Factors contributing to chronic increases in intra-abdominal pressure such as lifting, coughing or straining,
- Connective tissue disorders
- Damage to or weakness of the muscles

## ETIOLOGY

Pelvic organ prolapse occurs as a result of the following.

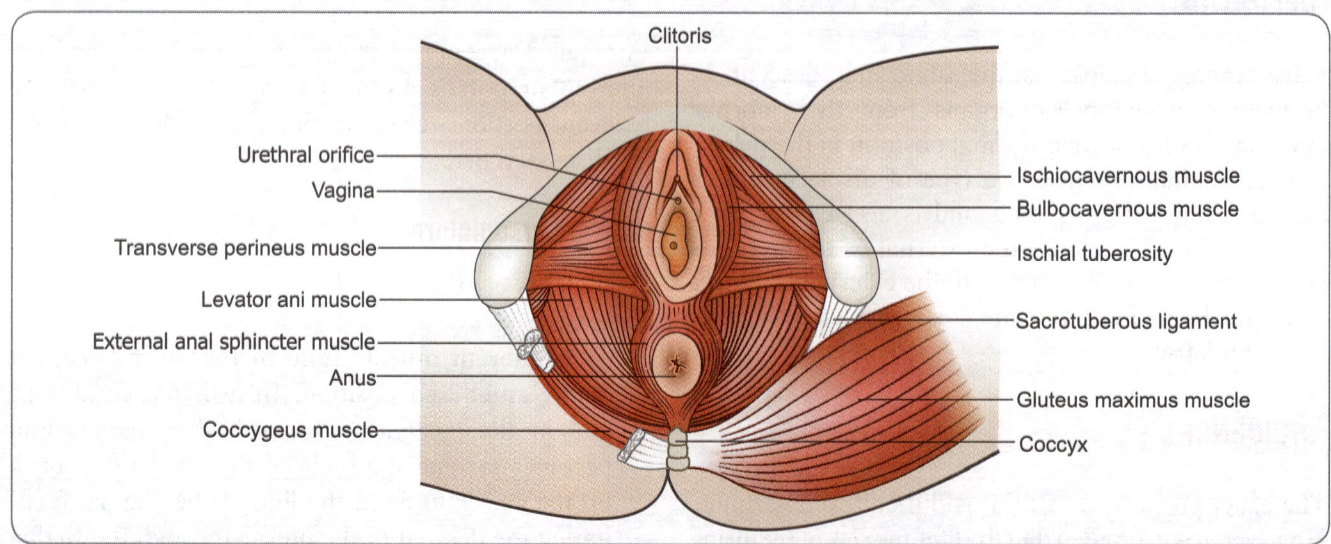


**Fig. 26.1** Muscles of the pelvic floor

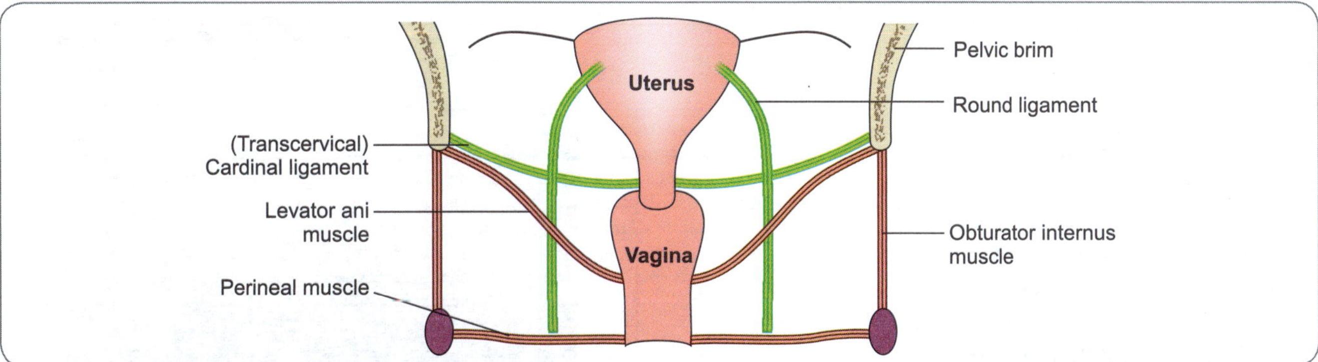


**Fig. 26.2** Diagrammatic representation of ligamentous and muscular supports of uterus

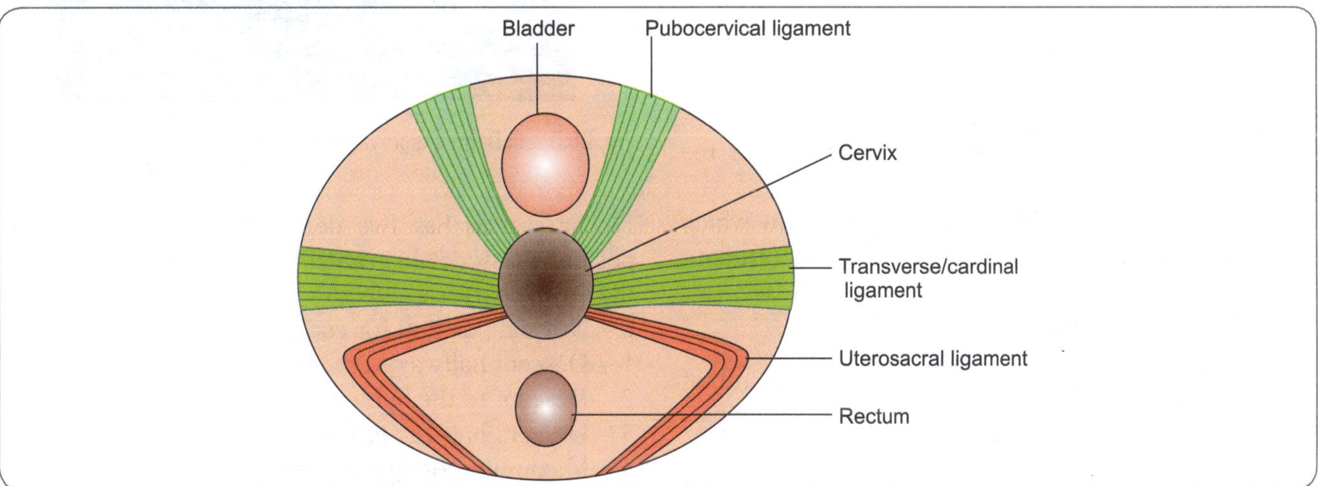


**Fig. 26.3** Ligamentous supports of uterus

**Inherited racial difference** It can be explained on the basis of differences in the pelvic architecture, quality of supporting pelvic muscles and connective tissues.

**Environmental and social factors** These factors may be contributing towards reproductive function and care, participation in hard physical labour and pelvic infections.

**Difficult childbirth** This causes excessive stretching and tearing of the endopelvic fascia and the levator muscles and perineal body. Partial pudendal and perineal neuropathies are also associated with labour. Impaired nerve transmission during pregnancy to the muscles of the pelvic floor may predispose them to decreased tone, leading to further sagging and stretching. Difficult deliveries, mismanaged labour, obstructed and prolonged labour, bearing down in incompletely dilated cervix, difficult instrumental deliveries, crude methods to remove placenta, etc. are responsible for POP. Considering these factors, multiparous women are at higher risk for genital prolapse.

**Menopause, genital atrophy and hypoestrogenism** These play important contributory roles in the pathogenesis of prolapse. However, the exact mechanisms are not completely understood.

Apart from the above-said major causes, the following conditions also contribute significantly to POP.

- Pelvic tumours
- Sacral nerve disorders
- Diabetic neuropathy
- Chronic medical conditions associated with increase in intra-abdominal pressure (e.g., obesity, chronic pulmonary disease, smoking, constipation)
- Rare abnormalities in connective tissue (collagen), such as Marfan disease
- Chronic lung diseases resulting from tobacco abuse
- Chronic bronchitis
- Neglected dystocia and traumatic vaginal delivery
- Excess weight gain
- Tight corsets
- Anal stenosis and chronic constipation
- Hard physical exertion and physical activities

Hence preventive strategies should always be implemented to prevent genital organ prolapse.

## CLASSIFICATION SYSTEMS

### I. Shaw's System

**A. Anterior vaginal wall defect**
1. Upper 2/3 cystocele
2. Lower 1/3 urethrocele

**B. Posterior vaginal wall defect**
1. Upper 1/3 enterocele
2. Middle 1/3 rectocele
3. Lower 1/3 deficient perineum

**C. Uterine prolapse**
1. Grade 0: Normal position
2. Grade 1 (or first degree): descent into vagina not reaching introitus
3. Grade 2 (or second degree): descent up to the introitus
4. Grade 3 (or third degree): descent outside the introitus
5. Grade 4 (or Procidentia): a condition in which the entire uterus comes outside the vulval outlet

### II. Jeffcoate's System

The grading for vaginal prolapse is the same as in that of the Shaw's system, but for uterocervical prolapse, the grading is different and is as follows:
1. First degree: descent into vagina not reaching introitus
2. Second degree: descent up to the introitus
3. Third degree or complete or general prolapse: Procidentia (Figs. 26.4 and 26.5).

### III. Baden-Walker System

The grade/degree is defined as the extent of prolapse for each structure noted on examination while the patient is straining.

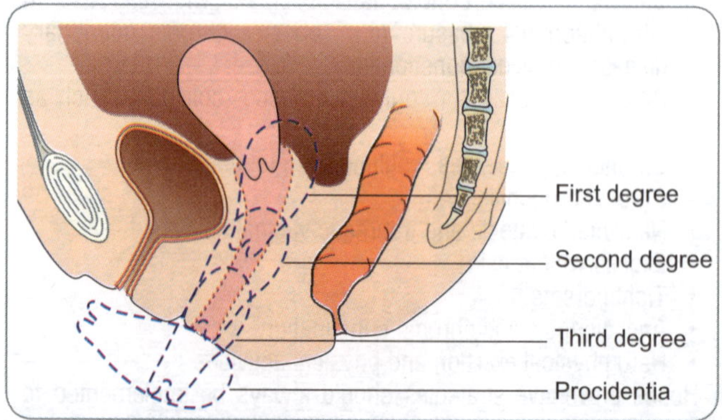


**Fig. 26.4** Degrees of uterine prolapse

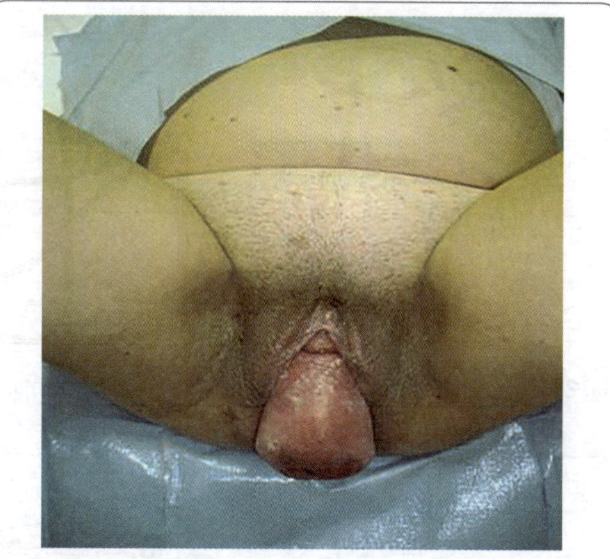

**Fig. 26.5** III Degree uterovaginal prolapse

The system has five degrees/grades. For urethra, posterior descent is graded, for other anatomic sites, the lowest part is graded:
0 – Normal position for each respective site
1 – Descent halfway to the hymen
2 – Descent to the hymen
3 – Descent halfway past the hymen
4 – Maximum possible descent for each site

### IV. POPQ Classification

**Pelvic Organ Prolapse Quantification System (POPQ)**

| Stage | Description |
|---|---|
| 0 | No prolapse anterior and posterior points are all −3 cm, and C or D is between −(Total vaginal length) and −(TVL-2) cm. |
| 1 | The criteria for stage 0 are not met, and the most distal prolapse is more than 1 cm above the level of the hymen (less than −1 cm). |
| 2 | The most distal prolapse is between 1 cm above and 1 cm below the hymen (at least one point is −1, 0, or +1). |
| 3 | The most distal prolapse is more than 1 cm below the hymen but no further than 2 cm less than TVL. |
| 4 | Represents complete procidentia or vault eversion; the most distal prolapse protrudes to at least (TVL-2) cm. |

#### Modifications of the POPQ system

***Simplified POPQ (S-POPQ)***

A simplified version of the POP-Q system (Fig. 26.6), which was developed by an international

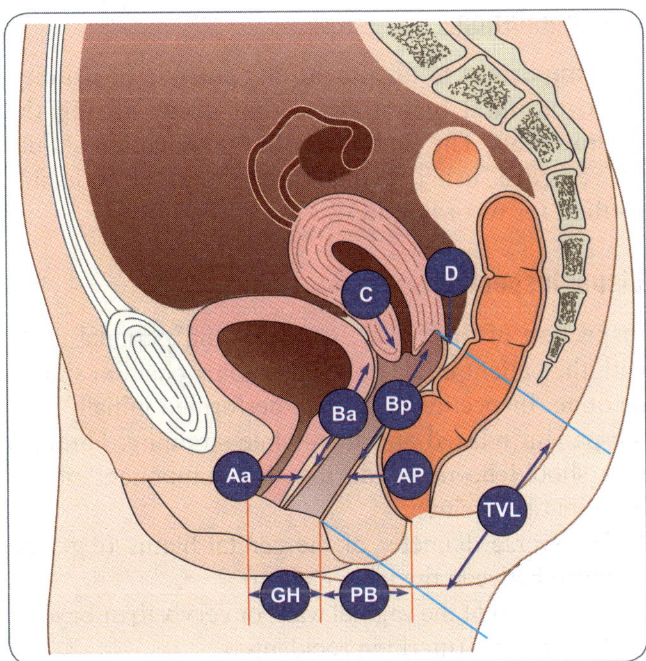


Fig. 26.6 Simplified POPQ system

group of investigators, has been proposed. Simple POPQ (S-POPQ) measures the anterior, posterior and up to two measurements of the apex, including both the cervix, in women who still have one, and posterior cul-de-sac. **It records the ordinal stage of the four measurements by estimating the distances involved.**

For measurement of the anterior wall, a point approximately 3 cm or halfway up the anterior vaginal wall is visualised, the woman is asked to strain, and the amount of descent is recorded. A similar process is carried out to estimate the descent of the posterior wall. Finally, a Sims speculum is utilised to record the descent of the apex of the vagina. The following definitions are used to stage the prolapse:

**Stage 1** Prolapse where the given point remains at least 1 cm above the hymenal remnants.

**Stage 2** Prolapse where the given point descends to the introitus, defined as an area extending from 1 cm above to 1 cm below the hymenal remnants.

**Stage 3** Prolapse where the given point descends greater than 1 cm past the hymenal remnants, but does not represent complete vaginal vault eversion or complete uterine procidentia.

This implies that at least some portion of the vaginal mucosa is not everted.

**Stage 4** Complete vaginal vault eversion or complete uterine procidentia. This implies that the vagina and/or uterus are maximally prolapsed with essentially the entire extent of the vaginal mucosa everted.

The S-POPQ has been validated against the original staging system of the POPQ and has been found to be highly correlative.

### *SLmax*

SLmax, also known as **maximum vaginal descent**, was introduced as a continuous value of vaginal support, which describes prolapse as a single-summary score. This measure is calculated as a single score for comparison of prolapse between populations and is not meant to replace the more detailed POPQ. SLmax simply represents the most distal presenting part of the vagina, in centimetres. The minimum value is −3 by definition, and the measure was shown to correlate well with POPQ measurements and results of the Pelvic Organ Prolapse Distress Inventory.

## CLINICAL EVALUATION

The points to be addressed in the clinical evaluation are

1. Age, desire to preserve reproductive and coital function, general medical status, past history of surgical corrections, symptoms and their impact on quality of life and then physical examination.
2. Decision on the correction will greatly depend on the degree of symptoms and its relationship with the clinical assessment.
3. The issue of rate of progression should be addressed as the management of rapidly progressive is different from that of slowly progressive prolapse.

A detailed history especially obstetric history is essential.

**Symptoms**

1. Protrusion of mass at vaginal introitus.
2. Often patients complain that there is a feeling as if "Everything is falling out."
3. The prolapsed becomes more prominent and hangs down further while standing and the symptoms are relieved by lying down.
4. Physical and psychological difficulty during intercourse.
5. Organ-specific complaints
   - cystocele—history of voiding difficulties including incontinence
   - rectocele—the need to use enema regularly for defecation
   - enterocele—chronic backache

## EXAMINATION

### Examination Components

Physical examination of women with POP includes the following components:

1. Visual inspection
2. Speculum examination
3. Bimanual pelvic examination
4. Rectovaginal examination
5. Neuromuscular examination

Each component of the examination is discussed in the sections below.

### Equipment

Instruments that are useful in assessment of pelvic prolapse include a

- Sims retractor (single blade speculum)
- Bivalve speculum that can be easily taken apart so that the anterior and posterior blades can be used separately to observe individual compartments of the vagina (anterior, posterior, apical).
- To make the measurements for the POPQ system, a ruler or a large cotton swab or sponge forceps marked in 1 cm increments is used.

### Patient Positioning

- Examination is performed in each position with the woman relaxed and then using valsalva maneuver* (to demonstrate the maximum degree of prolapse and delineating the compartment). The extent of prolapse visualised on examination should confirm the patient's description of bulging symptoms. If the severity of prolapse visualised does not correlate with the patient's description, the extent of the actual prolapse may be demonstrated to the patient by holding a hand-held mirror, so that she could appreciate the extent clearly by herself.

After examination in the **lithotomy** or **lateral** position, the examination is repeated with the **patient standing**. This position will best approximate the extent of prolapse that the patient experiences. In the standing position, the patient places one foot on a well-supported footstool. The examining gown is lifted slightly to expose the genital area during the examination.

*Valsalva maneuver is performed by attempting to forcibly exhale while keeping the mouth and nose closed.

### Documentation

**It is important to document any episode of urinary, fecal, or flatal incontinence that occur during the examination.** The findings of the examination should be recorded using a quantitative and reproducible method for recording POP.

### Visual Inspection

Inspection of the vulvar, perineal, and perianal areas with the patient in the dorsal lithotomy position should be done. Inspection should be performed initially with the patient relaxed and then while straining. Findings that should be noted during this component of the examination include:

1. Transverse diameter of the genital hiatus (e.g., the space between the labia majora)
2. Protrusion of the vaginal walls or cervix to or beyond the introitus (uterine procidentia)
3. Length and condition of the perineum
4. Rectal prolapse
5. In patients with prolapse to or beyond the hymen, the vaginal tissue is examined for ulceration like decubitus ulcer, which is due to chronic exposure of the cervix to the exterior and reduced blood supply.
6. Any other findings (e.g., skin or mucosal lesions) should be noted and evaluated appropriately.

### Speculum and Bimanual Examination

Prolapse of each anatomic compartment is evaluated as follows:

1. **Apical prolapse (prolapse of the cervix or vaginal vault)** A bivalve speculum is inserted into the vagina and then slowly withdrawn; any descent of the apex is noted.
2. **Anterior vaginal wall** A Sim's retractor or the posterior blade of a bivalve speculum is inserted into the vagina with gentle pressure on the posterior vaginal wall to isolate visualisation of the anterior vaginal wall.
3. **Posterior vaginal wall** A Sim's retractor or the posterior blade of a bivalve speculum is introduced the vagina with gentle pressure on the anterior vaginal wall to isolate visualisation of the posterior vaginal wall.
   - The terms anterior vaginal wall prolapse, posterior vaginal wall prolapse and apical prolapse are preferred to the terms "cystocele," "rectocele," and "enterocele" because vaginal topography does not reliably predict the location of the associated viscera in women with POP.

- To complete the exam, a bimanual examination is performed in order to evaluate any coexisting pelvic abnormalities.

## USING THE POPQ SYSTEM

As described earlier, all these points are taken together and these measurements can be used to produce a sagittal diagram of the prolapse.

During the examination, the maximum extent of prolapse is determined for each of the six points.

Maximal prolapse is defined by the following findings:
1. Vaginal wall becomes tight during straining
2. Traction on the prolapse causes no further descent
3. Patient confirms that protrusion is maximal

The maximal point of prolapse of each of the six points is then recorded in relation to a fixed point of reference, the anterior–posterior plane of the hymen.

**All measurements are expressed in centimetres**; increments of 0.5 cm can also be used, if clinically useful. A minus sign is used to designate a point that is proximal, or superior, to the hymenal plane (e.g., −3 cm), while points distal or inferior to the hymenal plane are preceded by a positive sign (e.g., +2 cm).

The measurements can be marked on line diagrams, noted on a grid or recorded in text form.

### POPQ Measurements

Each point is located by measuring along the vaginal wall or identifying the most dependent point of a prolapsed structure. The measurement is then taken of the distance from the point to the hymenal plane. The anatomic location of each point is as follows:

#### I. Anterior vaginal wall points

a) **Aa** is located in the midline of the anterior vaginal wall, 3 cm proximal to the external urethral meatus, corresponding approximately to the urethrovesical junction. The quantitative value of point Aa is anywhere from –3 to +3 cm from the hymenal plane, depending upon the extent of anterior wall prolapse.
b) **Ba** is the most distal (i.e., most dependent) position of any part of the anterior vaginal wall between point Aa and the vaginal cuff or anterior vaginal fornix. If there is no prolapse, point Ba is –3 cm by definition. In a woman with total post hysterectomy vault prolapse, Ba has a positive value equal to the distance between the vaginal apex and hymenal plane (so the quantitative value of point Ba can range from the most supported measurement −3, to the most prolapsed portion beyond the hymenal ring (this may exceed +3 cm).

#### II. Superior vaginal wall points

a) **C** is the most distal (i.e., most dependent) edge of the cervix or the leading edge of the vaginal cuff (post hysterectomy).
b) **D** is measured only in women with a cervix. It is the deepest point of the posterior fornix, corresponding approximately to where the uterosacral ligaments attach to the posterior cervix. Measuring this point distinguishes between suspensory failure of the uterosacral-cardinal ligament complex and cervical elongation: if point C is significantly more positive than point D (>4 cm), the cervix is elongated.

#### III. Posterior vaginal wall points

These are analogous to the two points on the anterior wall.

a. **Ap** is located in the midline of the posterior vaginal wall, 3 cm proximal to the posterior hymen. The quantitative value of point Ap is anywhere from –3 to +3 cm from the hymenal plane, depending upon the extent of posterior wall prolapse.
b. **Bp** is the most distal (i.e., most dependent) position of any part of the upper posterior vaginal wall between point Ap and the vaginal cuff or posterior vaginal fornix. If there is no prolapse, point Bp is –3 cm by definition. In a woman with total post hysterectomy vaginal prolapse, Bp has a positive value equal to the distance between the vaginal apex and hymenal plane (so the quantitative value of point Bp can range from the most supported measurement [−3], to the most prolapsed portion beyond the hymenal ring [this may exceed +3 cm]).
c. Total vaginal length (**TVL**) is measured by reducing point C or D to its most superior position (e.g., with a swab or ring forceps).
d. Genital hiatus (**gh**) is measured anterioposteriorly from the middle of the external urethral meatus to the posterior midline hymen. If the location of the hymen is obscured by a band of skin (usually from surgery or episiotomy repair), the firm tissue of the perineal body is the posterior margin of this measurement.

e. The perineal body (**pb**) is measured from the posterior margin of the genital hiatus to the mid-anal opening.

## ADDITIONAL EXAMINATION TECHNIQUES

### Simulated Apical Support

Repeating the speculum examination with simulated apical support (i.e., supporting the vaginal apex with a large cotton swab or ring forceps) approximates the results following apical prolapse repair. Reduction of apical prolapse temporarily corrects anterior and posterior vaginal wall prolapse in many women. This examination technique may help a clinician decide whether a vaginal pessary may be helpful or, in preoperative patients, whether to perform apical prolapse relapse repair.

### Inspection for Paravaginal Defects

Paravaginal defects occur when the anterior vaginal wall detaches from its lateral support, the arcus tendineus. The arcus tendineus is a line of connective tissue that runs from posterior (ischial spine) to anterior (symphysis pubis) anteriorly. Surgical repair of paravaginal defects is not typically performed as it does not improve surgical outcomes.

### Rectovaginal Examination

A rectovaginal examination is performed to diagnose an enterocele, differentiate between a high rectocele and an enterocele, assess the integrity of the perineal body and detect rectal prolapse. The best method for detecting an enterocele is to perform the rectovaginal exam with the patient standing; the small bowel can be palpated in the cul-de-sac between the thumb and forefinger.

### Neuromuscular Examination

**Neurologic evaluation** Neurological examination is helpful not only to rule out any neurological etiology but also to assess the strength of the pelvic floor muscles, which in turn would indicate the outcome of pelvic floor repair (vide infra).

i. **Lumbosacral dermatomes** Sensory function for light touch and sharp touch is performed using a small cotton swab and a sharp point. If sensory function is abnormal, more detailed neurologic testing may be warranted.

ii. **Sacral reflexes** To evaluate sacral nerve integrity, the **bulbocavernosus reflex** is elicited by gently tapping or squeezing the clitoris. The **anocutaneous reflex (anal wink sign)** is triggered by stroking the skin immediately surrounding the anus and observing a reflexive contraction of the external anal sphincter; this reflex should be elicited bilaterally. Sacral nerve route motor function is further evaluated by having the patient move the lower extremity; this includes active extension and flexion of the knee, ankle, and toes. Strength is assessed by having the patient move each joint against resistance. The patellar and plantar reflexes are also assessed.

**Pelvic floor muscle testing** To evaluate integrity and symmetry of the pelvic floor, the examiner should also note the presence of scarring, for example, due to episiotomy, and whether pelvic floor contraction pulls the perineum inward. Palpation through the vagina or rectum helps in assessing pelvic floor squeeze strength and levator muscle thickness. The tone and strength of the pelvic floor muscles can be assessed by asking the patient to contract the pelvic floor muscles around the examining fingers. Women with poor pelvic floor muscle function may benefit from pelvic physical therapy.

#### Guidelines to Assess Pelvic Floor Musculature

Guidelines have been published by the International Continence Society to assess pelvic floor musculature tone and four conditions have been defined:

i. **Normal** pelvic floor muscles are those which can voluntarily contract and relax,
ii. **Overactive** pelvic floor muscles are those which do not relax
iii. **Underactive** pelvic floor muscles are those which cannot voluntarily contract.
iv. **Non-functioning** pelvic floor muscles are when there is no pelvic floor muscle action palpable.

**Ancillary studies**

1. **Imaging** There are few clinical uses of imaging to evaluate the anatomic findings of prolapse. Imaging techniques are used for some aspects of evaluation of urinary or bowel functions.
2. **Dynamic magnetic resonance imaging** This is under investigation for use in identifying site-specific pelvic support defects, as well as for differentiating between a rectocele and an enterocele. However, there are no standardised criteria for use of this

modality for the diagnosis of POP and it is largely used for research purposes.

3. **Urinary tract evaluation** Urinary tract evaluation for women with prolapse is guided by an individual patient's complaints (e.g., incontinence, urinary retention). Studies may include testing for urinary tract infection, urinary incontinence, or urinary retention.
4. **Bowel function evaluation** Evaluation of anal incontinence or obstructive symptoms is important (e.g., constipation, incomplete emptying). Defecography may demonstrate an enterocele that was not detected on POPQ. Defecography, however, is not a routine test for prolapse.

## DIFFERENTIAL DIAGNOSIS

- In women with symptoms of a vaginal bulge or pelvic pressure, a pelvic mass should be excluded with pelvic examination, and if appropriate, imaging studies.
- Common conditions that may present with these symptoms include adnexal (e.g., benign ovarian cysts or ovarian cancer) and uterine masses (e.g., fibroids).
- Other conditions like periurethral cysts and cysts of the vaginal wall, diverticulum of the urethra, Gartner's cyst, infravaginal elongation of cervix (Fig. 26.7), polyps and chronic inversion of uterus should also be considered as possible differentials.

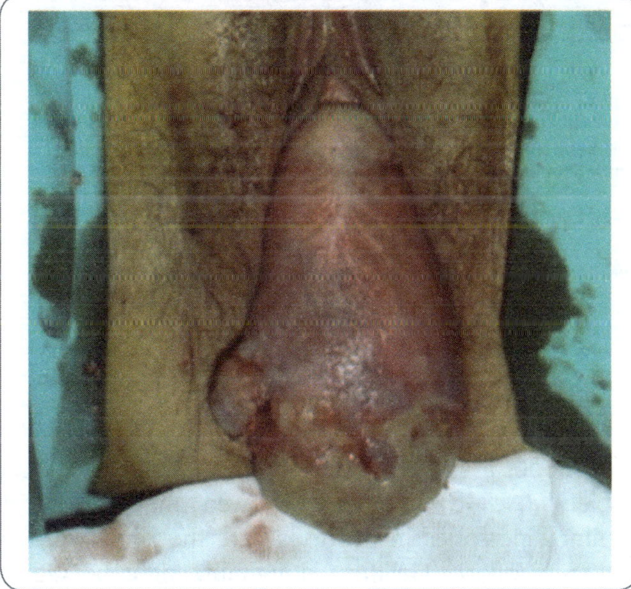

**Fig. 26.7** Infravaginal elongation of cervix (*Source:* 'Turhan N et al. Journal of Surgery Case Reports. 2014;5(8):513–15.)

## MANAGEMENT

### Medical Therapy

**Non-surgical (conservative) management of pelvic organ prolapse is recommended by the Agency for Health Care Policy and Research and ACOG Committee on Practice Bulletins and should be attempted before surgery**. It is safe and inexpensive, not usually associated with morbidity and mortality, minimally invasive, leads to high patient satisfaction, and may be used for patients awaiting surgery or patients who are not fit for surgical management.

**Pelvic muscle exercises** can improve muscle tone and stress urinary incontinence, but in any prospective, randomised trials, no evidence indicates that improvement of pelvic floor muscle tone leads to regression of pelvic organ prolapse.

**Vaginal support devices (pessaries)** are manufactured from medical-grade silicone and are safe, cost-effective, and minimally invasive options for treating patients with pelvic organ prolapse. A study of pessary use showed that 75% of urogynecologists used pessaries as first-line therapy for prolapse (Fig. 26.8).

#### Pessaries

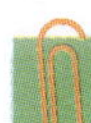

**Indications**

Pessaries can be used for both diagnostic and therapeutic purposes.

1. To relieve symptoms of prolapse
2. To relieve symptoms of stress incontinence
3. In preoperative evaluation of prolapse
4. As a temporary measure while waiting for surgery
5. To heal ulcers like decubitus ulcer by keeping the prolapse inside

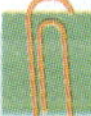

**Contraindications for Pessary Use**

- Lack of patient's ability to comply with follow-up and instructions (e.g., dementia)
- Vaginal fistulas
- Uterovaginal erosions
- Undiagnosed uterovaginal bleeding

Application of topical estrogen prior to pessary use, particularly if signs of hypoestrogenism (atrophic vaginitis) exist, serves good purpose. Once the pessary is in place, continued vaginal estrogen cream application (i.e., 1–2 times per week) or application of a vaginal estrogen ring

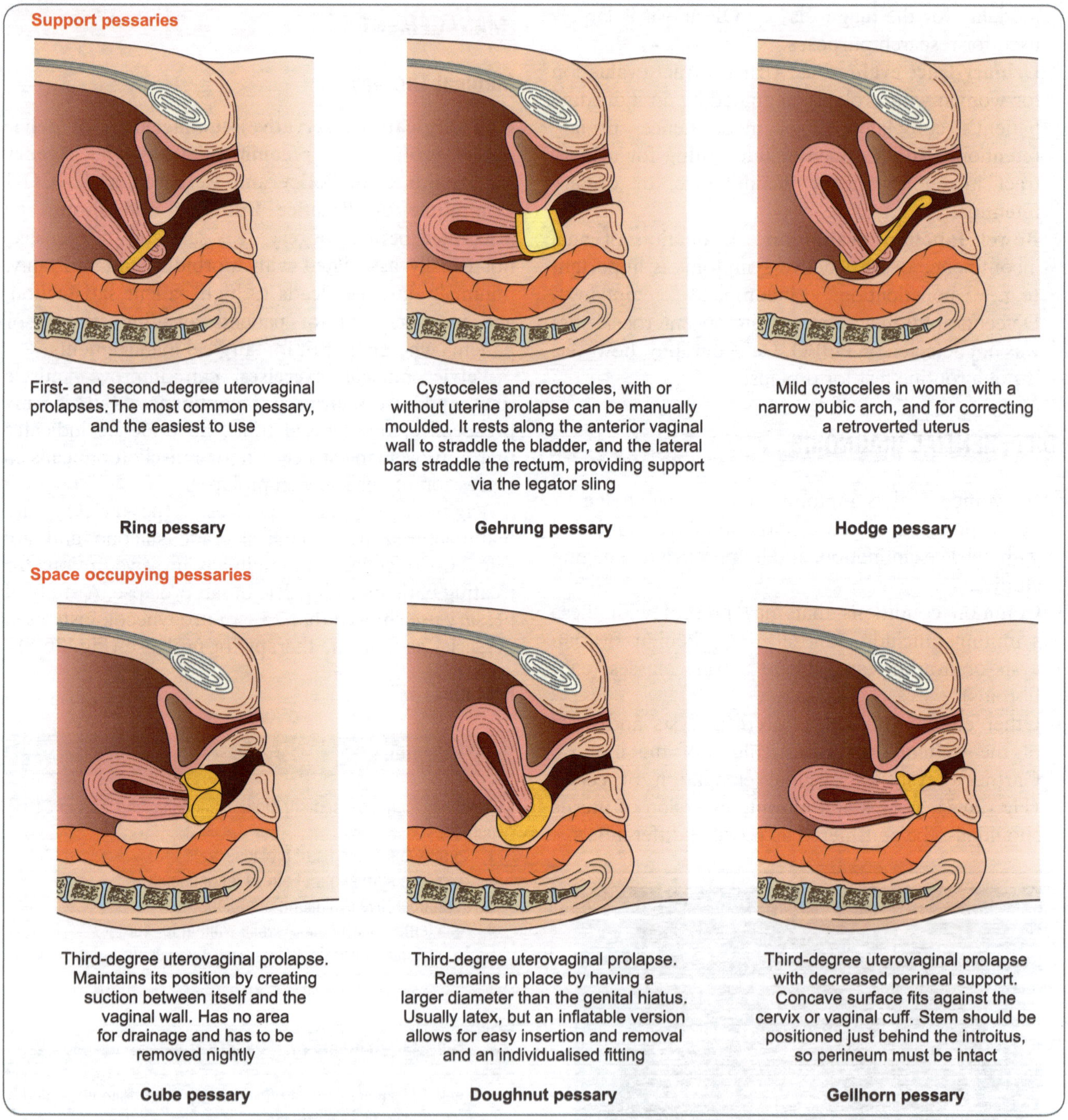

**Support pessaries**

First- and second-degree uterovaginal prolapses.The most common pessary, and the easiest to use

**Ring pessary**

Cystoceles and rectoceles, with or without uterine prolapse can be manually moulded. It rests along the anterior vaginal wall to straddle the bladder, and the lateral bars straddle the rectum, providing support via the legator sling

**Gehrung pessary**

Mild cystoceles in women with a narrow pubic arch, and for correcting a retroverted uterus

**Hodge pessary**

**Space occupying pessaries**

Third-degree uterovaginal prolapse. Maintains its position by creating suction between itself and the vaginal wall. Has no area for drainage and has to be removed nightly

**Cube pessary**

Third-degree uterovaginal prolapse. Remains in place by having a larger diameter than the genital hiatus. Usually latex, but an inflatable version allows for easy insertion and removal and an individualised fitting

**Doughnut pessary**

Third-degree uterovaginal prolapse with decreased perineal support. Concave surface fits against the cervix or vaginal cuff. Stem should be positioned just behind the introitus, so perineum must be intact

**Gellhorn pessary**

**Fig. 26.8** Different types of pessaries in placement

once every 3 months is indicated, unless estrogen is contraindicated. Vaginal erosions are indications for temporary pessary removal and treatment with topical estrogen.

### *Types of pessaries*

Many different types of pessaries (Fig. 26.9) can be used. Pessaries may be classified as

- Supportive (e.g., ring (Fig. 26.10)), or
- Space-occupying (e.g., doughnut, cube, inflatoball).

In 2000, a survey of the American Urogynecologic Society (AUGS) members showed that the most common pessaries in use today are the ring (with or without support), Gellhorn, doughnut, and cube. Other types are the Inflatoball (Milex Products, Inc., Chicago, Ill), and Smith, Hodge, Risser, and Shaatz pessaries.

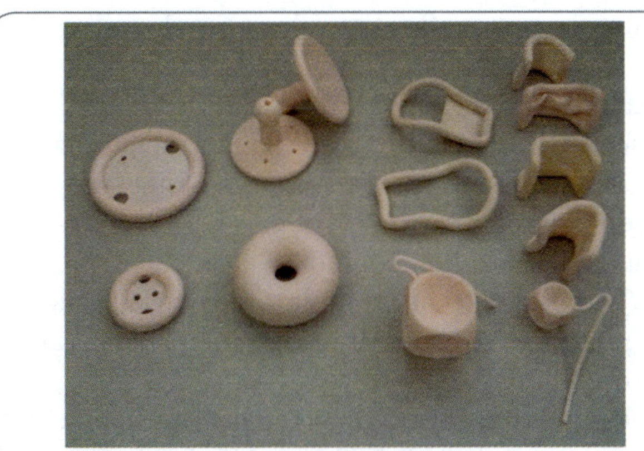

**Fig. 26.9** Different types of pessaries (*Source:* Wikimedia/©Huckfinne)

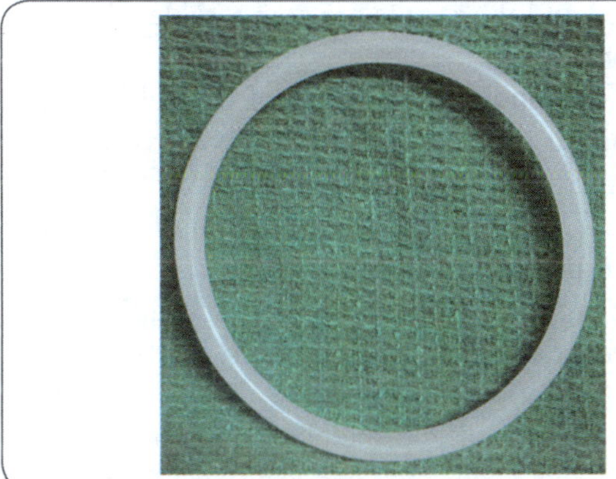

**Fig. 26.10** Ring pessary

Ring pessaries were used more successfully with stage II (100%) and stage III (71%) pelvic organ prolapse. The stage IV prolapse was most successfully treated with Gellhorn pessaries (64%). The Smith, Hodge, and Risser pessaries may help retrodisplacement of the uterus and should be used for patients with a well-defined pubic notch and an adequate vaginal width.

### *Factors of a good pessary*

- The smallest pessary that reduces pelvic organ prolapse should be used.
- A well-supported pessary should not be visible at the introitus.
- The patient should not feel vaginal pressure or discomfort while ambulating with the pessary in place.
- The ring pessary should fit snugly between the posterior fornix and the symphysis pubis. The pessary should not obstruct urinary flow.

A patient who is able to manipulate the pessary on her own may remove the pessary each night and replace it in the morning, or at least 1–2 times per week. If the pessary falls out with Valsalva maneuvers or with abdominal straining (e.g., constipation), a larger pessary or a different pessary type may be fitted. Vaginal odour and discharge are common and may be alleviated by the use of antibiotic pessaries after appropriate culture. Vaginal bleeding should always be investigated by inspection for vaginal erosions, and endometrial biopsy and Papanicolaou test.

### *Outcome following pessary insertion*

After a successful pessary fitting, 50% of patients will continue to use the pessary beyond the first year of use. The primary reasons for pessary discontinuation, in 40% of patients, were patient inconvenience and inadequate relief of symptoms. Women with more severe degrees of pelvic organ prolapse (stages III–IV) are more likely to continue pessary treatment and women with concomitant stress urinary incontinence symptoms and mild-to-moderate pelvic organ prolapse (stages I–II) are more likely to undergo surgery.

## Surgical Management

**Principle** The purpose of surgical management of POP is the correction of anatomical defects.

Surgical routes are through the vagina or abdomen and include laparotomy and the use of a laparoscope or robotic system

There are typical patterns of surgery:

1. Restorative surgery using the patient's endogenous supportive tissue.
2. Compensatory surgery using synthetic meshes or biological graft materials.
3. Obliterative surgery, which partially or totally closes the vagina.

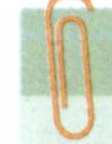

**Surgical Management**

**RESTORATIVE SURGERY**

*Cystocele*

Lateral cystocele

- Transvaginal paravaginal repair
- Retropubic paravaginal repair

Central cystocele

- Transvaginal anterior colporrhaphy
- Intra-abdominal anterior repair

Combination of lateral and central defects

- Transvaginal anterior repair and paravaginal repair
- Transabdominal anterior repair and paravaginal repair

*Rectocele*

High rectocele

Midvaginal rectocele

Low rectocele
OR
Lateral defect
Central defect
Apical defect
Perineal defect
- Traditional posterior colporrhaphy
- Defect-specific posterior repair

*Prolapse of the apical segment*
- Transvaginal approaches
  - Sacrospinous ligament fixation
  - Uterosacral vaginal vault suspension
  - Iliococcygeus suspension
  - Posterior intravaginal slingoplasty
- Abdominal sacrocolpopexy

*Enterocele*
- McCall culdoplasty
- Moschcowitz procedure
- Halban procedure

*Minimally invasive laparoscopic and robotic POP repair*
- Laparoscopy
- Robotic POP repair

**COMPENSATORY SURGERY**

**CONVENTIONAL SURGERIES FOR PROLAPSE**
- Fothergill's or the Manchester operation
- Vaginal hysterectomy with anterior colporrhaphy and posterior colpoperineorrhaphy (Ward–Mayo's operation)
- Operations for nulliparous prolapse
  - Shirodkar's method
  - Purandare's cervicopexy

**OBLITERATIVE SURGERY**
- Colpocleisis

### Restorative surgery

#### *I. Cystocele*

Anterior vaginal wall prolapse is defined as the descent of the anterior vagina such that the urethrovesical junction (a point 3-cm proximal to the external urethral meatus) or any anterior point proximal to this is less than 3 cm above the plane of the hymen. Cystocele is classified as a paravaginal defect (lateral, displacement), midline defect (central, distention), or transverse defect (apical) when the pubocervical fascia separates from the vaginal cuff or uterosacral ligaments or a combination of these defects.

**Grades of cystocele** Cystocele is graded as

**Grade 1** mild when the bladder droops only a short way into the vagina.

**Grade 2** the bladder sinks far enough to reach the vaginal introitus.

**Grade 3** occurs when the bladder bulges out through the opening of the vagina

A. **Lateral cystocele** Lateral cystocele is caused by the detachment of the pubocervical fascia and pubourethral ligaments from the arcus tendineus fasciae pelvis (ATFP). According to the mechanism of lateral cystocele, the purpose of the proposed operation is the correction of the relaxed or detached pubocervical and pubourethral ligaments.

   i. **Transvaginal paravaginal repair** The success rate of transvaginal paravaginal repair ranges from 82.5% to 98%.

   ii. **Retropubic paravaginal repair** This approach is recommended in the case of a Burch operation or total abdominal hysterectomy. The reported success rate of this procedure is from 85% to 98%. Recently, laparoscopic approach has been studied and the results are comparable with open surgery.

B. **Central cystocele** The cause of central cystocele is the failure of support by the pubocervical fascia at the midline of the anterior vaginal wall. The aim of surgical repair is the approximation of relaxed or separated pubocervical fascia.

   i) **Transvaginal anterior colporrhaphy** This procedure was developed by **Kelly** in 1913. Many variable modifications have been described. However, the basic principle is an approximation of the detached pubocervical fascia with 2–0 delayed absorbable sutures interruptedly. The cure rate has been reported to be up to 97%.

   ii) **Intra-abdominal anterior repair** In case of mild high central cystocele during an abdominal surgery such as hysterectomy, this procedure can be undertaken. After dissection between the bladder and vagina, wedge resection of the redundant vaginal wall is performed and interrupted or running sutures can be placed.

   Success rate for grade 1 cystocele was 89%. There was a considerable deterioration over time with failure rates of 30% after 2 years and 61% after 5 years.

C. **Combination of lateral and central defects** Most cystoceles include a combination of lateral and central defects. The purpose of surgery is the correction of associated defects.

   i) **Anterior colporrhaphy with paravaginal repair** Though this procedure can be performed as per anterior colporraphy mentioned previously, difficulties arise while performing paravaginal repair after anterior colporrhaphy. Different vector forces are applied on the pubocervical fascia; this is one reason why synthetic mesh or biological graft material is used for this procedure.

ii) **Transabdominal anterior repair and paravaginal repair** The transabdominal approach is not recommended for patients with only lateral and central cystocele.

For women with apparent or occult stress, urinary incontinence in association with advanced prolapse, placement of a midurethral mesh sling or **Burch procedure** results in continence rates higher than suburethral plication or paravaginal repair alone.

### *II. Rectocele*

**Definition** Posterior vaginal wall prolapse is defined as any descent of the posterior vaginal wall so that a midline point on the posterior vaginal wall 3 cm above the level of the hymen or any posterior point proximal to this point is less than 3 cm above the plane of the hymen. Posterior vaginal wall relaxation is caused by attenuation or site-specific tearing of the rectovaginal fascia, which results in herniation of the rectum and small intestine in approximately 40% of asymptomatic parous women.

**Classification** Rectoceles are subdivided by location and anatomical defects as low, midvaginal, or high rectocele.

- **High rectocele** is the result of defects in the cardinal/ uterosacral ligament complex.
- **Midvaginal rectocele** is caused by the weakening or detachment of the rectovaginal fascia from the ATFP.
- **Low rectocele** Separation of the perineal body at the level of rectovaginal fascia results in perineal descent or a low rectocele.

The other classifications of rectocele are according to the tearing portion of rectovaginal fascia:

- lateral defect
- central defect
- apical defect
- perineal defect

**Non-surgical treatments** consist of proper bowel training, following an active lifestyle, and eating an appropriate amount of dietary fibre to avoid constipation. Other non-surgical treatments include hormonal replacement therapy for menopausal women and vaginal pessary use.

**Indications** for surgery include having symptoms that respond well to surgery, including pelvic pressure, vaginal bulge and vaginal splinting for defecation, anatomic defects, or undergoing another POP surgery.

**Traditional posterior colporrhaphy** This procedure involves the plication of the pubococcygeus muscles across the anterior rectum as well as perineal body reconstruction.

**Complications** This procedure has complications such as severe postoperative pain, dyspareunia, vaginal stricture, fecal incontinence and sexual dysfunction, which have been reported to range from 18% to 27%. To prevent these complications, the repaired opening should accommodate two to three finger breadths, taking into account the fact that the levator ani and perineal muscles are relaxed from general anaesthesia and may further constrict postoperatively and undergo postmenopausal atrophy. The modified technique includes site-specific repair and midline fascial plication without levator plication.

The success rate of traditional posterior repair is reported to be from 78% to 97%, whereas that of midline fascial plication is from 79% to 92.1%.

**Defect-specific posterior repair** After separation between the vaginal epithelium and fibromuscular layer, insertion of a finger in the rectum makes the differentiation of site specific defects possible. Interrupted or running sutures with delayed absorbable sutures are utilised. Next, plicating fascia is used to cover the area with interrupted 2–0 delayed absorbable sutures. Afterwards, evaluation of the levator hiatus is performed and, in turn, narrowing of the levator hiatus with interrupted 1–0 delayed absorbable sutures is completed. If needed, perineal body reconstruction can be performed.

The success rate of site-specific repair ranges from 59% to 100%. Complications like constipation and dyspareunia occurs in 0% to 8% of patients.

**Graft material** may be used in both the traditional posterior colporrhaphy and the defect-specific technique in an attempt to strengthen the repair.

### *III. Prolapse of the apical segment*

**Definition** Prolapse of the apical segment of the vagina is defined as any descent of the vaginal cuff scar (after hysterectomy) or cervix below a point that is 2 cm shorter than the total vaginal length above the plane of the hymen.

Transvaginal and abdominal approaches are used according to patient status and co-morbidity.

1. **Transvaginal approaches**

A. **Sacrospinous ligament fixation**

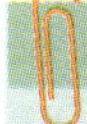

**Indication for Sacrospinous Ligament Fixation**

The main indication for sacrospinous ligament fixation is to correct total procidentia or posthysterectomy vaginal vault prolapse with an associated weak cardinal uterosacral ligament complex and to correct posthysterectomy enterocele.

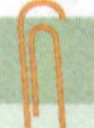

**Contraindication for Sacrospinous Ligament Fixation**

The contraindication for the procedure is a short vagina.

**Principle** The principle of this procedure is the fixation of the vaginal vault to the sacrospinous ligament with non-absorbable sutures.

The fixation site is typically the right sacrospinous ligament. However, bilateral fixation is performed in patients with recurrent vault prolapse and with the goal of restoring a vaginal axis and sexual life. The routes of entry to the sacrospinous ligament may be posterior and anterior. Usually, a unilateral, right-sided, posterior approach is preferred. The success rate is up to 96% and the common causes of failure are poor approximation of the vault to the ligament, i.e., the Suture Bridge and postoperative infection.

**Advantages** This procedure has advantages, including success rates comparable to abdominal procedures, the ability to repair concomitant pelvic floor defects, the absence of laparotomy, shorter hospital stays, and the preservation of vaginal length and function.

**Complications** The most common problem after this procedure is the high rate of postoperative cystocele, which approaches 20% to 33% resulting from the deviation of the vaginal axis. Other disadvantages include difficulty in exposing the ligament, the potential need for excessive tensioning during tying, injury risk to the pudendal or inferior gluteal vessels and sciatic or pudendal nerve, alterations in the vaginal axis, and vaginal narrowing.

B. **Uterosacral vaginal vault suspension**

**Routes** Uterosacral vaginal vault suspension can be performed intra-abdominally after hysterectomy. This procedure is a fixation of both lateral sides of the vaginal vault to the uterosacral ligament bilaterally.

The other route can be through the vagina. After vaginal hysterectomy, both sides of the vaginal vault are fixed to the uterosacral ligament. If this procedure is applied for vaginal vault prolapse, the uterosacral ligament must be identified by palpation. During the procedure, attention to the ureter is needed because the ureter runs through the lateral side of the uterosacral ligament. Thus, **after the surgery, cystoscopy must be performed to confirm ureteral efflux and to rule out bladder injury**.

The success rates are 95% to 98% within the first few years. It is recommended that native tissue repair be considered with priority for vaginal hysterectomy, and that mesh repair be considered for recurrent vault prolapse and for selective cases such as complete uterovaginal eversion.

C. **Iliococcygeus suspension**

**Principle** The principle of iliococcygeus suspension is the fixation of the vaginal vault to the fascia of the iliococcygeus muscle bilaterally.

**Indication** This procedure can be performed in cases where the uterosacral ligament is not identified or is of insufficient length to attach to the vaginal vault.

**Advantages** This procedure has the proposed advantages of decreasing neurovascular injury or postoperative cystocele. It has been reported that iliococcygeus suspension does not shorten the vaginal length, whereas sacrospinous ligament suspension does. This is one of the advantages of iliococcygeus suspension, because maintaining vaginal length is an important factor for the recurrence of POP and is also essential for coital function.

2. **Abdominal sacrocolpopexy** Lane first proposed abdominal sacrocolpopexy in 1962. The basic concept of the procedure is support of the vagina with a suspensory bridge connected to the anterior longitudinal ligament of the sacrum.

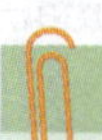

**Indications for Abdominal Sacrocolpopexy**

This procedure is indicated in patients with failed previous vaginal repair, in patients with isolated apical prolapse or enterocele, and in younger women with an active sexual life.

In this procedure, vaginal vault is fixed to the anterior longitudinal ligament of the sacral promontory with biological graft materials or synthetic mesh, preferably macroporous polypropylene mesh.

**Advantage** The procedure is more durable because of less paravaginal scarring and denervation and the fixation of the entire vaginal apical area by a permanent mesh to the stable ligament. The procedure maintains a maximal vaginal length and near-normal axis. If enterocele is present, the peritoneal cul-de-sac is closed with the **Halban or Moschcowitz procedure**.

**Abdominal sacrocolpopexy is considered the gold standard procedure for the surgical correction of vaginal vault prolapse based on numerous level 1 studies reporting its efficacy and long-term durability.**

**Complications** The complications of this procedure include vaginal erosion of the graft material or suture, intraoperative hemorrhage, postoperative ileus, and small bowel obstruction. Retroperitonealisation of the mesh is needed to prevent bowel complications.

### *IV. Enterocele*

**Definition** Enterocele is prolapse of the peritoneal cul-de-sac (the pouch of Douglas) with or without the bowel and is usually caused by apical or high posterior compartment defects.

Complete vaginal vault prolapse is accompanied by enterocele in 75% of patients. The surgery for enterocele is obliteration of the pouch of Douglas.

During the vaginal correction of the apical compartment, enterocele can be corrected. After identifying the sac of enterocele, the sac is opened, a finger is inserted into the sac, and the intestinal content is displaced back into the abdomen. One or two purse-string sutures are placed around the neck of the enterocele sac. Three sets of 0 synthetic absorbable sutures should be placed between the anterior rectal wall, the stump of the enterocele sac, and the uterosacral ligaments. The cure rate is reported to be almost 67%.

During intra-abdominal surgery, if enterocele is identified, McCall culdoplasty or the Moschcowitz or Halban procedure can be applied. In 1912, **Moschcowitz** described a procedure involving the obliteration of the pouch of Douglas with several horizontal circular, purse-string-type sutures, beginning at the most distal part of the enterocele. The **Halban** procedure is the occlusion of the pouch of Douglas with several sagittal sutures positioned along the pouch in a vertical direction and was described in 1912 by Halban. **McCall culdoplasty** is the plication of the uterosacral ligament in the midline. Two or three sutures are placed. There are many modifications of the procedures that are a combination of the McCall, Moschcowitz and Halban procedures.

### *V. Minimally invasive laparoscopic and robotic POP repair*

Minimally invasive adaptations of this procedure have been developed, initially as laparoscopic, and more recently as robotic surgery. Laparoscopic technique is basically the same as an open procedure and the indication is also the same.

**Advantages** However, the advantages of minimally invasive surgery, which include improved cosmetic aspects, reduced pain, short recovery time, low morbidity, and convenience of surgery, have led surgeons to perform more laparoscopic-based surgery in the field of POP. Most reports that compared open, laparoscopic and robotic POP surgeries with one another showed similar outcomes in cure rate, anatomic results, and complications except rate of satisfaction which was higher for the minimally invasive surgeries.

#### Compensatory surgery

Restorative surgical repairs of POP are associated with high failure rates. In particular, anterior vaginal wall prolapse may recur in 30% to 70% of patients after standard anterior colporrhaphy, whereas recurrence rates in the posterior compartment after posterior colporrhaphy are only 10% to 20%. In light of these high failure rates of the anterior compartment, vaginal surgery with **synthetic meshes** and **biological grafts** has been introduced.

**Tension-free vaginal kits** have been introduced to provide graft-augmented durable repair. The proposed advantages of the kits are a less invasive procedure, standardisation of technique, standardisation of the mesh, and ability to repair multiple compartments through a vaginal approach.

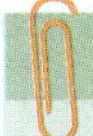

**Indications for Using Synthetic Mesh**

The indication of transvaginal mesh surgery for anterior compartment repair is the selection of patients who are at risk for native tissue failure and in whom the benefit of mesh use outweigh the risks. These groups include patients with recurrent prolapse, high-stage prolapse (POPQ stage III or IV), collagen disorders, and chronic stress to the pelvic floor.

#### Conventional surgeries for prolapse

#### *Fothergill's or the Manchester operation*

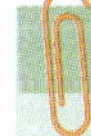

**Indication for Fothergill's Operation**

Fothergill's or the Manchester operation is ideal for uterovaginal prolapse with supravaginal elongation of the cervix.

The cervix is amputated to restore the normal length of the uterus. The lateral ligaments are shortened by separating them from the sides of the cervix and stitching them in front of it. This step not only lifts the uterus to its original position but also pulls the cervix backwards restoring anteversion.

If enterocele is present, it is opened, excised and supported by the uterosacral ligaments behind the amputated cervix.

### *Vaginal hysterectomy with anterior colporrhaphy and posterior colpoperineorrhaphy (Ward–Mayo's operation)*

**Indications for Ward–Mayo's Operation**

This is ideal for postmenopausal women with complete prolapse as the atrophic uterus does not provide a good anchor for the ligaments. It is also indicated for associated uterine pathology.

The essential part of the operation is the approximation of the stumps of the ligaments in the midline and the suspension of the vaginal vault to them.

### *Operations for nulliparous prolapse*

In these patients, vaginal procedures are inadequate as ligamentary and muscle supports are weak, and too much tightening of the vagina following excision of the vaginal walls interferes with coital function. Different abdominal sling operations for them have been described. They may be combined with anterior and posterior colporrhaphy, if necessary.

***Shirodkar's method*** A strip of mersilene tape is attached to the posterior aspect of the uterus close to the insertion of the uterosacral ligaments and passed subperitoneally around the rectum to be attached to the front of the anterior longitudinal lumbosacral ligament. On the left, it is attached to the psoas muscle to avoid pressure on the sigmoid and the vessels of the sigmoid mesocolon. The advantage of this method is that in addition to suspension, it increases the anteversion of the uterus and prevents herniation of the small bowels into the pouch of Douglas.

***Purandare's cervicopexy*** The abdomen is opened by a transverse incision, and two fascial strips are fashioned from the anterior rectus sheath and oblique aponeurosis. Each strip is pulled through the internal inguinal ring and is brought subperitoneally along the round ligament to the anterior surface of the cervix where it is fixed. The disadvantage of this method is that, in addition to suspension, the cervix is pulled anteriorly and the uterus falls back into the position of retroversion, in line with the vagina. The space behind the cervix is also widened, allowing the small bowels to prolapse into the pouch of Douglas.

### Obliterative surgery—colpocleisis

**Advantages** Colpocleisis has advantages in elderly patients with multiple co-morbidities and who do not desire sexual activity. This procedure has other advantages, such as a short operation time and the ease and safety of employing regional or local anaesthesia, minimising the uncommon complications of hemorrhage or nerve injury.

Traditionally called **Le Fort's operation and modified Le Fort's is called Godel's operation.**

These procedures include partial or total colpocleisis and colpectomy. In the absence of a uterus, either complete colpocleisis or colpectomy can be performed, whereas the presence of the uterus necessitates partial colpocleisis, which creates two lateral channels to allow uterine drainage. The most commonly described technique for partial colpocleisis is a variation of the operation originally described by LeeFort in 1977.

Other simplified procedures include a rectangular incision of the anterior vaginal wall from 2 cm below the external urethral meatus to the bladder neck until the pubocervical fascia is identified. In the same manner, the posterior vaginal wall, which is exactly opposite the site of anterior incision is also exposed and the tissues are dissected out until the prerectal fascia is exposed. Interrupted 2-0 absorbable sutures are made on the dependent vaginal wall. This procedure can be performed under local anaesthesia and on an outpatient basis.

## RECAP

- Uterovaginal prolapse is a type of displacement of uterus and vaginal walls and is also called pelvic organ prolapse.
- Supports of the uterus—The inherent muscle tone of the uterus keeps it in the anteflexed position. In asthenic conditions and in the postpartum period, the myometrium becomes lax and the body of the uterus falls back on the cervix to lie in the line of the vagina, facilitating the descent of the uterus through the vagina on straining.
- The two levator ani muscles covered by a dense layer of pelvic fascia constitute the pelvic floor. This is pierced in the midline by the urethra, the vagina and the rectum.

- The levator ani muscles consist of three parts, the pubococcygeus, the iliococcygeus and the ischiococcygeus. The iliococcygeus and ischiococcygeus form the lateral part of the pelvic floor and do not directly support the pelvic viscera. The pubococcygeus is the most important part.
- Ligaments supporting the uterus—uterosacral ligaments, transverse cervical ligaments, Mackenrodt's ligaments (also called cardinal ligaments), pubo-vesico-cervical ligament
- Risk factors include pregnancy, childbirth, factors contributing to chronic increases in intra-abdominal pressure such as lifting, coughing or straining, connective tissue disorders and damage to or weakness of the muscles.
- Pelvic organ prolapse occurs as a result of inherited racial difference. environmental and social factors, difficult childbirth, menopause, genital atrophy and hypoestrogenism, pelvic tumours, sacral nerve disorders, and diabetic neuropathy.
- Chronic medical conditions associated with increase in intra-abdominal pressure (e.g., obesity, chronic pulmonary disease, smoking, constipation).
- Marfan disease, chronic lung diseases, chronic bronchitis, neglected dystocia and traumatic vaginal delivery, excess weight gain, tight corsets, anal stenosis, chronic constipation and hard physical exertion and physical activities also contribute to POP.
- Classifications—Shaw's system, Jeffcoate's, Baden-Walker system, POPQ classification
- Clinical evaluation—Age, desire to preserve reproductive and coital function, general medical status, past history of surgical corrections, symptoms and their impact on quality of life and then physical examination.
- Decision on the correction will greatly depend on the degree of symptoms and its relationship with clinical assessment.
- Issue of rate of progression should be addressed as the management differs in rapidly progressive and slowly progressive prolapse.
- Examination components—Visual inspection, Speculum examination
- Bimanual pelvic examination, Rectovaginal examination, Neuromuscular examination.
- Differential diagnosis: Common conditions that may present with these symptoms include adnexal (e.g., benign ovarian cysts or ovarian cancer) and uterine masses (e.g., fibroids). Other conditions like periurethral cysts and cysts of the vaginal wall, diverticulum of the urethra, Gartner's cyst, infravaginal elongation of cervix, polyps and chronic inversion of uterus should also be considered as possible differentials.
- Management involves medical therapy and surgical management. Medical Therapy is by pelvic muscle exercises and vaginal support devices (pessaries). Many different types of pessaries can be used. Pessaries may be classified as supportive (e.g., ring), or space-occupying (e.g., doughnut, cube, Inflatoball). The most common pessaries in use today are the ring (with or without support), Gellhorn, doughnut and cube.
- Surgical management is by restorative surgery using the patient's endogenous supportive tissue, by compensatory surgery using synthetic meshes or biological graft material or by obliterative surgery, which partially or totally closes the vagina.
- Conventional surgeries for prolapse include Fothergill's or the Manchester, Vaginal hysterectomy with anterior colporrhaphy and posterior colpoperineorrhaphy (Ward–Mayo's operation) and Operations for nulliparous prolapse which include Shirodkar's method and Purandare's cervicopexy.
- Obliterative surgery involves colpocleisis.
- The treatment modality should be chosen according to the patient's medical status, anatomic defects, balance between the benefits and risks, patient's preference, and the surgeon's experience. If the surgeon and patient choose compensatory surgery with synthetic meshes, informed consent should be obtained in consideration of mesh-related complications.

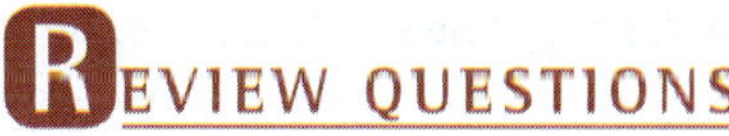

## REVIEW QUESTIONS

### Long-Answer Question

Discuss the muscular and ligamentous supports of the uterus and their role in the development of pelvic organ prolapse.

### Short-Answer Questions

1. Write short notes on abdominal sacrocolpopexy.
2. What are the indications and contraindications for use of pessaries in uterovaginal prolapse.

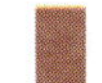

### MCQs

**1. Which is the action of transverse cervical ligaments?**

a) Keeps the uterus anteverted
b) Supports the cervix and the bladder
c) Forms the central point of the perineum
d) Helps prevent the descent of the uterus whenever there is increased intra-abdominal pressure

**2. Which is a surgery for nulliparous prolapse?**
   a) Colpocleisis
   b) Shirodkar's method
   c) Ward–Mayo's operation
   d) Manchester operation

**3. Enterocele is caused by**
   a) Weakening or detachment of the rectovaginal fascia
   b) Defects in the cardinal/uterosacral ligament complex
   c) Apical or high posterior compartment defects
   d) Separation of the perineal body at the level of rectovaginal fascia

**4. Uterosacral vaginal vault suspension is**
   a) The fixation of the vaginal vault to the fascia of the iliococcygeus muscle bilaterally
   b) The support of the vagina with a suspensory bridge connected to the anterior longitudinal ligament of the sacrum
   c) The fixation of the vaginal vault to the sacrospinous ligament with non-absorbable sutures
   d) The fixation of both lateral sides of the vaginal vault to the uterosacral ligament bilaterally

**Further Reading**

ACOG Committee on Practice Bulletins–Gynecology. ACOG Practice Bulletin No. 85: Pelvic organ prolapse. Obstet Gynecol. 2007;110:717.

Barber MD, Kuchibhatla MN, Pieper CF, Bump RC. Psychometric evaluation of 2 comprehensive condition-specific quality of life instruments for women with pelvic floor disorders. Am J Obstet Gynecol. 2001;185:1388.

Barber MD, Lambers A, Visco AG, Bump RC. Effect of patient position on clinical evaluation of pelvic organ prolapse. Obstet Gynecol. 2000;96:18.

Brubaker, L, Norton, P. Current clinical nomenclature for description of pelvic organ prolapse. Journal of Pelvic Surgery. 1996;2:257.

Bump RC, Mattiasson A, B, K, et al. The standardization of terminology of female pelvic organ prolapse and pelvic floor dysfunction. Am J Obstet Gynecol. 1996;175:10.

Elkadry EA, Kenton KS, FitzGerald MP, et al. Patient-selected goals: a new perspective on surgical outcome. Am J Obstet Gynecol. 2003;189:1551.

Hall AF, Theofrastous JP, Cundiff GW, et al. Interobserver and intraobserver reliability of the proposed International Continence Society, Society of Gynecologic Surgeons, and American Urogynecologic Society pelvic organ prolapse classification system. Am J Obstet Gynecol. 1996;175:1467.

Hullfish KL, Bovbjerg VE, Steers WD. Patient-centered goals for pelvic floor dysfunction surgery: long-term follow-up. Am J Obstet Gynecol 2004;191:201.

Mahajan ST, Elkadry EA, Kenton KS, et al. Patient-centered surgical outcomes: the impact of goal achievement and urge incontinence on patient satisfaction one year after surgery. Am J Obstet Gynecol. 2006;194:722.

Maher C, Feiner B, Baessler K, Schmid C. Surgical management of pelvic organ prolapse in women. Cochrane Database Syst Rev. 2013:CD004014.

Manonai J, Mouritsen L, Palma P, et al. The inter-system association between the simplified pelvic organ prolapse quantification system (S-POP) and the standard pelvic organ prolapse quantification system (POPQ) in describing pelvic organ prolapse. Int Urogynecol J. 2011;22:347.

Muir TW, Stepp KJ, Barber MD. Adoption of the pelvic organ prolapse quantification system in peer-reviewed literature. Am J Obstet Gynecol. 2003;189:1632.

Nygaard I, Barber MD, Burgio KL, et al. Prevalence of symptomatic pelvic floor disorders in US women. JAMA. 2008;300:1311.

Treszezamsky AD, Rascoff L, Shahryarinejad A, Vardy MD. Use of pelvic organ prolapse staging systems in published articles of selected specialized journals. Int Urogynecol J. 2010;21:359.

Vierhout ME, Stoutjesdijk J, Spruijt J. A comparison of preoperative and intraoperative evaluation of patients undergoing pelvic reconstructive surgery for pelvic organ prolapse using the Pelvic Organ Prolapse Quantification System. Int Urogynecol J Pelvic Floor Dysfunct. 2006;17:46.

# CHAPTER 27

# Disorders of the Urinary System

**AT A GLANCE**

Applied Anatomy of Bladder and Urethra
Histology of the Urinary Bladder
Innervation of Bladder and Urethra
Physiology of Micturition
Congenital Abnormalities
Infections
Cystitis
Non-gonococcal Urethritis
Pyelonephritis
Urinary Tract Lesions in Genital Prolapse
Changes in the Urinary Tract in Endometriosis and Benign Pelvic Tumours
Changes in the Urinary Tract due to Malignant Pelvic Growths
Common Urinary Symptoms
Urinary Incontinence
Types
Stress Urinary Incontinence (SUI)
Treatment of Stress Incontinence
Management
Urge Incontinence
Mixed Incontinence

Disorders of the urinary system include heterogeneous conditions like congenital anomalies, inflammatory and traumatic lesions including urinary fistulae and stress incontinence of urine. Some of these acquired lesions may be due to or as a result of associated gynecological conditions and hence are of interest to us.

## APPLIED ANATOMY OF BLADDER AND URETHRA

The **bladder** is a hollow structure which can expand to accommodate up to 300–500 mL of urine. The smooth muscle of the bladder is known as detrusor muscle. This muscle is arranged in three layers, spiral, longitudinal, and circular bundles.

The **urethra** is a tube-like structure which is 2.5 to 4 cm long in the female. It empties through the external urethral meatus situated about 2–3 cm posterior to the clitoris. The urethra consists of a muscular layer and a mucosal layer. There are two layers, the inner longitudinal layer and outer circular layer which in turn is surrounded by a circular layer of skeletal muscle forming the sphincter urethrae or rhabdosphincter. Apart from this, at the junction of the middle and upper third, there are two strips of skeletal muscles known as **urethrovaginal sphincter** and **compressor urethrae**. **These three muscles together provide constant tonus to the urethra to maintain urinary continence** (Fig. 27.1).

There is also an **internal urethral sphincter** made up of smooth muscle bundles passing on either side of the urethra, though they do not encircle the urethra. Further along the urethra is a sphincter of skeletal muscle, the sphincter of the membranous urethra (external urethral sphincter).

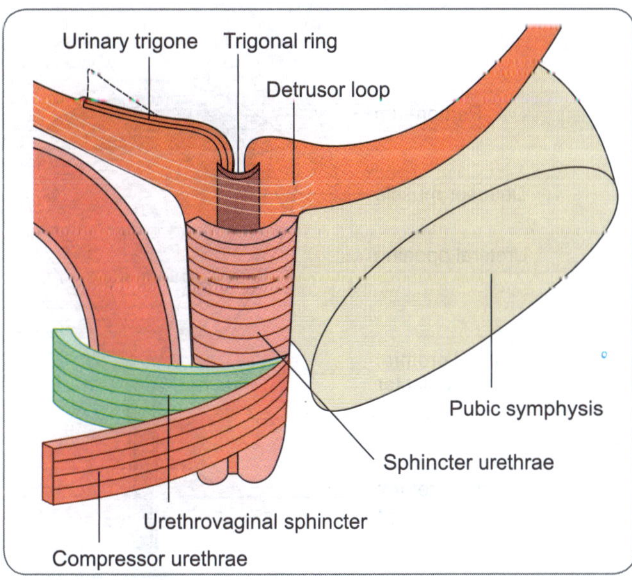


**Fig. 27.1** Urethral support

## HISTOLOGY OF THE URINARY BLADDER

The bladder epithelium is transitional epithelium (Fig. 27.2). It contains a superficial layer of dome-like cells and below that multiple layers of stratified cuboidal cells. When the bladder is fully distended, the superficial cells become squamous (flat) and the stratification of the cuboidal cells is reduced in order to provide lateral stretching.

## INNERVATION OF BLADDER AND URETHRA

The innervation is from both the lumbar and sacral spinal cord, with the fibres of the sympathetic nervous system being contributed by the former and the fibres of the parasympathetic nervous system contributed by the latter (Fig. 27.3).

The **sympathetic nerves (T11–T12 hypogastric nerve)** relax the bladder but constrict the internal sphincter. This results is filling of the bladder.

On the other hand the **parasympathetic nerves (S2–S4 pelvic nerve)** constrict the bladder but relax the internal sphincter. This results is emptying of the bladder (urination).

The external urinary sphincter is supplied by the **somatic nerve (pudendal nerve motor fibres of S2–S4)** which keeps the external sphincter constricted facilitating voluntary control of urination.

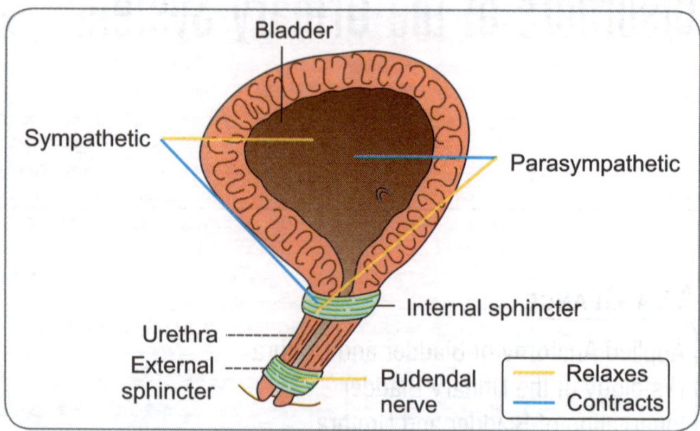


**Fig. 27.3** Innervation of the bladder and urethra

## PHYSIOLOGY OF MICTURITION

In healthy individuals, the process of micturition has two phases:

i. **Storage phase** During the storage phase the sympathetic fibres from T11-T12 keep the bladder relaxed and constrict the internal sphincter. This results in filling of the bladder. When the bladder is filled up to 150–200 ml, the first sensation of bladder filling reaches the higher centres through the afferent impulses via S2-S4 fibres.

ii. **Voiding phase** When it is possible to urinate, the parasympathetic fibres through pelvic nerve (S2-S4) contract the bladder and relax the internal sphincter. The external sphincter under the somatic

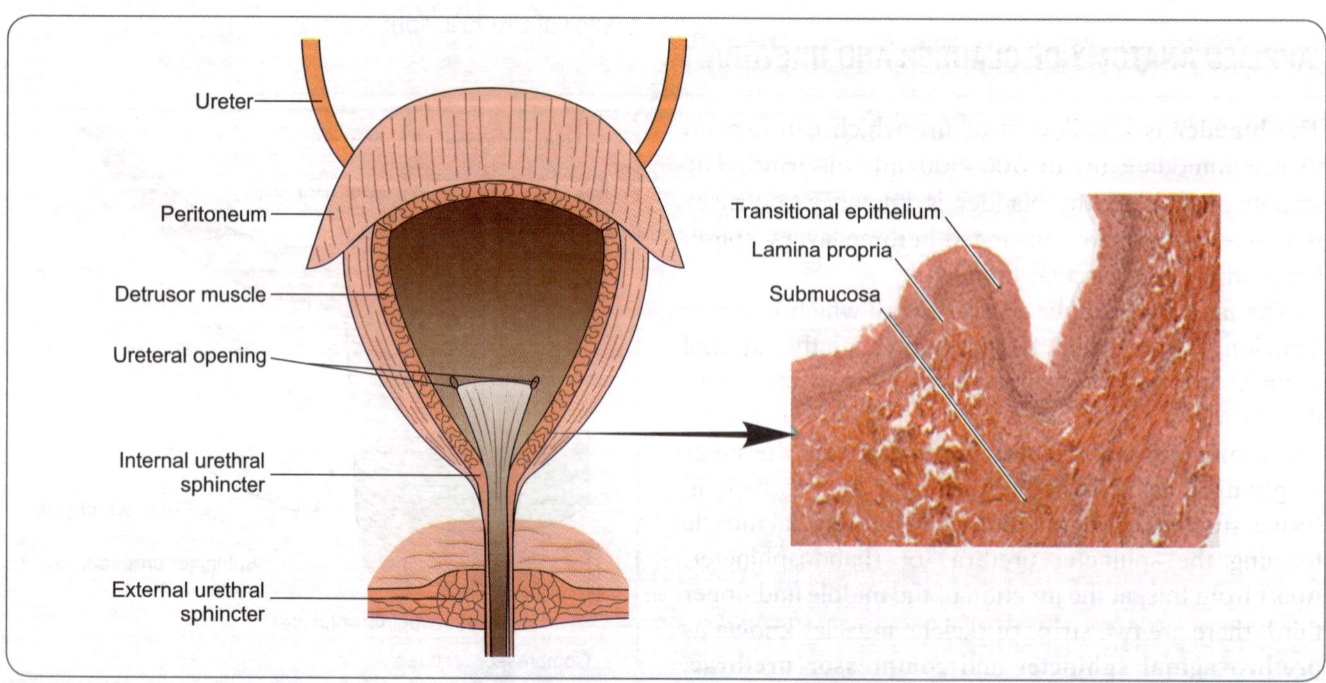


**Fig. 27.2** Anatomy of the female bladder, showing transitional epithelium as well as part of the wall in a histological cut-out

control of pudendal nerve is consciously relaxed during micturition.

## CONGENITAL ABNORMALITIES

Some of the congenital disorders of the urinary tract are the following.

### *Ectopia vesicae*

This is a rare congenital anomaly wherein the notable defect is the protrusion of the bladder wall through a defect in the anterior abdominal wall. This may be associated with a split pelvis.

### *Ureteric abnormalities*

These are more common than ectopia vesicae. The abnormalities encountered in the ureter include:

- **Ectopic ureter** Ureter, instead of it regular insertion at trigone of the bladder, may get inserted into some other location like urethra or even the vagina in its distal third.
- **Bifid ureters** The upper pole and lower pole ureters join proximal to the bladder
- **Double ureters** The two ureters, one from the upper pole and another from the lower pole enter the bladder separately.
- **Ureterocele** This is the ballooning of the ureter where it enters the bladder. It is necessary to rule out other anomalies of the urinary system.
- **Accessory and aberrant ureter** The accessory ureter is always connected with the upper pole of the kidney. It crosses posterior to the main ureter and may be injured in pelvic operations. This ureter opens into the anterolateral wall of the vagina, and the patient complains of continuous dribbling of urine due to the congenital ureterovaginal fistula.

### *Absence of one kidney*

This condition is associated with the unilateral absence of the Mullerian duct as in uterus unicornis.

### *Pelvic kidney*

This may be located at the pelvic brim or the sacro-iliac joint and may be mistaken for a gynecological tumour. It may lead to hydronephrosis and may obstruct labour.

## INFECTIONS

Urinary tract infection (UTI) is the most common bacterial infection in the female. Because of the anatomy, UTI is more common in women than in men. The infection from the urethra has the potential to reach the bladder and then ascend up even to the kidneys. This is facilitated by the short length of the urethra, the proximity of the rectum to the moist vulva and sexual intercourse.

### Cystitis

This is the most common of the UTIs in the female.

#### Signs and symptoms

- Painful micturition
- Strangury
- Fever with chills may be encountered in cystitis, though it is more common in pyelonephritis
- Bloodstained urine

**The pain in cystitis is characteristically present at the end of urination unlike in urethritis where it is present at the beginning of urination.**

**Etiology** The most common infecting organism is *E. coli* in 50–60% of infections. The other organisms which could be isolated in urine culture include streptococci, *B. proteus*, *Pseudomonas* and, occasionally, *M. tuberculosis*.

#### Treatment

**Diagnosis and Treatment** The current consensus is to treat uncomplicated acute bacterial cystitis with a short course of antibiotics and not to wait for investigation reports.

However, nearly 50% of women with uncomplicated cystitis would develop recurrent cystitis. These women come under the category of complicated cystitis. In such women who develop complicated or recurrent infections or with persistent or new symptoms during treatment, urinalysis and culture are recommended. Urinary microscopy has the advantage of identifying both pyuria and bacteriuria.

Treatment consists of appropriate antibiotics according to the sensitivity reports. The commonly used antibiotics include the following:

| Drug | Dose | Condition to be treated |
|---|---|---|
| Ciprofloxacin | 250 mg bd × 3 days | Uncomplicated cystitis |
| Ofloxacin | 200 mg bd × 3 days<br>200 mg bd × 10 days | Uncomplicated cystitis<br>Complicated cystitis |
| Amoxicillin-clavulanate A | 500 mg bd × 3–7 days | |

### Non-gonococcal Urethritis

This condition is caused by *Chlamydia trachomatis.* Doxycycline 100 mg thrice daily for 7 days is the treatment of choice.

### Treatment

**Treatment for pyelohephritis**

| Type | Infection | Drug | Dosage |
|---|---|---|---|
| Mild | Gram negative | Oral Ciprofloxacin | 500 mg bd for 7 days |
| | | Oral Norfloxin | 400 mg bd for 7 days |
| | Gram positive | Amoxicillin-clavulanic acid | 875/125 mg bd for 7 days |
| Severe intravenous therapy for 24–48 hours or till the fever subsides followed by oral therapy for 7–14 days. | Gram negative | Ciprofloxacin Cefotaxime (Claforan) | 400 mg bd 1 to 2 g two to four times daily |
| | Gram positive | Piperacillin-tazobactam | 3.375 g every 6 hours |

## Pyelonephritis

Acute uncomplicated pyelonephritis is divided into mild and severe forms. In the mild variety, there is no nausea or vomiting, the leucocyte count is normal and there may be fever, which, if present, is only a low-grade one. On the contrary, the severe form presents with vomiting, dehydration, sepsis and fever. There is usually lower urinary tract infection, back pain and tenderness in the renal area.

# URINARY TRACT LESIONS IN GENITAL PROLAPSE

In major degrees of genital prolapse of long duration, there is hypertrophy of the bladder wall, hydroureter and hydronephrosis due to the kinking of the ureters at the crossing by the uterine arteries. These changes are reversible following the surgical treatment for prolapse.

## Changes in the Urinary Tract in Endometriosis and Benign Pelvic Tumours

In 30–50 per cent of women with large ovarian tumours, fibroids or broad ligament tumours there may be exertion of pressure on the ureters, which displaces them resulting in hydroureter and hydronephrosis. There may be kinking of the ureter due to endometriosis and occasionally cyclical hematuria is a condition in which there is bloody urination during menstruation. This occurs in endometriosis of the bladder.

## Changes in the Urinary Tract due to Malignant Pelvic Growths

These changes may be due to new growth or sequelae of radical surgery and radiation.

In cervical carcinoma, depending on the stage of the disease, cystoscopy may show transverse ridges or bulging due to the tumour, hyperemia, edema of the bladder base bullous edema and in advanced cases, ulceration or even a vesicovaginal fistula.

The urethra may be encroached upon, occluded or ulcerated by direct extension of carcinoma of the cervix or the vulva. In cervical cancer, the ureters may be compressed due to parametrial infiltration or sometimes by radiation fibrosis depending on the stage of the disease. The pre-treatment intravenous pyelography may show hydroureter and hydronephrosis in about 6–10 per cent in Stage I, about 20 per cent in Stage II and 50 per cent in cases of advanced cervical carcinoma.

# COMMON URINARY SYMPTOMS

Some of the common urinary complaints encountered in gynecological practice are:

### *Frequency of micturition*

The common causes of frequency of micturition are pyelonephritis, cystitis, diabetes and any pressure on the bladder, like early pregnancy, an ovarian tumour or a myoma.

### *Difficulty in micturition*

This symptom may be seen in all conditions leading to the retention of urine, which include the following.

a) Prolapse of the uterus with a large cystocele. When the patient strains, there is increased pouching of the bladder with most of the urine collected below the level of the internal urinary meatus.
b) Bladder calculi
c) Pelvic hematocele

### *Painful micturition*

This is caused by cystitis (including post-radiation cystitis), urethritis, caruncle and partial or complete prolapse of the urethra. Prolapse of the urethra is mostly seen in postmenopausal women when it gives rise to painful micturition. On examination, the urethral mucosa appears reddish and bleeds easily. This condition has to be distinguished from a urethral caruncle.

### *Retention of urine*

This condition is often seen in the following.

a) Operations on the vagina and the perineum: Fothergill's operation, vaginal hysterectomy or sometimes even after an episiotomy; it can also occur in Wertheim's operations, due to the stripping of the nerve supply to the bladder.
b) Hematocolpos.
c) Impacted pelvic tumours such as ovarian tumours or an anterior cervical myoma.
d) Neurological causes as in spinal cord lesions.

### *Incontinence of urine*

This is considered in detail in this chapter.

## URINARY INCONTINENCE

**Definition** Urinary incontinence is defined as any involuntary leakage of urine. According to the International Continence Society guidelines, urinary incontinence is a symptom, a sign and a condition.

### Types

Urinary incontinence is of two types (Fig. 27.4).

1. **True incontinence** This type of incontinence occurs when there is continuous involuntary discharge of urine as in urinary fistulae. These fistulae may be congenital or acquired, and depending on the organ involved, may be vesicovaginal or ureterovaginal.
2. **False incontinence** In this, there is involuntary leakage of urine only under certain conditions:
   a) When there is involuntary leakage of urine (whether a few drops or in spurts) during coughing, sneezing or under conditions of stress it is called stress incontinence. This is usually due to
      – **Urethral hypermobility** where the urethra shifts positions due to an increase in abdominal pressure or
      – **Intrinsic sphincter** deficiency which is the inability to effectively seal off the sphincter.
   b) On the other hand, in **urge incontinence** there is a marked urgency to pass urine and before the person can reach the lavatory there is escape of urine. It is more common than stress incontinence. The vesical sphincter is normal but there is trigonitis or cystitis.
   c) **Detrusor dyssynergia** This is due to spinal injury or multiple sclerosis, often mistaken for stress incontinence.
   d) **Functional incontinence** It is the inability due to reasons other than urinary tract dysfunction or neurological causes (e.g., delirium, psychiatric disorders, urinary infection, impaired mobility).
   e) In bladder neuropathies such as syphilis, multiple sclerosis and spinal injuries, there is the **overflow type of incontinence of urine**.
   f) Increased intra-abdominal pressure with pregnancy or a tumour may also cause temporary stress incontinence in some women.

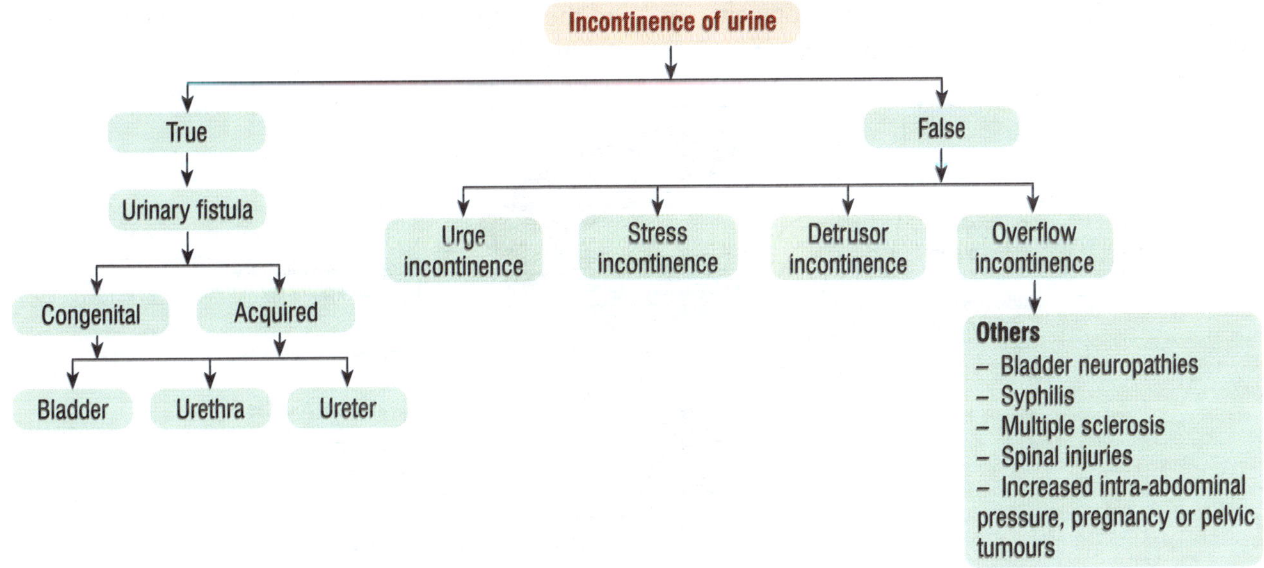


**Fig. 27.4** Types of urinary incontinence

## STRESS URINARY INCONTINENCE (SUI)

In stress urinary incontinence (SUI), there is involuntary leakage of small amounts of urine through an intact urethra and bladder due to the increase in the intra-abdominal (and consequently intravesical) pressure during coughing, laughing, sneezing, lifting or in severe cases even while walking. It is a distressing symptom. The patient does not voluntarily disclose it during history-taking unless specifically asked about this disability.

### Classification of SUI

The female SUI can be sub-categorised into:

**Type I** Loss of urine without urethral hypermobility. This is considered the mild form.

**Type II** Loss of urine due to urethral hypermobility. This is also known as genuine stress urinary incontinence (GSUI).

**Type III** It is defined as urine leakage occurring from an intrinsic sphincter deficiency (ISD).

**Etiopathology** Normally when a person coughs, the urethral pressure exceeds the bladder pressure and prevents the escape of urine. The urethral pressure is about 100 cm of water compared to 40–60 cm of intravesical pressure. When this mechanism is altered and the intravesical pressure exceeds intraurethral pressure, SUI results.

Stress incontinence could be due to:

1. Childbirth injury to the bladder-control mechanism
2. Menopausal atrophy of the supports of the bladder and urethra
3. Congenital defects like poor development or innervations of the pelvic or urethral supports
4. Scarring following surgery in the region of the bladder
5. A cystocele being associated with a urethrocele.

The most important structures involved in controlling micturition are the involuntary vesical sphincter (which consists of two opposing loops of muscle at the bladder neck), the pubovesicocervical fascia and to some extent the anterior fibres of the puborectalis. The voluntary sphincter of the urethra has only an accessory role (Fig. 27.5).

As long as these supporting structures are efficient and the bladder neck is kept in its normal position with the posterior urethrovesical (PUV) angle maintained at 100°, there is continence of urine.

Normally, this angle is abolished only during micturition (Fig. 27.6). But when the supporting structures are damaged or weakened, there is loss of the PUV angle even at rest or on coughing, resulting in stress incontinence.

Weakness of the internal sphincter and the fascial supports results in the escape of urine on coughing or sneezing. To achieve urinary continence, these supports have to be strengthened and the PUV angle restored.

**Diagnosis**

***History taking and clinical examination*** The history should be taken carefully, to distinguish stress incontinence from other types of incontinence (Table 27.1). An appraisal of the past obstetric experience and of previous pelvic surgery should also be made. Presence of any of the factors mentioned above in the etiopathology should be carefully elicited while taking the history.

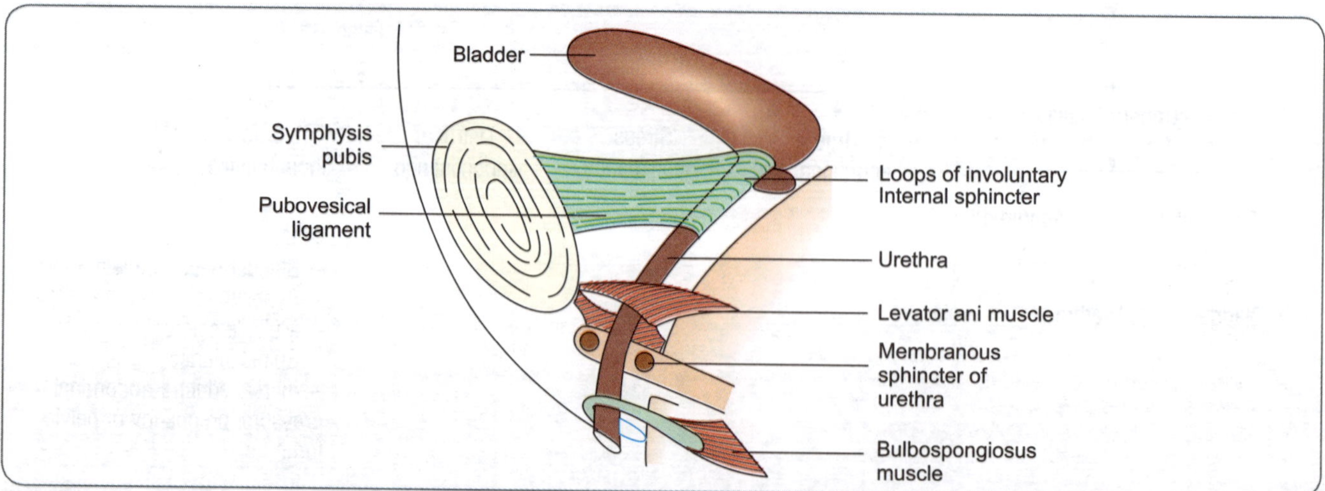


**Fig. 27.5** The anatomy of bladder neck and urethra showing the important structures involved in controlling micturition

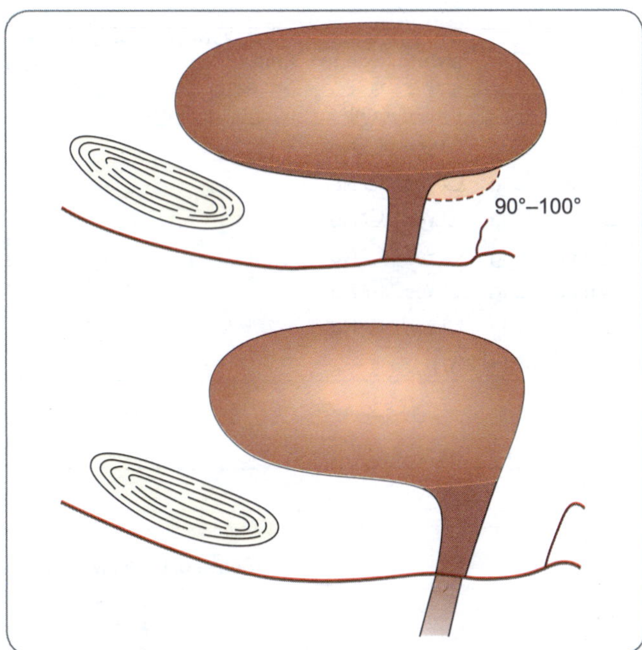


Fig. 27.6 The bladder before and during micturition

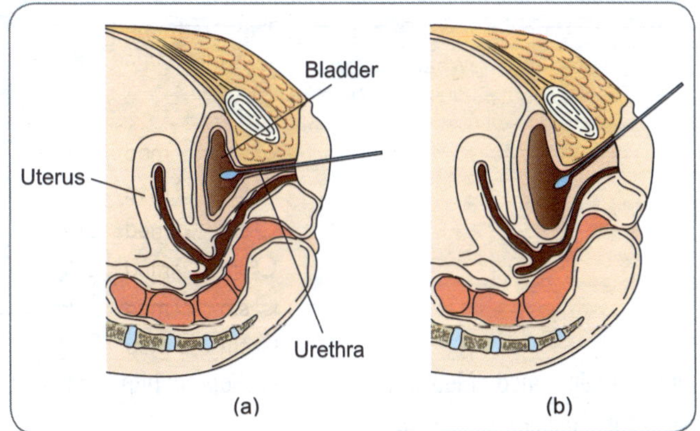


Fig. 27.7 Q-tip test

1. **Pelvic and neurological examination** Here, relaxation of the supports of the urethra and bladder neck, scarring of the anterior vaginal wall and any other associated pelvic disease are looked out for. Neurological causes (e.g. multiple sclerosis, Parkinson's disease) that could be responsible for urinary incontinence should be ruled out.
2. The following factors should be specifically asked for and noted:
   a. Duration of the complaint and its progression
   b. Frequency of incontinence and its progression
   c. Volume of urine lost (small/large quantity)
   d. Triggers for incontinence
3. For demonstration of stress incontinence, the patient has to be examined with a full bladder, in the lithotomy position and while standing. In mild cases, the ejection of urine is present only when she raises the intra-abdominal pressure in the standing posture.

### Investigations

1. **Urine analysis and culture** This is to rule out cystitis and other urinary infections.
2. **Q-Tip test** is performed to assess the angle of urethra (Fig. 27.7). It is performed by inserting a cotton swab into the urethra and making the patient perform Valsalva manoeuvre. Urethral hypermobility is indicated by an angle of excursion of more than 30°.
3. **Voiding diary** This gives information about the number of voids, the amount of urine leaked and the events during 24 hours (Fig. 27.8).
4. **Residual urine** This can be measured either by ultrasound or catheterisation. More than 200 mL of residual urine is indicative of reduced bladder function.

When these investigations fail to suggest the type of incontinence further investigation is required.

1. **Cystometrogram** The intravesical and urethral pressure are recorded with the bladder filled artificially (Fig. 27.9). This again helps to distinguish stress incontinence from other types of urinary incontinence.
2. **Lateral cysto-urethrography** This radiographic investigation is very helpful in confirming the diagnosis and also in identifying the type of repair needed (Fig. 27.10). The anatomic deformity may show the following.
   a) Posterior urethrovesical (PUV) angle is lost or obliterated even at rest.
   b) There is a descent and funneling of the bladder neck.
   c) In some cases, there is a rotational (backward and downward) type of deviation in the urethral axis.
3. **Video cysto-urethrography** gives better information about bladder function.
4. **Bonney's vesical neck elevation test** This test indicates whether surgery would be beneficial to the patient. With the patient in the lithotomy position, the bladder is filled up and the patient is asked to cough when there is escape of urine. The examiner then places two fingers, one on either side of the urethra at the urethrovesical junction. Upward pressure is exerted against the subpubic angle and at the same time the patient is asked to cough. If no urine escapes during this procedure, the surgery is likely to be beneficial.
5. **Cystoscopy** and **urethroscopy** These are done to eliminate any primary pathology in the bladder or urethra.

| Date | Time | Drinks | | Trips to the bathroom How much urine? (Select one) | Leaks How much? (Select one) | Did you feel a strong urge to go? (Select one) | What were you doing at the time? Sneezing, exercising, lifting coughing, having sex, etc. |
|---|---|---|---|---|---|---|---|
| | | What kind? | How much? | | | | |
| | | | | O sm O med O lg | O sm O med O lg | O Yes O No | |
| | | | | O sm O med O lg | O sm O med O lg | O Yes O No | |
| | | | | O sm O med O lg | O sm O med O lg | O Yes O No | |
| | | | | O sm O med O lg | O sm O med O lg | O Yes O No | |
| | | | | O sm O med O lg | O sm O med O lg | O Yes O No | |
| | | | | O sm O med O lg | O sm O med O lg | O Yes O No | |

sm : Small; med : Medium; lg : Large; (*Source:* http://remendiumlabs.com/bladder-diary/)

**Fig. 27.8** Voiding diary sample

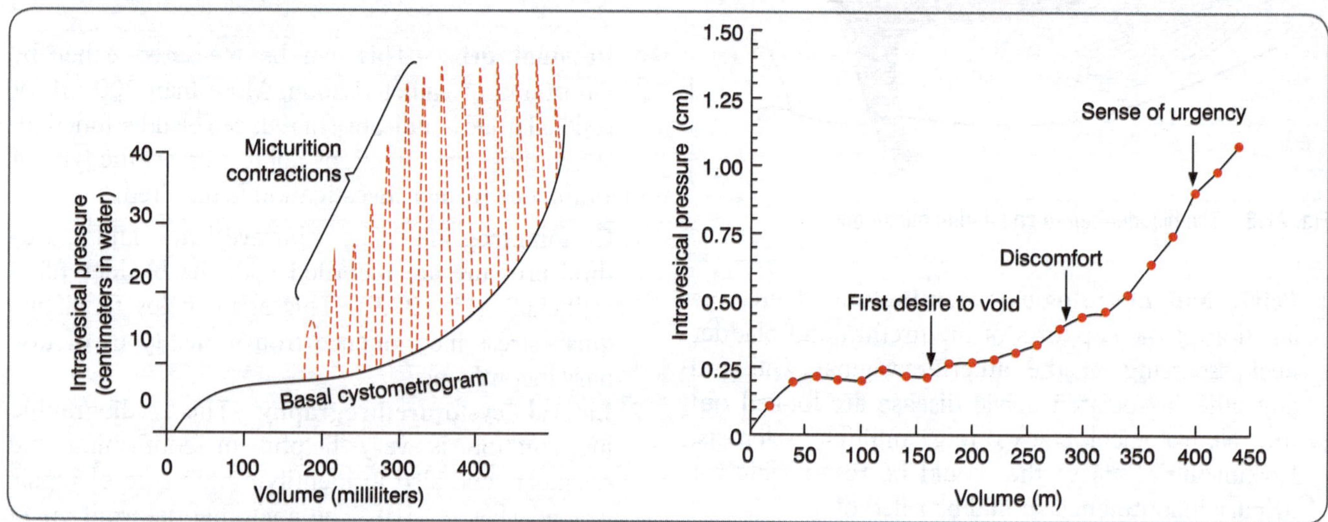


**Fig. 27.9** A normal cystometrogram

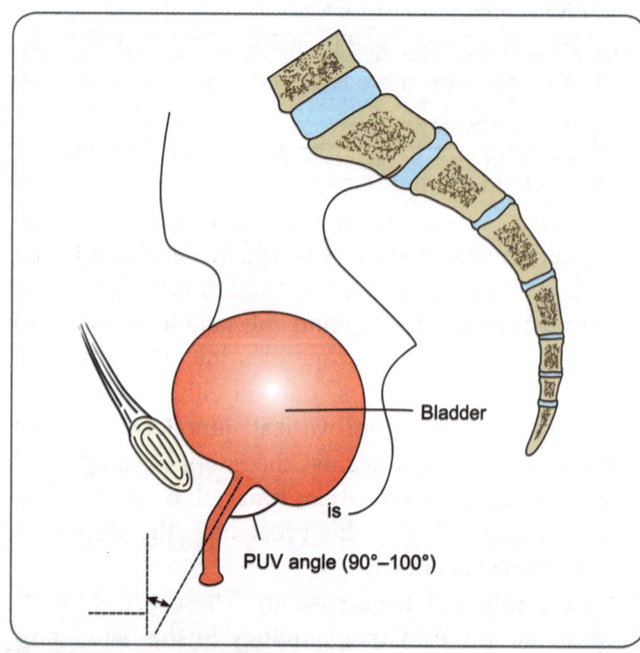


**Fig. 27.10** A lateral cysto-urethrograph

### Differential Diagnosis of SUI

1. True incontinence
2. Urge incontinence
3. Detrusor dyssynergia
4. Overflow incontinence
5. Cystitis or calculi
6. Neurological disorders like tabes dorsalis, disseminated sclerosis and spinal cord injury

**Table 27.1** Differences between urge and stress incontinence

| Urge incontinence | Stress incontinence |
|---|---|
| 1. A large amount of urine is usually passed. | The quantity of urine escaping is small, sometimes a few drops. |
| 2. The patient is aware of passing urine and the bladder may be completely emptied. | It is preceded by the rise of intra-abdominal pressure like coughing, sneezing or laughing. |
| 3. There is a time lag between the trigger and leakage. | Leakage is instant. |

| 4. Routine urine examination and culture may suggest urinary infection. | There may be no evidence of urinary infection. |
|---|---|
| Cystometry and urodynamic study confirm the diagnosis. | |

## Treatment of Stress Incontinence

***Prophylaxis*** Delay in the second stage of labour must be avoided by timely interference. There should be no undue pressure anteriorly over the bladder neck area by the fetal head in the course of the delivery.

## Management

I. Medical (conservative or non-surgical)
II. Surgical

### I. Medical treatment

#### *Pelvic floor exercises*

Kegel stresses the value of physiotherapy and has devised a set of pelvic floor exercises which can be done by voluntary contraction or by electrical stimulation. The women should voluntarily contract the pelvic floor muscles many times a day. This has been found to be more effective than placebo.

#### *Bio-feedback therapy*

These are behavioural techniques to measure physiological signals like muscle tension.

#### *Vaginal cones/pessaries*

Specific pessaries (Fig. 27.11) to treat incontinence have been devised particularly in patients with pelvic organ prolapse, who also have incontinence. They act by providing support to the bladder neck.

#### *Pharmacotherapy*

Pharmacotherapy has a minor role in the management of SUI. It aims at improving urinary frequency, nocturia, urgency and urge incontinence. Pharmacotherapy is more useful in women with mixed urinary incontinence (vide infra).

**Imipramine** is a tricyclic antidepressant (TCA) which has alpha adrenergic action. Since the urethra has larger amount of alpha adrenergic receptors, the drug can be tried.

**Estrogen cream** as well as **oral estrogen** have been used over a period of time. It has been shown to increase the urethral blood flow and also alpha adrenergic receptor sensitivity. Topical estrogen cream application is particularly useful in menopausal and older women where there is atrophy of the external genitalia. In spite of all this, no consensus has been reached on the beneficial effect of estrogen on the lower urinary tract. However, it can be used, particularly when there is associated menopausal symptom.

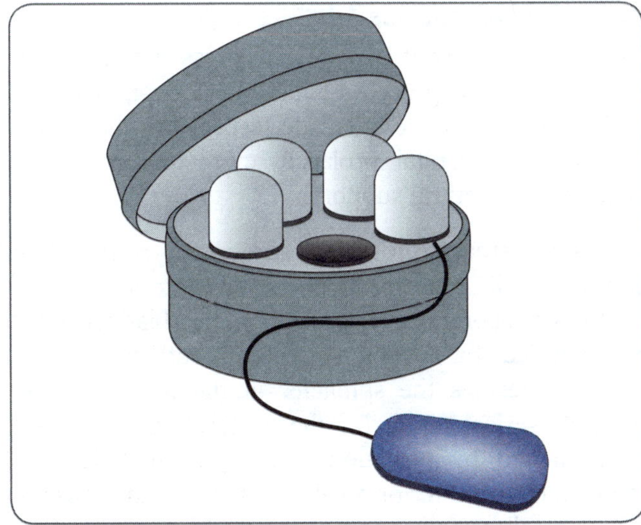

**Fig. 27.11** Weighted vaginal cones

Another drug that is being investigated in the management of SUI is Duloxetine, which is a selective serotonin reuptake inhibitor (SSRI). Initial studies have shown a promising trend.

#### *Electrical stimulation*

This can be used in those women who are not compliant with pelvic floor exercises. Electrical simulation is used to improve the tone of levator ani muscles.

#### *Behavioural approach*

Behavioural training includes bladder training and prompted voiding. Frequent and timed voiding is recommended in women with SUI. Though it could be very useful in young women, it may not be easy in elderly patients.

### II. Surgical treatment

Though non-surgical methods are useful, for severe incontinence and in those whose quality of life is greatly altered by the problem of incontinence, surgery is the best option. The various surgeries are based on elevating and supporting the bladder neck and urethra. Surgery could be by the vaginal or abdominal route depending on the choice of surgery.

### *A. Vaginal operations*

In over 80 per cent of cases of stress incontinence, vaginal corrective procedures like anterior colporrhaphy and urethroplasty are adequate, especially when there is associated genital prolapse, cysto-urethrocele or laxity of the urethral supports.

**a. Kelly's operation** This surgery is very often combined with anterior colporraphy (anterior repair). In Kelly's operation (Fig. 27.12), the bladder neck is identified by means of Foley's catheter in the bladder. Besides the sphincter at the bladder neck, the pubovesical fascia (or the urethral supports) are strengthened by placation. The cystourethrocele is reduced by the anterior repair and it also reinforces the pubovesical fascia support of the bladder and urethra. The Kelly's placation of the urethra is primarily meant to decrease the urethral diameter. However, this surgery is slowly losing its prime place in the management of stress incontinence.

### *B. Abdominal operations*

#### Vesico-urethral suspension or cysto-urethropexy (or the Marshall–Marchetti–Krantz operation)

**Indications**

i) Stress incontinence associated with some other pelvic pathology which requires laparotomy.
ii) Stress incontinence with urethral axis deviation (Type II)
iii) Failure to restore urinary continence with vaginal surgery alone

This is an extraperitoneal procedure where the bladder neck and the urethra are first mobilised through the space of Retzius and are then attached to the periosteum of the symphysis pubis by means of a series of sutures (Fig. 27.13). The bladder and the urethra are thus suspended upwards and forwards restoring the PUV angle.

**Stamey–Pereyra procedure** In this endoscopic procedure, the bladder neck is elevated by nylon sutures tied to the rectus sheath. It gives relief in 80 per cent of cases. But long-term follow-up showed recurrences in 15–20 per cent due to infection or breakage of the nylon. It is quicker to perform than the colposuspension.

**The sling operation** Here, after the necessary dissection to mobilise the bladder neck, the vesico-urethral junction is supported by means of a sling (a band of fascia or synthetic non-absorbable ribbon) by the abdominal route (**Millin's operation**) or the abdominovaginal route (**Aldridge's operation**).

**Tension-free vaginal tape procedure (TVT)** This is a minimally invasive suburethral sling procedure. This procedure is done through the vaginal route with two small incisions on the lower abdomen. It uses polypropylene mesh tapes attached to needles (Fig. 27.14). The needle is introduced via the endopelvic fascia on one side and advanced into the retropubic space of Retzius. It should be ensured that the needle is close to the posterior wall of the pubic symphysis. The needle is brought out on the anterior abdominal wall close to the pubic symphysis. Before attempting on the

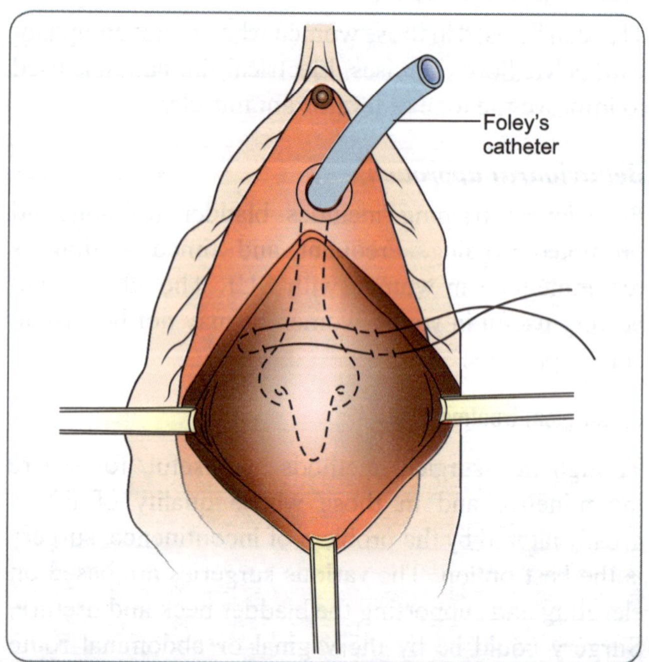


**Fig. 27.12** Kelly's operation for urinary stress incontinence

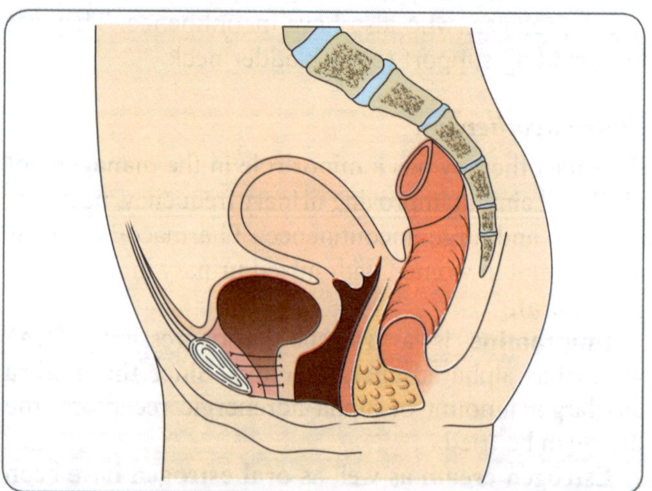

**Fig. 27.13** Marshall–Marchetti–Krantz operation for urinary stress incontinence

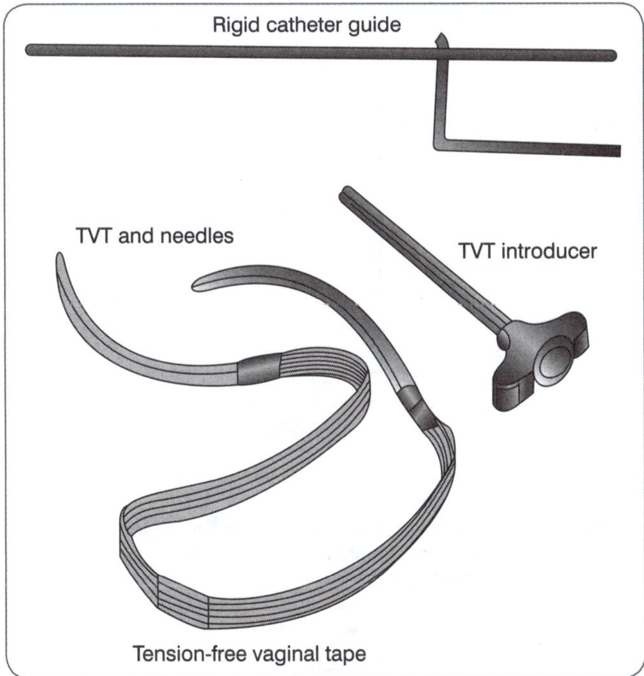


**Fig. 27.14** Tension-free vaginal tape (TVT)

other side, a cystoscopy is performed to make sure that there is no bladder or urethral injury. The procedure is repeated on the other side. The needles should be cut and the tape tied with sufficient tension to ensure that there is no leakage of urine. The success rate has been claimed to be around 85%.

**Transobturator tape sling (TOT)** This is almost like the TVT described above. The tape is passed through the obturator membrane rather than the bladder and space of Retzius (Fig. 27.15). The tape is fixed to the thigh in its antero-mediolateral aspect. This is safer than TVT and the results are comparable.

The Burch colposuspension is performed by securing the full thickness of the vaginal wall, excluding the mucosa, to the ileopectineal line of Cooper's ligament. This is the most suitable operation for young patients without much prolapse.

**Laparoscopic colposuspension** Since the introduction of laparoscopic colposuspension surgery for urinary incontinence in the early 1990s, it has undergone many technical variations, materials, different types of mesh and suture materials. The main advantages of laparoscopic colposuspension are minimal hospital stay and lesser pain. However, there is still no clear evidence that laparoscopic colposuspension is better than open colposuspension. It needs further study.

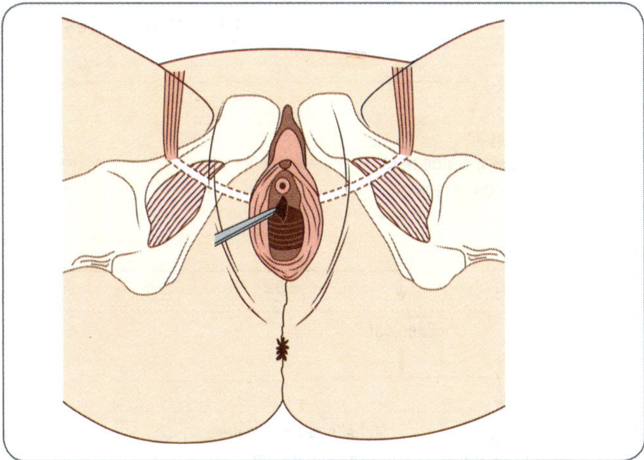

**Fig. 27.15** Transobturator sling

Fig. 27.16 summarises the management approach for SUI.

## URGE INCONTINENCE

Urge incontinence is a condition in which there is involuntary loss of urine when there is a sudden uncontrollable urge to urinate. It is also known as **overactive bladder.** The affected women may also have an urge to urinate frequently and also wake up often in the night to urinate. Urge incontinence could be a result of detrusor myopathy or neuropathy or due to a combination of both.

**Treatment of urge incontinence** Bladder drill, psychosomatic support, treatment for urinary tract infection with reassurance help in curing this condition.

**Drugs** Anticholinergic drugs act at the level of detrusor muscle by competitively inhibiting acetylcholine at the muscaranic receptors. The commonly used drugs of this group are: oxybutynin, tolterodine, and fesoterodine.

Imipramine is also being used in urge incontinence, particularly when it is associated with SUI.

Solifenacin, trospium chloride and darifenacin are selective muscarinic-receptor antagonists which are being tried.

Sacral neuromodulation is a technique using a pulse generator and electrical leads to modulate bladder and pelvic floor innervation.

## MIXED INCONTINENCE

When symptoms of both stress and urge incontinence are noted together, it is often called mixed incontinence.

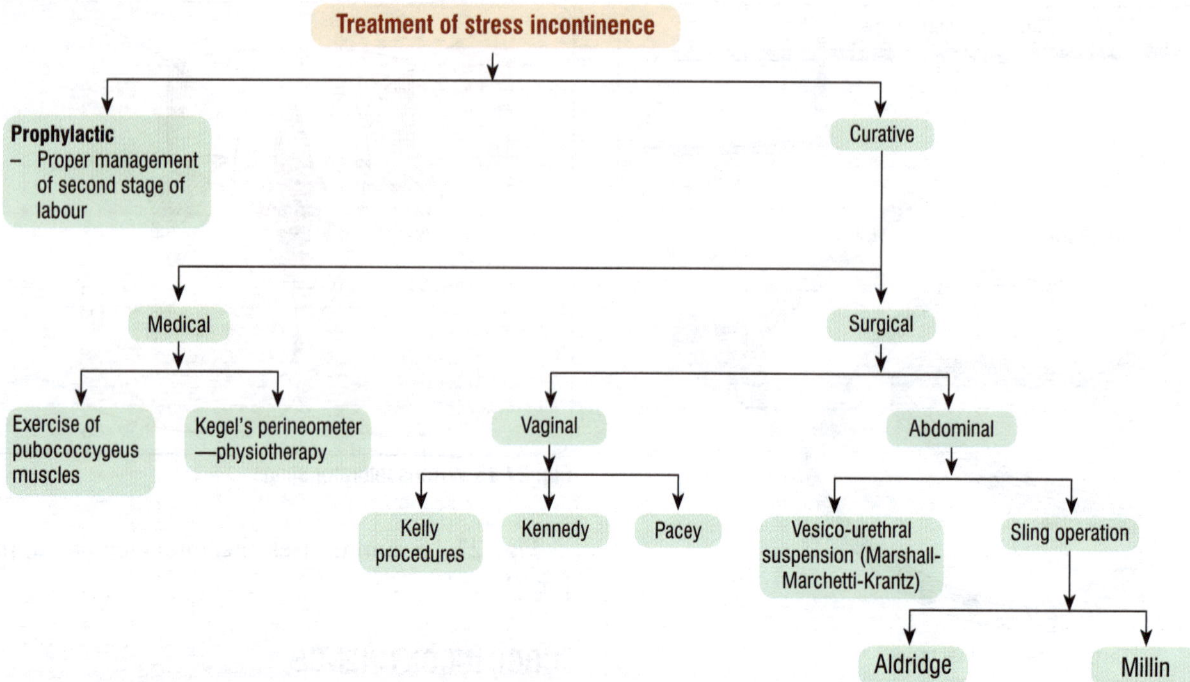


**Fig. 27.16** Management approach for SUI

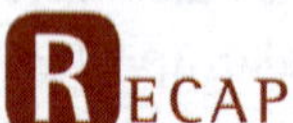

## RECAP

- The bladder is a hollow structure which can expand to accommodate up to 300–500 mL of urine.
- The smooth muscle of the bladder is known as detrusor muscle.
- The urethra is a tube-like structure which is 2.5 to 4 cm long in the female. It empties through the external urethral meatus situated about 2–3 cm posterior to the clitoris. The urethra consists of a muscular layer and a mucosal layer.
- There is also an internal urethral sphincter made up of smooth muscle bundles passing on either side of the urethra, though they do not encircle the urethra.
- Further along the urethra is a sphincter of skeletal muscle, the sphincter of the membranous urethra (external urethral sphincter).
- The sympathetic nerves (from T11-T12- hypogastric nerve) relax the bladder but constrict the internal sphincter. This results in filling of the bladder.
- On the other hand the parasympathetic nerves (S2-S4- pelvic nerve)) constrict the bladder but relax the internal sphincter. This results in emptying of the bladder (urination).
- The external urinary sphincter is supplied by the somatic nerve (pudendal nerve- motor fibres of S2-S4) which keeps the external sphincter constricted facilitating voluntary control of urination.
- Congenital abnormalities: ectopia vesicae, ectopic ureter, double ureters, ureterocele, accessory and aberrant ureter, absence of one kidney, pelvic kidney
- Infections: cystitis, non-gonococcal urethritis, pyelonephritis
- Common urinary symptoms: frequency of micturition, difficulty in micturition, painful micturition, retention of urine
- Urinary incontinence is defined as any involuntary leakage of urine.
- True incontinence: This type of incontinence, occurs when there is continuous involuntary discharge of urine by the patient as in urinary fistulae.
- In false incontinence, there is involuntary leakage of urine only under certain conditions.
- False incontinence includes stress incontinence, urge incontinence, detrusor dyssynergia, functional incontinence and over-flow type of incontinence.

- SUI—Etiopathology: Childbirth injury to the bladder control mechanism, menopausal atrophy of the supports of the bladder and urethra, congenital defects like poor development or innervations of the pelvic or urethral supports, scarring following surgery in the region of the bladder, a cystocele being associated with a urethrocele.
- The differential diagnosis of SUI are true incontinence, urge incontinence, detrusor dyssynergia, overflow incontinence, cystitis or calculi, and neurological disorders like tabes dorsalis, disseminated sclerosis and spinal cord injury.
- Medical treatment: Pelvic floor exercise, bio-feedback therapy, vaginal cones/pessaries, hormone therapy, electrical stimulation and behavioural training
- Surgical treatment includes vaginal operations and abdominal operations.
- Vaginal operations—Kelly's operation
- Abdominal operations—Vesico-urethral suspension or cysto-urethropexy or the Marshall–Marchetti–Krantz operation, Stamey–Pereyra procedure
- The sling operation—Tension-free vaginal tape procedure, transobturator tape sling
- Laparoscopic colposuspension
- Urge incontinence is a condition in which there is involuntary loss of urine when there is a sudden uncontrollable urge to urinate. It is also known as overactive bladder.
- Treatment of urge incontinence: oxybutynin, tolterodine, imipramine, solifenacin, trospium chloride and darifenacin
- Sacral neuromodulation

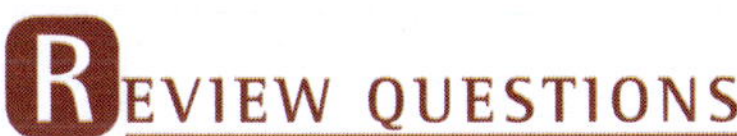

## REVIEW QUESTIONS

### Long-Answer Question

Define stress urinary incontinence. Discuss the signs and symptoms, diagnosis and sling operation for stress urinary incontinence.

### Short-Answer Questions

1. Briefly describe the innervations of the bladder and how it facilitates micturition.
2. Give an account of management of pyelonephritis.

### MCQs

**1. Oxybutynin and Tolterodine are used in**
a) Stress incontinence b) Urge incontinence
c) Cystitis d) Pyelonephritis

**2. Ectopia vesicae is a condition in which**
a) The bladder protrudes through a defect in the anterior abdominal wall
b) The urethra protrudes through a defect in the anterior abdominal wall
c) The ureters protrude through a defect in the anterior abdominal wall
d) The bladder protrudes through a defect in the posterior abdominal wall

**3. Kelly's operation for stress urinary incontinence is a/an**
a) Abdominal procedure b) Vaginal procedure
c) Sling operation d) Laparoscopic procedure

**4. In which of these conditions is there a time lag between the trigger and leakage of urine?**
a) Functional incontinence b) Detrusor dyssynergia
c) Urge incontinence d) Pyelonephritis

**Further Reading**

Berek J, editor. Berek & Novak's Gynecology. 15th ed. New York: Wolters Kluwer; 2012.
Edmonds K, editor. Dewhurst's textbook of obstetrics and gynecology. 8th ed. New Jersey: John Wiley & Sons, Ltd; 2012.
Hoffman B, Schorge J, Schoffer J, Halvorson L, Bradshaw K, Cunningham F. William's Gynecology. 2nd ed. New York: McGraw-Hill; 2012.

# Chapter 28

# Genitourinary Fistula

## At a Glance


Etiology
Classification of Genitourinary Fistula
Vesicovaginal Fistula (VVF)
- Incidence
- Classification of VVF
- Etiology
- Signs and Symptoms
- Diagnosis
- Differential Diagnosis
- Treatment
- Surgical Management

Ureterovaginal Fistula (UVF)
- Signs and Symptoms
- Examination
- Treatment

Ureteric Injuries in Gynecology
- Common Sites of Ureteric Injury
- Pathological Conditions Likely to Predispose a Woman to Ureteric Injuries
- Surgical Procedures Likely to Cause Ureteric Injuries
- Types of Ureteric Injury
- Signs and Symptoms
- Management


## INTRODUCTION

Urinary fistulae are seen in 0.5 per cent of gynecological admissions. The most common type seen in hospitals in the developing countries is the vesicovaginal fistula. Other varieties of urinary fistulae are vesicocervical, urethrovaginal, vesicouterine and ureterovaginal fistulae (Fig. 28.1).

**Definition** **Urinary fistula can be defined** as an abnormal opening in an organ of the urinary tract or an abnormal connection between a urinary tract organ and another nearby organ like the vagina.

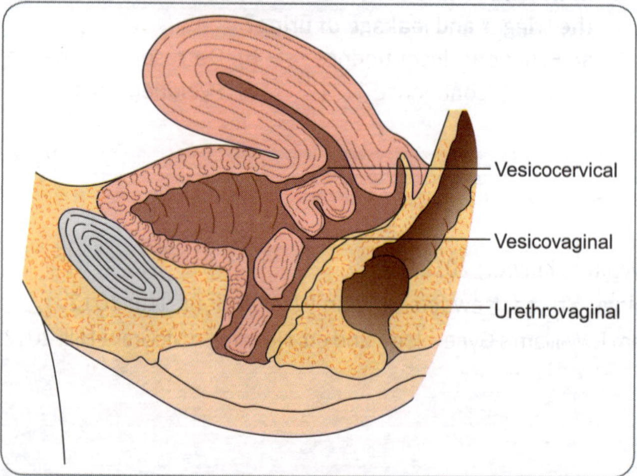


**Fig. 28.1** Different types of urinary fistulae

## ETIOLOGY

Genitourinary fistula could be due to any of the following causes, viz., obstetric, surgical or other causes. Figure 28.2 gives the etiology and the classification of urinary fistulae.

## CLASSIFICATION OF GENITOURINARY FISTULA

There is no single, well-accepted classification system for the genitourinary fistula. One method of classification is based on anatomic consideration and as shown in Table 28.1.

**Table 28.1** Classification of genitourinary fistula based on anatomic consideration

| | Urinary system | | |
|---|---|---|---|
| | Ureter | Bladder | Urethra |
| Vagina | Ureterovaginal | Vesicovaginal | Urethrovaginal |
| | Vesicoureterovaginal | | |
| Cervix | Ureterocervical | Vesicocervical | Urethrocervical |
| Uterus | Ureterouterine | Vesicouterine | — |

(*Source:* William's Gynecology. 2nd ed. Page 678)

## VESICOVAGINAL FISTULA (VVF)

This is the most common cause of true incontinence of urine, in India and other developing countries.

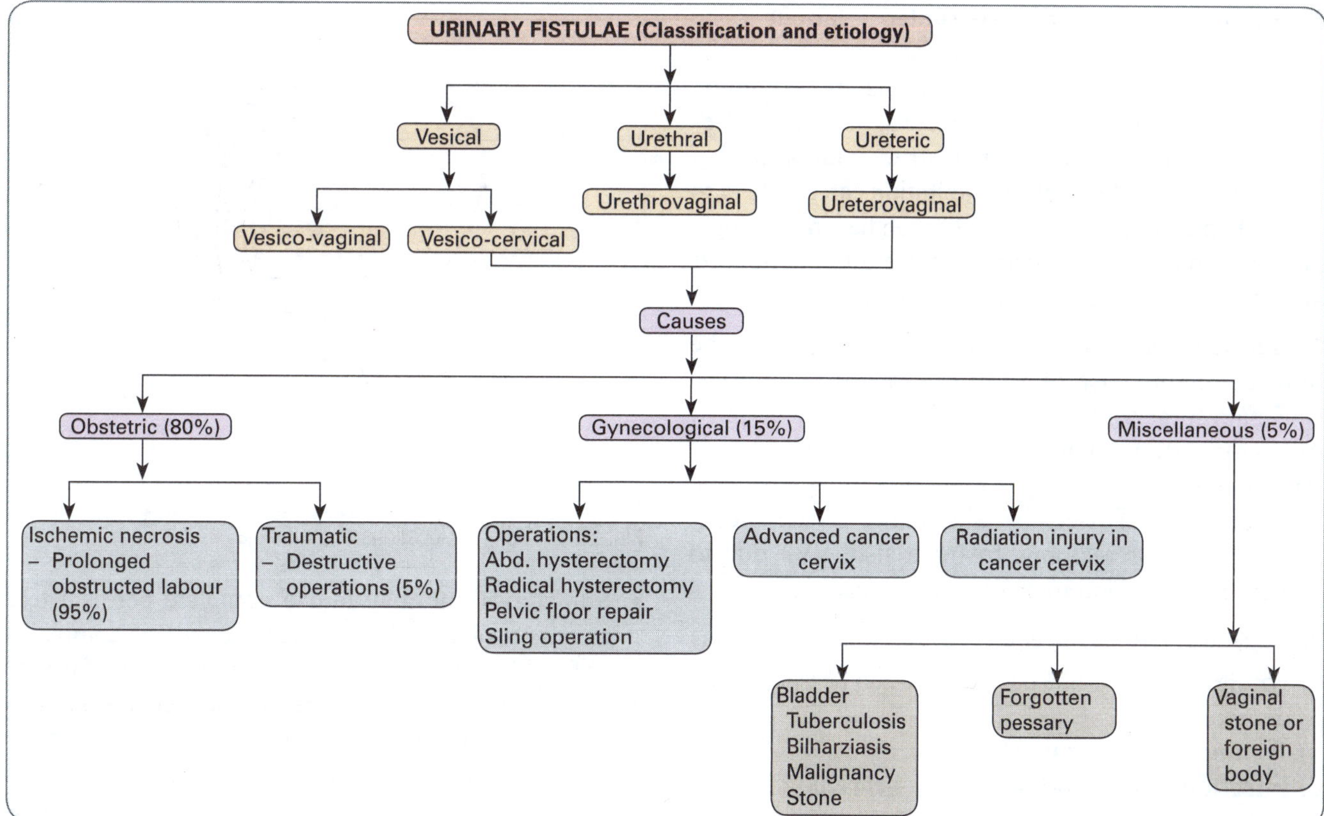


**Fig. 28.2** Etiology and classification of urinary fistulae

## Incidence

There is no definite study on the incidence of VVF. In one study the incidence in Maharashtra and Karnataka were found to be 0.86 and 2.6 respectively (BMC Pregnancy and Childbirth, 2013).

## Classification of VVF

Though many classification have come, the most commonly used classification is based on the area of the vagina where the fistulous opening is seen. High-vaginal is close to the vault and low vaginal is close to the urethra.

| | |
|---|---|
| High-vaginal | when found proximally in the vagina |
| Low-vaginal | when noted distally |
| Mid-vaginal | when identified centrally |

Post hysterectomy VVF are usually high-vaginal.

An alternative classification was given by Elkins et al. in 1999 (Table 28.2).

A more detailed classification was introduced in 2004 by Goh.

**Table 28.2** An alternative classification of vesicovaginal fistula (Elkins et al 1999)

| Classification | Description |
|---|---|
| Simple | Fistula measures 2 to 3 cm and is located near the cuff (supratrigonal)<br>Patient with no prior radiation or malignancy<br>Vaginal length is normal |
| Complicated | Patient with prior radiation therapy<br>Pelvic malignancy is present<br>Vaginal length is shortened<br>Fistula measures 3 cm<br>Fistula is distant from cuff or has trigonal involvement |

Source: William's Gynecology. 2nd ed. Page 678

## Etiology

### Congenital VVF

This is uncommon and only few cases are reported in literature.

### Acquired VVF

Obstetric trauma is the most common cause of acquired VVF in the developing countries. This occurs due to any of the following causes or a combination of them:

**1. Prolonged and/or obstructed labour** The prolonged compression of the fetal head over the bladder base leads to ischemic necrosis and sloughing of the devitalised area in the vesicovaginal septum resulting in VVF. Similarly faulty instrumentation during destructive procedures like decapitation can also lead to VVF. Of late, female genital mutilation has increasingly become the cause of obstetric fistulae due to attempts at delivering through a narrow introitus.

**2. Surgical causes** Trauma during surgery is the most common cause of VVF in developed countries. The main surgery responsible for VVF is hysterectomy. An earlier study demonstrated that the chance of VVF due to hystercetomy is more due to laparoscopic hysterectomy followed by abdominal hysterectomy and vaginal hysterectomy. In India also, VVF due to surgery is the second most common cause.

**3. Causes of rare occurrence** The other rare causes are:

a) **Foreign bodies**—like a long forgotten pessary, bladder stone.
b) **Trauma**—direct trauma.
c) **Infection and inflammation**—chronic inflammatory lesions like lymphogranuloma venereum and urinary tuberculosis.
d) **Radiation therapy**—leads to tissue necrosis due to endarteritis resulting in fistula formation.
e) **Malignancy**—VVF and rectovaginal fistula are not uncommon in cancer cervix as a consequence of tissue necrosis.

## Signs and Symptoms

- The patient complains of **continuous dribbling of urine** following a difficult delivery or gynecological surgery.
- Due to constant leakage of urine, there is **excoriation of the vulva.**
- On examination of the external genitals, there might be **vulvitis** and leakage of urine.
- On separating the labia, in some cases a large fistula with prolapsed bladder mucosa can be seen as a **red, velvetty, tender mass.**
- A digital examination will reveal the fistula mostly in the middle of the anterior vaginal wall. Depending on its location, the fistula may be midvaginal, juxtacervical (close to the cervix) or juxtaurethral (Fig. 28.3).
- In obstetric fistulae, the patient may complain of secondary amenorrhea of hypothalamic origin.
- In about 5–10 per cent of cases, there may be a foot-drop caused by prolonged compression of the sacral nerve roots by the fetal head during labour.

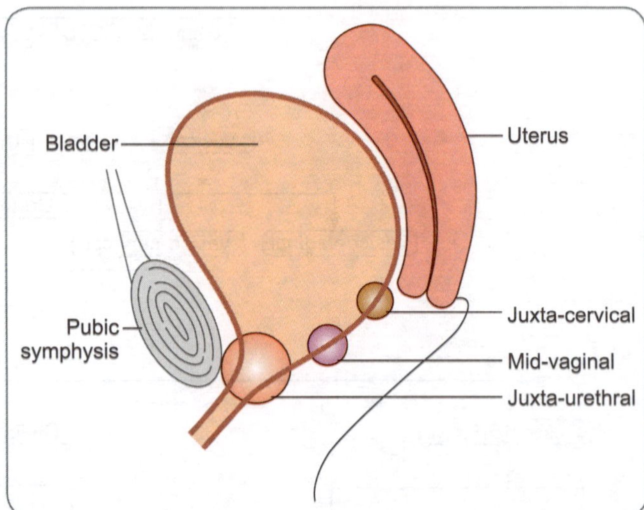


**Fig. 28.3** Different locations of the fistula

- Sometimes one may find a complete perineal tear or a rectovaginal fistula when the patient complains of fecal incontinence besides incontinence of urine.
- Rarely, one may find other associated lesions like vesical or vaginal calculus, genital prolapse or separation of symphysis pubis.

## Diagnosis

From the history and vaginal examination findings, a diagnosis can be made easily.

### History

A thorough history and physical examination is mandatory in the diagnosis of VVF. History of past obstetric events, prior surgeries, past history of fistula and its repair, malignancy and radiation therapy should be carefully elicited and documented.

### Examination

- In cases of small fistulae, the patient may have to be examined in the lithotomy position or sometimes in the knee chest position to visualise the fistula and the amount of scarring around it. A metal catheter passed through the external urinary meatus into the bladder would come out through the fistula into the vagina, confirming that it is a VVF (Fig. 28.4). Incidentally, this also helps to establish the urethral patency in these cases.
- **Methylene blue test** In small fistulae or in doubtful cases, the methylene blue test (or the three-cotton-swabs test (Fig. 28.5)) is done. The patient is placed in the lithotomy position and three cotton swabs are placed in the vagina: one at the vault, the second

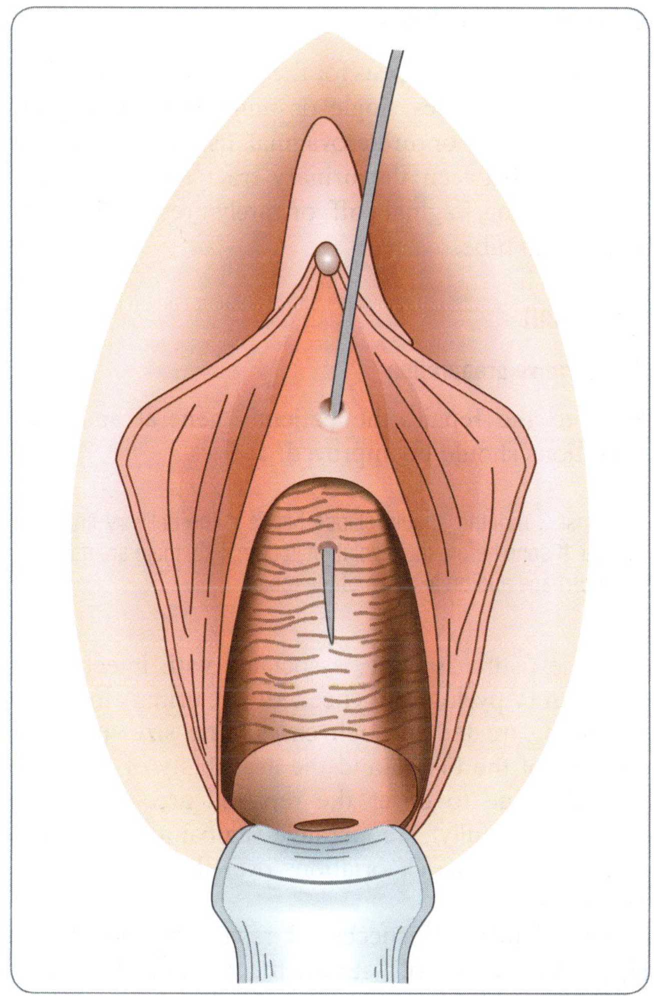
Fig. 28.4 Catheter coming out through the fistula

below this and the third just within the vaginal introitus. The methylene blue solution is then injected into the bladder by means of a catheter. After 15–20 minutes, these swabs are examined. If the lowest one is blue and the others are dry, it is due to urethral incontinence or urethrovaginal fistula; if the middle one is stained, it is a VVF. If the top one is wet with urine but not stained blue, then it is a case of ureterovaginal fistula.

It must always be remembered that there might be more than one fistulous tract and merely identifying one fistula should not be taken as the final diagnosis.

- **Cystourethroscopy examination** has become a routine in the diagnosis of genitourinary fistula (Fig. 28.6). This investigative modality enables one to localise the fistula, assess the ureteral orifices and their proximity to the fistula, study the bladder mucosa and also look for any other fistulous tract.

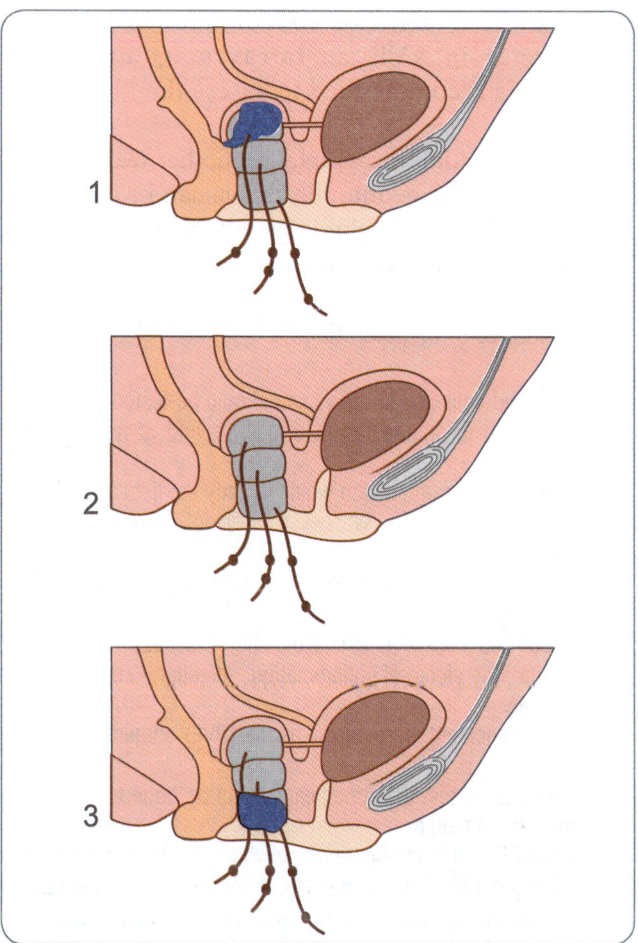

Fig. 28.5 Three-swab test 1. Discolouration of topmost or middle swab indicates vesicovaginal fistula; 2. Wetting of the topmost swab but no discolouration indicates ureterovaginal fistula; 3. Discolouration of lowermost or middle swab indicates urethrovaginal fistula.

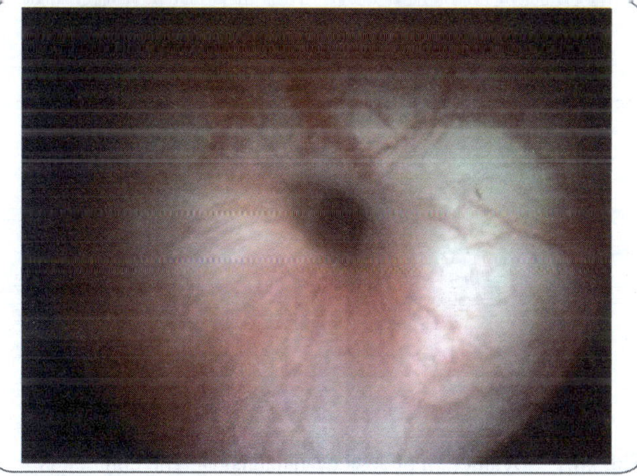
Fig. 28.6 Cystoscopic view of vesicovaginal fistula (*Source:* Image reprinted with permission from Medscape Drugs & Diseases (http://emedicine.medscape.com/), 2017, available at: http://emedicine.medscape.com/article/452934-overview.)

- Since there might be concomitant involvement of ureter in VVF, an **intravenous urography (IVU)** is recommended to assess the kidney and ureter.
- Voiding cystourethrography is another technique by which the leakage into the vagina can be confirmed (Fig. 28.7). It also helps in identifying the number of fistulous tracts and their location.

**Summary of Investigations**

1. Any fluid collected in the vagina should be tested for urea, creatinine to ensure the fluid is urine and is not due to vaginitis.
2. Cystoscopic examination would identify the fistula.
3. IVU is performed whenever ureteric involvement is suspected.
4. Urine is tested for culture and sensitivity and appropriate treatment.
5. A detailed vaginal examination should assess the tissue status like signs of inflammation, infection, edema and mobility.
6. Any associated rectovaginal fistula (RVF) should be ruled out.
7. Three-swab test described earlier can be done to confirm the type of fistula.
8. Colour Doppler ultrasonography with contrast media of the urinary bladder has been tried in cases where cystoscopic evaluation is suboptimal, such as in those patients with severe bladder wall changes like bullous edema or diverticula.
9. Routine examination for any surgical procedure would form a part of the investigations.

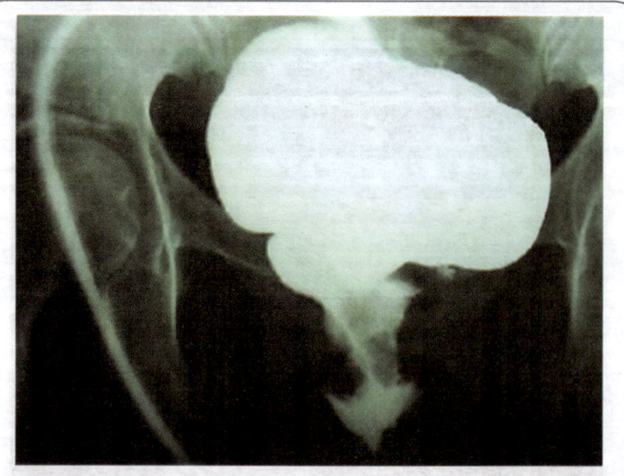

**Fig. 28.7** Cystogram of vesicovaginal fistula. The contrast is seen flowing from the bladder into the vaginal canal. (*Source:* Image reprinted with permission from Medscape Drugs & Diseases (http://emedicine.medscape.com/), 2017, available at: http://emedicine.medscape.com/article/452934-overview.)

## Differential Diagnosis

The differential diagnosis for the discharge of urine into the vagina includes single or multiple vesicovaginal, urethrovaginal, or ureterovaginal fistulae and fistula formation between the urinary tract and the cervix, uterus, vagina, vaginal cuff, or rarely ureteral fistula to a Fallopian tube.

## Treatment

### Preoperative preparation

Prior to the repair, the patient's general and local conditions should be improved.

At least 3 months should elapse between the delivery and the repair. If done before the involution is complete, there are risks of hemorrhage and breakdown of the repair.

If the fistula is large, associated with infection or stone, an IV pyelogram is needed. The urinary infection has to be treated in such cases. The size, position, mobility of the fistula and the availability of adequate vaginal tissue to cover the repaired area should be assessed carefully. Preoperative vaginal application of zinc cream to the excoriations over the vulva may be necessary.

The chances of successful repair depend on the site, size, number of fistulae, the amount of scarring or proximity to the bone, associated lesions (such as a rectovaginal fistula) and the number of previous attempts at surgical closure. With good surgical technique and, more important, careful postoperative nursing, 90 per cent of these fistulae can be closed successfully at the first attempt.

### Prophylactic treatment

To prevent urinary fistulae of obstetric origin, it is essential to provide good prenatal care, screen out high-risk cases, especially those where cephalopelvic disproportion or malpresentation is suspected or diagnosed, and be vigilant during labour. Instead of a prolonged or difficult vaginal delivery, a cesarean section is preferred. Whenever there is evidence of prolonged pressure on the bladder by the fetal head as in prolonged or obstructed labour, bladder drainage for 5 to 7 days after delivery would minimise the chances of the development of urinary fistulae. During gynecological surgery, care should be taken to avoid injury to the bladder, ureter and the urethra.

#### Conservative treatment

In some instances, spontaneous closure of small fistulae has been reported following prolonged catheterisation and drainage. **However if the fistula has not closed within 4 weeks, it is unlikely to do so.** A trial of conservative therapy may be taken up if it could be instituted early and the fistula is small.

Fibrin sealant has also been used more as a surgical adjunct. It needs more elaborate usage and study.

### Surgical Management

The following are the different methods of repair in cases of VVF:

a. Vaginal repair is the method of choice in most cases.
b. Transperitoneal or transvesical methods of abdominal repair are reserved for fistulae which are located high up (as in the vesicouterine type) and are not accessible from below or when the primary repair surgery has failed.
c. Diversion of the urinary stream into the sigmoid (ureterosigmoidostomy) or into an isolated loop of ileum is the last resort in large irreparable fistulae.
d. **Laparoscopic method** This technique is being tried in some places. The procedure requires a skilled laparoscopic surgeon and a unit. It is being attempted as an alternative to abdominal repair in cases where the fistula is high or close to the ureters or is difficult to approach by the vaginal route.
e. Colpocleisis or closure of the vagina may be necessary in some cases of VVF and RVF due to radiation injury. This operation is extremely rare, as the vagina has to be completely shut down. Healing is also difficult in these cases.

**Surgical Principles for Best Results**

- Ensuring adequate healing of the fistula and the surrounding tissues
- Good exposure
- Ensuring complete tissue mobilisation all around
- Total excision of the fistulous tract
- Suturing using appropriate suture material without tension
- Complete hemostasis and maintaining good blood supply at the surgical site
- Meticulous postoperative care

#### Vaginal method of repair

Marion Sims (1852) of the USA was a pioneer in the repair of VVF. He devised special instruments like Sims' speculum to visualise the fistula and the silver wire to close it after paring the edges of the fistula. The two well known vaginal methods of repair are the **flap-splitting method** and **Latzko technique**.

**Advantages** The advantages of vaginal repair over abdominal method are:

- Short operating time
- Reduced blood loss
- Lesser morbidity compared to other methods leading to shorter hospital stay (Wang, 1990). The transvaginal route also allows the use of ancillary equipment, such as ureteral stents.

#### *Flap-splitting method*

The patient is placed in the lithotomy position and the fistula is well exposed and made accessible with an episiotomy or **Schuchardt's paravaginal incision**. The labia are sutured and the cervix is pulled down with a vulsellum. An incision is made encircling the fistula and the margins are dissected to separate the bladder flap from the vaginal wall (Fig. 28.8a, b). After mobilising it well to avoid any tension and after obtaining hemostasis, the margins of the fistulae are fixed by stay sutures to facilitate the closure. The bladder margins are approximated with interrupted sutures avoiding the bladder mucosa with 3/0 atraumatic suture material. A second layer of sutures is now applied to reinforce it (Fig. 28.8c). The bladder is finally tested with methylene blue to see whether there is any leakage. The vaginal edges are then brought together by interrupted sutures (Fig. 28.8d).

#### *Latzko technique*

This has been likened to a partial colpocleisis. The fistulous tract is not excised and the most proximal portions of the anterior and posterior vaginal walls apposed to close the defect. This partially obliterates the upper vagina. The main disadvantage of this method is that the vaginal depth is obliterated and hence it may not be suitable where this is already compromised.

The bladder is continuously drained for 2 weeks, with care being taken to see that it is not blocked at any time. The patient is given a non-residual diet, urinary antiseptics and antibiotics during this period. After 2 weeks, the catheter is removed, and the patient is encouraged to pass urine frequently on her own. She is discharged a week later with the advice to avoid intercourse for the next three months and to report to the hospital when she is pregnant next. The delivery following a successful repair of a VVF should be by an elective cesarean section to avoid recurrence of the fistula.

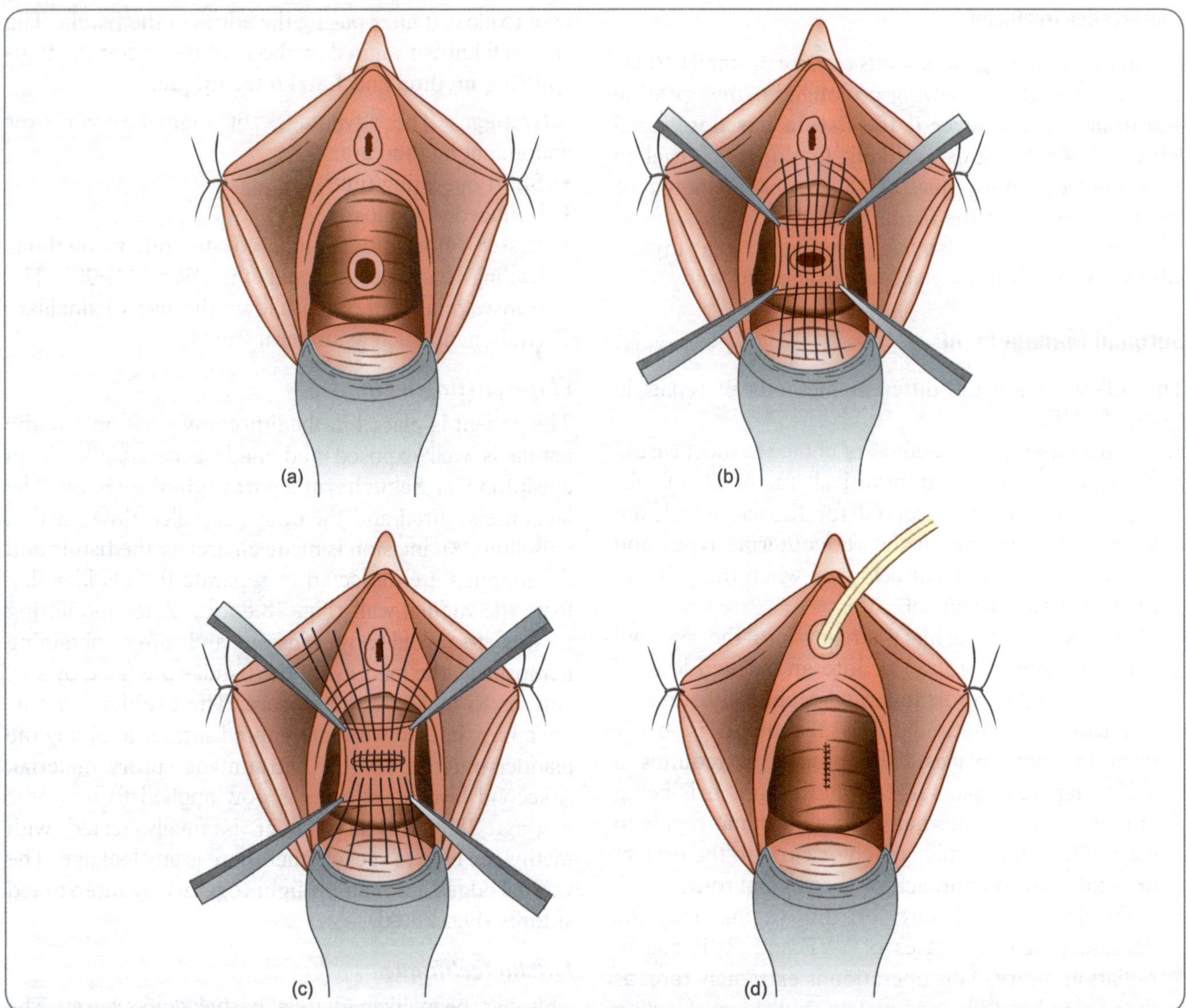


**Fig. 28.8** Repair of vesicovaginal fistula: a. A circular incision is made around the fistula. b. After reflecting the vaginal mucosa, the edges of the bladder opening are sutured with interrupted catgut which avoids the bladder mucosa. c. A second layer of reinforcing sutures is applied before testing for leakage with methylene blue solution. d. The vaginal mucosa is finally closed with interrupted sutures and the bladder drain is kept for two weeks.

### Transvesical or transperitoneal methods of abdominal repair

The **transvesical suprapubic approach** is preferred by genitourinary surgeons for the very high fistula which is inaccessible by the vaginal route.

A **transperitoneal operation** should be performed again in case of combined VVF and high RVF when colostomy can be done together with repair of VVF.

**In combined fistulae (VVF and RVF), it is best to repair both at the same sitting, with the VVF done first.** If the RVF is high, large and difficult to close, a temporary colostomy is made initially, the VVF is repaired first and the RVF repair attempted later. The colostomy is finally closed after both the fistulae have been successfully repaired.

### Laparoscopic repair

This was first introduced in the 1990s. Not many cases are being attempted by this approach.

### Diversion of the urinary stream

In cases of large irreparable fistulae or when repeated attempts at repair fail, urinary continence can be restored by diverting the urinary stream into the sigmoid colon or into an isolated ileal loop. This may be needed in 2–3 per cent of cases of bladder fistulae. For this procedure there should be good anal sphincter control.

After additional investigations of the kidney function including IV pyelography, the abdomen is opened, the lower ends of the ureters are isolated and transplanted into the sigmoid colon by the **modified Coffey technique**. The complications are ascending infection of the kidney from the bowel and hyperchloremic acidosis due to absorption of electrolytes from the urine by a large mucosal surface of the colon. To avoid these complications, urologists presently prefer implantation of the ureters into an isolated loop of the terminal ileum, one end of which is closed and the other opened to the outside as an ileostomy.

Figure 28.9 summarises the broad outlines that can be used in the treatment of VVF.

## URETEROVAGINAL FISTULA (UVF)

### Signs and Symptoms

When there is a ureterovaginal fistula, the patient complains of dribbling of urine continuously but there is some residual urine in the bladder.

### Examination

- **History** The patient has a history of a recent surgery, usually an abdominal hysterectomy.
- The speculum examination shows that dribbling is from the vaginal vault.
- The methylene blue test (with three cotton swabs in the vagina) described earlier helps to distinguish a ureterovaginal fistula from the vesicovaginal variety.
- Chromocystoscopy and intravenous pyelography should be done to confirm the affected side and also to confirm that the excretory function of the kidney is within normal limits.

### Treatment

This is mainly prophylactic to avoid injury to the ureter during surgery. When the ureterovaginal fistula occurs, it may heal spontaneously in a few cases. If it persists for 4 to 6 weeks, the uretero-neocystostomy is done preferably by the extraperitoneal approach.

Other fistulae like urethrovaginal fistula, vesicocervical and vesicouterine fistulae are fortunately very rare. Urethrovaginal fistula can occur due to obstructed labour or following surgery for urethral diverticulum; vesicocervical and vesico-uterine fistula can occur following cesarean section. The details of their repair is beyond the scope of this book. However, they are repaired on the basis of fistula repair mentioned above preferably by the vaginal route.

## URETERIC INJURIES IN GYNECOLOGY

Injury to the ureter occurs in 0.5 per cent of major gynecological surgery and is a serious complication.

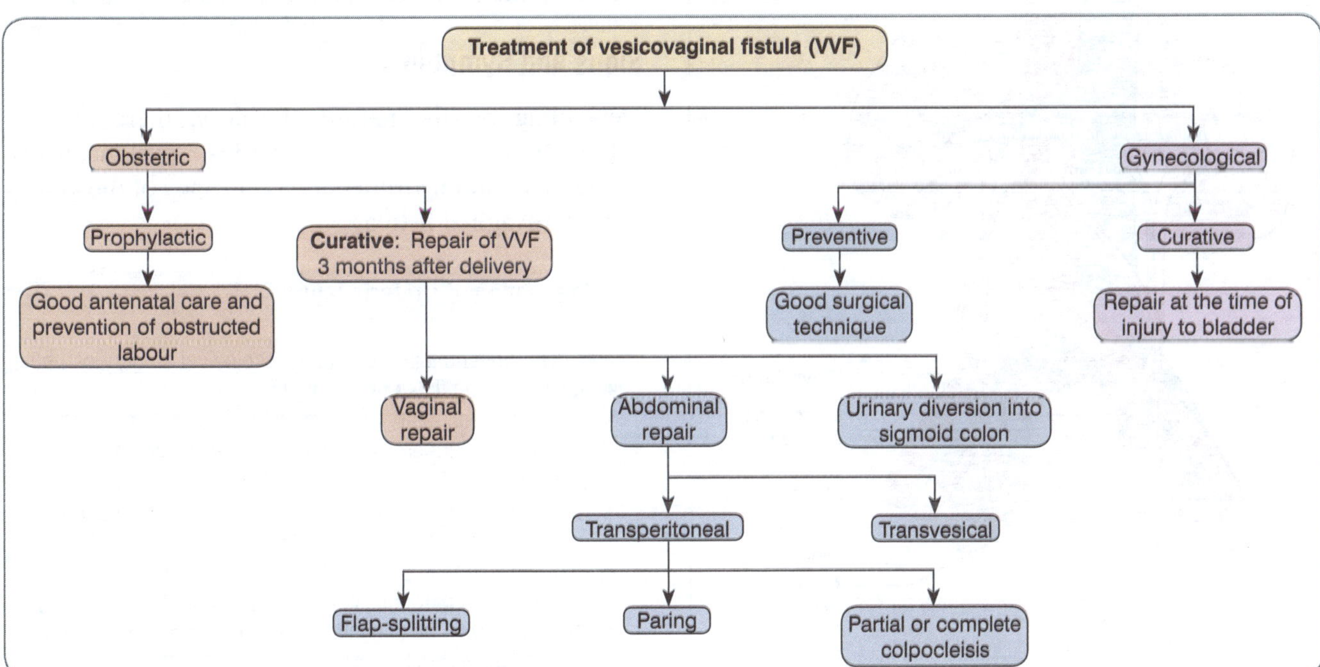


**Fig. 28.9** Broad outlines for the treatment of VVF

**Definition** A significant ureteral injury is defined as any recognised or unrecognised iatrogenic trauma to the ureter that prevents it from functioning properly or effectively (Bradley Fields Schwartz).

## Common Sites of Ureteric Injury

The common sites of ureteric injury are depicted in Fig. 28.10.

## Pathological Conditions Likely to Predispose a Woman to Ureteric Injuries

Certain pathological conditions may cause displacement or distortion of the ureters exposing them to risk of injury.

These are

- broad ligament and cervical myomata
- endometriosis
- broad-ligament cysts
- large ovarian tumours
- tubo-ovarian masses
- carcinoma of the genital tract, in particular, cervix

## Surgical Procedures Likely to Cause Ureteric Injuries

The following gynecological operations may expose the ureters to the risk of injury.

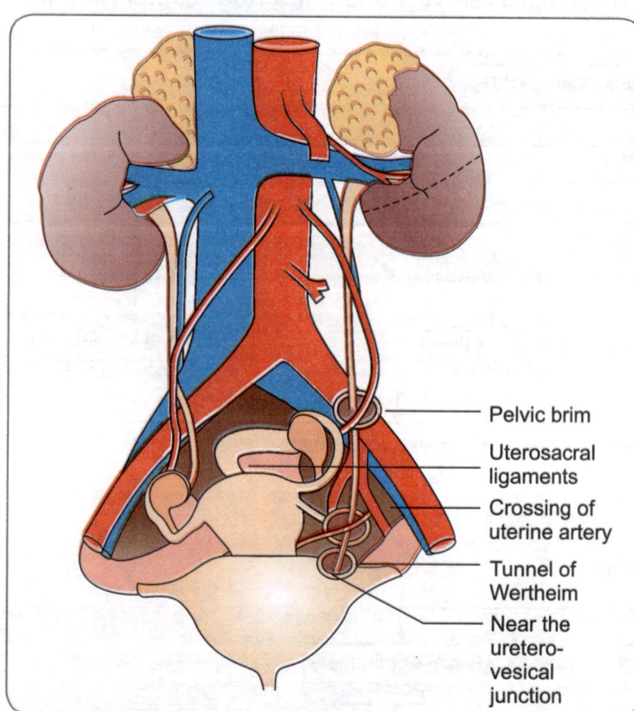


**Fig. 28.10** Common sites of ureteric injury

1. **Total hysterectomy** The most common site of injury is near the internal os when the ureter is close to and crossed over by the uterine artery. When this vessel is clamped, it may be injured. **The left ureter is more liable to injury than the right.**

2. **Presacral neurectomy** The ureters may be injured as they cross the common iliac arteries.

3. **Radical hysterectomy (Wertheim's operation)** This procedure is notorious for ureteric injury for which over-dissection of the ureter or accidental injury is most often responsible. Here, the ureters may be injured directly or indirectly (when the blood supply is interfered with).

4. During removal of the tubo-ovarian masses or chocolate cysts, the ureter may be damaged in the ovarian fossa or near the infundibulopelvic ligament.

5. During **vaginal hysterectomy**, the risk of ureteric trauma is less, but it may be caught in the sutures on one or both sides during surgery for genital prolapse.

Figure 28.11 lists the various causes and types of ureteric injuries in gynecological surgery.

## Types of Ureteric Injury

This may be **transection, laceration, clamping, ligation** or **perforation by a needle.**

The ureteric injury may be **direct, accidental** or **indirect**, due to the stripping of its vascular coat.

## Signs and Symptoms

Depending on the nature of injury, there may be extravasation of urine, peritonitis, pyelonephritis, hydroureter and hydronephrosis, atrophy of the kidney or ureterovaginal fistula.

### Prevention of Ureteric Injury

With care, ureteric injury during gynecological surgery can be avoided by taking these precautions:

- In broad ligament tumours or in radical surgery, a preoperative urological study including an IV urogram is indicated.
- In a laparotomy, the ureters should be inspected and palpated to see if there is any displacement.
- In broad ligament tumours, the tumour should be mobilised or enucleated before ligating the ovarian or uterine vessels.
- Working within the capsule of the fibroid is another method of avoiding ureteral injury.
- No structure should be cut without first identifying it.

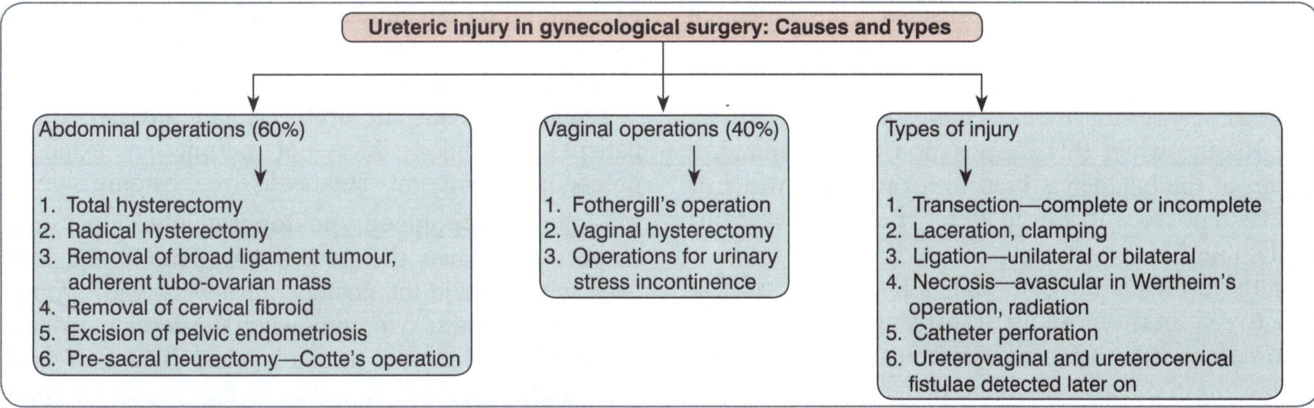


**Fig. 28.11** Causes and types of ureteric injuries in gynecological surgery

- In tubo-ovarian masses and myomas, one should keep close to the pathology during the dissection.
- During radical surgery, the blood supply to the ureter should be preserved, preferably the branch it receives from the internal iliac artery. It should not be stripped of its vascular sheath. The gynecologist must always have a healthy respect for the ureters.

## Management

**During surgery** When ureteric injury is recognised during an operation, the primary procedure is first completed. Then, depending on the site and type of injury, a suitable corrective step is adopted (Fig. 28.12).

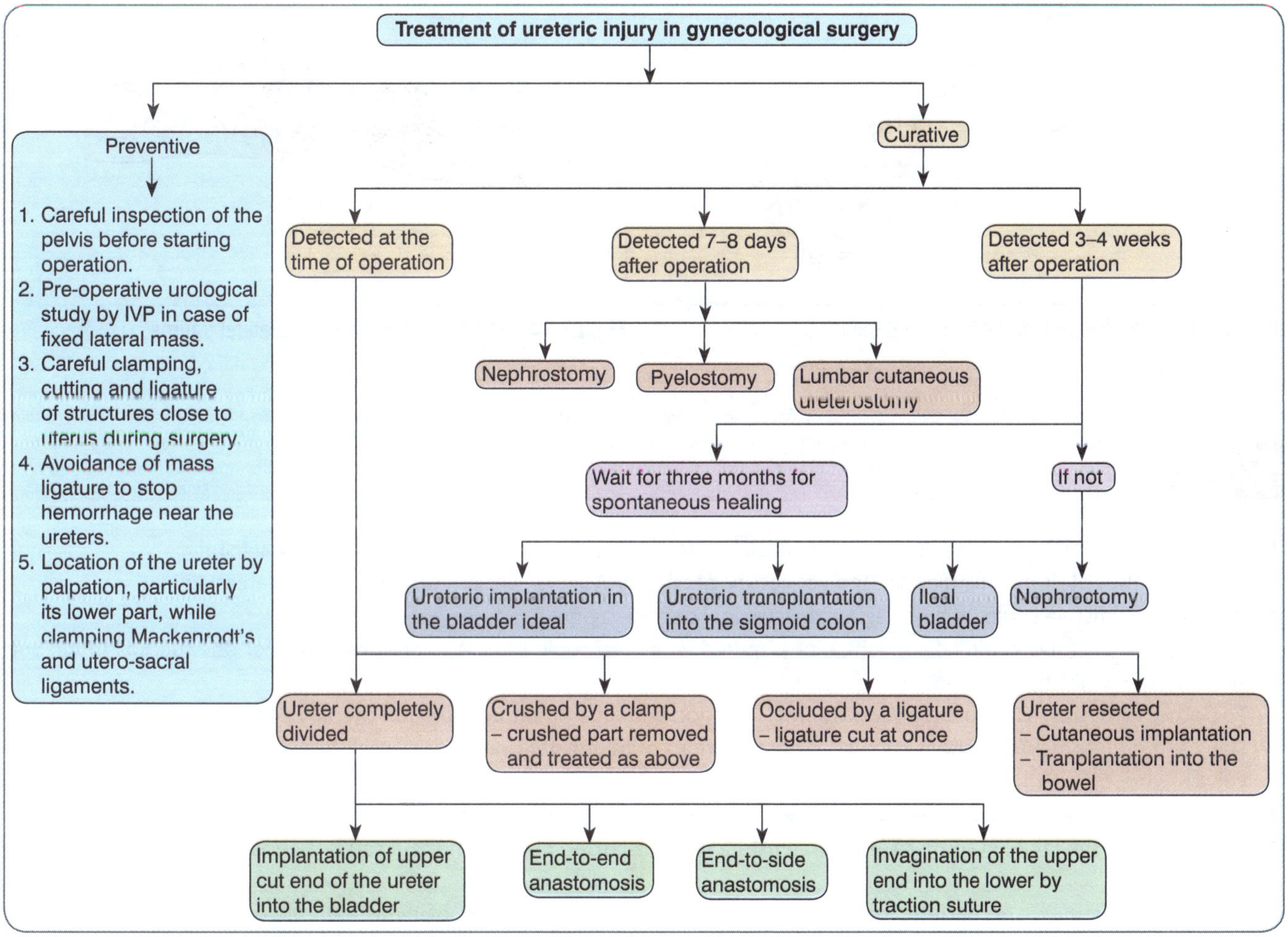

**Treatment of ureteric injury in gynecological surgery**

Preventive
1. Careful inspection of the pelvis before starting operation.
2. Pre-operative urological study by IVP in case of fixed lateral mass.
3. Careful clamping, cutting and ligature of structures close to uterus during surgery.
4. Avoidance of mass ligature to stop hemorrhage near the ureters.
5. Location of the ureter by palpation, particularly its lower part, while clamping Mackenrodt's and utero-sacral ligaments.

Curative

Detected at the time of operation

Detected 7–8 days after operation

Detected 3–4 weeks after operation

Nephrostomy

Pyelostomy

Lumbar cutaneous ureterostomy

Wait for three months for spontaneous healing

If not

Ureteric implantation in the bladder ideal

Ureteric transplantation into the sigmoid colon

Ileal bladder

Nephrostomy

Ureter completely divided

Crushed by a clamp – crushed part removed and treated as above

Occluded by a ligature – ligature cut at once

Ureter resected – Cutaneous implantation – Tranplantation into the bowel

Implantation of upper cut end of the ureter into the bladder

End-to-end anastomosis

End-to-side anastomosis

Invagination of the upper end into the lower by traction suture

**Fig. 28.12** Treatment of ureteric injury in gynecological surgery

a. If the ureter is cut close to the bladder, it is reimplanted into the bladder or a uretero-neocystostomy is done without any tension. If necessary, the bladder and ureter may be mobilised to achieve this without tension.

   Rarely, when this mobilisation is inadequate, a flap of the bladder is used to form a tube which is anastomosed with the cut ureter **(Boari's operation)** (Fig. 28.13).

b. If the ureter is cut at a higher level, the choice is between anastomosis or transplantation. The end-to-end anastomosis may result in stricture; end-to-side anastomosis is therefore better (Fig. 28.14).

c. If the ureter is clamped, the clamp is removed, the crushed part is resected and treated by one of the methods described earlier.

**Ligation of the cut ureter is not advised.** If the patient's condition does not permit an extended procedure, a temporary cutaneous ureterostomy is done.

**In injury recognised postoperatively** One may suspect this when the patient has pain in the loin, fever with rigor in the postoperative week with prompt subsidence of these symptoms when she develops urinary incontinence due to a ureterovaginal fistula. If both ureters are ligated, there will be anuria, and pyelostomy or nephrostomy are indicated as an emergency. The ureters can be reimplanted into the bladder later on.

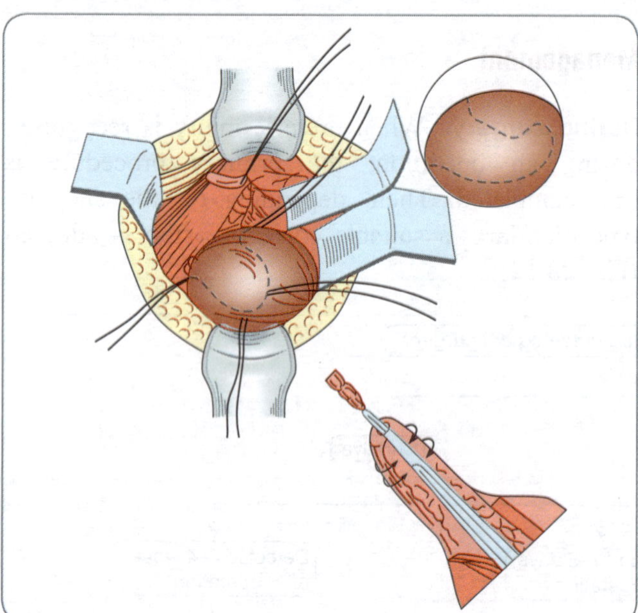

**Fig. 28.13** Boari flap procedure in ureteral trauma

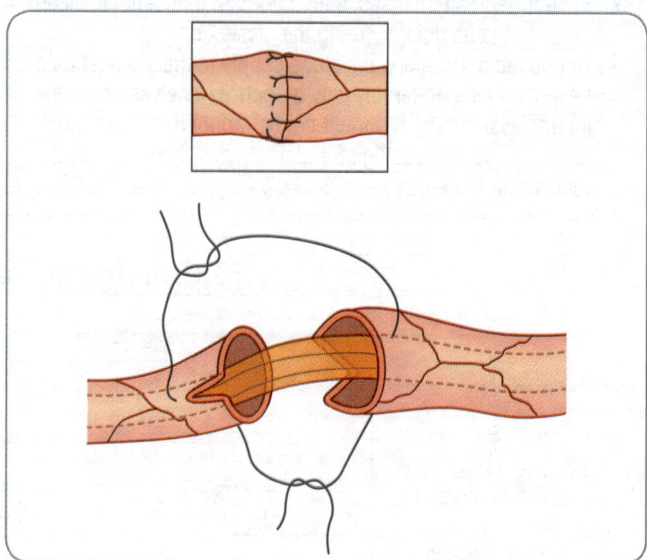

**Fig. 28.14** Ureteroureterostomy in ureteral trauma

## RECAP

- The most common type of fistula seen in hospitals in the developing countries is the vesicovaginal fistula.
- Other varieties of urinary fistulae are the vesicocervical, urethrovaginal, vesicouterine and the ureterovaginal.
- Vesicovaginal fistula could be high vaginal, low vaginal or mid-vaginal.
- Genitourinary fistulae could be congenital or acquired. Acquired could be due to prolonged and/or obstructed labour, and surgical causes like hysterectomy.
- The other rare causes are foreign body, trauma, infection and inflammation, radiation therapy and malignancy.
- Signs and symptoms: The patient complains of continuous dribbling of urine due to which there might be excoriation of the vulva.
- On examination of the external genitals, there is vulvitis and leakage of urine.
- On separating the labia, in some cases a large fistula with prolapsed bladder mucosa can be seen as a red, velvetty, tender mass.
- In obstetric fistulae, the patient may complain of secondary amenorrhea of hypothalamic origin, foot drop caused by prolonged compression of the sacral nerve roots by the fetal head during labour, complete perineal tear or a

rectovaginal fistula, other associated lesions like vesical or vaginal calculus, genital prolapse or separation of symphysis pubis.

- History of past obstetric events, prior surgeries, past history of fistula and its repair, malignancy and radiation therapy should be carefully elicited and documented.
- In small fistulae or in doubtful cases, the methylene blue test (or the three-cotton-swabs test) is done.
- Cystourethroscopy, intravenous urography (IVU) and voiding cystourethrography are other investigative modalities.
- Colour Doppler ultrasonography with contrast media of the urinary bladder has been tried.
- The differential diagnosis for the discharge of urine into the vagina includes single or multiple vesicovaginal, urethrovaginal, or ureterovaginal fistulae and fistula formation between the urinary tract and the cervix, uterus, vagina, vaginal cuff, or (rarely) ureteral fistula to a Fallopian tube.
- Treatment: Preoperative preparation: Prior to the repair, the patient's general and local conditions should be improved.
- At least 3 months should elapse between the delivery and the repair. If done before the involution is complete, there are risks of hemorrhage and breakdown of the repair.
- If the fistula is large, associated with infection or stone, an IV pyelogram is needed.
- The urinary infection has to be treated in such cases. The size, position, mobility of the fistula and the availability of adequate vaginal tissue to cover the repaired area should be assessed carefully.
- Preoperative application of zinc cream to the excoriations over the vulva may be necessary.
- Prophylactic treatment: To prevent urinary fistulae of obstetric origin, it is essential to provide good prenatal care, screen out high-risk cases, especially those where cephalopelvic disproportion or malpresentations are present, and be vigilant during labour.
- Conservative Treatment: In some instances, spontaneous closure of small fistulae has been reported following prolonged catheterisation and drainage.
- Fibrin sealant has also been used.
- Curative treatment: Vaginal repair—flap-splitting method and Latzko technique.
- Transvesical or transperitoneal methods of abdominal repair: The transvesical suprapubic approach is preferred by genitourinary surgeons for the very high fistula which is inaccessible by the vaginal route.
- Diversion of the urinary stream: In cases of large irreparable fistulae or when repeated attempts at repair fail, urinary continence can be restored by diverting the urinary stream into the sigmoid colon or into an isolated ileal loop.
- Laparoscopic method—not much attempted.
- A significant ureteral injury is defined as any recognised or unrecognised iatrogenic trauma to the ureter, which prevents it from functioning properly or effectively.
- Pathological conditions likely to predispose a woman to ureteric injuries are broad ligament and cervical myomata, endometriosis, broad ligament cysts, large ovarian tumours, tubo-ovarian masses and carcinoma of the genital tract, in particular, cervix.
- Surgical procedures likely to cause ureteric injuries are total hysterectomy, presacral neurectomy, radical hysterectomy, during removal of the tubo-ovarian masses or chocolate cysts, during vaginal hysterectomy.
- Ureteric injury may be transection, laceration, clamping, ligation or perforation by a needle.
- The ureteric injury may be direct, accidental or indirect, due to the stripping of its vascular coat.
- Depending on the nature of injury, there may be extravasation of urine, peritonitis, pyelonephritis, hydroureter and hydronephrosis, atrophy of the kidney or ureterovaginal fistula.
- Management options are reimplantation into the bladder or a uretero-neocystostomy, Boari's operation and anastomosis or transplantation.

## REVIEW QUESTIONS

### Long-Answer Question

Enumerate the etiology of vesicovaginal fistula. How is it diagnosed? What are the vaginal methods of repair of the vesicovaginal fistula?

### Short-Answer Questions

1. Discuss the management of ureteric injury in gynecological surgery.
2. How is methylene blue test (three-swab test) performed? How do you interpret the results of the same?

## MCQs

1. **Most common type of genitourinary fistula in the developing countries is**
   a) Vesicocervical fistula
   b) Vesicouterine fistula
   c) Urethrovaginal fistula
   d) Vesicovaginal fistula
2. **In three-swab test (methylene blue test) if the lowest swab is coloured blue, it is suggestive of**
   a) Vesicovaginal fistula
   b) Vesicouterine fistula
   c) Ureterovesical fistula
   d) Urethrovaginal fistula
3. **In which of the following conditions is diversion of the urinary stream not indicated?**
   a) Large irreparable fistulae
   b) Failure of repeated attempts at repair
   c) As a routine in vesicovaginal fistula
   d) Malignancy of the bladder
4. **The treatment of choice in ureterovaginal fistula is**
   a) Uretero-neocystostomy
   b) Ureteroureterostomy
   c) Latzko technique
   d) Flap-splitting method

**Further Reading**

Berek J, editor. Berek & Novak's Gynecology. 15th ed. Philadelphia: Wolters Kluwer; 2012.

Das Gupta S. Urological problems in gynaecology. Postgraduate obstetrics and gynaecology. 3rd ed. Menon MKK, Devi PK, Rao KB, editors. Madras: Orient Longman; 1986. 482 p.

Green TH. Gynaecology: essentials of clinical practice. 3rd ed. Boston: Little Brown; 1977.

Hoffman BL, Schorge JO, Bradshaw KD, Halvorson LM, Schaffer JI, Corton MM, editors. William's Gynecology. 3rd ed. New York: McGraw-Hill Education; 2016.

Lawson JB, Stewart DB. Obstetrics and gynaecology in the tropics. London: Edward Arnold; 1967.

Rao KB. Genital fistulae. Postgraduate obstetrics and gynecology. 3rd ed. Menon MKK, Devi PK, Rao KB, editors. Madras: Orient Longman; 1986. 497 p.

Report of a RCOG Meeting 1994. Urinary incontinence. Br J Obstet Gynecol. 1994; 101:1094–6.

Stanley A. Surgery of female incontinence. Stanton and Terango, editors. Springer Verlag; 1980. 77 p.

# Chapter 29

# Radiological Investigations in Gynecology

## At a Glance


Principles of Ultrasound
Transabdominal Sonography (TAS)
Transvaginal Sonography (TVS)
 Method of Transvaginal Scanning
Transrectal and Transperineal Sonography
Saline Infusion Sonography (SIS) or Sonohysterography
Doppler Study
Limitations for Transvaginal Sonography
Clinical Applications
 Uterus
 Ovary
Computed Tomography (CT) in Gynecology
 Disadvantages of CT Scan
Magnetic Resonance Imaging (MRI)
 MRI in Gynecology
Positron Emission Tomography (PET) Imaging


Gynecological ultrasound deals with the application of medical ultrasonography for the visualisation of female pelvic organs and related structures. Ultrasound was introduced in the field of medicine by Ian Donald in the 1950s mainly for obstetric practice. It has come a long way from being a static visualisation to the present real time 2D, 3D and even 4D ultrasound along with Doppler facilities.

## PRINCIPLES OF ULTRASOUND

The use of ultrasound in medicine was developed from **SONAR (sound navigation and ranging) systems** that were used to detect submarines. Ultrasound uses the principle of **inverse piezoelectric effect**. This refers to the phenomenon that occurs when pressure is applied to the surface of piezoelectric crystals; the mechanical pressure produces an electric current. Inversely, when an electric pulse is applied to piezoelectric material, a mechanical wave is produced and this mechanical wave is the ultrasound beam.

An **ultrasound scanner** is made up of transducer(s) which contain piezoelectric crystals. When excited by an electric pulse, the crystals generate ultrasonographic waves which pass from the ultrasound transducer into the tissues in their path. When these waves meet a tissue interface, they are reflected back to the transducer and converted into an electric signal which is processed and digitalised as an ultrasound image on the monitor.

**Sound is the orderly transmission of mechanical vibrations through a medium.** The number of vibrations that occur per second is known as the frequency and is measured in hertz (Hz). 1 Hz is 1 cycle/second. The human ear can detect frequencies in the range of 20 Hz to 20,000 Hz (20 kilohertz). Sound above this range is known as **ultrasound**. Most medical diagnostic equipment have a range of 1–10 megahertz (MHz); 1 MHz is 1,000,000 cycles/second.

The penetration of a high-frequency wave is limited. Therefore, high-frequency probes are used to examine nearer structures, while lower frequency probes are used to study tissues in depth. **A transvaginal transducer (TVS)** (Fig. 29.1) uses a frequency of 5 to 15 MHz, while **transabdominal transducers (TAS)** (Fig. 29.2) use a frequency of 2 to 6.5 MHz.

A dense structure, like bone, appears white on the screen (**echogenic**), while fluid appears black (**anechoic**);

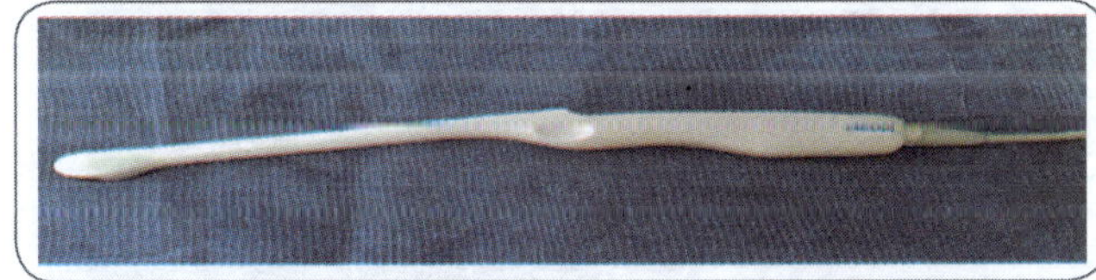

**Fig. 29.1** Vaginal transducer

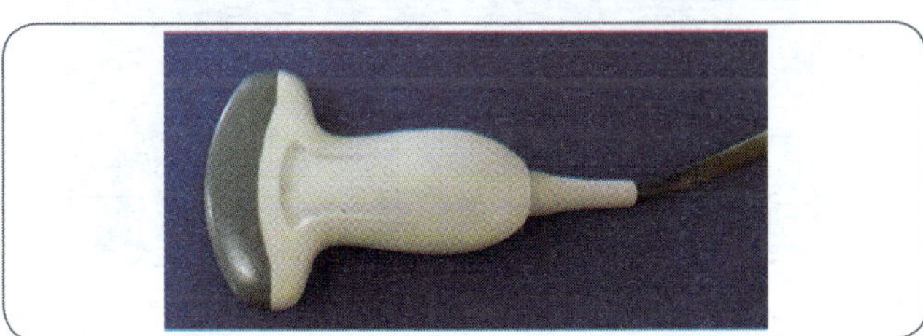

**Fig. 29.2** Abdominal transducer

this happens when an entire wave is transmitted and none is reflected. Structures made up of a few echoes are referred to as being **echo-poor** or **hypoechoic**.

In gynecological examination, transvaginal route is preferred to transabdominal route. This is true in almost all gynecological conditions except when the suspected pathology is large and is expected to extend the uterus out of the pelvis, as in large leiomyoma. The transvaginal route has a higher resolution and is also in close proximity to the scanned structures, which enhances the details. The other advantage of the transvaginal route is that there is no need for a full bladder as an acoustic window as in transabdominal route.

## TRANSABDOMINAL SONOGRAPHY (TAS)

Transabdominal sonography is usually performed with a curved 3–5 MHz transducer. The advantage of TAS is its ability to visualise the entire pelvic organs, which also delineates the relationship between the pelvic organs to one another.

The bladder acts as an acoustic window and improves the transmission of ultrasound waves (Fig. 29.3).

## TRANSVAGINAL SONOGRAPHY (TVS)

Transvaginal sonography uses a 5–10 MHz transducer. The probe is placed in the vaginal fornices, in close proximity to the pelvic organs thereby providing better image details and quality. Unlike TAS screening, there is no need for a full bladder.

### Method of Transvaginal Scanning

Transvaginal scanning is performed in the midsagittal plane (Fig. 29.4). This view clearly demonstrates the uterine fundus, isthmus and the cervix. It is also easy to measure the uterine length in this view. The midsagittal view also facilitates the measurement of endometrial thickness. It is important to look for any hitherto unknown anomalies of the uterus, cervix and adnexa while performing ultrasound examination.

Vaginal probe can also be used for exerting gentle pressure on the uterus and adnexa to elicit any tenderness, particularly in conditions like endometriosis and PID. Care should be taken not to exert too much pressure and produce discomfort and pain to the patient.

## TRANSRECTAL AND TRANSPERINEAL SONOGRAPHY

These techniques are not commonly used and their use is restricted to study of the pelvic floor, particularly in urogynecology. 3-D imaging has been found to be better and less troublesome to the patient than transrectal or transperineal sonography.

## SALINE INFUSION SONOGRAPHY (SIS) OR SONOHYSTEROGRAPHY

This was first introduced in the late 1970s for studying the endometrial cavity in greater detail. Before introducing the catheter into the uterine cavity, TVS is done. **Care should be taken not to touch the fundus of the uterus with**

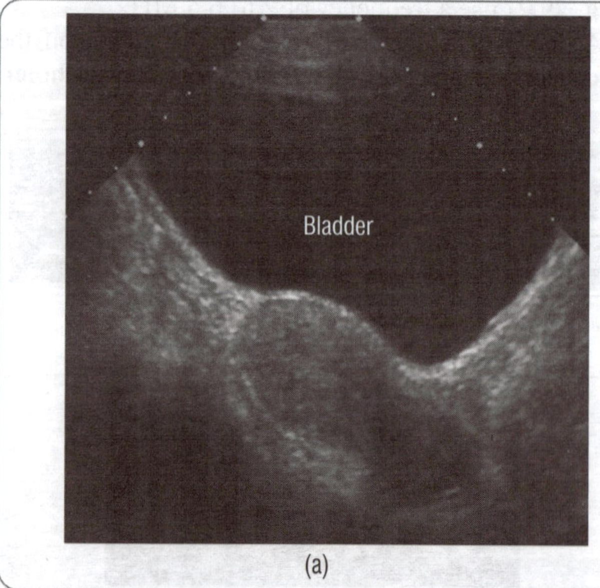


(a)

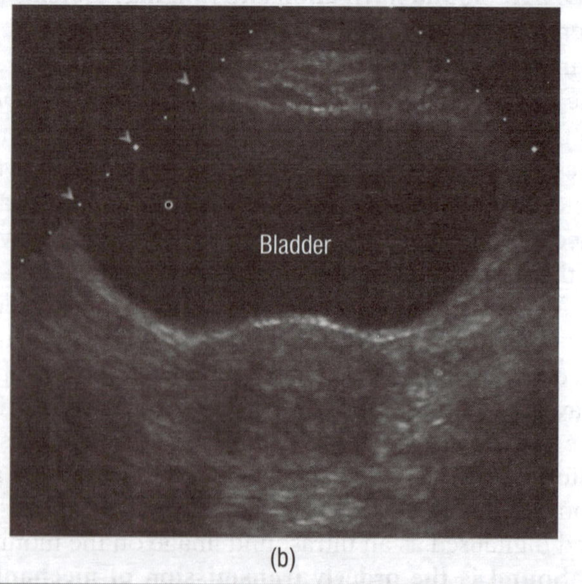


(b)

**Fig. 29.3** Transabdominal scan: Sagittal and transverse view of normal uterus (*Source:* Radiology Key, Reproduced with permission)

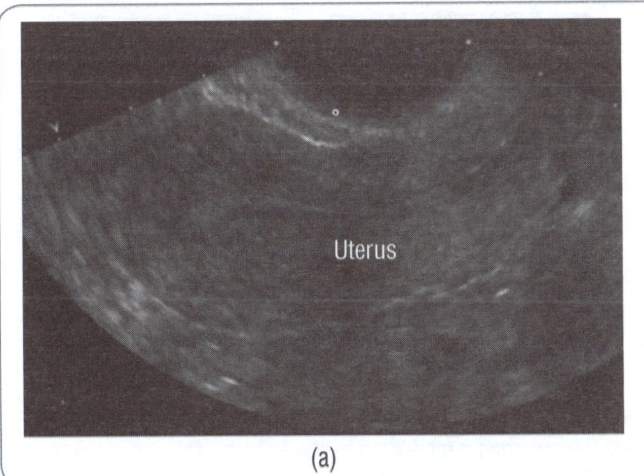


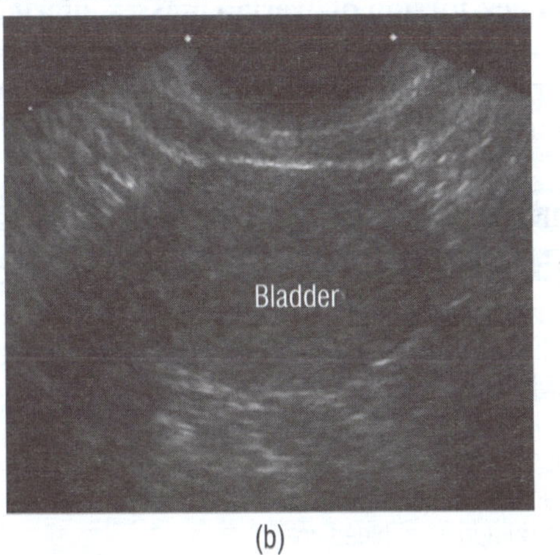


**Fig. 29.4** Transvaginal scan: Sagittal and transverse view of normal uterus (*Source*: Radiology Key, Reproduced with permission)

**the advancing catheter as this may produce vasovagal attack**. After introducing the catheter, the TVS probe is introduced and 20–30 mL of sterile saline is introduced. As the saline is being introduced, the uterine cavity and the endometrium are visualised (Fig. 29.5). This visualisation is done in various planes to obtain a comprehensive study of the uterus and endometrial cavity. After the procedure, the catheter is withdrawn.

## DOPPLER STUDY

Doppler shift is a principle of physics according to which, when sound waves strike a moving target, their frequency is changed proportional to the velocity and direction of the moving target. This principle is used to determine the rate and volume of blood flow through different vessels. The waveforms of different vessels are studied, and based upon the systolic and diastolic blood flow, various indices are calculated (Fig. 29.6).

Both TAS and TVS can be used for this technique. Resistance Index (RI) and pulsatility index (PI) are the commonly calculated arterial waveform parameters.

Colour Doppler study is used in gynecology for identifying the direction and velocity of the blood flow. This is used for identifying **ectopic pregnancy, ovarian**

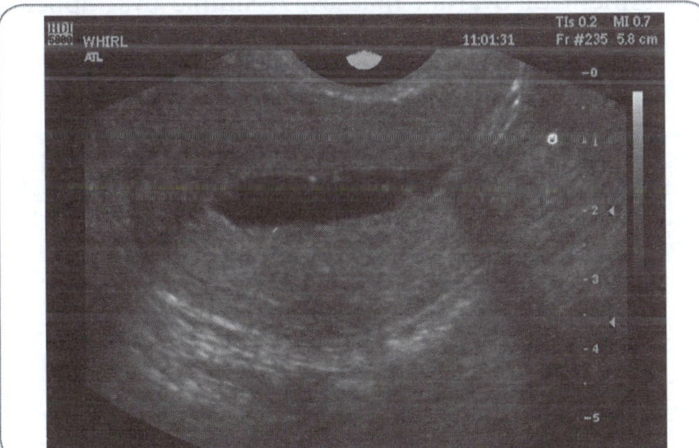


**Fig. 29.5** Saline infusion sonography showing normal uterus and endometrial cavity (*Source*: Chizen, D, Pierson, R, Glob. libr. women's med.)

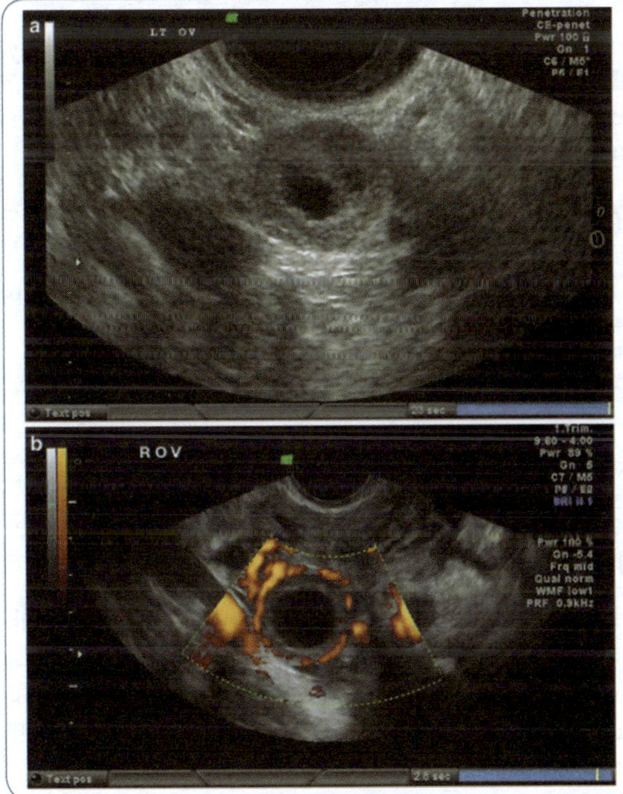


**Fig. 29.6** Colour Doppler of corpus luteum cyst (*Source*: Radiology Key, Reproduced with permission)

**malignancy, torsion of ovarian masses, uterine masses like leiomyoma and endometrial pathology.** Power Doppler is also another technique of Doppler flow study, mainly used for identifying endometrial pathology.

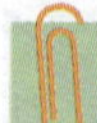

### Common Indications for Ultrasound Examination in Gynecology

- To assess amenorrhea (non-pregnant)
- In the assessment of heavy menstrual bleeding
- Pelvic pain
- PCOS
- Suspected leiomyoma
- Suspected adenomyosis
- Postmenopausal bleeding
- Endometriosis
- Infertility workup including follicular study
- Ovum aspiration
- Suspected uterine anomalies
- Ovarian pathology
- Endometrial thickness
- Localisation of an intrauterine contraceptive device
- Suspected ectopic pregnancy
- Study of the surrounding organs

The list is not complete and pelvic ultrasound is used more exhaustively.

## LIMITATIONS FOR TRANSVAGINAL SONOGRAPHY

There are few limitations to transvaginal sonography. The absolute limitations are imperforate hymen and refusal by the patient. The relative contraindications include a virgin or strictured introitus.

## CLINICAL APPLICATIONS

The normal dimensions of the uterus and ovaries are as follows:

| Organ | Dimension |
|---|---|
| Uterus | 7.5 cm long, 5 cm wide and 2.5 cm thick |
| Ovary | 3.5 cm long, 2.5 cm wide and 1.5 cm thick<br>After menopause ovaries measure 2 × 1.5 × 1 cm |

### Uterus

**Fibroid Uterus** The fibroids appear as solid, well-defined masses with hypoechoic periphery (Fig. 29.7).

**Adenomyosis** The uterine contour is regular in shape and the myometrium is asymmetrically thickened with heterogeneous areas (Fig. 29.8).

**Congenital anomalies of the uterus** Anatomical anomalies of the uterus are clearly diagnosed by transvaginal ultrasonography (Fig. 29.9). However, the anatomical defects are visualised better by 3D ultrasound.

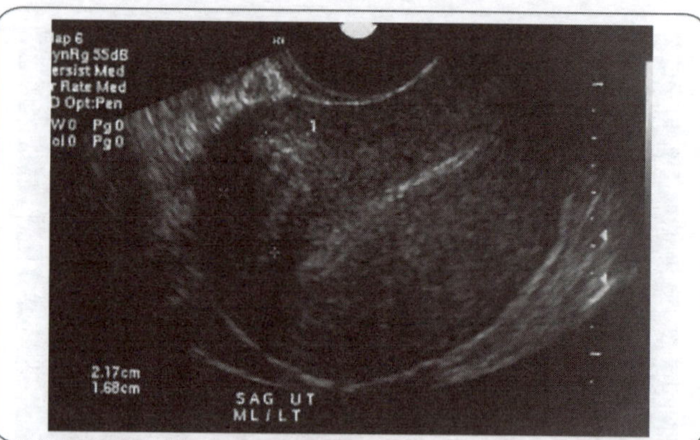


**Fig. 29.7** Intramural myoma (*Source*: Neuwirth, R, Moritz, J, Glob. libr. women's med.)

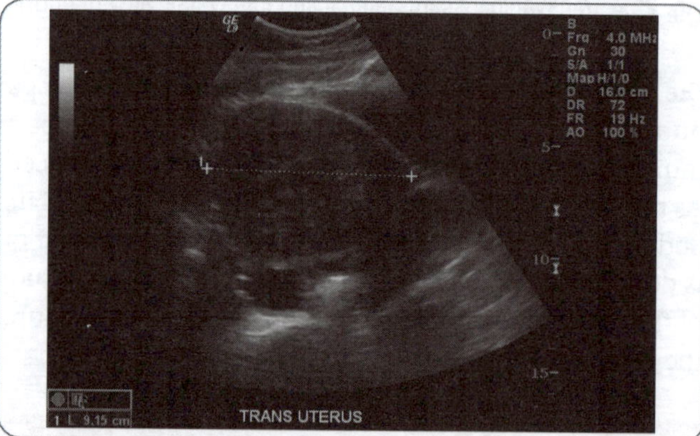


**Fig. 29.8** Adenomyosis (*Source*: WikiDoc)

### Ovary

Ultrasound is the main sonographic evaluation in the assessment of ovarian masses. A simple cyst appears

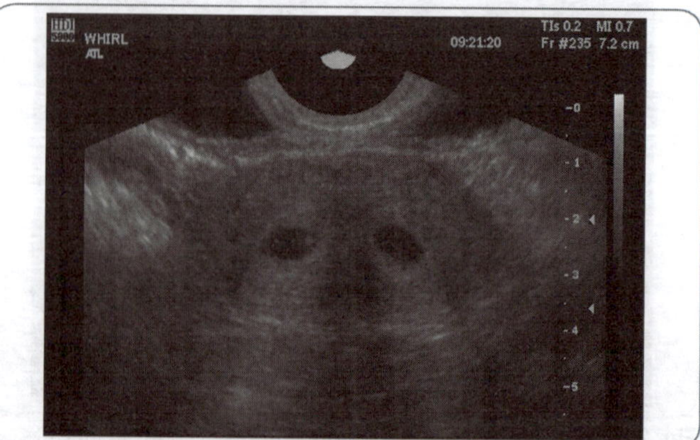


**Fig. 29.9** Bicornuate uterus (*Source:* Chizen, D, Pierson, R, Glob. libr. women's med.)

as a smooth-walled cystic mass without any internal echoes. But in contrast, a complex ovarian abscess shows thickened septations and may even demonstrate fluid-filled pockets (Fig. 29.10).

The other pathology that could be diagnosed are hydrosalpinx (Fig. 29.11), identification of intrauterine device (Fig. 29.12) where the thread is not palpated.

Ultrasound has come a long way from the static mode to B mode real time scan and from transabdominal to transvaginal scan. Transvaginal scan is better for the gynecological study since it can assess the structures in closer proximity than transabdominal scan. The introduction of Doppler study has helped in the study of blood flow and in identifying neovascularisation, which helps in detecting neoplasia. 3D scan has further enhanced the quality of diagnosis. Ultrasonography is being used in therapeutic procedures also. 4D ultrasound and compression sonography are further improvements for better diagnostic and therapeutic applications.

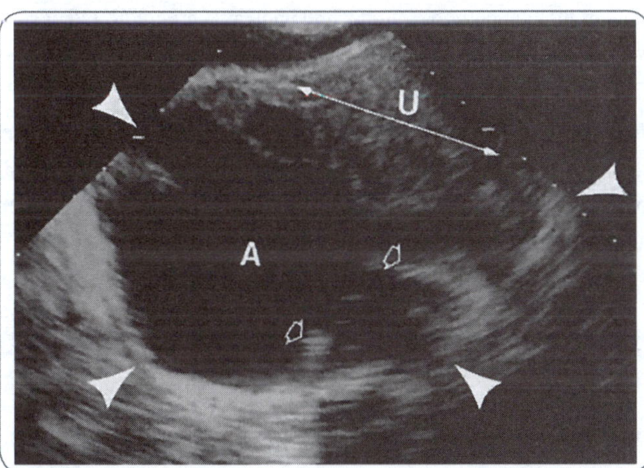


**Fig. 29.10** Transverse transabdominal scan of right tubo-ovarian abscess. Scan depicts uterus (U) and abscess (A). Small open arrowheads show irregularity of the abscess wall. Large white arrowheads show the borders of the abscess. (*Source:* Wade, R, Bliss, S, Glob. libr. women's med.)

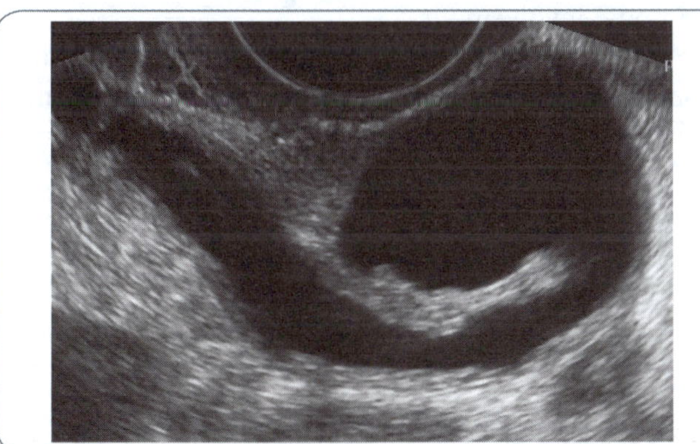

**Fig. 29.11** Left hydrosalpinx (*Source:* Wkimedia/©Ekem)

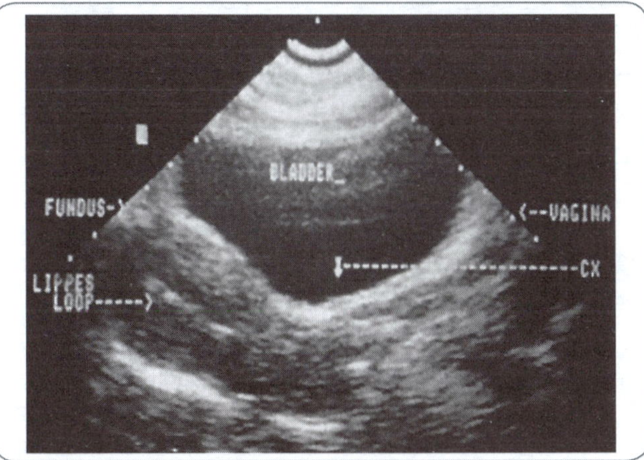


**Fig. 29.12** Intrauterine device. Transabdominal scan depicting Lippes loop in situ, cervix (CX), fundus, bladder, and vagina (*Source:* Wade, R, Bliss, S, Glob. libr. women's med.)

## COMPUTED TOMOGRAPHY (CT) IN GYNECOLOGY

Computed tomography is an X-ray-based investigation in which 2D axial images are provided for analysis. These images are called slices of the area covered. The advancement of CT scan is spiral CT which is a multichannel helical CT. Contrast CT can also be performed where indicated. **In gynecology, CT is mainly used as an additional tool for diagnosing malignancy and its extent** (Fig. 29.13).

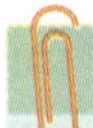

### Indications for CT in Gynecology

1. **Malignancy**
   - Cancer Cervix
   - For indentifying extent of local lesion and local recurrence
   - Parametrical infiltration and lymph node enlargement
   - Endometrial cancer
   - For assessing myometrial infiltration
   - Ovarian cancer—size of the tumour
   - Lymph node involvement
   - Distant metastasis
2. **Benign conditions**
   - When other imaging modalities do not clearly identify the lesion.

### Disadvantages of CT Scan

Radiation exposure is the major disadvantage of CT scan. Similarly lymph nodes of less than 2 cm size may be missed by CT scan. The risk of allergic reaction to contrast is a potential hazard.

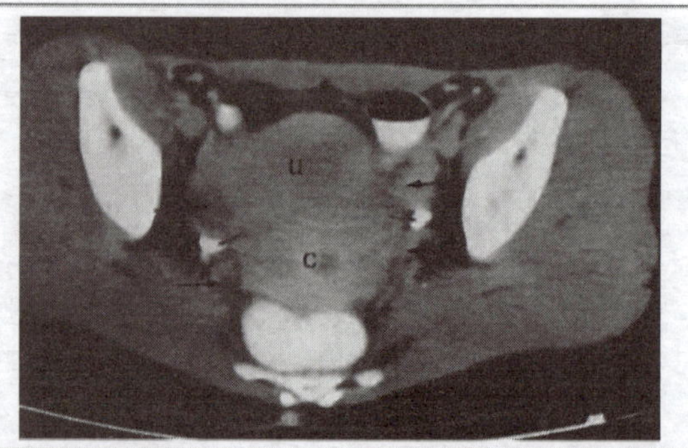


**Fig. 29.13** Cervical carcinoma with invasion of the parametria. CT scan of the pelvis shows inhomogeneous and enlarged cervix (c) with irregular soft-tissue densities extending into the parametria (long arrows), without invasion of the pelvic sidewalls. The periureteral fat planes are partially obliterated by tumour (short arrows), but the ureters are not obstructed (u, uterus). (*Source:* Source: Abu-Yousef, M, Pelsang, R, et al, Glob. libr. women's med.)

## MAGNETIC RESONANCE IMAGING (MRI)

In this technique, images are constructed based on the radio frequency signal emitted by hydrogen nuclei in a strong magnetic field. The radio frequency signals have a relaxation time known as T1 relaxation time (Longitudinal) and T2 relaxation time (Transverse).

### MRI in Gynecology

An MRI of a normal female pelvis is shown in Fig. 29.14. MRI is very useful in the diagnosis of the following conditions.

**Leiomyoma** MRI is the most accurate method for evaluating leiomyoma. This method is very helpful in mapping leiomyoma. Magnetic Resonance Imaging guidance of focused ultrasound (MRgFUS) therapy is being used as a treatment for fibroids.

**Adenomyosis** MRI has been found to be as good as USG or even better in diagnosing adenomyosis.

**Congenital anomalies** MRI has been found to be better in diagnosing congenital anomalies than conventional techniques.

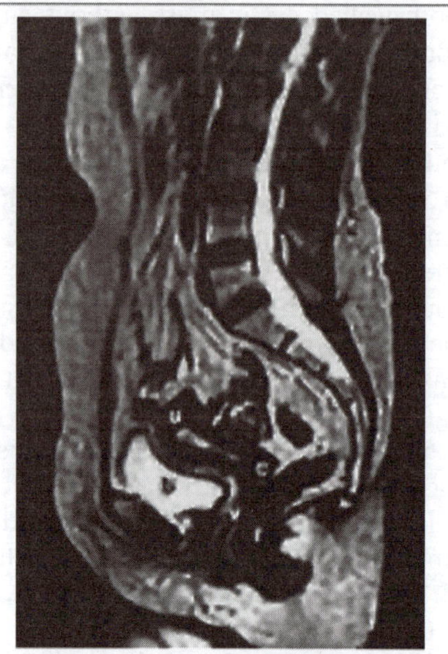

**Fig. 29.14** T2-weighted MRI of a normal female pelvis; sagittal view of the uterine body, cervix, and vagina. (*Source:* Abu-Yousef, M, Pelsang, R, et al, Glob. libr. women's med.)

**Adnexal masses, endometrial lesions and malignancies** Cervical cancer, endometrial cancer, ovarian malignancies can all be diagnosed with better accuracy by using MRI.

## POSITRON EMISSION TOMOGRAPHY (PET) IMAGING

PET scan uses short-life radiochemical compounds for identification of malignancy or other conditions. The most common PET tracer used is Fluoro Deoxy Glucose (FDG). FDG-PET has been found to be very effective for initial staging of cancer cervix and has both therapeutic and prognostic benefits. It has been found to be equally effective in diagnosing other malignancies and nodal involvement.

PET scan can also be used for postoperative monitoring of endometrial and ovarian cancer patients.

## RECAP

- Sound is the orderly transmission of mechanical vibrations through a medium.
- The number of vibrations that occur per second is known as the frequency and is measured in hertz (Hz). 1 Hz is 1 cycle/second.

- The human ear can detect frequencies in the range of 20 Hz to 20,000 Hz (20 kilohertz). Sound above this range is known as ultrasound.
- A transvaginal transducer (TVS) uses a frequency of 5 to 15 MHz, while transabdominal transducers (TAS) use a frequency of 2 to 6.5 MHz.
- A dense structure, like bone, appears white on the screen (echogenic), while fluid appears black (anechoic); this happens when an entire wave is transmitted and none is reflected. Structures made up of a few echoes are referred to as being echo-poor or hypoechoic.
- In gynecological examination, transvaginal route is preferred to transabdominal route.
- Transabdominal sonography is usually performed with a curved 3–5 MHz transducer. The advantage of TAS is its ability to visualise the entire pelvic organs, which also delineates the relationship between the pelvic organs to one another. The bladder acts as an acoustic window and improves the transmission of ultrasound waves.
- The transvaginal probe is placed in the vaginal fornices, in close proximity to the pelvic organs thereby providing better image details and quality.
- Transrectal and transperineal techniques are not commonly used and their use is restricted to study of the pelvic floor, particularly in urogynecology. 3D imaging has been found to be better and less troublesome to the patient than transrectal or transperineal sonography.
- Saline Infusion Sonography (SIS) or sonohysterography is useful for studying the endometrial cavity is greater detail.
- Doppler shift is a principle of physics according to which, when sound waves strike a moving target, their frequency is changed proportional to the velocity and direction of the moving target. This principle is used to determine the rate and volume of blood flow through different vessels.
- Colour Doppler study is used in gynecology for identifying the direction and velocity of the blood flow. This is used for identifying ectopic pregnancy, ovarian malignancy, torsion of ovarian masses, uterine masses like leiomyoma and endometrial pathology.
- Common indications for ultrasound examination in gynecology include amenorrhea (non-pregnant), heavy menstrual bleeding, pelvic pain, PCOS, suspected leiomyoma, suspected adenomyosis, postmenopausal bleeding, endometriosis, infertility workup including follicular study, ovum aspiration, suspected uterine anomalies, ovarian pathology, endometrial thickness, localisation of an intrauterine contraceptive device, suspected ectopic pregnancy and study of the surrounding organs.
- Computed tomography is an X-ray-based investigation in which 2D axial images are provided for analysis.
- It can be used for diagnosing malignant conditions like cervical cancer, endometrial cancer, ovarian cancer and their extent of spread and also benign conditions.
- Disadvantages of CT scan include radiation exposure, lymph nodes of less than 2 cm size may be missed and risk of allergic reaction to contrast.
- In Magnetic Resonance Imaging (MRI), images are constructed based on the radio frequency signal emitted by hydrogen nuclei in a strong magnetic field.
- MRI can be used for diagnosing leiomyoma, adenomyosis, congenital anomalies of uterus, adnexal masses, endometrial lesions and malignancies.
- PET scan uses short-life radiochemical compounds for identification of malignancy or other conditions.
- The most common PET tracer used is Fluoro Deoxy Glucose (FDG).
- FDG-PET has been found to be very effective for initial staging of cancer cervix and has both therapeutic and prognostic benefits.
- It has been found to be equally effective in diagnosing other malignancies and nodal involvement.

# REVIEW QUESTIONS

## MCQs

**1. Which of these is not a limitation for transvaginal sonography?**

a) Imperforate hymen
b) Refusal by the patient
c) Strictured introitus
d) Absence of full bladder

**2. Saline Infusion Sonography (SIS) is done using**

a) Transvaginal probe
b) Transabdominal probe

c) Transrectal probe
d) Any of the probes mentioned above

**3. Transvaginal probe uses a frequency of**

a) 2 to 6.5 MHz.
b) 5 to 15 MHz
c) 20–25 MHz
d) 0.5–1.5 MHz

**4. In ultrasound image fluid appears as**

a) Black (anechoic)
b) White (echogenic)
c) Hypoechogenic
d) No definite echo pattern

# CHAPTER 30

# Endoscopy in Gynecology

**AT A GLANCE**

Laparoscopy
Surgical Technique
Hysteroscopy
Hysteroscope
Newer Endoscopic Techniques
Salpingoscopy
Falloposcopy
Complications of Newer Techniques

Gynecological endoscopy is a surgical discipline which uses optical instruments to help in the diagnosis and management of the most frequent female disorders and pathologies such as infertility problems, vaginal bleeding or endometrial polyps among others. **Gynecological endoscopy employs laparoscopy and hysteroscopy for these purposes.**

Endoscopy was reported by Phillip Bozzini way back in 1805. With the advancement in technology and availability of better equipment like high-resolution cameras, video laparoscopy, electrical and laser energy, it has become popular in the last few decades. It allows minimal handling of tissues, avoids abdominal scar and hence causes less postoperative morbidity.

## LAPAROSCOPY

Laparoscopy provides minimal invasive option for women to undergo various gynecological surgeries. Initially it was used as a diagnostic and sterilisation procedure. With advancement in robotic techniques, surgeons are enabled to perform more complex procedures. But to improve patient safety, surgeon should appropriately select the patients.

### Surgical Technique

The procedure is performed in the operation theatre under aseptic precautions. Usually general anaesthesia is preferred. The patient is placed in semi-lithotomy or deep Trendelenburg position. Abdomen, perineum and vagina are painted and draped. Bladder is catheterised and the findings are reconfirmed by bimanual examination. A uterine manipulator is introduced through the cervical canal for manipulation to visualise the uterus, tubes and ovaries.

#### Pneumoperitoneum

- A sub-umbilical incision of 1.25 cm is made and the **Veress needle is introduced at an angle of 45°** into the peritoneal cavity. The correct placement of Veress needle is verified by
  a. *Syringe barrel test* Normal saline is aspirated with 10 mL syringe. The saline is then pushed and aspiration is done. This ensures that the tip is not misplaced in a blood vessel or viscera. The fluid cannot be withdrawn if the needle placement is correct.
  b. *Hanging drop method* A small volume of sterile normal saline is placed on top of the Veress needle. The saline drops into the peritoneal cavity due to negative intraperitoneal pressure. This confirms proper placement of the Veress needle.
  c. *Intraabdominal pressure* (<10 mm of Hg) on the insufflator with free flow of gas.
- Port of entry: The most common sites are (Fig. 30.1):
  - At the umbilicus (most common)
  - Palmer's point (on left midclavicular line)
  - Suprapubic (2–4 cm above the pubic symphysis).
- Introduction of primary trocar and cannula:
  - The abdominal wall is lifted and the trocar with the cannula is inserted through the same incision.
  - The direction of insertion is the same as that of the veress needle directing towards the pelvis. There is escape of gas once the trocar is in the peritoneal cavity.

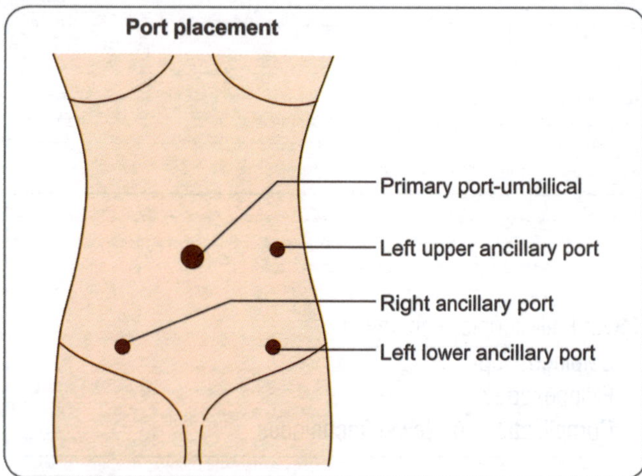


**Fig. 30.1** Port placement

- To avoid blind insertion and to reduce the risk of injury, open laparoscopy (Hasson's technique) is followed especially in patients with previous surgeries, failed entry with closed technique, large cystic mass, pediatric cases and women with early pregnancy. Complications can occur in 0.5% of cases, mainly bowel injury. Few disadvantages of this technique are difficulty in maintaining pneumoperitoneum due to escape of gas and longer time for the procedure.
- After ensuring proper placement of the canula, the trocar is removed and the laparoscope is introduced.

- Secondary trocar insertion:
  - It is done under direct vision.
  - Secondary port is required in both diagnostic and operative procedures.

  Common sites include:
  - Flank: 3–4 cm lateral to medial umbilical ligament.
  - Lateral to lateral margin of rectus abdominis muscle.
  - Suprapubic region.

Recently ***single port access laparoscopy*** is performed using a single 2–3 cm incision around the umbilicus and multiple instruments are introduced into the peritoneal cavity. It is mainly used for cosmetic purposes and is technically challenging.

| **Basic Instruments** | **Accessory Instruments** |
|---|---|
| • Telescope: 4–12 mm, Angle: 0–30° | • Grasping forceps |
| • Veress needle | • Scissors |
| • Trocar and cannula | • Blunt probe |
| • Light source | • Suction/Irrigation cannula |
| • Monitor | • Monopolar/Bipolar cautery |
| • Insufflator | • Monopolar hook |
| | • Myoma screw |

**Indications** Laparoscopy is used for both diagnostic and therapeutic purposes. The common indications are:

- Infertility
  - to check uterus, tubes and ovaries for any pathology (Fig. 30.2)
  - to rule out peritoneal pathology like endometriosis
  - Tubal patency by chromotubation (Fig. 30.3)
  - Prior to tuboplasty for feasibility
- Pelvic endometriosis (Fig. 30.4)
  - Diagnosis and staging of the disease
  - Laparoscopic cystectomy in chocolate cyst

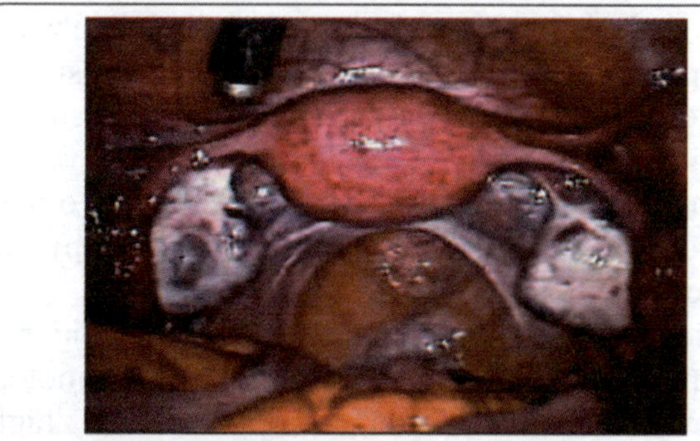

**Fig. 30.2** Normal pelvic organs

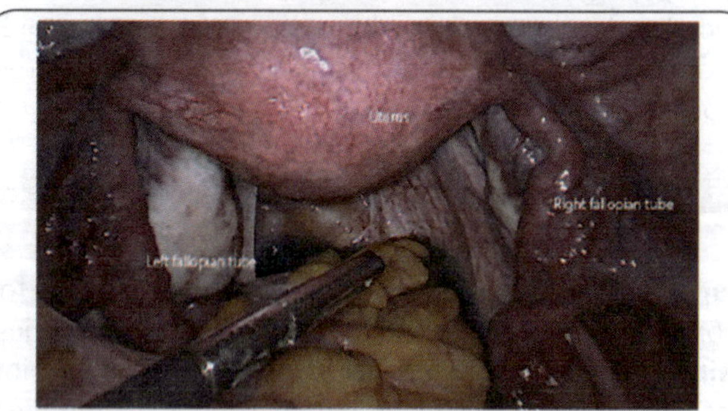


**Fig. 30.3** Laparoscopic chromotubation

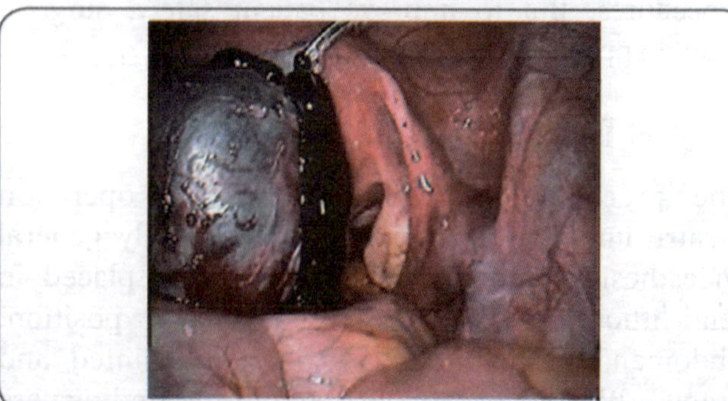

**Fig. 30.4** Endometrioma

- Ablation of endometriotic spots
- Adhesiolysis (Fig. 30.5)

- Chronic pelvic pain—LUNA (Laparoscopic uterosacral nerve ablation)
- Pelvic inflammatory disease
- Ectopic pregnancy—in hemodynamically stable patients
  - Salpingostomy
  - Salpingectomy—partial/total
  - Pelvic tuberculosis
- Uterine malformations (Fig. 30.6)
  - Septal resection
  - Fibroid—laparoscopic myomectomy (Fig. 30.7)
  - Adenomyosis

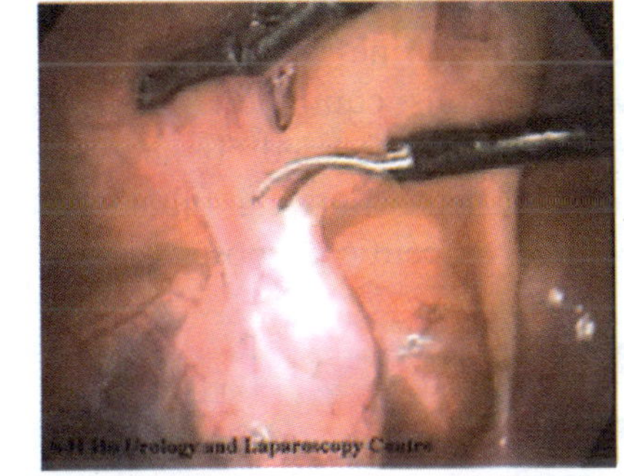

**Fig. 30.5** Adhesiolysis

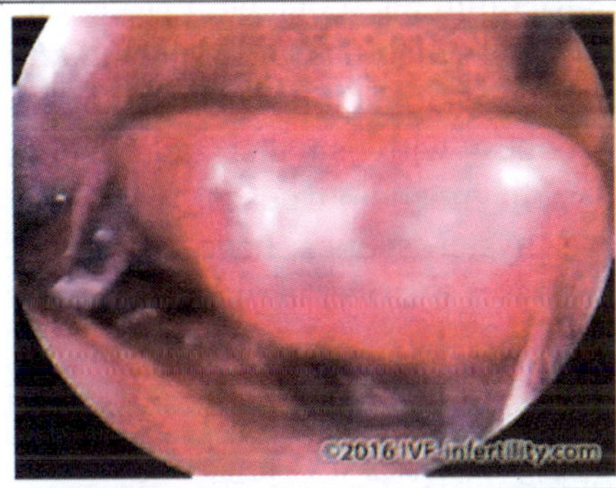


**Fig. 30.6** Uterine anomaly

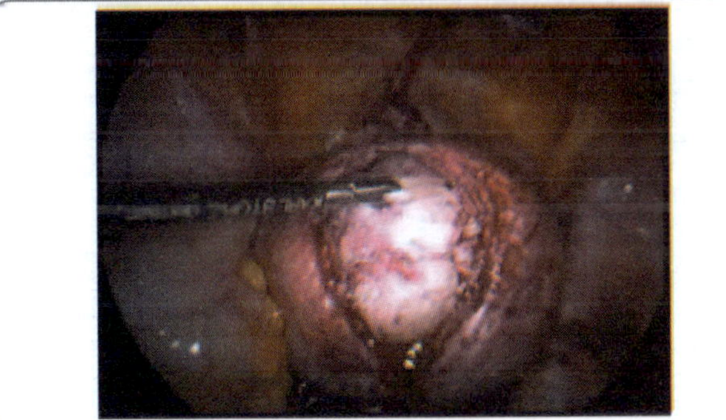

**Fig. 30.7** Laparoscopic myomectomy

- Ovarian complications
  - Ovarian cyst—laparoscopic cystectomy (Fig. 30.8)
  - Cyst aspiration
  - Ovarian drilling
  - Ovarian tumours—benign/malignant
  - Staging of the disease
  - Retroperitoneal lymph node dissection
  - Second look laparoscopy
- Vault prolapse—sacrocolpopexy

***Contraindications*** The contraindications include

- women on anticoagulation therapy
- those with severe cardiopulmonary disease
- hemodynamically unstable patient
- pregnant women with pregnancy > 16 weeks
- those who have significant hemoperitoneum
- women with advanced malignancy
- in large abdominal tumour since the risk of injury by instruments is more

Laparoscopy also has its own advantages and disadvantages.

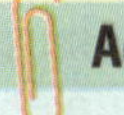

**Advantages and Disadvantages of Laparoscopy**

| Advantages of laparoscopy | Disadvantages of laparoscopy |
|---|---|
| • Early ambulation<br>• Shorter hospital stay<br>• Less postoperative pain and need of analgesia<br>• Reduced blood loss<br>• Less adhesion formation<br>• Less abdominal scar, i.e., cosmetic value. | • Prolonged operation time—depends on case selection, experience of surgeon<br>• Long learning curve<br>• Visceral injuries<br>• Need for sophisticated instruments<br>• Hemorrhage<br>• Expensive |

With regular use and experience, laparoscope is a safe technique. However, it has its own complications like any other surgical procedure.

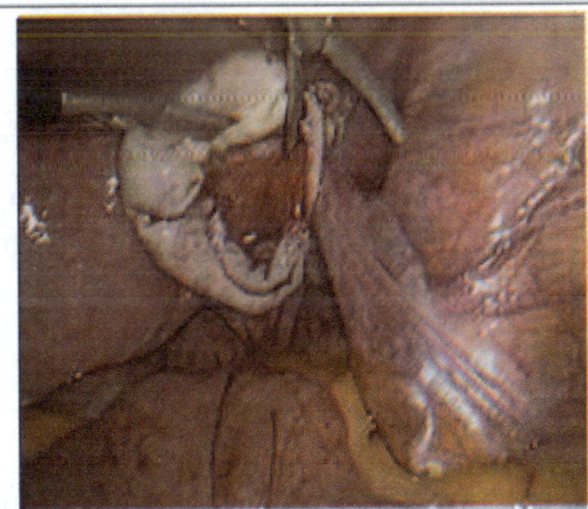

**Fig. 30.8** Laparoscopic cystectomy

*Major complications* Reported incidence of major complications varies from 5–15%. They include the following:

- **Cardiopulmonary arrest**—an anaesthetic complication
- **Gas embolism** can occur
  - with use of air
  - accidental insertion of Veress needle or trocar in vessels. This dreaded complication can be avoided by ensuring correct placement of Veress needle.
- **Hemorrhage** can occur due to
  - epigastric vessel injury during trocar insertion.
  - injury to aorta, IVC, iliac vessels and mesenteric vessels by sharp instruments.
  - Inadequate sealing of vessels by energy source.

The injuries mentioned above can be avoided by following the proper technique for trocar insertion.

If there is uncontrolled hemorrhage, laparotomy is required.

- **Visceral injuries**—due to cautery burns, sharp instruments. They may go unnoticed intraoperatively and manifest clinically as peritonitis after 24 hours with abdominal distension and vomiting. These bowel injuries may require laparotomy, resection and end-to-end anastomosis.
- **Sepsis** can be avoided by proper aseptic precautions and administration of broad-spectrum antibiotics.
- **Carbon dioxide** used during insufflations can cause acidosis, arrhythmia, cardiac arrest.

**Other complications** include

- Surgical emphysema
- Hematoma
- Postoperative adhesions—less common due to less handling of tissues
- Hernia—at portal site, though rare
- Metastatic cancer reported at the portal sites
- Failed procedure
  - Due to adhesions
  - Uncontrollable hemorrhage
  - Extensive pelvic lesion

This requires conversion to laparotomy. Hence pre-operatively, consent should be taken for laparotomy also to avoid medico-legal issues.

### Newer developments

#### *Robotic-assisted laparoscopic surgery*

A surgical robot is a computer-controlled device that can be programmed to aid the positioning and manipulation of surgical instruments. Surgical robotics is typically used in laparoscopy rather than in open surgical approaches. The goal of robot-assisted laparoscopic surgery is to help surgeons improve patient care by converting procedures that would have otherwise been performed by laparotomy into minimally invasive procedures.

Robot-assisted laparoscopic surgery has all of the advantages of minimally invasive surgery, includes less postoperative pain, smaller and possibly more cosmetically appealing incisions, shorter hospital stay, shorter recovery time, and faster return to work.

## HYSTEROSCOPY

Hysteroscopy was first performed in 1869 by Pantaleoni for visualising the uterine cavity (Fig. 30.9). With the availability of various equipment, many therapeutic procedures can be performed. It allows endoscopic view of endometrial cavity and tubal ostia for both diagnostic and therapeutic purposes.

### Hysteroscope

#### Rigid hysteroscope

- A rigid hysteroscope is commonly used for both diagnostic and therapeutic procedures. It consists of a rigid 3 to 4 mm telescope with Hodgkin's rod lens optical system which has wide viewing angle from 0 to 70° and fibre-optic illumination cable.
- Hysteroscopes with smaller diameter are used mainly for diagnostic purposes.
- Operative hysteroscopes have an added sheath, which increases the overall diameter.

### Equipment

- Hysteroscope
- Light source
- Video camera system
- Uterine distension equipment

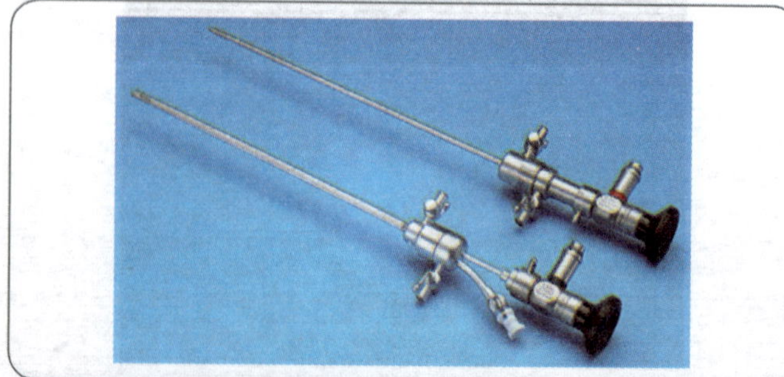

**Fig. 30.9** Hysteroscope

#### Flexible hysteroscope

- Flexible hysteroscopes have the advantage of deflectable tips which can move in a range of 120–160°.
- This facility helps in easy maneuvering in irregularly shaped endometrial cavities.
- It is suitable for in-office procedures as it causes less intraoperative pain.
- But optical view is less clear than rigid hysteroscope.

### Distension Media

- Distension media is essential for distension of uterine cavity and separation of the uterine walls thereby providing a panoramic view. Both liquid and gaseous media are used.
  - Carbon dioxide is the commonly used gas. It is soluble in blood and is safe. It can be used for diagnostic purposes but it can obscure the vision in the presence of blood.
  - ***Liquid media*** is preferred for operative purpose and include
    a) ***Low-viscosity electrolyte fluids*** like normal saline and Ringer's lactate which are isotonic fluids. They are used for diagnostic hysteroscopic procedures. As they conduct current and dissipate energy, they cannot be used with monopolar energy source.
    b) ***Low-viscosity electrolyte-poor fluids*** are 1.5% glycine, 3% sorbitol and 5% mannitol. They are non-conducting and can be used with monopolar energy source. The main problems with these fluids are fluid overload with hyponatremia, hypokalemia and hypoosmolality. These increase the risk of cerebral edema and death. Among them, normal saline, glycine 1.5% are commonly used.

### Technique

- It is usually performed in the pre-ovulatory phase when endometrium is thin and bleeding is less likely to occur.
- It can be performed under local anaesthesia (paracervical block) and sedation, but operative hysteroscopy requires regional or general anaesthesia.
- The patient is placed in the lithotomy position and the findings are reconfirmed by bimanual examination.
- The cervix is dilated if required, especially for operative procedures.
- Hysteroscope is progressively advanced with the distension of uterine cavity under direct vision.
- Endocervical canal, endometrial lining, uterine cavity and both the tubal ostia are visualised for any pathology (Figs. 30.10 and 30.11).

#### *Normal appearance of endometrium*

- Follicular phase—Endometrium looks pale and thin with smooth surface, the glands are not seen easily, and there is minimal vascularisation.
- Ovulatory phase—Endometrium is edematous, and glands are seen.
- Luteal phase—Endometrium is pink, glands are seen, and there is increased vascularity with edema.

### Indications for hysteroscope

- Congenital malformation of the uterus:
  - Confirms septate uterus or bicornuate uterus (Fig. 30.12). It should be combined with laparoscopy. Laparoscopically, in septate uterus, fundus is seen whereas in bicornuate uterus, fundus is not visualised.

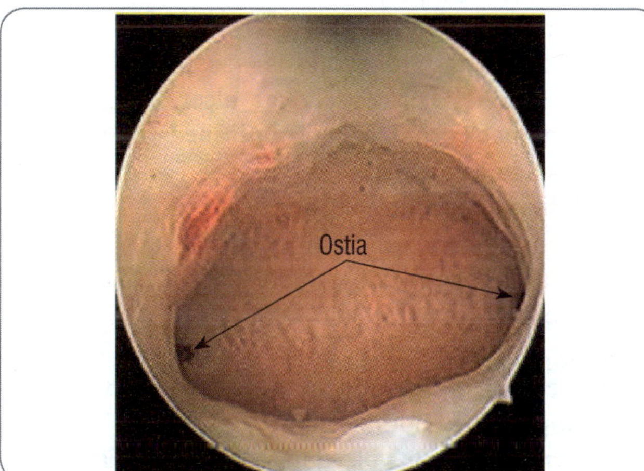


**Fig. 30.10** Hysteroscopic appearance of both ostia

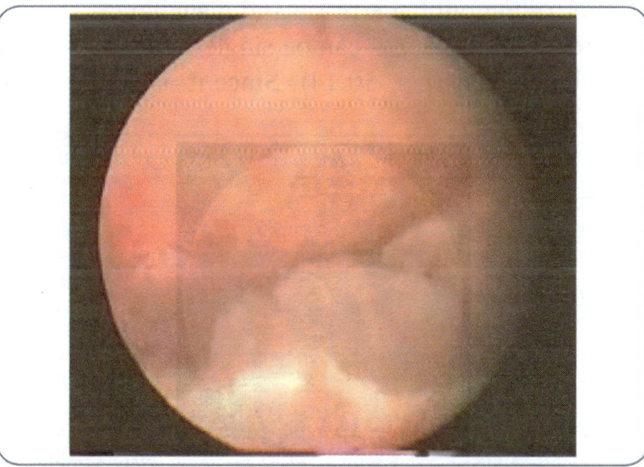

**Fig. 30.11** Endometrial cavity as seen through hysteroscope

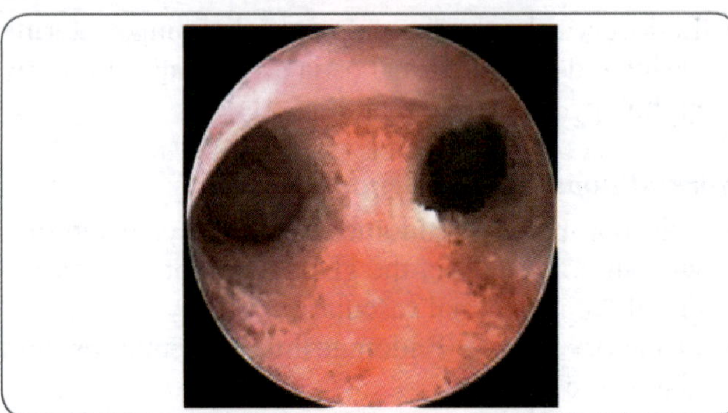
**Fig. 30.12** Uterine septum

Septum can be cut with scissors, cautery, laser or resectoscope.

- Endocervical
  - Allows visualisation of endocervical lining in dysplasia and carcinoma in situ.
  - Allows visualisation of the extent of neoplasm so that biopsy from suspicious areas can be taken.
  - Allows visualisation and removal of the endocervical polyp.
- Endometrial
  - Endometrial tuberculosis—suspected in the presence of caseous areas, ulcers, tubercles in endometrial lining and confirmed by biopsy of suspicious areas.
  - Asherman syndrome
- Confirms the presence of synechiae and the type (whether flimsy/fibrous) and extent of adhesions.
- Can release the adhesions (Fig. 30.13) in the same sitting. Post procedure IUCD insertion for 3 months and estrogen therapy prevent re-adhesions by developing the endometrium.
- Abnormal uterine bleeding—can be diagnosed. AUB can be treated by trans-cervical resection of endometrium (TCRE) in perimenopausal women after ruling out hyperplasia and malignancy.
- Endometrial polyp—can be single/multiple, senile/pedunculated (Fig. 30.14). Since it is due to the folds of endometrium in hyperplasia, polyps are more prominent in the luteal phase. It can be differentiated from fibroid polyp by its firm consistency and pale nature.
- Submucous fibroid (Fig. 30.15)—Type 0 (pedunculated) and type I fibroid with less than 50% intramural location can be removed using resectoscope or by morcellation. It can be performed either in single or two sittings.
- Endometrial hyperplasia and carcinoma—can confirm the diagnosis by biopsy of suspicious areas.
- Hysteroscopic tubal sterilisation can be done using sclerosing agents, cautery or ESSURE.
  ESSURE is a coil device (Fig. 30.16) inserted hysteroscopically into the proximal section of the Fallopian tubes. It causes local chronic tissue inflammatory response and tissue growth, which in turn occlude the lumen. This is documented by HSG at the end of 3 months post surgery.
- IVF programme as a part of endometrial cavity evaluation, in patients with recurrent implantation failure and recurrent pregnancy loss.
- Falloposcopy—to study the mucosa, feasibility of tubal cannulation and adhesiolysis.

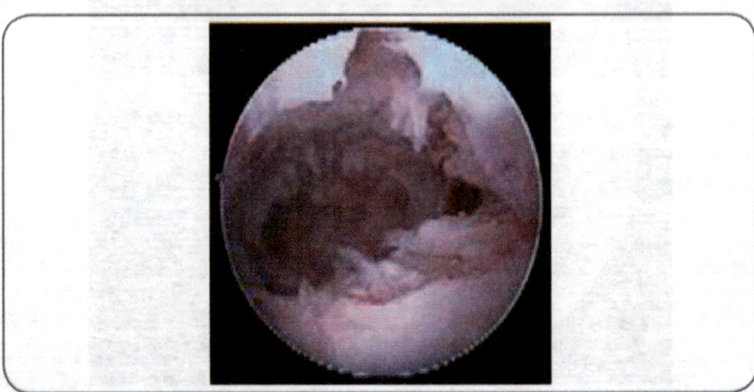
**Fig. 30.13** Hysteroscopic adhesiolysis

### Contraindications

1. Infection
2. Pregnancy

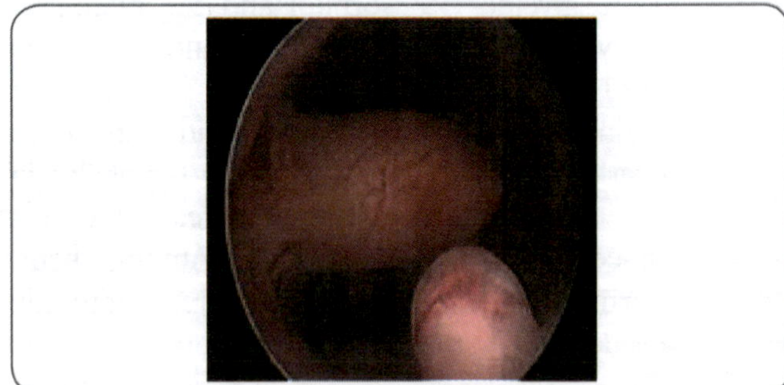
**Fig. 30.14** Endometrial polyp

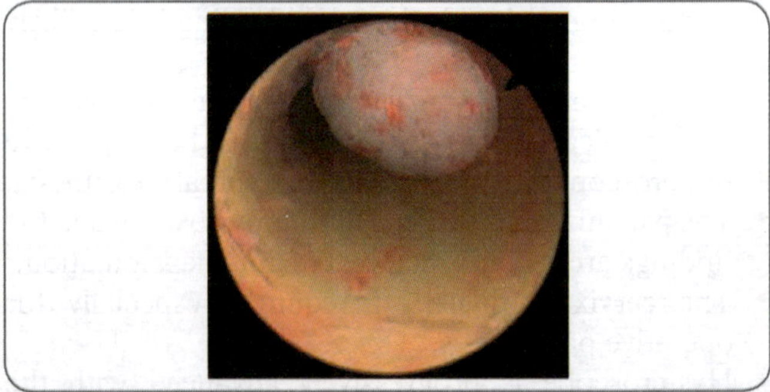
**Fig. 30.15** Submucous fibroid

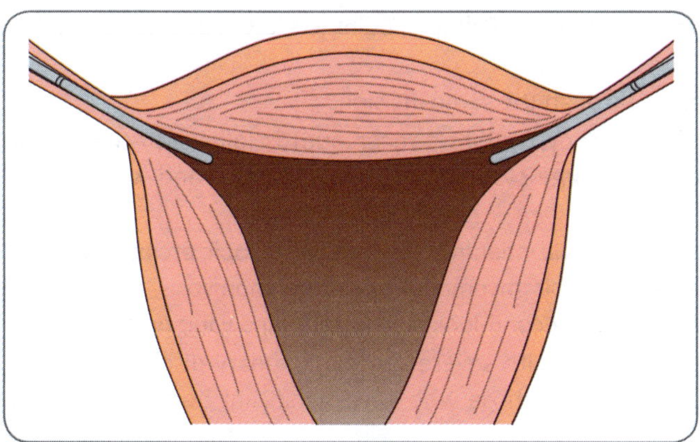

**Fig. 30.16** Essure

3. During menstruation
4. Anaesthesia risk—cardiopulmonary disorder

### Complications

- Anaesthesia complications
- Uterine perforation
  - Incidence varies from 1 to 10%, occurs mostly during insertion of hysteroscope through the cervix.
  - **Should be suspected when the uterine wall collapses with poor visibility**.
  - Can be managed by observation, laparoscopic coagulation of the bleeding or laparotomy depending on the severity.
- Injury—thermal injury to bowel when cautery or laser is used and delayed diagnosis worsens the morbidity.
- Hemorrhage—occurs in 1–2%
  - Can be minimised by performing the surgery in preovulatory phase or by thinning the endometrium by hormones prior to TCRE.
  - More common when the distension is reduced and intrauterine pressure drops.
  - Can be controlled by distending the uterine cavity with Foley's catheter and distending the balloon with 30 mL of saline for 24 hours for hemostasis.
- Infection—can be prevented by prophylactic broad-spectrum antibiotics.
- Embolism with carbon dioxide
  - Avoided by using proper instruments and setting the pressure to < 100 mm Hg.
- Fluid overload
  - Occurs if proper check is not kept with inflow and outflow and leads to pulmonary edema.
  - Occurs in 4% of cases if deficit of fluid is >1000 mL and electrolyte imbalance can occur.

## NEWER ENDOSCOPIC TECHNIQUES

### Salpingoscopy

- A fine 1 mm diameter salpingoscope is introduced through the fimbrial end of the Fallopian tube through laparoscopy and the lumen is distended with saline.
- Can be performed to study the damage to mucosa and feasibility of tuboplasty.
- Flattening of mucosa, adhesions and mucous polyp can be visualised.

### Falloposcopy

- This is performed hysteroscopically to visualise the tubal pathology in the cornual and interstitial regions of the Fallopian tube.

### Complications of Newer Techniques

- Perforation
- Infection
- Damage to tubal mucosa

Endoscopic surgery is helpful in many ways. But the patient selection should be proper, the surgeon should be well versed with the technique and should recognise the complications and manage them early. It is also imperative that the surgeon does not hesitate to convert to laparotomy when indicated.

## RECAP

- Gynecological endoscopy is a surgical discipline which uses optical instruments to help in the diagnosis and management of the most frequent female disorders and pathologies such as infertility problems, vaginal bleeding or endometrial polyps.
- The procedure is performed in the operation theatre under aseptic precautions.
- The patient is placed in semi-lithotomy or deep Trendelenburg position.
- A sub-umbilical incision of 1.25 cm is made and Veress needle is introduced at an angle of 45° into the peritoneal cavity.

- The most common sites or ports of entry are at the umbilicus (most common), Palmer's point (on left midclavicular line) or suprapubic (2–4 cm above the pubic symphysis).
- Abdominal wall is lifted and the trocar with the cannula is inserted through the same incision.
- To avoid blind insertion and reduce the risk of injury, open laparoscopy (Hasson's technique) is followed especially in patients with previous surgeries, failed entry with closed technique, large cystic mass, pediatric cases and women with early pregnancy.
- Indications include infertility, pelvic endometriosis, chronic pelvic pain, pelvic inflammatory disease, ectopic pregnancy, pelvic tuberculosis, uterine malformations including septal resection, laparoscopic myomectomy and adenomyosis, laparoscopic ovarian cystectomy, cyst aspiration, ovarian drilling, staging of the disease, second-look laparoscopy, and vault prolapse.
- The contraindications include women on anticoagulation therapy, those with severe cardiopulmonary disease, hemodynamically unstable patient, pregnant women with pregnancy > 16 weeks, those who have significant hemoperitoneum, women with advanced malignancy and in large abdominal tumour.
- Advantages are early ambulation, shorter hospital stay compared to laparotomy, decreased postoperative pain and reduced need for analgesia. The other advantages are reduced blood loss, minimal adhesion formation compared to laparotomy and the cosmetic effect due to small abdominal scar.
- The disadvantages include prolonged surgery and this depends on the experience of the surgeon and the case selection. It also has a long learning curve.
- Major complications are cardiopulmonary arrest, gas embolism, hemorrhage, visceral injuries and sepsis.
- Robotic Assisted Laparoscopic Surgery—A surgical robot is a computer-controlled device that can be programmed to aid the positioning and manipulation of surgical instruments.
- Hysteroscopy allows endoscopic view of endometrial cavity and tubal ostia for both diagnostic and therapeutic purposes.
- Both rigid and flexible hysteroscopes are available.
- Carbon dioxide is commonly used as distension media. Liquid media include low-viscosity electrolyte fluids like normal saline and Ringer's lactate which are isotonic fluids and low-viscosity electrolyte-poor fluids like 1.5% glycine, 3% sorbitol and 5% mannitol.
- It is usually performed in the pre-ovulatory phase when the endometrium is thin and bleeding is less likely to occur.
- Endocervical canal, endometrial lining, uterine cavity and both the tubal ostia are visualised for any pathology.
- Hysteroscopic tubal sterilisation is done using sclerosing agents, cautery or ESSURE.
- Salpingoscopy involves a fine 1 mm diameter salpingoscope being introduced through the fimbrial end of the Fallopian tube through laparoscopy and the lumen is distended with saline.
- It can be performed to study the damage to mucosa and feasibility of tuboplasty.
- Falloposcopy is performed hysteroscopically to visualise the tubal pathology in the cornual and interstitial regions of the Fallopian tube.

## REVIEW QUESTIONS

### Long-Answer Question

How is pneumoperitoneum created prior to laparoscopy? What are the methods to assess the correct placement of the Veress needle?

### MCQs

**1. Which is not a contraindication for laparoscopy?**
a) Women on anticoagulation therapy
b) Women with small fibroid
c) Hemodynamically unstable patient
d) Women with pregnancy more than 16 weeks

**2. Which is a disadvantage of laparoscopic surgery?**
a) Early ambulation b) Small incision
c) More chances of visceral injury
d) Minimal adhesion formation

**3. ESSURE is a**
a) Hysteroscopic tubal sterilisation technique
b) Laparoscopic tubal sterilisation technique
c) Open method of tubal sterilisation
d) Open method for creating pneumoperitoneum

**4. Falloposcopy is performed through**
a) Laparoscope b) Colposcope
c) Hysteroscope d) Abdominal route

# Chapter 31

# Operative Gynecology

## At a Glance

Preoperative Preparation
Pre-operative Investigations
Vaginal Procedures
Abdominal Procedures
Antibiotic Prophylaxis
Anaesthesia
Suture Material
Consent for Surgery
Thromboprophylaxis
**Vaginal Operations**
Minor Vaginal Surgical Procedures
Dilatation and Curettage
Endometrial Aspiration
Operations on the Cervix
Cervical Punch Biopsy
Removal of the Cervical Polyp
Operations on the Vulva
Operations for Bartholin's Cyst
Major Vaginal Surgical Procedures
Anterior Colporrhaphy for Cystocele and Urethrocele
Posterior Colpoperineorrhaphy for Rectocele
Amputation of the Cervix
Fothergill's or the Manchester Operation
Vaginal Hysterectomy with Anterior Colporrhaphy and Posterior Colpoperineorrhaphy (Ward–Mayo's Operation)
**Operations for Nulliparous Prolapse**
Shirodkar's Method
Purandare's Cervicopexy
**Abdominal Surgeries**
Surgical Anatomy of Anterior Abdominal Wall
Types of Incisions
Hysterectomy
Classification
Total Abdominal Hysterectomy
Radical Abdominal Hysterectomy (Wertheim's Operation)
Operations on the Adnexa
Salpingectomy
Salpingo-oophorectomy
Postoperative Care

## PREOPERATIVE PREPARATION

A proper and careful preoperative preparation is an integral part of surgery and is as important as surgical intervention. It is helpful to both the patient and the surgeon. The patient should be thoroughly investigated with reference to her general condition and fitness for the procedure. Previous admission in the same facility for similar or any other complaint should be reviewed along with old records of surgery and anaesthesia, if any.

### Pre-operative Investigations

The following routine investigations are done for all patients.

- Urine analysis for albumin, sugar and deposits
- Complete blood count (CBC) which includes hemoglobin (Hb), total and differential white cell count, red cell count (RBC), ESR and peripheral smear study if she is anemic
- Bleeding and clotting time and when these are altered, coagulation profile including platelet count serum fibrinogen, prothrombin time (PT), activated partial thromboplastin time (aPTT) and international normalised ratio (INR)
- Blood grouping and Rh typing
- Blood urea, sugar (fasting and postprandial sugar in known diabetics and wherever necessary), serum creatinine
- X-ray chest
- ECG

Other investigations may be done as per the individual need.

**Except in emergency situations, the preop target Hb should be 11 g.** A history of allergy or sensitivity to drugs, the type of drugs currently or recently used, including cortisone (and other steroidal hormones), hypotensives or antituberculous agents should be elicited and recorded. If the patient is diabetic or obese, it is advisable to control the diabetes or to advise the patient to lose some weight before taking her up for surgery.

**Routine use of enema is not encouraged.** Instead, the patient is asked to take a light dinner early the previous evening and a laxative is given in the night. In cases of minor surgery, the patient is asked to empty the bladder just before the procedure. **Unnecessary catheterisation should be avoided to prevent urinary infection.**

## Vaginal Procedures

- Before undertaking a vaginal procedure, pre-existing vaginitis should be treated. An antiseptic vaginal plug is necessary before surgery in cases of polyps or cervical growths.
- In cases of genital prolapse with a thin atrophic mucosa and ulcers, local application of estrogenic cream promotes healing. If the prolapse is edematous and irreducible, the foot of the bed should be slightly elevated to reduce the congestion. Glycerine-magnesium sulphate dressing would help in reducing the edema. Similarly decubitus ulcers, usually seen in prolapse uterus should be managed by keeping the prolapse reduced by using a vaginal plug soaked in acriflavine or normal saline.

## Abdominal Procedures

The abdomen has to be prepared meticulously by shaving and cleaning first with soap and water and later with an antiseptic solution. A sterile towel is wrapped over the prepared area. There is no need for routine use of Ryle's tube. The bladder should be kept empty during major surgical procedures by inserting an indwelling catheter like Foley's catheter and connecting it to a urine collection bag.

## Antibiotic Prophylaxis

Antibiotic prophylaxis is recommended (Table 31.1) in most of the gynecological procedures particularly in hysterectomies and in surgeries with frank sepsis and pus.

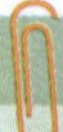

### Classification of Surgical Wound

Class I/Clean
Class II/Clean-Contaminated
Class III/Contaminated
Class IV/Dirty-Infected

(Modified from Centers for Disease Control and Prevention. Guideline for Prevention of Surgical Site Infection, 1999)

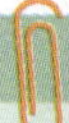

### Recommendations for Antibiotic Prophylaxis

The following are the recommendations for antibiotic prophylaxis by various societies:

1. Women undergoing abdominal or vaginal hysterectomy
2. Women undergoing laparoscopic hysterectomy or laparoscopically assisted vaginal hysterectomy
3. The choice of antibiotic for hysterectomy should be a single dose of a first-generation cephalosporin. If patients are allergic to cephalosporin, clindamycin, erythromycin, or metronidazole should be used.
4. Prophylactic antibiotics should be administered 15 to 60 minutes prior to skin incision. No additional doses are recommended.
5. If an open abdominal procedure lasts longer than 3 hours or the blood loss is more than 1.5 litres, an additional dose of antibiotic is given after 3–4 hours of the initial dose.

(Modified from ACOG Practice Bulletin, No. 104 and SOGC Clinical Practice Guideline No. 275).

**Table 31.1** Common drugs used for antibiotic prophylaxis, and their dosage

| Drug | Dose |
|---|---|
| Cefazolin | 1–2 g IV |
| Cefotaxime | 1 g IV |
| Metronidazole | 500–1000 mg IV |
| Doxycyxline | 100 mg oral bd × 5 days |

IV: Intravenous route; bd: Twice daily

## Anaesthesia

**All cases should be assessed by the anesthesiologist with regard to fitness for surgery and the type of anaesthesia required.** The anesthetic and surgical risks vary according to the patient and the nature of surgery proposed. Pre-anesthetic assessment based on **American Society of Anesthesiologists' Classification of Physical Status** always helps to grade the cases (Table 31.2).

**Table 31.2** American Society of Anesthesiologists (ASA) classification

| Class | Criteria |
|---|---|
| ASA Class 1 | A normal healthy patient |
| ASA Class 2 | A patient with mild systemic disease |
| ASA Class 3 | A patient with severe systemic disease |
| ASA Class 4 | A patient with severe systemic disease that is a constant threat to life |
| ASA Class 5 | A moribund patient who is not expected to survive without the operation |
| ASA Class 6 | A declared brain dead patient whose organs are being removed for donor purposes |

The addition of "E" denotes Emergency surgery (*Source:* ASA PHYSICAL STATUS CLASSIFICATION SYSTEM Last approved by the ASA House of Delegates on October 15, 2014 )

**It is also necessary to arrange for adequate amounts of compatible blood.** The anesthetist should also advise on premedication or any special preparation needed before surgery.

The most preferred anaesthesia is spinal anaesthesia. Where spinal anaesthesia could not be given or when the anesthetist feels general anaesthesia is better the same is given. For short procedures, intravenous anaesthesia is the preferred anaesthesia. Preoperative and postoperative monitoring are essential.

## Suture Material

There are two types of suture material: absorbable and non-absorbable. These are listed in Table 31.3.

**Table 31.3** Suture material

| Absorbable suture material | Non-absorbable suture material |
|---|---|
| Plain catgut (not used nowadays in gynecological surgeries) | Cotton (not used) |
| Chromic catgut | Silk |
| Polyglycolic acid suture (Dexon) | Polymer of ethylene glycol and terephthalic acid (Dacron) |
| Polyglactin 910 (Vicryl) | Polypropylene (Prolene) |
| | Nylon (Ethilon) |

The size of the suture material in indicated by a number. Suture materials of smaller size are indicated with a 0 after the number. In microsurgical procedures in gynecology like tubal recanalisation, the suture material used will be of size, 5–0 or 6–0. During abdominal or vaginal hysterectomy, the surgeons prefer 1 or 2 chromic catgut where the suture material is of a larger size.

### Common Errors in Suture Use

- Repeated knots do not provide additional strength. On the other hand, they increase the size of the foreign body (suture material) and can even loosen the suture.
- When monofilament suture material like nylon or prolene are held by instrument, they lose their tensile strength by 50%.
- Holding the needle near its eye or where the suture material is attached can cause needle and suture breakage.

## Consent for Surgery

An **informed consent** should be obtained, in writing, from the patient and one of her relatives/ attendants for any surgery whether it is a minor or a major procedure. ***In the case of minor girls and mentally affected women, the consent from her legal guardian is essential.*** The informed consent should consist of the type of the procedure that is planned, the need for the procedure, alternate procedures/methods available, if any, for the same condition, the benefits of the surgery, the risks involved in the procedure including risks of anaesthesia, consent for additional procedures that may become necessary during the course of the surgery (e.g., hysterectomy when the initial procedure planned was myomectomy, laparotomy when the initial procedure planned was laparoscopy, removal of ovaries when indicated during the procedure, etc.), and consent for blood transfusion. Apart from these, any other risk factor in the individual patient and surgery should be included in the consent form.

## Thromboprophylaxis

Venous thromboembolism (VTE) and pulmonary embolism (PE) are two dreadful conditions which could have a fatal outcome in postoperative patients. With changing lifestyle and increase in obese population, VTE and PE have become cause for concern in Indian women also. Thromboprophylaxis is done preoperatively and it may have to be continued postoperatively. Gynecological surgery patients are traditionally divided into 4 categories as detailed in Table 31.4, and the need for thromboprophylaxis depends on the risk group they belong to.

**Table 31.4** Traditional Risk Classification for Gynecologic Surgery*

| Risk level | Definition |
|---|---|
| Low | Surgery lasting < 30 minutes in patients < 40 years with no additional risk factors |
| Moderate | Surgery lasting < 30 minutes in patients with additional risk factors; surgery lasting < 30 minutes in patients aged 40–60 years with no additional risk factors; major surgery in patients < 40 years with no additional risk factors |
| High | Surgery lasting < 30 minutes in patients >60 years or with additional risk factors; major surgery in patients >40 years or with additional risk factors |
| Highest | Major surgery in patients >60 years plus prior VTE, cancer, or molecular hypercoagulable state |

*Modified from ACOG Practice Bulletin No. 84: Prevention of deep vein thrombosis and pulmonary embolism. *Obstet Gynecol*. Aug 2007;110(2 Pt 1):429-40. [PMID: 17666620].

Additional risk factors may be due to co-morbid conditions like diabetes, hypertension, previous VTE, etc.

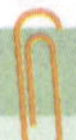

**ACOG Recommendation for Thromboprophylaxis**

| Risk | Precaution |
|---|---|
| Patients at very low risk for venous thromboembolism (< 0.5%) (ACOG low risk) | Early ambulation |
| Patients at low risk for venous thromboembolism (approximately 1.5%) (ACOG moderate risk) | IPC (Intermittent pneumaric compression devices) placed before the initiation of surgery and continued until the patient is fully ambulatory |
| **Patients at moderate risk for venous thromboembolism (approximately 3%) (ACOG high risk) but not at high risk for bleeding complications** | LMWH (Low molecular weight heparin) or dalteparin 2,500, antifactor-Xa units or enoxaparin 40 mg administered subcutaneously 12 hours before surgery and once a day postoperatively until discharge<br>LDUH (Low dose unfractionated heparin) or unfractionated heparin (5,000 units) administered subcutaneously 2 hours before surgery and every 12 hours after surgery until discharge<br>IPC placed before the initiation of surgery and continued until the patient is fully ambulatory<br>IPC placed before the initiation of surgery and continued until the patient is fully ambulatory |
| Patients at moderate risk for venous thromboembolism (approximately 3%) (ACOG high risk) and at high risk for bleeding complications | LMWH or dalteparin 2,500, antifactor-Xa units or enoxaparin 40 mg administered subcutaneously 12 hours before surgery and once a day postoperatively until discharge. |
| Patients at high risk for venous thromboembolism (approximately 6%) (ACOG high risk) but not at high risk for bleeding complications | LDUH (grade 2B) or unfractionated heparin (5,000 units) administered subcutaneously 2 hours before surgery and every 12 hours after surgery until discharge |

It is to be noted that IPC may not be available at all places and LMWH use may be restricted by cost constraints. Based on these recommendations, decision on appropriate therapy should be taken by the surgeon and the patient after discussion.

# VAGINAL OPERATIONS

## MINOR VAGINAL SURGICAL PROCEDURES

The common minor vaginal operations are described below.

### Dilatation and Curettage

Popularly referred to by its abbreviations 'D and C', this is the most common minor gynecological operation.

**Indications** The indications are mentioned in individual conditions. The basic indications are:

- Evaluation of abnormal uterine bleeding
- Removal of retained products of conception
- For removal of a uterine polyp
- In an attempt to remove an intrauterine device

**Though a minor operation, D and C is always performed under anaesthesia.**

**Procedure**

1. The patient is asked to empty her bladder before anaesthesia.
2. The field of operation is cleaned with antiseptic solution and sterile drapes are put on.
3. A vaginal examination is done to confirm the size and position of the uterus and the condition of the adnexae.
4. Sims' vaginal speculum is inserted and held by an assistant.
5. The anterior lip of the cervix is caught by a vulsellum and the cervix is cleaned again with an antiseptic swab.
6. Gentle traction is applied on the vulsellum to pull on the cervix as the uterine sound is inserted to find out the length and direction of the uterine cavity.
7. Dilatation of the cervix is done with a graded metal cervical dilator (Matthews–Duncan's). The tip of the dilator is dipped in K-Y jelly or an antiseptic cream and starting from the lowest number, the cervix is dilated sufficiently (Matthews–Duncan's No. 12) to admit the sharp end of the curette. The width of the curette gives an idea of how much dilatation is needed.
8. The curette is then introduced and the endometrium is scraped stopping just short of the feeling of a grating sensation.

9. The cervix is then swabbed with a sterile swab or an antiseptic.
10. The endometrial curettings obtained are collected in a vial containing 10% formalin solution and sent to the histopathologist. The vial should be labelled correctly with the patient's name, register number and age. A brief clinical history (including the date of the last menstrual period), the physical findings and the provisional diagnosis should also be provided for the pathologist's information.

**Possible problems** There may be

1. Difficulty in passing the uterine sound, in an acutely anteflexed uterus.
2. Difficulty in dilatation of the cervix due to the spastic or organic rigidity of the cervix. In such cases, dilatation should be slow and deliberate. It may be necessary to keep a dilator for a few minutes before passing on to the next. Occasionally one may have to go back to the previous dilator before proceeding further.

#### Complications

1. **Laceration of the cervix** This is not uncommon and can be prevented by careful and gradual dilatation. If torn, a few catgut sutures may be needed.
2. **Hemorrhage from a torn cervix or injury to the cervical branch of the uterine artery** This follows laceration or lack of care during dilatation. The bleeding may be arrested by sutures.
3. **Perforation of the uterus** This is a rare but important complication. It can be prevented by a routine preoperative vaginal examination and by care, gentleness and steadiness during the dilatation. Its occurrence is diagnosed by the abnormal mobility of the dilators into the uterine cavity and loss of resistance during dilatation. **When a perforation is recognised, the operation is immediately stopped.** The patient is observed for bleeding and the pulse rate is recorded regularly. In most cases, with careful observation and conservative treatment with prophylactic antibiotics, the perforation heals by itself. If the patient is hemodynamically stable, a laparoscope can be used to visualise the perforation and bleeding. This is not resorted to as a routine. In a rare case, in the presence of tachycardia or deteriorating general condition suggesting internal hemorrhage, a laparotomy is done and the perforation is sutured.
4. **Pelvic infection or PID** This can be avoided by asepsis and antiseptic precautions during D and C. It is unfortunate indeed if pelvic infection should supervene a diagnostic curettage done for infertility.
5. **Habitual midtrimester abortions** Such abortions due to an incompetent internal os may be a sequelae of indiscriminate forcible dilatation of the cervix.

### Endometrial Aspiration

Endometrial aspiration using Pipelle has the advantage of not requiring any anaesthesia, thereby making it an office procedure. The pipelle used is shown in Fig. 7.5. The other instruments that are being used are Novak Curette and Tao Brush.

## OPERATIONS ON THE CERVIX

### Cervical Punch Biopsy

The punch biopsy is performed in cases of suspected cervical disease such as chronic endocervicitis (erosion), non-healing ulcers and malignancy. It is advisable to perform the biopsy under colposcopic guidance. However, when colposopy facility is not available, Lugol's iodine can be applied to the cervix, the suspicious areas identified and then biopsy taken from those places.

### Removal of the Cervical Polyp

Small multiple mucus polypi are twisted off with a sponge-holding forceps. It is advisable to do the dilatation and curettage also in these cases to prevent their recurrence. The material collected should always be subjected to histopathological examination to rule out malignancy.

## OPERATIONS ON THE VULVA

### Operations for Bartholin's Cyst

**Excision** An elliptical incision is made on the mucous membrane over the labia minora which is distended due to the cyst. The cyst is gradually enucleated from the surrounding tissue by blunt dissection. If the cyst is adherent and cannot be dissected easily, sharp dissection may be done with a pair of Mayo scissors to take the cyst out from its bed.

If during the dissection, the cyst wall ruptures, it should be dissected out from the surrounding tissue.

Care must be taken to stop the bleeding from beneath the cyst. To ensure proper hemostasis, the cavity may be closed with tiering sutures with No. 0 chromic catgut. Finally the mucosa is sutured by interrupted sutures.

**Marsupialisation** This is a simpler technique and avoids many of the complications of excision of the cyst. A vertical incision is made on the vaginal mucosa over the centre of the cyst. After opening the cyst wall, the contents are drained. The lining of the cyst is everted and sutured with vaginal mucosa with No. 00 chromic catgut by interrupted sutures.

A portion of the cyst wall may be removed. Drains and packs are not necessary.

## MAJOR VAGINAL SURGICAL PROCEDURES

### Anterior Colporrhaphy for Cystocele and Urethrocele

A triangular flap of the redundant vaginal wall with its base towards the cervix and its apex near the urethral orifice is marked out and dissected off the bladder and urethra (Fig. 31.1).

The bladder is separated from the cervix by snipping the uterovesical attachment in the mid-line, and pushed upwards. The lateral extensions of this attachment bleed briskly and must be ligated.

The vesicovaginal fascia within the cut edges of the vagina are stitched together in the midline to support the bladder (Fig. 31.2).

The vaginal wall is finally closed with interrupted sutures.

**Fig. 31.1** Line of incisions for vaginal operations for genital prolapse. (a) Incision for anterior colporrhaphy; (b) Incision encircling the cervix for Manchester operation and vaginal hysterectomy.

### Posterior Colpoperineorrhaphy for Rectocele

A triangular flap of the posterior vaginal wall with its base at the vulval orifice and apex above the level of the rectocele is separated from the rectum and excised (Fig. 31.3).

When there is an enterocele, the dissection is carried up to the cervix and the pouch of Douglas exposed, opened and the redundant peritoneum excised. The peritoneum is closed and supported by approximating the uterosacral ligaments.

The rectovaginal fascia is next approximated in the midline to support the rectocele from above downwards.

The edges of the levator ani are brought together in the midline recreating the perineal body and tightening the urogenital opening.

The vaginal walls are then stitched, followed by the superficial perineal muscles and skin.

These two procedures are rarely carried out for cystocele and/or rectocele without concomitant descent of the uterus. For uterine prolapse, Fothergill's

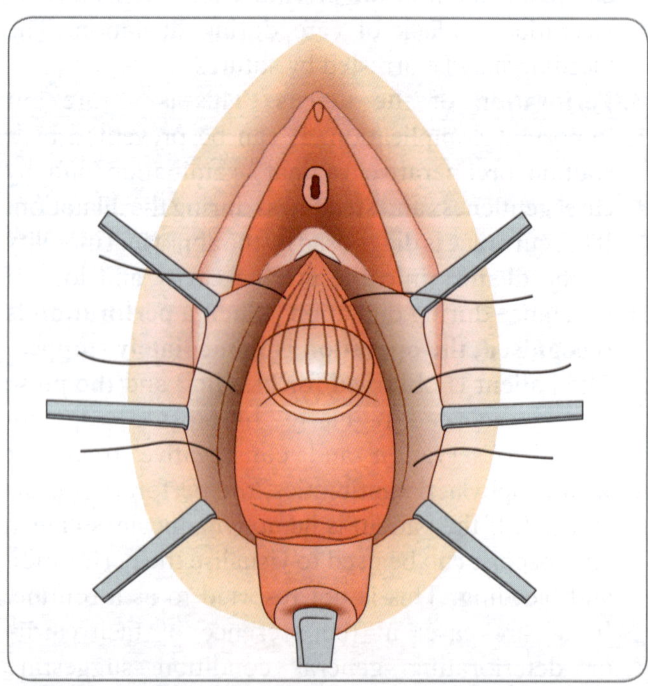

**Fig. 31.2** Repair of cystocele. Note the supporting sutures in the vaginal fascia after pushing up the bladder.

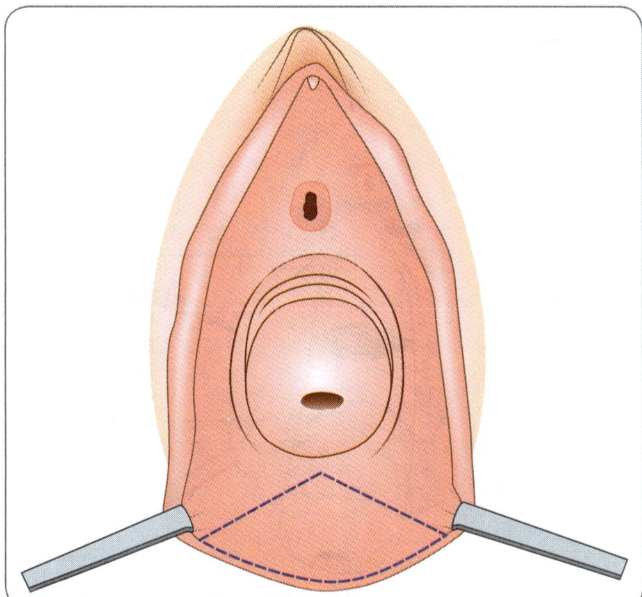

Fig. 31.3 Incision for posterior colpoperineorrhaphy

(Manchester) operation or vaginal hysterectomy combined with anterior colporrhaphy and/or posterior colpoperineorrhaphy are performed.

## Amputation of the Cervix

This is usually done under anaesthesia for elongation of cervix and as part of the Fothergill's operation. The procedure is as follows:

i. The speculum is introduced.
ii. The cervix is dilatated and a curettage done.
iii. The anterior lip of the cervix is held with a pair of vulsella.
iv. A uterine sound is passed and the extent of elongation of the cervix is noted.
v. After determining the area through which the amputation has to be done, a circular incision is made on the mucosa, anteriorly and posteriorly. Two flaps are made, one anteriorly and another posteriorly. The incision should be started at a varying distance below the imaginary plane of division.
vi. After reflecting the flaps upwards until the plane of division of the cervix is reached, the cervix is incised throughout in a transverse way.
vii. Two thick catgut mattress stitches are put in the lateral portion of the stump of the cervix. These should take sufficient bites of the cervical tissues and must control the hemorrhage from the lateral descending branches. These stitches are very important not only to prevent primary and reactionary hemorrhage but also secondary hemorrhage indirectly.
viii. The last step is covering the stump, that is, the flaps, anteriorly and posteriorly with stitches known as **Sturmdorf sutures** through the middle of the apex of the flaps and through the cervical canal. A knot is tied about 1 cm above the newly formed lips of the cervix anteriorly and posteriorly (Fig. 31.4).

## Fothergill's or the Manchester Operation

Fothergill's or the Manchester operation is ideal for uterovaginal prolapse with supravaginal elongation of the cervix. The cervix is amputated to a length of three to three and a half inches.

### Fothergill's Points

There are four Fothergill's points:

1. The first point is just below the urethral orifice
2. The second is placed posteriorly in the midline about 2½ inches from the external os
3. Third and the fourth are the two lateral points

The lateral ligaments are shortened by separating them from the sides of the cervix and stitching them in front of it. This step not only lifts the uterus to its original position but also pulls the cervix backwards restoring anteversion.

If enterocele is present, it is opened, excised and supported by the uterosacral ligaments behind the amputated cervix.

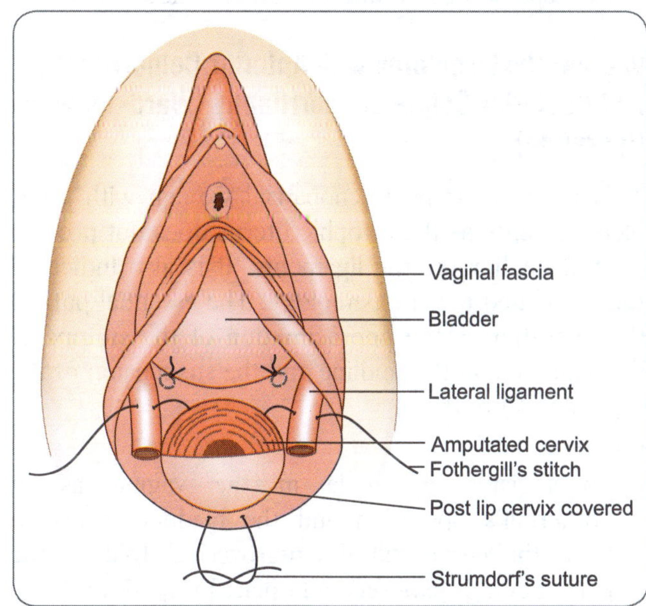


Fig. 31.4 Fothergill's or the Manchester operation. Note Fothergill's stitch as well as the Sturmdorff suture.

**Steps of the operation** The cervix is dilated to prevent cicatrisation later. The incision is started in the anterior vaginal wall and extended around the cervix posteriorly.

After separating the bladder from the cervix, the lateral ligaments are clamped and sutured. The cervix is amputated as detailed above.

Fothergill's stitch is applied starting at the lateral angle of the vagina on the right, passed successively through the stump of the right lateral ligament, the anterior surface of the cervix, the stump of the left lateral ligament, and finally the lateral angle of the vagina on the right side. The suture is tied at the end of the operation.

If an enterocele is present, it is managed as in the section on posterior colpoperineorraphy.

The posterior lip of the cervix is covered by placing a stitch in the midpoint of the posterior vaginal flap and drawing it out through the cervical canal onto the posterior surface of the cervix and the posterior vaginal flap on either side. This is called a **Sturmdorff suture** (Fig. 31.4).

A similar stitch is used to cover the anterior lip of the cervix with the anterior ends of the vaginal flap.

The bladder is suspended and the vagina closed as in anterior colporrhaphy. Fothergill's stitch is tied last after elevating and pushing back the cervix into the vagina.

In young women desiring children, amputation of the cervix is avoided if the supravaginal elongation of cervix is not too marked and the prolapse is limited to the first or second degree while carrying out all the other steps of the operation (Hunter's modification).

## Vaginal Hysterectomy with Anterior Colporrhaphy and Posterior Colpoperineorrhaphy (Ward–Mayo's Operation)

This is ideal for postmenopausal women with complete prolapse as the atrophic uterus does not provide a good anchor for the ligaments. It is also indicated for associated uterine pathology. The essential part of the operation is the approximation of the stumps of the ligaments in the midline and the suspension of the vaginal vault to them.

### Steps

a. An incision is made in the vagina as in Fothergill's operation and the bladder separated from the cervix till the uterovesical fold of the peritoneum is exposed and opened (Fig. 31.5).
b. Posteriorly the pouch of Douglas is opened and the redundant peritoneum excised.

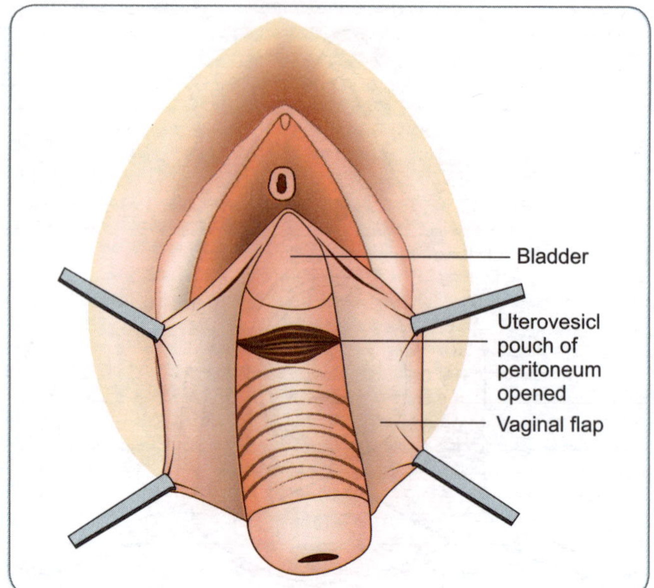


**Fig. 31.5** Vaginal hysterectomy — Step 1: Opening the uterovesical pouch of peritoneum after pushing up the bladder

c. The uterus is now attached to the lateral walls by the lateral and uterosacral ligaments, the uterine artery in the lower part of the broad ligament and the Fallopian tube, the round ligament and the ovarian ligaments in the upper part (Fig. 31.6). Each of these structures is clamped, cut and tied on either side.
d. The peritoneum is now closed with purse-string sutures commencing anteriorly near the bladder and picking up the stumps first on one side, the posterior peritoneum as high up as possible and, finally, the stumps on the opposite side.
e. Each stump is approximated to its counterpart on the other side in the midline and the sutures

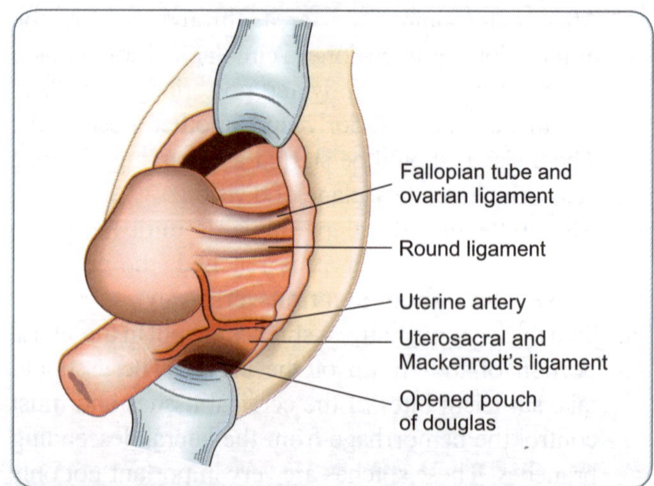


**Fig. 31.6** Vaginal hysterectomy — Step 2: The uterus is now attached laterally by its ligaments and other structures shown

drawn out of the vagina to suspend it to the stumps (Fig. 31.7). The uterovesical fold of the peritoneum is included in the uppermost stump comprising the Fallopian tubes and the ovarian ligaments and the posterior peritoneum included with the stumps of the uterosacral ligaments.

f. Anterior colporraphy and posterior colpoperineorraphy are carried out as described earlier.

Currently site-specific repairs find favour with the gynecologists. These are described in Chapter 26.

## Operations for Nulliparous Prolapse

In these patients, vaginal procedures are inadequate as ligamentary and muscle supports are weak, and too much tightening of the vagina following excision of the vaginal walls interferes with coital function. Different abdominal sling operations for them have been described. They may be combined with anterior and posterior colporrhaphy, if necessary.

### Shirodkar's Method

A strip of mersilene tape is attached to the posterior aspect of the uterus close to the insertion of the uterosacral ligaments and passed subperitoneally round the rectum to be attached to the front of the anterior longitudinal lumbosacral ligament. On the left, it is attached to the psoas muscle to avoid pressure on the sigmoid and the vessels of the sigmoid mesocolon. The advantage of this method is that in addition to suspension, it increases the anteversion of the uterus and prevents herniation of the small bowels into the pouch of Douglas.

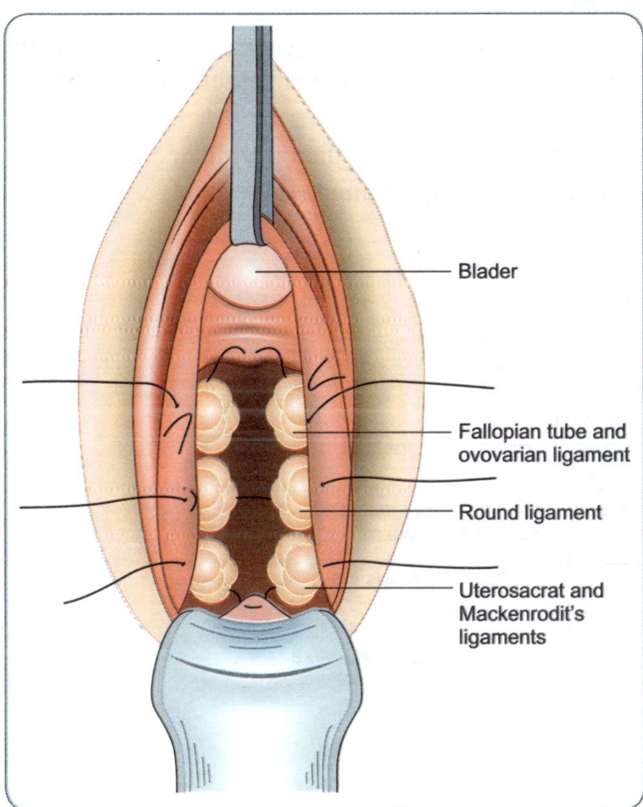


**Fig. 31.7** Vaginal hysterectomy — Step 3: Approximation of stumps in midline

### Purandare's Cervicopexy

The abdomen is opened by a transverse incision, and two fascial strips are fashioned from the anterior rectus sheath and oblique aponeurosis. Each strip is pulled through the internal inguinal ring and is brought subperitoneally along the round ligament to the anterior surface of the cervix where it is fixed. The disadvantage of this method is that, in addition to suspension, the cervix is pulled anteriorly and the uterus falls back into the position of retroversion, in line with the vagina. The space behind the cervix is also widened, allowing the small bowels to prolapse into the pouch of Douglas.

# ABDOMINAL SURGERIES

## SURGICAL ANATOMY OF ANTERIOR ABDOMINAL WALL

The structures in the anterior abdominal wall (Fig. 31.8) are the skin, the superficial fascia, the rectus sheath (anterior layer), the rectus muscle, including the pyramidalis muscle at the lower part of the abdomen just above the symphysis pubis; the anastomosis between the branches of superior and inferior epigastric vessels, the posterior layer of the rectus sheath which is deficient at the lower part, the fascia transversalis, and the parietal peritoneum.

### Types of Incisions

There are different types of incisions (Fig. 31.9) used in gynecological surgery, and they are as follows:

#### Vertical incisions

***a. Midline***

**Advantages**

- It is a comparatively simple, quick and bloodless entry into the abdomen.

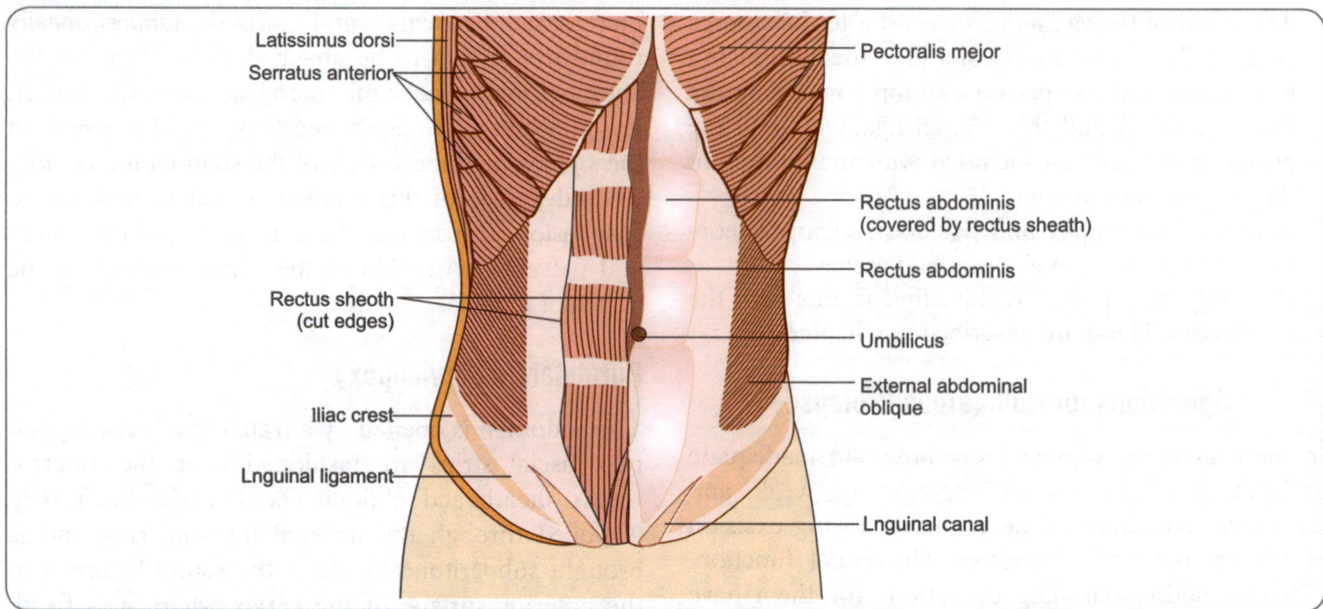


**Fig. 31.8** Structures of the anterior abdominal wall

- It can be extended easily by encircling the umbilicus with good access to the upper abdomen.

### Disadvantage

- Increased risk of wound dehiscence and incisional hernia.

### *b. Paramedian (right or left)*

With this incision, as the rectus sheath is cut lateral to the linea alba, the incidence of ventral hernia is decreased.

### Disadvatages

- Possibility of damage to the rectus muscle due to powerful retraction.
- Exposure may not be as good as with the midline incision.
- Risk of more bleeding as the perforating branches of the epigastric vessels are frequently damaged.
- More time-consuming than the midline incision.
- The scar may be asymmetrical.

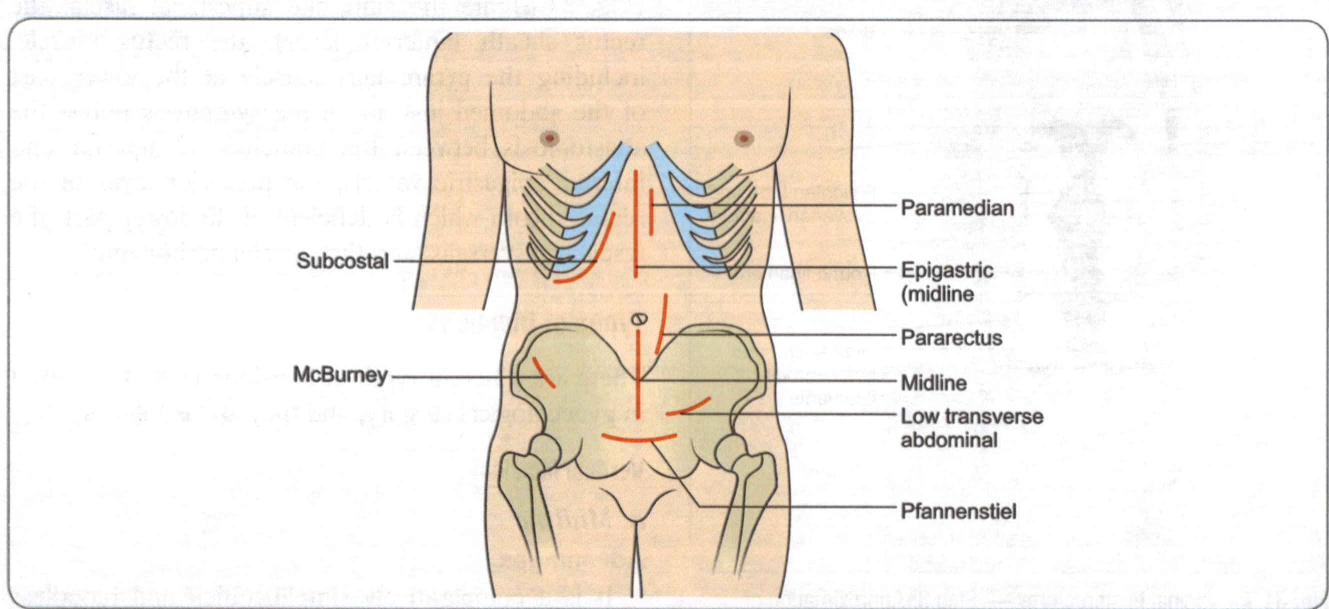


**Fig. 31.9** Types of abdominal incisions

If there is a previous midline scar the paramedian incision should be avoided to prevent two vertical incisions lying side by side with a devascularised area of skin in between.

**Tension in all longitudinal incisions is 30 times greater than that in transverse incisions.** When put on strain, longitudinal incisions tend to open along all their layers including the skin.

### Transverse incisions

#### Advantages

- They are more anatomical.
- When strained, they tend to close and therefore the chances of dehiscence and herniation are much less.
- Usually there is quick wound-healing and strong union due to good blood supply.
- Ambulation can be achieved easily as the patient is more comfortable and convalescence is smoother.
- There are fewer postoperative respiratory complications.
- The incidence of wound infection, hematoma, and wound breakdown are much less. It is also excellent from the cosmetic point of view.

#### Disadvantages

- The exposure is limited. Comparatively, midline structures are better exposed but lateral pelvic dissection is problematic.
- Access to the upper abdomen is not possible.
- It is more time-consuming.
- There is a slightly increased amount of bleeding from dissecting the fat and rectus fascia.

a. **The Pfannenstiel incision** This is a semi-lunar incision made just above the pubic symphysis. The incision on the fascia is at right angles to that on the peritoneum. The incidence of dehiscence is very low. It is possible to extend the incision by transversely splitting the body of the rectus muscle.

b. **The Maylard incision** This is also a transverse incision but placed at a higher level than the Pfannenstiel incision. The rectus muscle and parietal peritoneum are divided transversely for better exposure. The inferior epigastric vessels should be ligated to avoid a hematoma developing under the rectus muscle. The exposure of the lateral pelvic wall in this incision is good but access to the upper abdomen is limited.

c. **The Cherney incision** This is an incision at the tendinous insertion of the rectus and the pyramidalis muscle. It is used for the exposure of the retropubic space of Retzius, for example, in the Marshall–Marchetti–Krantz procedure or in the vesicourethral suspension for stress incontinence of urine.

### Oblique incisions

a. **The grid iron incision** On the right side, McBurney's incision is made for appendicectomy and on the left side a similar incision is made for pelvic colostomy. The risk of hernia is very small but the exposure is inadequate especially in obese women. **This is made only when the diagnosis is certain.**

b. **The Rutherford–Morrison incision (muscle-cutting incision)** This is a modification of McBurney's incision where the incision can be extended, medially splitting the internal oblique and the transversalis muscles. It may be extended downwards if necessary. It is suitable for the extraperitoneal drainage of a pelvic abscess or for exposure of the ureter and external iliac vessels. In cases of difficulty in appendicectomy with McBurney's incision, this modification is useful. Its disadvantage is the risk of incisional hernia but this can be minimised if the muscles are properly sutured.

## HYSTERECTOMY

**Definition** Hysterectomy is the operative removal of the uterus with or without the cervix, by the abdominal or the vaginal route.

- **Total hysterectomy** If the cervix is also removed, the operation is called total hysterectomy.
- **Subtotal hysterectomy** When the cervix is left behind, it is known as subtotal hysterectomy.

**Indications** The indications are mentioned in individual chapters. The major indications are

- Abnormal uterine bleeding when other methods of management fail or the patient is not willing for other options
- Myoma uterus when other methods of management fail or the patient is not willing for other options
- Uterine malignancy
- When there is adnexal pathology in a post/perimenopausal woman along with the removal of adnexa, uterus is usually removed.
- Subtotal hysterectomy is done in younger women in whom hysterectomy has to be done
- Subtotal hysterectomy is also done when cervix could not be removed due to dense adhesions and inapproachability and in obstetric hysterectomy.

Whenever there is any adnexal pathology, in all perimenopausal women and in all cases of pelvic malignancy, a bilateral salpingo-oophorectomy is performed along with the removal of the uterus. In a younger patient, when the uterus is removed, if the adnexa are healthy, the ovaries are conserved for their endocrine function.

## Classification

1. **Abdominal hysterectomy** also known as **type I** hysterectomy total or subtotal, with or without adnexectomy.
2. **Modified radical hysterectomy or Wertheim's operation or type II hysterectomy** This includes removal of the entire uterus with the cervix, both tubes and ovaries, the upper two-thirds of the vagina, the parametrial, paravaginal and paracervical cellular tissue along with the pelvic lymph nodes. It is done for cancer of the cervix Stage Ib and Stage II.
3. **Radical hysterectomy or type III hysterectomy** This was the original radical hysterectomy described by Meigs.

The various indications for hysterectomy are described in the respective chapters.

## Total Abdominal Hysterectomy

**Procedure** The abdomen is opened by a low transverse (Pfannenstiel) or right paramedian incision, the latter being preferred in patients with large tumours, in ovarian malignancy or in PID, for better exposure and exploration. The pelvic and abdominal viscera are carefully examined as soon as the peritoneal cavity is opened. Usually, at this point the patient is placed in a slight Trendelenburg position so that the bowels can gravitate away from the field of operation before they are packed out with a moist abdominal roller pack.

1. Traction is now applied on the fundus of the uterus with a vulsellum forceps (or a myoma screw in multiple fibroids). In cases of endometrial malignancy, this should not be done; instead, two clamps are applied on the medial ends of both the tubes to prevent spillage.
2. The ovarian ligaments on both sides are clamped with two pairs of clamps. If the tubes and ovaries have to be removed, the clamps are applied to the infundibulopelvic ligament taking care to avoid injury to the ureters. The tissues clamped are cut and ligated.
3. The round ligaments are next cut between the two clamps about 3–4 cm from their attachment to the uterus and the cut ends are ligated (Fig. 31.10).
4. The uterus is then put on the stretch by pulling the vulsellum upwards and backwards so as to expose the uterovesical fold of the peritoneum. This loose fold is now picked up and incised transversely from the proximal cut end of one round ligament to the other (Fig. 31.11). The vesical peritoneum with the bladder is now gently separated, with the finger or gauze, from the cervix in the midline as much as possible and again on the sides.
5. **Clamping the uterine vessels** The uterus is now held to one side, and the loose areolar tissue of the broad ligament is pushed down till the uterine vessels

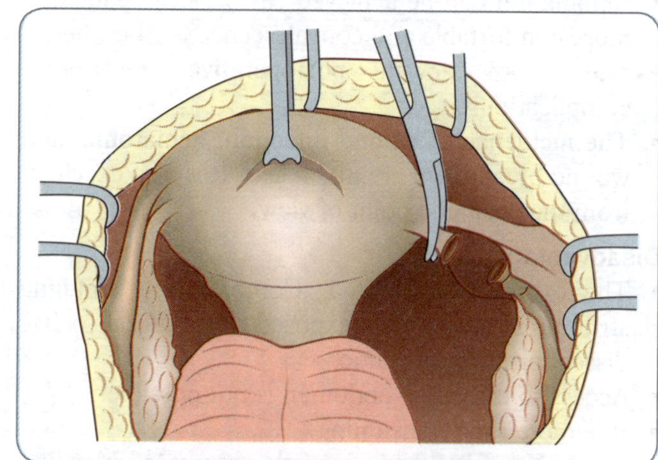

**Fig. 31.10** Abdominal hysterectomy. Note the clamps on the round ligaments. The isthmial portion of the tube and the ovarian ligaments are cut and sutured.

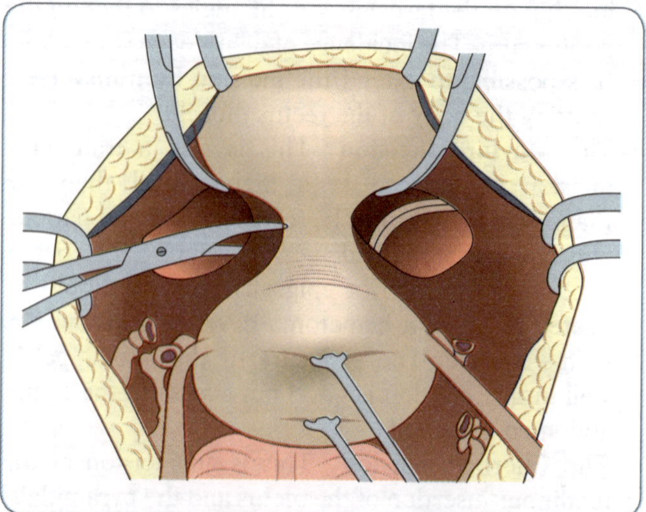

**Fig. 31.11** Abdominal hysterectomy. The uterovesical fold of the peritoneum is picked up and cut transversely.

are reached close to the uterocervical junction. These vessels are then clamped on either side with a curved Kocher's forceps directed medially, cut and sutured securely (Fig. 31.12). At this stage injury to the ureter should be avoided by applying the clamps as close to the uterus as possible. Then the stump cut and ligated. The uterus is then pulled to the opposite side and the procedure is repeated on that side.

6. The uterus is then pulled forwards to expose the posterior wall. This step is often skipped but cutting the posterior peritoneum and pushing the uterosacrals help in better mobilisation of uterus. The posterior serosal surface over the cervix is incised between the two uterosacral folds. The uterosacrals are clamped, cut and tied with 0 chromic catgut and pushed down along with the peritoneum of the pouch of Douglas (Fig. 31.13).
7. The bladder has now been pushed well out in the midline and the sides. The uterus is then pulled to one side, and the cardinal ligaments are cut between two clamps close to and parallel to the cervix, and tied. After doing the same on the opposite side, the uterus is pulled up and, by palpation with the thumb and fingers, it is made certain that the lower end of the cervix is reached (Fig. 31.14).
8. The bladder is well retracted; two Allis forceps are applied to the anterior vaginal wall just below the cervix, and the vaginal vault is opened with a No. 11 blade. The vagina is cut all round, taking care to clamp the vaginal angles with Kocher's forceps (Fig. 31.15). The uterus is now completely removed with care taken to see that posteriorly the rectum is well pushed out by a moist pad or manually by the assistant. The vagina is cleaned with a piece of gauze soaked in antiseptic solution and held on a long forceps.
9. The vagina is closed by a pair of mattress sutures at either angle and the vault is closed by interrupted sutures. Nowadays, continuous sutures are being applied to close the vault. To prevent vault prolapse, the stumps of the round ligaments, the infundibulopelvic ligaments and the uterosacrals are fixed to the vaginal angle on either side (Fig. 31.16).

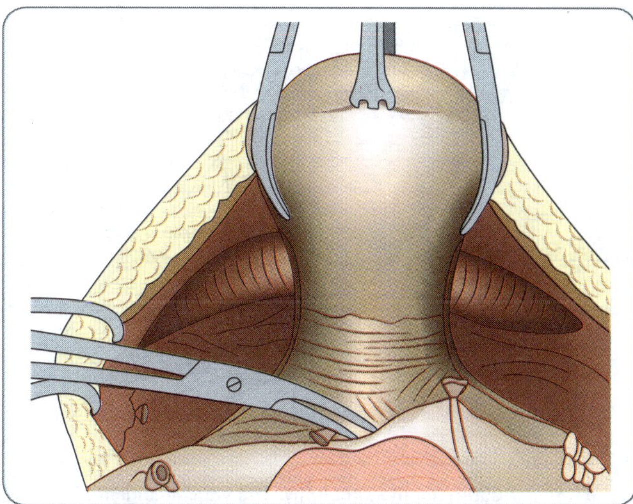

**Fig. 31.13** Abdominal hysterectomy. The uterosacral folds have been cut and ligated. The posterior serosal surface is reflected.

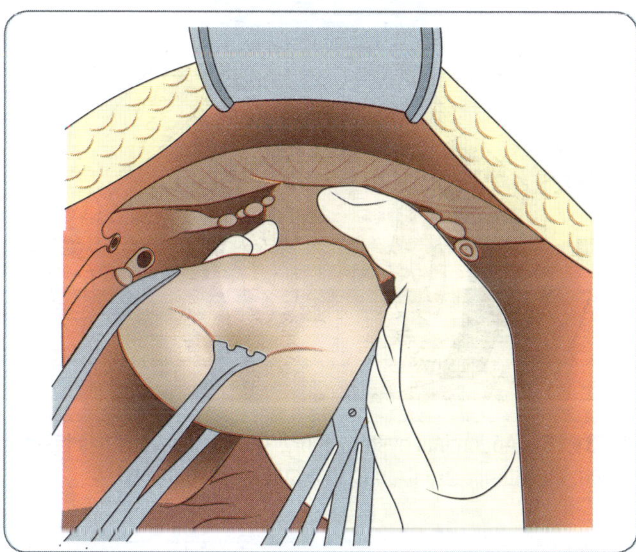

**Fig. 31.14** Abdominal hysterectomy. The uterus is pulled up as the surgeon makes sure that the lower end of the cervix is reached.

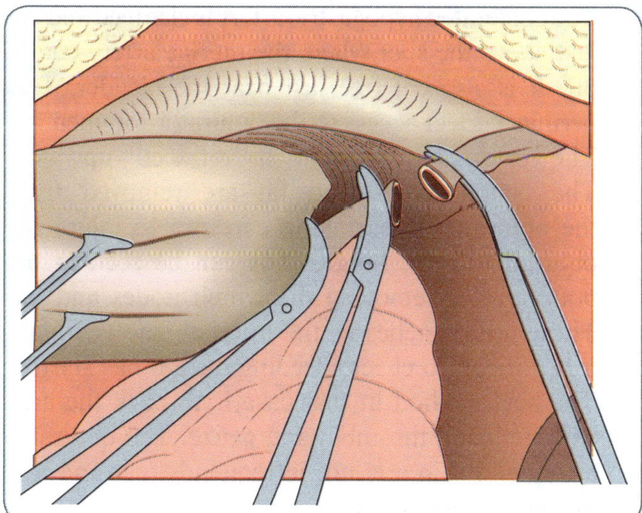

**Fig. 31.12** Abdominal hysterectomy. The uterine vessels are clamped and cut close to the uterocervical junction.

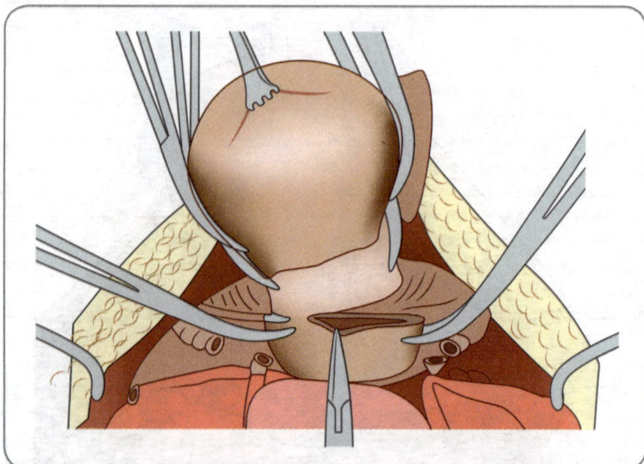

**Fig. 31.15** Abdominal hysterectomy. The vaginal angles are clamped and the vagina is cut around to remove the uterus.

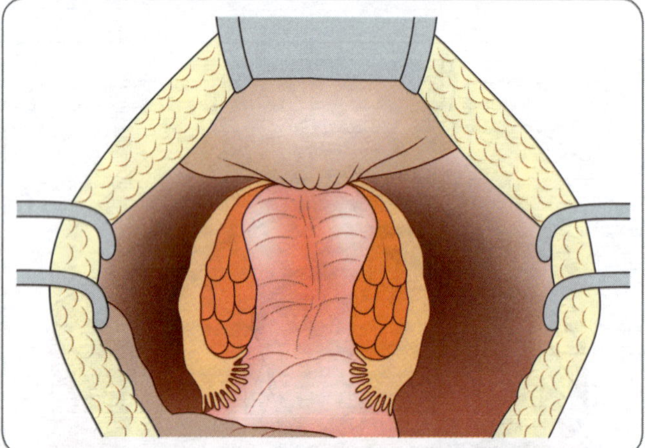

**Fig. 31.16** Abdominal hysterectomy. The vaginal vault has been closed; the stumps are fixed to the vault and peritonised.

10. The raw area is now peritonised by suturing the vesical peritoneum with that of the pouch of Douglas.
11. The peritoneum is mopped clean. The appendix is visualised and removed if necessary. The abdominal pack and pads are taken out and the count is verified. The abdomen is closed in layers.

The specimen is now examined, sectioned and any gross pathology noted before sending it for histologic examination.

## Radical Abdominal Hysterectomy (Wertheim's Operation)

### Procedure

1. Abdomen is opened preferably with a vertical incision. Maylord"s muscle cutting incision may also be used if a transverse incision is desired.
2. After opening the abdomen, the different viscera, particularly the liver and the aortic nodes, are palpated. The pelvic organs are also palpated to check their operability.
3. The round ligament is cut and tied as far laterally as possible. The infundibulopelvic ligament of the same side is clamped and cut as far as possible taking care to see that the ureter is not injured. The bladder peritoneum is cut and the bladder is pushed down to some extent by cutting the pubocervical fascia.
4. The broad ligament is opened up by joining the cut margin of the round ligament and the infundibulopelvic ligament. By pulling the uterus up and to the left, the common iliac artery and the bifurcation of the aorta are exposed. The ureter can now be easily seen crossing the common iliac artery, running down towards the bifurcation of the iliac vessels and inside the curve of the pelvis towards the bladder.
5. The dissection is started at the common iliac artery just below the bifurcation of the aorta. It is then carried from above downwards but the ureter is not dissected away. Care must be taken not to injure the common iliac vein. The psoas muscle which is located lateral and parallel to the iliac vessels is cleaned, taking care not to injure the genitofemoral or genitocrural nerves. The dissection is carried down the entire length of the external iliac artery, and the vein is easily seen and cleaned. About 1–2 cm below the bifurcation of the common iliac, there is a hypogastric branch to the ureter. This vessel should be preserved.
6. The obliterated hypogastric artery is clamped and cut just above the spot where the uterine artery comes off. It is also cut free just near the bladder. This permits perfect access to the obturator foramen.
7. The external iliac vein is retraced upwards. The lymph nodes and fat are removed from the obturator fossa taking care not to injure the obturator nerve. Large veins can be seen at the bottom after removing the lymph nodes and fat. These are branches of the internal iliac vein, and it is difficult to check bleeding once it has started. The best method in that case is to pack the area with gelfoam, thrombin and gauze. The obturator artery and vein are, not infrequently, cut and tied during the operation.
8. The medial end of the uterine artery is now retracted medially towards the uterus, and is

dissected down to the ureteric tunnel which runs around the lower cervix and the upper vagina. The tunnel is opened, and the ureter is freed and followed up to its entrance into the bladder. After this, a considerable portion of the parametrium is exposed.

On the left side of the pelvis, this becomes slightly more difficult because the mesentery of the sigmoid colon runs across the common iliac artery and vein. Here the sigmoid must be pushed upward and medially giving access to the common iliac artery and the same dissection is carried out.

9. The uterus is now pulled forward over the symphysis. The peritoneum of the pouch of Douglas is cut, and the vagina is separated from the rectum by cutting the uterosacral ligaments.
10. After cleaning out the pararectal region, clamps are placed on the parametrium, as far laterally as possible, and cut. The bladder is then further freed as far as possible down on the vagina to give perfect exposure to about three-fourths of the vagina.
11. Curved clamps are placed at the lateral angle of the vagina which is then cut, and the whole mass is removed.
12. The vagina is closed by interrupted sutures, and the whole operated area is inspected. The anterior and posterior peritoneal edges are finally approximated by continuous sutures, and the abdomen is closed in layers.

## OPERATIONS ON THE ADNEXA

### Salpingectomy

**Indication** The chief indication for the removal of the tube is tubal gestation.

**Procedure** The uterus is held up and the offending tube is elevated between the thumb and the index finger to expose the tubal mesentery. Two clamps are now applied close to the tube (to avoid injuring the ovarian artery), and the tissue between these clamps is cut. Two more clamps are then applied over the isthmial region of the tube, and another pair over the mesosalpinx between the tube and the ovary. The tube is elevated and then cut along its mesenteric attachment and also at the isthmial end (Fig. 31.17). The clamps are now replaced by interrupted mattress sutures. The sutured area is finally covered over by the peritoneum or the round ligament. The opposite tube is examined, and the peritoneum is cleaned before the closure of the abdomen.

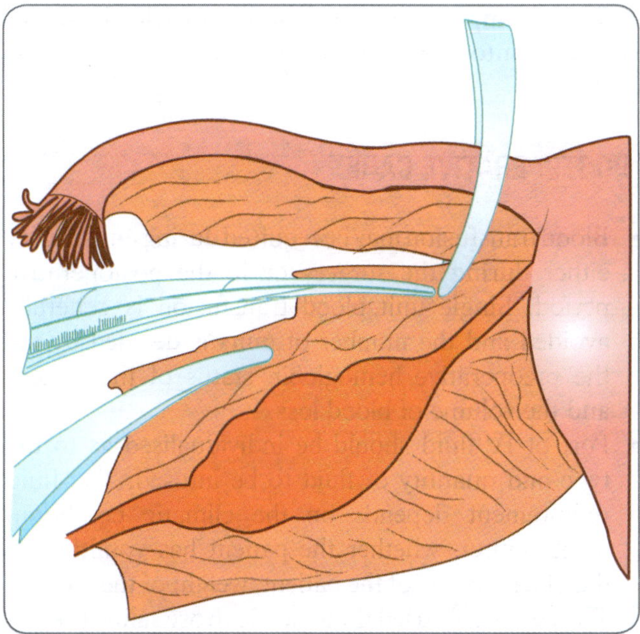

**Fig. 31.17** Salpingectomy. Two clamps are joined just below the tube and two more pairs over the isthmial region as the tube is resected.

### Salpingo-oophorectomy

**Indication** Salpingo-oophorectomy is done mostly in cases of unilateral disease of the tube and ovary, for example, in salpingo-oophoritis or tubo-ovarian mass and in benign unilateral ovarian tumours. If the lesions are bilateral, total hysterectomy with bilateral salpingo-oophorectomy is preferred.

**Procedure**

1. The uterus is held up and the diseased tube and ovary are separated from the surrounding adhesions and mobilised well. The adnexa of the affected side are lifted up to expose the infundibulopelvic ligament which is clamped in two places and cut. The ovarian artery is thus ligated.
2. Two more clamps are now placed close to the uterus over the isthmial portion of the tube and the ovarian ligament and the structures between these clamps are cut.
3. The broad ligament below the ovary now needs to be clamped and cut so as to facilitate the removal of the diseased tube and ovary.
4. These clamps are then replaced by mattress or interrupted sutures.

The stump of the infundibulopelvic ligament is buried into the peritoneum and the abdomen is closed.

## POSTOPERATIVE CARE

- Blood transfusion may be required during any surgery either during the surgery or in the postoperative period. Single unit blood transfusion is generally avoided and the number of units is decided by the the preoperative hemoglobin status of the patient and the volume of blood loss.
- Port of IV fluid should be individualised as to the type and quantity of fluid to be infused. The fluid requirement depends on the climatic condition, urine output, whether the patient has vomiting or diarrhea, the age of the patient, weight of the patient, The commonly used fluids are dextrose saline (DNS) and lactated Ringer (RL) solution. The standard regimen is 40 mL/hr for 24 hours. Pain control could be pre-emptive or after the pain sensation is felt. Pre-emptive analgesia is based on the fact that the pain should be controlled before it is felt by the patient. Whenever epidural anaesthesia is used during surgery, the same epidural route could also be used for pain control. The commonly used drugs for postoperative pain control are inj. pentazocine or inj. tramadol. These drugs are usually given in 4–8 hourly intervals. The dose and frequency should be individualised.
- Most patients are able to pass urine on their own 10–12 hours after surgery. If they are unable to do so, they are catheterised after taking all the aseptic precautions. A prerenal cause for oliguria should be ruled out by increasing the fluid input when there are no contraindications for doing so. Following radical surgery for carcinoma of the cervix (to combat atony of the bladder), and following repair of the bladder fistula, continuous drainage of the bladder is required for a longer duration.
- During the first day or two, ileus may be expected and therefore the oral intake of fluids is restricted to small sips of water. Once the bowel sounds are heard on auscultation of the abdomen, oral fluids are started. When paralytic ileus occurs, the initial management is to avoid oral fluids, continue IV fluids and monitor the patient's condition. Electrolyte study may be necessary in these patients.
- Usually from the third or the fourth postoperative day, the patient is able to have a normal, solid diet.
- Routine postoperative enema is not required as most patients have bowel movement on their own. In a few cases a laxative or a rectal suppository may be needed.
- Postoperative shock following gynecological surgery is usually due to internal hemorrhage. Hence before completing the surgery, it should be ensured that perfect hemostasis is secured. Sometimes due to a fall in BP, there may not be any bleeding at the end of the surgery but bleeding will start once the BP picks up. Hence it is the duty of the surgeon and the anaesthetist to make sure that the patient in normotensive, and hemostasis is adequate.
- Hemorrhage may not be visible outside even after vaginal surgery. **Any unexplained, persistent, postoperative tachycardia should warn the surgeon as to the possibility of internal hemorrhage.** Fall of BP, abdominal distension all appear later in hemorrhage. Examination of the vagina following vaginal surgery for bleeding and ultrasound examination of the abdomen would reveal excessive intraperitoneal fluid collection (sometimes with internal echoes) suggesting hemoperitoneum. USG-guided paracentesis would reveal the nature of the fluid and when internal hemorrhage is confirmed, laparotomy with adequate blood is usually required. Hemorrhage following vaginal surgery needs to be explored under anaesthesia in the operation theatre and the bleeding could be secured either vaginally or may require laparotomy.

**Postoperative Complications**

The postoperative complications following major gynecological surgery are

1. Shock
2. Reactionary hemorrhage
3. Paralytic ileus
4. Pelvic peritonitis/abscess
5. Pelvic cellulitis
6. Secondary hemorrhage from the vaginal vault
7. Thrombophlebitis
8. Pulmonary embolism

## RECAP

- A proper and careful pre-operative preparation is an integral part of surgery and is as important as surgical intervention.
- Except in emergency situations, the pre-op target Hb should be 11 g.
- Antibiotic prophylaxis is recommended in most of the gynecological procedures particularly in hysterectomies and in surgeries with frank sepsis and pus.
- Pre-anaesthetic assessment based on American Society of Anesthesiologists' Classification of Physical Status always helps to grade the cases.
- It is also necessary to arrange for adequate amounts of compatible blood.
- There are two types of suture material: absorbable and non-absorbable.
- The size of the suture material is indicated by a number. Suture materials of smaller size are indicated with a 0 after the number.
- An informed consent should be obtained, in writing, from the patient and one of her relatives/attendants for any surgery whether it is a minor or a major procedure. In the case of minor girls and mentally affected women, the consent from her legal guardian is essential.
- Thromboprophylaxis is done pre-operatively and it may have to be continued postoperatively.
- The need for thromboprophylaxis depends on the risk group they belong to.
- The common minor vaginal operations are dilatation and curettage, endometrial aspiration, cervical punch biopsy, removal of the cervical polyp, operations for Bartholin's cyst.
- Major vaginal surgical procedures are anterior colporrhaphy for cystocele and urethrocele, posterior colpoperineorrhaphy for rectocele, amputation of the cervix, Fothergill's or the Manchester operation, vaginal hysterectomy with anterior colporrhaphy and posterior colpoperineorrhaphy (Ward–Mayo's operation), operations for nulliparous prolapsed.
- Surgical anatomy of anterior abdominal wall: The structures in the anterior abdominal wall are the skin, the superficial fascia, the rectus sheath (anterior layer), the rectus muscle, including the pyramidalis muscle at the lower part of the abdomen just above the symphysis pubis; the anastomosis between the branches of superior and inferior epigastric vessels, the posterior layer of the rectus sheath which is deficient at the lower part, the fascia transversalis, and the parietal peritoneum.
- Types of incisions: vertical incisions, midline, paramedian (right or left).
- Transverse incisions: The Pfannenstiel incision, The Maylard incision, The Cherney incision
- Oblique incisions: The gridiron incision, The Rutherford–Morrison incision (muscle-cutting incision).
- Hysterectomy: Abdominal hysterectomy, Modified Radical hysterectomy or Wertheim's operation or type II hysterectomy, Radical hysterectomy or type III hysterectomy.
- Operations on the adnexa: Salpingectomy. Salpingo-oophorectomy.
- Postoperative care: Whenever blood transfusion is required, it may be given on the table or soon after, depending on the blood loss.
- Following laparotomy, the patient is given fluids and electrolytes intravenously depending on individual needs.
- Pain control could be pre-emptive or after the pain sensation is felt. Pre-emptive analgesia is based on the fact that the pain should be controlled before it is felt by the patient.
- Most patients are able to pass urine on their own 10–12 hours after surgery. If they are unable to do so, they are catheterised after taking all the aseptic precautions.
- During the first day or two, ileus may be expected and therefore the oral intake of fluids is restricted to small sips of water
- Usually from the third or the fourth postoperative day, the patient is able to have a normal, solid diet.
- Postoperative shock following gynecological surgery is usually due to internal hemorrhage. Hence before completing the surgery, it should be ensured that perfect hemostasis is secured. Sometimes due to a fall in BP, there may not be any bleeding at the end of the surgery but bleeding will start once the BP picks up.
- Hemorrhage may not be visible outside even after vaginal surgery. Any unexplained, persistent, postoperative tachycardia should warn the surgeon as to the possibility of internal hemorrhage.

# REVIEW QUESTIONS

## Long-Answer Question

Discuss the steps of anterior colporrhaphy and posterior colpoperineorrhaphy surgeries.

## Short-Answer Questions

1. Briefly discuss the recommendation for thromboprophylaxis.
2. Discuss the operation for Bartholin's cyst.

## MCQs

**1. Which of the following is not an indication for amputation of the cervix?**
   a) Elongation of cervix
   b) Nulliparous prolapse
   c) Stress incontinence
   d) All of the above

**2. Operations for nulliparous prolapse are the following except**
   a) Vaginal hysterectomy
   b) Shirodkar's operation
   c) Purandare's cervicopexy
   d) Khanna's sling operation

**3. Which incision is commonly used in abdominal hysterectomy?**
   a) Subcostal
   b) McBurney
   c) Epigastric
   d) Pfannenstiel

**4. Which is a non-absorbable suture material?**
   a) Plain catgut
   b) Polypropylene
   c) Polyglycolic acid suture
   d) Polygalactin 910

**Further Reading**

Hawkins J, Hudson CN. Shaw's textbook of operative gynecology. Indian edn. BI-Churchill Livingstone; 1993.
Monaghen JM. Bonney's gynecological survey. London: Bailliere and Tindal; 1986.
Rock JA, Thompson JD. Te Linde's operative gynecology. 8th ed. New York: Lippincott; 1996.

# Chapter 32

# Pain in Gynecology

**At a Glance**

Anatomical Considerations
Chronic Pelvic Pain (CPP)
Etiopathology
History and Importance
Backache

Pain is an important gynecological problem because of its frequency and the diversity of its causes. In about 40 per cent of cases, it may be of gynecological origin but in the rest it is due to orthopedic, urologic, neurologic and other factors.

## ANATOMICAL CONSIDERATIONS

The vulva is richly supplied with nerves, mainly the pudendal (S2, S3 and S4), the ilio-inguinal (LI) and the genitofemoral (L1 and L2) nerves. The pudendal nerve supplies the clitoris, the posterior aspect of the labia and the perineum. There is no unanimity of opinion regarding the nerve supply of the pelvic viscera. The sympathetic nerve supply is derived from T11, T12, L1 and L2 to form the 'presacral nerve' or the plexus which along with the parasympathetic from the pelvic nerve (S2, S3 and S4) supplies through the hypogastric ganglia, the uterus, cervix, vagina, bladder and the rectum.

The nerve supply to the ovary is from T12. As the T11–L1 segments are responsible for uterine sensation, spinal or epidural anaesthesia to this level is necessary for pain relief in labour or in cesarean section.

The uterus is not sensitive to cutting. In cervicitis, the sensory fibres of the parasympathetic S2, S3 and S4 may cause referred pain to the mid-sacral region. The cervix does not tolerate stretching or dilatation but can be biopsied or cauterised without anaesthesia. The bladder is relatively insensitive after Wertheim's operation as its nerve supply is stripped during surgery. There is some pain when the ovary is stretched by follicular distension but none when it is gradually distended by a tumour. It is sensitive to compression as can be made out when prolapsed ovaries are palpated during a bimanual pelvic examination.

## CHRONIC PELVIC PAIN (CPP)

CPP is seen in about 5–10 per cent of patients and is responsible for 10–20 per cent of diagnostic laparoscopies and 10 per cent of hysterectomies.

**Definition** The American College of Obstetrics and Gynecology (ACOG) defines chronic pelvic pain (CPP) as **continuous or non-cyclical pelvic pain of longer than 6 months duration, which localises to the anatomic pelvis, abdominal wall at or below the umbilicus, lumbosacral back, or the buttocks and is of sufficient severity to cause functional disability or lead to medical care.**

Nearly 4% of women are thought to have ongoing CPP.

### Etiopathology

Pain in gynecology is multifactorial and causes may be broadly divided into two groups: gynecological, and non-gynecological.

#### Gynecological causes of pain

a. **Early pregnancy**—abortion (spontaneous or induced) and ectopic gestation (acute or chronic).
b. **Menstrual disorders**—dysmenorrhea (spasmodic, congestive or membranous); ovulation pain at mid-cycle; premenstrual tension; hematometra due to congenital or acquired causes.
c. **Iatrogenic causes**—intrauterine contraceptive devices.

d. **Functional causes**
   i. primary dysmenorrhea in the adolescent age group;
   ii. dyspareunia which may be functional or due to organic causes. Dyspareunia may be superficial, at the introitus, (caruncle, bartholinitis) or deep-seated as in cervicitis, endometriosis or prolapsed ovaries.

e. **Inflammatory conditions**—acute or chronic PID, adnexitis, pelvic cellulitis, pelvic abscess.

f. **Neoplasms**
   i. benign—adenomyosis, endometriosis, myoma (depending on size, site, location, degeneration or vascular changes) and ovarian tumours (due to torsion, rupture or in rare cases, infection);
   ii. malignant pelvic neoplasms where pain is late due to infiltration into neighbouring organs and nerves.

g. **Vascular lesions**
   - Pelvic congestion syndrome, usually when a woman in the third or fourth decade complains of dysmenorrhea or dyspareunia and leucorrhea. There is no cervicitis but generalised pelvic tenderness on examination. Unnecessary surgery, often resorted to in such cases, must be avoided.
   - Thrombophlebitis of the pelvic veins following surgery, delivery or abortion may give rise to low fever, and pain in the lower abdomen and legs. There is a risk of thromboembolism in some of these patients.

h. **Residual ovary syndrome** In this the pain is often due to ovaries left behind during a hysterectomy. Most of these patients complain of dyspareunia or chronic lower abdominal pain. Laparoscopic examination may show cystic ovaries, hydrosalpinx, adhesions or, rarely, malignancy.
   i. In ***remnant ovarian syndrome*** a part of the ovary might have been left behind especially in surgery for pelvic endometriosis or PID and causes constant or cyclic lower abdominal pain.

### Non-gynecological causes of pain

a. **Enterocolic or mesenteric** in origin caused by appendicitis, intestinal obstruction, diverticulitis, hernia or postoperative adhesions.

   Pain due to adhesions could be a distressing symptom and the etiology is very often diagnosed late. The adhesion scoring group (1994) has brought out a comprehensive system for scoring of adhesions. This could be used as a tool for further evaluation of adhesions.

**Adhesion Score**

| | |
|---|---|
| Severity | 0: None<br>1: Filmy, avascular<br>2: Dense and/or avascular<br>3: Cohesive |
| Extent of total area or length | 0: None<br>1: ≤25%<br>2: 26–50%<br>3: >50% |

   It may be acute, subacute or chronic depending on the stage of the disease.

b. **Urologic**—urethral caruncle, urethritis, cystitis, perivesical abscess, pyelonephritis or ureteral colic.

c. A **low backache**, a symptom very common in women. It may be postural, fibromuscular or bony in origin. Fibromyositis, spondylitis, spondylo-listhesis, disc lesions and sacralisation of the fifth lumbar vertebra are important causes.

d. **Functional** in origin, when no obvious lesion is found, but organic causes must always be ruled out before this diagnosis is arrived at.

## History and Importance

In each case one has to ascertain from the patient whether the pain is sudden or gradual; whether it is related to food, the menstrual pattern, exercise, injury, childbirth or surgery; whether it is localised, referred or spreading; whether it is dull or dragging, spasmodic, colicky, constant or intermittent.

- Sudden severe pain is due to torsion, rupture, hemorrhage or perforation of a viscus or tumour.
- When there is sudden and severe pain associated with collapse and pallor in a young patient complaining of atypical amenorrhea (or having an IUCD), a disturbed ectopic gestation has to be thought of. The movement of the cervix is painful in such a case and ultrasound, laparoscopy (when she is stable) and culdocentesis often help to confirm the diagnosis.
- The pain at a level higher than the iliac crests may not be of pelvic origin.
- Similarly the pain on moving the joints, radiating pain down the thigh, is not of pelvic origin except in advanced cervical cancer.

## Backache

The backache over the sacrum is probably due to pelvic disease.

If the backache is above or below a line drawn through the lowest part of the costal margin, it is probably postural.

- In genital prolapse of a major degree, the overstretched uterosacrals give rise to a 'dragging' sacral pain which grows worse as the day wears on but is relieved by rest.
- Coccydynia may be caused by fracture or dislocation of the coccyx during childbirth or a fall in the sitting position.
- During pregnancy, due to a hormonal relaxation of the joints, most women complain of a low backache.
- Low backache may also be occupational in origin (lifting heavy loads incorrectly), or may be due to bad posture, an unsuitable mattress, obesity or abnormality of the knees or feet. Most backaches arise in the back and not in the pelvis.

### Management

**History** Eliciting a proper history and carrying out a thorough examination are necessary before initiating therapy. One should consider age, parity, duration and type of pain; its relation to menstruation, micturition, intestinal and other symptoms. The date of the last menstrual period is useful when dealing with complications of pregnancy.

**Examination** A detailed examination including a bimanual pelvic and rectal examination indicates whether or not the pain is of gynecological origin.

**Investigations** In selected cases, urinalysis, culdocentesis, radiography (including the barium meal series), ultrasonography, or CT scan are useful in diagnosing the causative lesion.

**Procedures**

- Endoscopy is useful in the diagnosis and management of pelvic pain.
- On laparoscopy, there may be pelvic lesions like PID, endometriosis, ovarian lesions like PCOD or ovarian malignancy. Often, there may not be any pelvic pathology at all. In some cases, one may find adhesions which may be flimsy or thick and vascular.
- Hysteroscopy may reveal a submucous myomatous polyp or a septate uterus.

**Differential diagnosis** Ectopic pregnancy, appendicitis, salpingitis, ruptured corpus luteum with hemorrhage, ruptured endometrial cyst, pyelitis and septic abortion are some of the conditions which have to be considered in differential diagnosis. **When in doubt, depending on the patient's general condition, it is better to do a laparoscopy or a laparotomy.**

**Treatment** Once a diagnosis is established, the cause has to be treated.

1. Analgesics are useful in relieving pain in dysmenorrhea or threatened abortion, but no habit-forming drugs should be used. The commonly used analgesics are the following.
   **Non-steroidal anti-inflammatory drugs (NSAIDs)** Mefanemic acid is a commonly used drug with minimal side effects and good response. The initial dose for acute pain is 500 mg, followed by 250 mg/day. The other NSAIDs—Naproxen and Ibuprofen—are also used.
   **Opioid analgesics** Acetaminophen can be used in a maximum dose of 4 g/day.
2. Appropriate antibiotics in adequate doses are indicated in PID and urinary infection. Urine culture and sensitivity tests are useful here.
3. Hormones have a place in the management of dysmenorrhea, endometriosis and premenstrual tension (*see* individual chapters).
4. Psychological assurance is adequate in some cases of primary dysmenorrhea, premenstrual tension and dyspareunia.

**Surgical treatment** This will be necessary depending upon the lesion.

- In hematometra, the pent-up blood has to be drained from below.
- The pus also has to be let out by colpotomy in cases of pelvic abscess.
- In chronic cervicitis, antibiotics and cryotherapy are required.
- Laparotomy (with adnexectomy) is necessary for tubal pregnancy, twisted ovarian cysts and tubo-ovarian masses.
- Hysterectomy is indicated in most cases of myoma, adenomyosis or bilateral tubal disease.
- The role of conservative surgery in endometriosis and myoma has been discussed elsewhere.

  In a doubtful abdominal condition, assistance from a surgical colleague is extremely useful.

For pain relief in advanced malignancy, drugs and other procedures may be needed, as discussed elsewhere.

Pain is a symptom and not a lesion. However, it is not advisable to treat only the symptom. It is essential that an early diagnosis is established, if necessary in consultation with an orthopedic specialist, urologist or a psychiatrist.

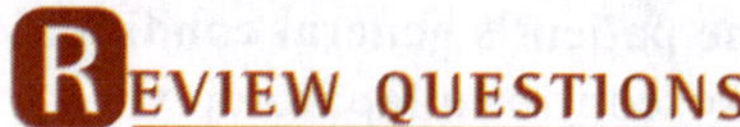

## REVIEW QUESTIONS

### Long-Answer Question

Define chronic pelvic pain. What are the common causes of chronic pelvic pain? Discuss the scoring system for adhesions.

### Further Reading

Drife JC. Pelvic pain syndrome. Br J Obstet Gynecol. 1993; 100: 508–9.

Hoffman B, Schorge J, Schoffer J, Halvorson L, Bradshaw K, Cunningham F. William's Gynecology. 2nd ed. New York: McGraw-Hill; 2012.

Premila S. Chronic pelvic pain. Obstetrics and gynecology for postgraduates. vol. 2. Ratnam SS, Rao KB, Arulkumaran S, editors. Madras: Orient Longman; 1994. 359–368 pp. 2 vol.

Report of a RCOG meeting. Pelvic pain. Br J Obstet Gynecol. 1995;102:580–582.

# Contraception

**At a Glance**


Mode of Action of Conception
Medical Eligibility Criteria
Methods of Fertility Control
**Temporary Methods**
1. Fertility Awareness Methods (Natural family planning methods)
   a. Rhythm Method or Calendar Method
   b. Basal Body Temperature (BBT) Method
   c. Billings's Method or Cervical Mucus Method or Ovulation Method
   d. Symptothermal Methods
   e. Coitus Interruptus or Withdrawal Method
   f. Lactational Amenorrhea Method (LAM)
2. Barrier Method of Contraception
   In Female
   In Male
3. Intrauterine Contraceptive Devices (IUCD)
   Types of Intrauterine Contraceptive Devices
4. Oral Contraceptives
5. Injectible Contraceptive
   Progesterone-Containing Compounds
   Injectables Containing a Combination of Estrogen and Progesterone
6. Implants
   Types
   Mechanism of Action of Implants
Hormonal Contraceptive Vaginal Rings
Transdermal Contraceptive Patch
**Permanent Contraceptive Methods**
1. Female Sterilisation
   A. Postpartum Sterilisation
   B. Laparoscopic Sterilisation
   C. Mini-lap Sterilisation
   Failure Following Sterilisation
   Reversibility Following Sterilisation
2. Male Sterilisation
   A. Non-scalpel Vasectomy
3. Emergency Contraception
   Methods of Emergency Contraception
Contraception and Cancer


Population explosion is one of the leading challenges the world faces today. Since independence (1947), the population of India has more than doubled and is 1.252 billion now (2013 census). It is growing at the rate of over 2 per cent per year and is directly responsible for increased poverty, unemployment, malnutrition and deforestation. Overpopulation is a global problem but mainly concerns the developing world. In India, due to the efforts made to contain the population explosion, the birth and death rates are 21.6 and 7.0 respectively (SRS 2013). This is in contrast to the birth rate of 28.6 and the death rate of 9.2 reported for the year 1994.

The global total fertility rate (TFR) has declined from 4.9 in 1963 to 2.36 in 2010–15. This has been possible due to better family health education and increased acceptance of effective fertility control methods. In the last 30 years, contraceptive acceptance has more than doubled especially in developing countries. **In India only 10 per cent of the population used contraception in 1960 compared to 45 per cent in 1990. The use of contraceptives rose to 59.8 percent by 2015.**

## MODE OF ACTION OF CONCEPTION

For conception to occur the sperms deposited in the vagina should find their way up the uterus to the outer parts of the Fallopian tube and one of them should succeed in fertilising the ovum released at ovulation. This fertilised ovum should be transported by tubal motility to the uterus and remain there to grow into the fetus. Fertility control or contraception may be effected by bringing about the following (Fig. 33.1):

1. **Suppression of ovulation** at the hypothalamic or pituitary levels by hormonal contraception.
2. **Suppression of spermatogenesis** by hormones or prevention of sperm deposition in the vagina by the use of condoms or through vasectomy.
3. **Preventing the union** of the ovum and sperm by producing a block, or ligation of the tube.
4. **Interfering with tubal motility** or **ovum transport** by intrauterine devices or hormones.

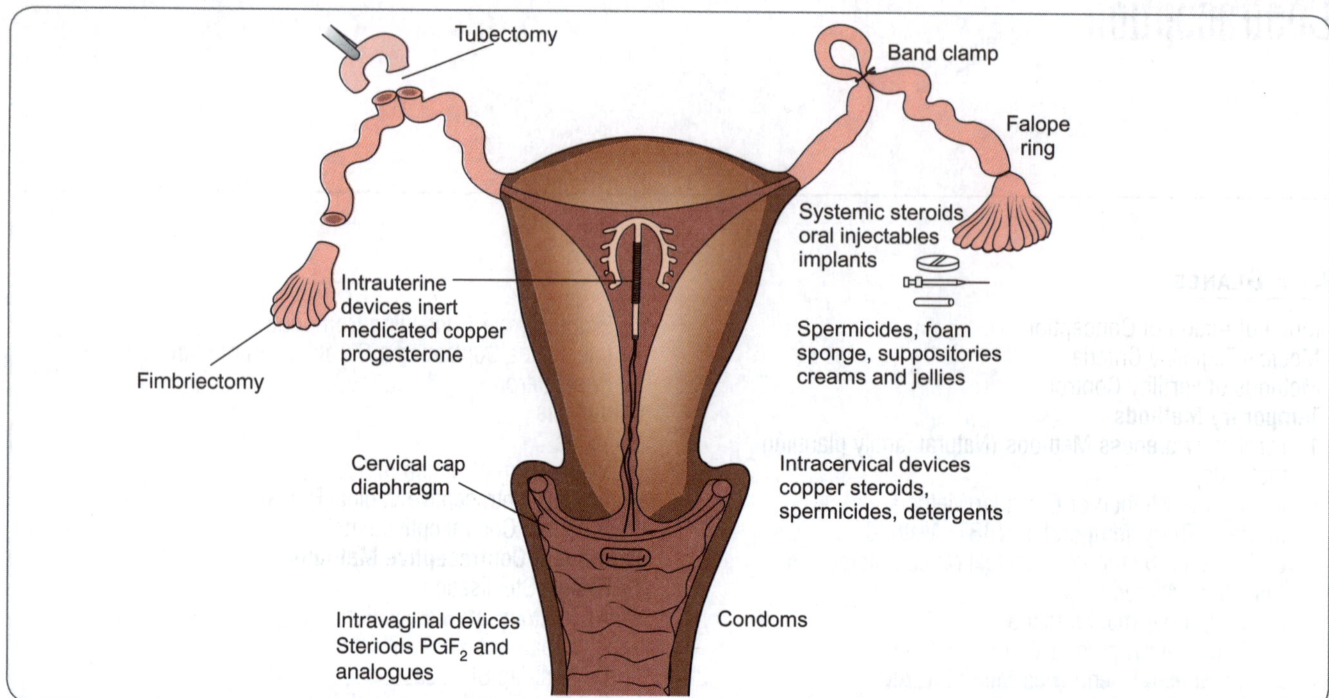


**Fig. 33.1** Different methods of contraception

5. **Preventing the implantation** of the fertilised ovum by causing changes in the endometrium by intrauterine devices or by oral pills.
6. **Preventing sperm migration** through the cervix by increasing the viscosity of the cervical mucus by hormonal contraception.
7. **Luteolysis** of the corpus luteum of the ovary by antiprogesterone.
8. **Disruption of the early zygote** by immunological or other means, by antifertility vaccines.

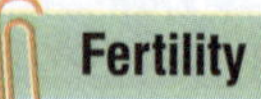

**Fertility Control**

Suppression of ovulation
Suppression of spermatogenesis
Preventing the union of the ovum and sperm
Interfering with tubal motility or ovum transport
Preventing the implantation of the fertilised ovum
Preventing sperm migration
Luteolysis of the corpus luteum
Disruption of the early zygote

## MEDICAL ELIGIBILITY CRITERIA

Medical eligibility criteria are a set of guidelines published by WHO which helps in decision-making as to the suitability of a particular method to the client.

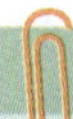

**Eligibility Criteria for Reversible Contraceptives**

Contraceptive methods are organised into four categories:

1. Methods in which there is no restriction on the use of the contraceptive method.
2. Methods in which the advantages of using the method generally outweigh the theoretical or proven risks.
3. Methods in which the theoretical or proven risks usually outweigh the advantages of using the method.
4. Methods in which there would be an unacceptable health risk if the contraceptive method is used.

While Category 1 indicates that the method is suitable for all, Category 4 indicates that it is not suitable under particular conditions/circumstances. Categories 2 and 3 indicate relative contraindications. Category 2 indicates that the method can generally be used, but careful follow-up is required, whereas Category 3 indicates that the method is best avoided unless no other method is available.

## METHODS OF FERTILITY CONTROL

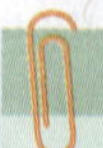

**Methods of Fertility Control**

I. **Temporary contraceptive methods**
   1. **Fertility awareness methods (Natural family planning methods)**
      – Rhythm method

- Basal body temperature
- Billings method
- Symptothermal method
- Coitus interruptus or withdrawal method
- Lactational amenorrhea method (LAM)

2. Barrier methods of contraception
   - Female
   - Male
3. **Intrauterine contraceptive devices**
4. **Oral contraceptives**
5. **Injectable contraceptives**
6. Implants
7. Vaginal rings
8. Transdermal contraceptive patch

II. **Permanent contraceptive methods**

1. **Female sterilisation**
   - Postpartum sterilisation
   - Laparoscopic sterilisation
   - Minilap sterilisation
2. **Male sterilisation**
   - Non-scalpel vasectomy
3. **Emergency contraception**

## TEMPORARY METHODS

## 1. FERTILITY AWARENESS METHODS (NATURAL FAMILY PLANNING METHODS)

### a. Rhythm Method or Calendar Method

Avoidance of coitus during the period of maximum fertility is one of the oldest methods of contraception. It is based on the assumption **(Ogino–Knaus theory)** that in a woman with regular cycles, ovulation takes place on the 14 ± 2 days before the onset of the next period and that the ovum, if it is not fertilised, seldom survives for more than 48–72 hours. **Therefore, if coitus is restricted to the ten days prior to menstruation and the first three or five days after, conception is less likely to occur (failure rate is 9–10 per 100 woman years).**

**Contraindication** This method is not suitable for those with irregular cycles.

### b. Basal Body Temperature (BBT) Method

This method is based on the fact that after ovulation, the progesterone level in the blood rises, increasing the basal metabolic rate (BMR) and causing a rise in temperature by 0.5°F to 0.8°F in the luteal phase; sometimes there is a drop of 0.2°F just before the rise. **The temperature has to be taken as soon as waking up, before doing any other chore.** The impracticality of such a technique and the fact that the exact timing of ovulation cannot be predicted makes it unpopular. Failure rate is 11 per 100 woman years.

### c. Billings's Method or Cervical Mucus Method or Ovulation Method

Owing to hormonal change, particularly the effect of estrogen on the cervix at about the time of ovulation, a scant and thick preovulatory cervical discharge changes in character to a profuse transparent watery slippery discharge which can be drawn or stretched out into a thread **(spinnbarkeit test)** between two fingers, this is designated as the peak day and intercourse is avoided. Failure rate is 3 per 100 woman years.

### d. Symptothermal Methods

This is a combination of BBT and changes in the cervical mucus secretion. When there is a rise in BBT of 0.5°F along with copious, watery cervical mucus, it indicates an unsafe period for coitus. Failure rate of this method is 2 per 100 woman years.

### e. Coitus Interruptus or Withdrawal Method

Coitus interruptus is another time-worn method which also gives rise to a significant number of failures, apart from the stress and strain on both the man and the woman.

### f. Lactational Amenorrhea Method (LAM)

It is based on the fact that lactation protects against ovulation. For this method to be effective, three conditions have to be fulfilled, namely,

1. The mother has not started her periods after delivery.
2. The baby is fully breastfed, fed day and night and often. The baby must be breastfed at least every four hours during the day and at least every six hours during the night.
3. The baby is less than six months of age. It is based on the principle that elevated levels of prolactin inhibit pulsatile secretion of GnRH leading to anovulation.

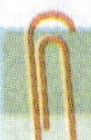

**Natural Family Planning Methods**

**Advantages**
1. No physical side effects
2. Natural menstruation is not affected
3. No financial cost involved
4. Culturally and socially acceptable
5. Does not need follow-up

**Disadvantages**
1. Needs commitment, motivation, training and the co-operation of both partners.
2. They are less effective.
3. Do not protect against STDs and HIV.

## 2. BARRIER METHOD OF CONTRACEPTION

### In Female

The traditional methods of contraception used by men or women were designed to prevent the entry of live sperm into the cervical canal. For this to be achieved, two conditions have to be fulfilled:
1. Direct insemination of the vagina/cervix during ejaculation must be made impossible.
2. Any sperm deposited in the vagina must be immobilised before it can reach the cervix.

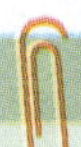

**Barrier Method of Contraception**

For the greatest protection, therefore, two elements should be used:
1. A mechanical barrier protecting the external os and
2. A dose of chemical spermicide in the vagina.

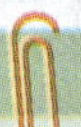

**Barrier Methods Used by Women**

Diaphragm
Cervical cap
Female condom
Spermicides

#### A. Diaphragm

It is a soft latex cup that covers the cervix. The rim contains a firm, flexible spring that keeps the diaphragm in place. It comes in different sizes and requires training before fitting it properly. **It should not be inserted before six hours of coitus and should not be left behind for more than six hours after coitus.** This method of contraception is not completely reliable without the addition of a chemical spermicide. The most satisfactory spermicides, for use with a cap, are made in the form of pastes, creams and jellies. **The cap should be smeared both inside and outside with the spermicide.**

##### *1. The Dutch cap (diaphragm)*

This type consists of a thin rubber dome attached to a circular metal, rubber-covered rim which may be a flat watch-spring or a coil of thin wire (Fig. 33.2). The cap is placed with the dome upwards or downwards diagonally across the vagina with the diameter of the rim fitting snugly between the symphysis pubis and the face of the sacrum. The diaphragm is held in position partly by the tension of the spring and partly by the muscles of the vagina. **For it to be used effectively, however, there must be a reasonably intact perineum and good tone in the muscles of the vagina.**

##### *2. Vault cap (Dumas cap)*

This is a suction cap, shaped like a bowl with a thick rim and a thick centre (Fig. 33.3). The rim clings to

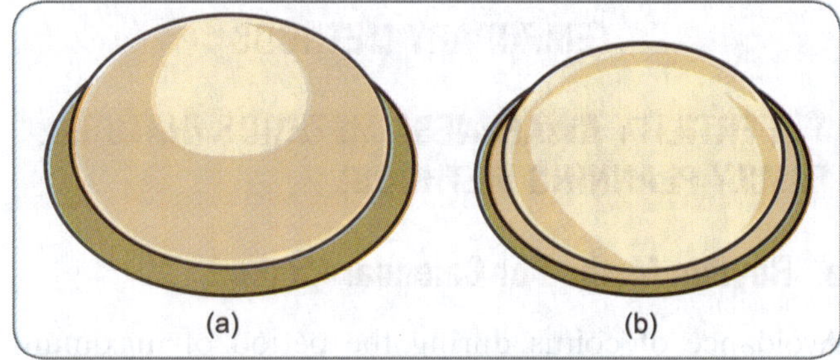


**Fig. 33.2** Types of vaginal diaphragm. (a) Coil spring type; (b) Flat spring type.

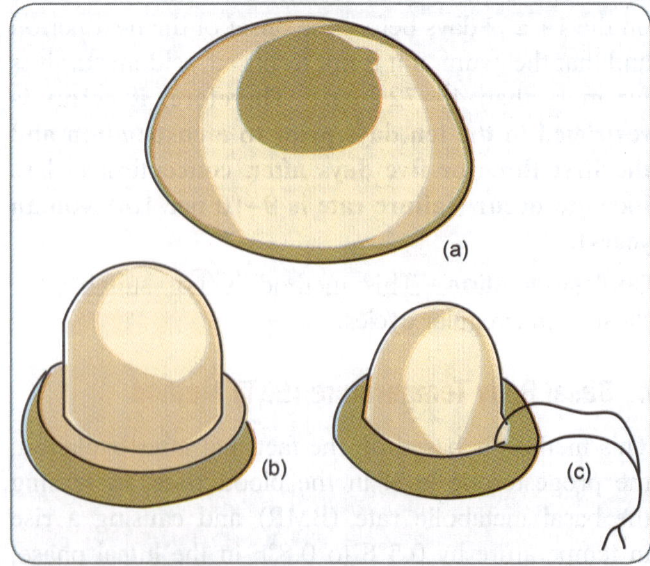


**Fig. 33.3** Types of cervical caps. (a) Vault (dumas) cap; (b) Cervical cap; (c) Vinule cap.

the vaginal roof covering the cervix. It is made either of plastic or rubber. **A vault cap can be used only in women with a moderately short cervix, short enough to be completely contained in the bowl.**

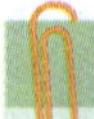

**Timing**

Diaphragm users should be given the following instructions.

- The diaphragm should be inserted no earlier than six hours prior to sexual intercourse.
- Spermicide cream or jelly should be placed in the dome of the diaphragm prior to insertion.
- The diaphragm should be left in place for approximately six hours (but no more than 24 hours) after coitus.

**Care of the diaphragm** After removal, the diaphragm should be washed with soap and water, rinsed and dried.

### B. Cervical cap

It is shaped like a thimble with a raised rim and is made of rubber or plastic. It covers the cervix to its base.

**Criteria for use**

- The size of the circular rim should fit the circumference of the cervix closely.
- It is suitable only for cervices that do not taper.
- The cervix must be long enough to protrude well into the bowl of the cap.
- It must be healthy and so situated in the vagina that it is accessible to the woman's fingers.

It is also made in different sizes—small, medium, large and extra large.

### C. Female condom

The female condom is a pouch made of polyurethane which lines the vagina. An internal ring in the closed end of the pouch covers the cervix and an external ring remains outside the vagina, partially covering the perineum. It works by forming a barrier that keeps sperms out of the vagina, thereby preventing pregnancy. It also prevents harmful microbes in the semen, on the penis, or in the vagina from infecting the other partner.

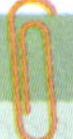

**Important Features of the Female Condom**

- It is prelubricated with silicone; hence spermicide need not be used.
- It should be an effective barrier against STDs.
- High cost and acceptability are major problems.

### D. Spermicides

Many inexpensive varieties of spermicidal preparations are now available. They are harmless and fairly effective. They are easy to use; so help from a doctor or nurse is not required. However, they have the disadvantage of having to be inserted shortly before coitus. The risk of pregnancy when a chemical alone is used is greater than when the chemical is combined with a mechanical barrier. Modern spermicides contain surface active agents that damage the sperm cell membranes. The agents currently used are nonoxynol 9, octoxynol 9 and benzalkonium chloride. Most preparations contain 60–100 mg of these agents in various applications.

Chemical contraceptives are manufactured in the following forms:

#### *1. Foam tablets*

They dissolve in the presence of moisture with the formation of carbon dioxide foam and release the active spermicide into the vagina.

#### *2. Creams, pastes, jellies*

These are contained in metal or plastic tubes with screw-on caps. Applicators are available for deposition in the vagina.

#### *3. Aerosols*

These are pastes or creams compressed into strong containers with a gas.

The foam is released by pressure on a release valve into an applicator from which it is injected into the vagina.

## In Male

### Male Condom

The condom is an effective contraceptive method as well as a protector against STDs. **It is the only barrier method that can be used by men. The male condom is the only one proven to be effective against HIV infection.** Most condoms are made of latex; polyurethane and silicone rubber condoms are also manufactured. Latex condoms are 0.3–0.8 mm thick. Sperms that are 0.003 mm in diameter cannot penetrate condoms. Prospective users need instructions if they are to avoid pregnancy and STDs.

## 3. INTRAUTERINE CONTRACEPTIVE DEVICES (IUCD)

The copper-bearing intrauterine device (IUD) is a small, flexible plastic frame with copper sleeves or wire

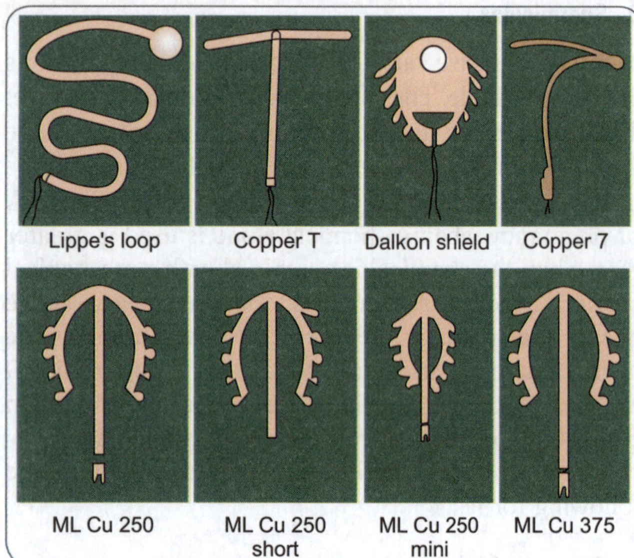


Fig. 33.4 Types of intrauterine devices

around it. A specifically trained healthcare provider inserts it into a woman's uterus through her vagina and cervix. Almost all types of IUDs have one or two strings, or threads, tied to them. The strings hang through the cervix into the vagina. It works primarily by causing a chemical change that damages sperm and egg before they can meet.

The IUCD has now come into great prominence as a very effective method of preventing conception. Over the last few decades, there has been a lot of development in this field.

## Types of Intrauterine Contraceptive Devices

The various types of intrauterine devices are shown in Fig. 33.4.

### Unmedicated IUDS

The Lippe's loop is a polyethylene device in the shape of a double 'S' with a small polyethylene filament protruding through the cervix to facilitate identification. It is not being used any more in routine contraceptive practice.

### Copper IUDS

#### *Copper-T device*

As stated earlier, various types of devices of varying shape and size are available. The 'T' device of Tatum was originally introduced with a view to providing a design which could best adapt itself to the uterine cavity even when it is contracted maximally. Results of preliminary investigations showed that the 'T' device gave rise to a much lowered expulsion rate and bleeding complications as compared to others. However, the pregnancy rate was higher. Because of the lower incidence of side effects with the 'T' device and its antifertility properties, the idea of using the 'T' device as a carrier for copper emerged, and thus, the Copper-T device emerged. The one that is now recommended for use in India is the **Copper-T 380A.** Copper-T 380A has a surface area of 380 $mm^2$ of copper wire wound round the vertical stem of the device. It has a long lifespan of 10 years. The failure rate ranges from 0.6 to 0.8.

**Side effects and complications** The side effects of IUD are as follows:

1. Menorrhagia is the most important side effect and is seen in 5–15 per cent of the acceptors. The menstrual blood loss in some women increased by almost 100 per cent with an inert IUD compared to 50 per cent with a Copper-T. With a progesterone device, however, the menstrual blood loss is less than normal.
2. Breakthrough bleeding (BTB)
3. Colicky pain
4. Pelvic Inflammatory Disease (PID) occurs in 1–2 per cent of IUD users. Its incidence is greater in young nulliparous women, in those with a previous history of PID or STD and in those with multiple sex partners.
5. Leucorrhea
6. Perforation of the device through the uterus resulting in translocation may occur in one in 1500–5000 cases. This risk is greater in postpartum insertions and also with the 'push out' technique of insertion (Lippe's loop) rather than with the 'withdrawal' method (Copper-T).

### Advantages and disadvantages

1. The advantages of the IUD are that it is economical, effective and Copper T-380 A can be used for 10 years. Levonorgestrel IUD (Mirena) is effective for five years.
2. It does not need sustained motivation as for oral contraceptives, and can be used during lactation, or after medical termination of pregnancy (MTP).
3. It is reversible, and fertility is restored soon after its removal.
4. The disadvantages are mainly bleeding, expulsions (sometimes without the acceptor's knowledge), and the fact that it is not self-administered. Bleeding is an important cause of IUD removal. Its exact cause is not known. The new frameless device has not helped in reducing bleeding.

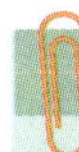

### Contraindications for the use of the IUD

The contraindications are:
1. An intrauterine pregnancy or a suspicion of it,
2. In pelvic inflammatory disease (PID),
3. A history of ectopic gestation,
4. In cases where there have been previous expulsions,
5. A double uterus.

### Hormone-releasing IUDs

These intrauterine devices contain progesterone in the device. The **Progestasert** (Fig. 33.5a) contains a reservoir of 38 mg of progesterone and releases progesterone at a rate of 65 microgram per day. Progestasert is not freely available. The **LNG-20** (Fig. 33.5b) contains 52 mg levonorgestrel, which is released at the rate of 20 microgram per day. The lifespan of LNG 20 is 5 years and it is being used successfully in dysfunctional uterine bleeding, simple hyperplasia, adenomyosis and fibroids.

#### *Mechanism of action*

Progesterone-releasing IUDs add the endometrial action of the progesterone to the foreign body reaction. The endometrium becomes decidualised with atrophy of the glands.

The progesterone IUD probably has two mechanisms of action:
1. Inhibition of implantation and inhibition of sperm capacitation and survival
2. Thickening of the cervical mucus, creating a barrier to sperm penetration

#### *Follow-up*

The woman should be educated to feel the thread after each period and report if the thread is missing.

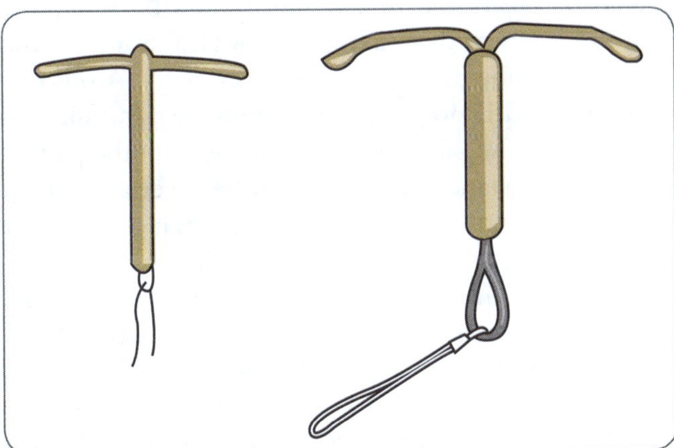

**Fig. 33.5** Hormone-releasing IUDs. (a) Progestasert; (b) LNG 20.

### Indications for Removal of IUD

- expiry of the device,
- PID,
- pelvic pain,
- menopause and
- suspected malignancy.

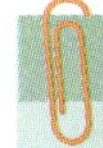

### Fertility Control

1. **Unmedicated IUDs** Lippe's loop, saf-T-coil, Chinese single coil ring, Chinese double-coiled ring (Mahua ring) and Ota ring.
2. **Copper IUDs** Copper 7, Copper T 200, Multiload copper 250, Multiload copper 375, Copper T 380A, Copper T 380 Ag, Copper T 380S, Nova T and Copper T 220C.
3. **Hormone-releasing IUDs** Progesterone IUD (Progestasert) and Levonorgestrel IUD (Mirena, LNG 20).

## 4. ORAL CONTRACEPTIVES

The ovulation-inhibiting effects of progesterone, estrogen and testosterone have been known since 1934. But it was only in 1955 that the value of these steroids as anti-fertility agents was recognised, when Pincus and Rock presented data on ovulation inhibition by progesterone taken orally in the cycle 'day 5 to day 24' regimen, as well as some preliminary data on the use of norethynodrel as an ovulation inhibitor. In 1956, the first contraceptive field trials using norethynodrel was started in San Juan, Puerto Rico.

Oral contraceptives have been used in two forms:
- Combined (Combined Oral Contraceptives COC)
- Sequential

In the **COC**, each tablet consisting of a highly potent, orally active, synthetic estrogen (either ethinyl estradiol or mestranol) is combined with an orally active progestogen. Progestogen compounds of widely varying potency are in use. Broadly speaking, most progestational compounds used in oral contraceptives belong to the 19-norethisterone derivatives group. They include norethisterone, norethynodrel, lynoestrenol and ethynodiol diacetate. The compounds in the group are somewhat estrogenic, probably because they are metabolised to estrogenic compounds. They are the most powerful ovulation inhibitors and have the most marked hemostatic effect on uterine bleeding of endocrine origin. The tablets are taken daily, beginning on the fifth day of the menstrual cycle for 20–22 days and resumed on the fifth day of the subsequent cycle or after seven days. Some preparations have inert tablets or tablets containing iron to fill in the gaps so that the patient takes a pill a day continuously which saves the bother of remembering day five of the next cycle. This is of particular value to those with poor education.

In the usual **sequential regimen**, estrogen alone is taken for 15 or 16 days, beginning on the fifth day of a menstrual cycle, and is followed by estrogen plus progestogen for five days.

**Types of Contraceptive Pills**

Three types of pills are now used in contraception.
1. Combination pills containing both estrogen and progestogen
2. The sequential regimen: estrogens 14–16 days and progestogen added in the last 5–6 days
3. Progestogens only: this is known as the 'mini pill' or progestogen-only pill (POP)

Though the pharmacology of these compounds is beyond the scope of this book, it has been observed that during the last few years, many pills of the same compounds have been found to be effective in preventing ovulation at a much smaller dose.
1. The **first-generation** oral contraceptives had 50 μg or more of ethinyl estradiol.
2. The **second-generation** oral contraceptives contain 30 μg or 35 μg of ethinyl estradiol with progesterones, such as levonorgestrel, norgestimate and other members of the norethindrone family.
3. The **third-generation** oral contraceptives contain desogestrel or gestodene with 20 μg or 30 μg ethinyl estradiol.
4. **Low-dose** oral contraceptives contain less than 50 μg of ethinyl estradiol.

### *Mechanism of action*

The mode of action of the pills is mainly by suppressing ovulation by inhibiting gonadotropin secretion. The progestational agent in the pill primarily suppresses the luteinising hormone (LH), while the estrogenic component suppresses follicle stimulating hormone (FSH) secretion. OCs make the endometrium unfit for implantation. The cervical mucus becomes scanty and viscous, which impairs sperm transport.

### Non-contraceptive benefits of oral contraceptives

- Less risk of endometrial and ovarian cancer
- Regular menstrual cycles.
- Probably less endometriosis, benign breast disease, rheumatoid arthritis and increased bone density.

### Side effects

1. The common **minor** side reactions which are encountered mostly in the early cycles are
- nausea,
- vomiting,
- breakthrough bleeding,
- increase in weight,
- breast tenderness,
- headache and
- increased vaginal discharge.

These are more common in the first cycle and with persistent and continued medication, drop to insignificant levels after the third cycle.

2. The **serious** side effects are
- thrombosis and
- embolism

**Contraindications for OC Pills**

A few rare conditions are known to be aggravated by oral contraceptive administration.
1. These are certain acquired or hereditary defects of hepatic excretory function including Dubin–Johnson and Rotor syndromes.
2. Women who have experienced idiopathic recurrent jaundice of pregnancy redevelop jaundice if given oral progestogens.
3. Oral contraceptives should be prescribed with caution in those with a history or suspicion of carcinoma of the generative organs and breasts,
4. Present or past history of liver disease.

In the presence of cardiovascular disease, the adverse consequences of sodium and fluid retention have to be considered. Thromboembolic disease, varicose veins, cerebrovascular accidents, certain ophthalmological manifestations and psychic depressive states may be considered as contraindications.

### Prescribing oral contraceptives

Before prescribing an oral contraceptive, a detailed history should be taken and the woman should be submitted to a thorough medical and gynecological examination, ideally including a study of vaginal cytology. **A pill can be prescribed if no contraindications are found.** It is possible that the pill prescribed may not suit the patient in the first instance. This fact can be ascertained only after its use for a while. In that case, changing to another pill of a different composition often helps.

**It is now advised that it is safer to use 'pills' containing not more than 30 ¬g of estrogen.** Such pills now available are **Mala-D** (dl-norgestrel 0.5 mg + ethinyl estradiol 30 μg), **Mala-N** (norethisterone acetate 1.0 mg + ethinyl estradiol 30 μg), **Marvelon, Lyndiol**, and so on. It is also useful to choose the one containing the smallest effective dose of progestogen, in the presence of cardiovascular disease. The adverse consequences of sodium and fluid retention have to be considered.

### *Progesterone-only pill or mini pill or POP*

Pills that contain very low doses of a progestin do not contain estrogen, and so can be used throughout the period of breastfeeding and by women who cannot use preparations with estrogen. These pills work primarily by thickening for cervical mucus, disrupting the menstrual cycle and preventing ovulation. Among the large number of progestogens studied so far, norethindrone and its acetate, norgestrel, lynestrenol, quingestanol acetate, ethynodiol diacetate and megestrol acetate have been favourably reported, though each has its own drawbacks.

From the various studies that have been published, pregnancy rates vary from 0.8–2.5 per 100 women users. In a large majority, discontinuation is due to an unacceptable bleeding pattern.

#### Side effects of progesterone-only pills

- Menstrual disturbances
- Delay in return of menstruation in breastfeeding women (lengthened postpartum amenorrhea)
- Frequent, prolonged bleeding
- Infrequent, irregular bleeding
- Amenorrhea
- Nausea
- Headaches
- Mood changes
- Dizziness
- Abdominal pain
- For women who are not breastfeeding, enlarged ovarian follicles
- Govt. of India, under the National Family Planning Programme, has introduced oral contraceptive Centchroman as Chhaya and injectable DMPA in the name of Antara as part of the contraceptive basket of choice.

#### Centchroman (Ormeloxifene) (Chhaya)

Centchroman (Ormeloxifene) is a non-steroidal, non-hormonal once a week oral contraceptive pill. It acts as selective estrogen receptor modulator (SERM).

For initiation of the Centchroman (Ormeloxifene), the first pill is to be taken on the first day of period (as indicated by the first day of bleeding) and the second pill three days later. This pattern of days is repeated through the first three months.

Starting from fourth month, the pill is to be taken once a week on the first pill day and should be continued on the weekly schedule regardless of her menstrual cycle.

**Medical Eligibility Criteria for Centchroman (Ormeloxifene)**

Women with following conditions should not use Centchroman (Ormeloxifene):

- Polycystic ovarian disease
- Cervical hyperplasia
- Recent history of clinical evidence of jaundice or liver disease
- Severe allergic states

  Chronic illnesses such as tuberculosis, renal disease.

  Centchroman (Ormeloxifene) possesses no effect on platelet aggregation, lipid profile and HDL cholesterol. It can be safely used by lactating mothers.

## 5. INJECTABLE CONTRACEPTIVE

### Progesterone-Containing Compounds

These are depot medroxyprogesterone acetate (DMPA) and norethindrone enanthate (NET-EN).

#### Depot medroxyprogesterone acetate (DMPA)

Depo-Provera (DMPA) comes as microcrystals suspended in an aqueous solution. The correct dose for contraceptive purposes is 150 mg intramuscularly (gluteal or deltoid) every three months. The circulating level of progestin is high enough to effectively block LH surge and inhibit ovulation. It also acts by thickening the cervical mucus and altering the endometrium.

The injection should be given within the first seven days of the current menstrual cycle; otherwise, a backup method is necessary for one week. The injection must be given deeply in the muscle by the Z-track technique and not massaged. In terms of efficacy, this method is equal to sterilisation.

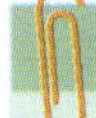

**Contraindications for Injectable Contraceptives**

***Absolute***

1. Women with unexplained genital bleeding
2. Severe coagulation disorders
3. Previous sex steroid-induced liver adenoma

***Relative***

1. Liver disease
2. Severe cardiovascular disease.

### Norethindrone enanthate

This is given in a dose of 200 mg intramuscularly every two months. This progestin acts in the same way as Depo-Provera and has the same disadvantages/ effects.

DMPA can be given both by the intramuscular route and also by the subcutaneous route.

Injectable contraceptive (DMPA) is an aqueous suspension of microcrystal for depot injection of pregnane 17 alpha-hydroxyprogesterone, a derivative of medroxyprogesterone acetate. It is given deep intra-muscular every three months (one dose = one vial of 150 mg, aqueous suspension of DMPA)

Effectiveness depends on timing of first injection, taking injections regularly on time, the injection technique and post injection care.

### *Problems with progesterone-only compounds*

Major problems are irregular menstrual bleeding, breast tenderness, weight gain and depression. Up to 25% of patients discontinue usage in the first year due to menstrual problems.

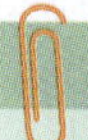

#### Side Effects of Injectable Contraceptives

**Side effects of DMPA**: Changes in bleeding patterns

**First three months**
- Irregular bleeding
- Prolonged bleeding

**At one year**
- Amenorrhea
- Infrequent bleeding
- Irregular bleeding

**Side effects of NET-EN**
- Fewer days of bleeding in the first six months and are less likely to have no monthly bleeding after one year than DMPA
- Weight gain
- Headache
- Dizziness
- Abdominal bloating and discomfort
- Mood changes
- Less sex drive
- Loss of bone density

### Injectables Containing a Combination of Estrogen and Progesterone

This combination is given to overcome the problem of irregular menstrual bleeding.

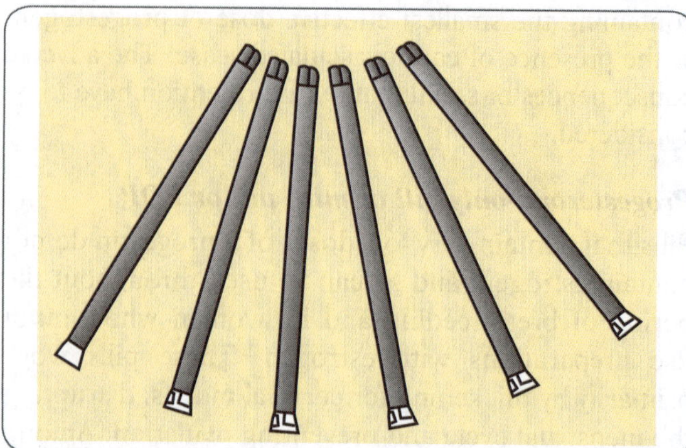

Fig. 33.6 Norplant

### Cyclo-Provera or cyclofem

This consists of 25 mg depot medroxyprogesterone acetate and 5 mg estradiol cypionate. It is administered monthly as a deep intramuscular injection. This method is as effective as Depo-Provera, but is not associated with menstrual irregularity.

The method is rapidly reversible.

## 6. IMPLANTS

The subdermal implant system is a long-acting, low-dose, reversible, progestin-only method of contraception. Insertion and removal of these implants has to be done by the physician. Single-rod implants are easier to insert and remove compared to the set of six capsules.

### Types

Different types of implants have been in use. These include:

- Norplant containing six capsules or rods
- Jadelle and Norplant-2 containing two rods
- Implanon containing one rod

### Norplant

The Norplant system consists of six capsules containing a total of 216 mg of levonorgestrel (each capsule contains 36 mg of levonorgestrel).

Each capsule measures 34 mm in length with a 2.4 mm outer diameter. The capsules release approximately 85 µg of levonorgestrel per 24 hours during the first 6–12 months of use. The rate declines gradually to 50 µg by 9 months and 30 µg per day for the remaining duration of use. The system delivers a sustained level of levonorgestrel for a long time (up to 7 years), though the use is approved for five years.

### Norplant-2

This consists of two levonorgestrel rods (Fig. 33.6). Each rod measures 43 mm in length and 2.5 mm in diameter; it contains 75 μg of the drug and releases the drug at the same dose as the six capsules.

### Implanon

This is a long-acting single-rod subdermal implant. The rod measures 4 cm in length and 2 mm in diameter. The core of the implant contains 68 mg of crystalline etonogestrel, dispersed in a matrix of ethylene vinyl acetate copolymer. The initial release rate is 60–70 μg per day and declines to 25–30 μg at the end of the third year. Its use is recommended for 3 years.

## Mechanism of Action of Implants

These implants cause a sustained release of progestin which inhibits ovulation and thickens the cervical mucus, like Depo-Provera.

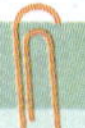

**Side Effects of Implants**

The side effects include menstrual disturbance and weight gain.

## HORMONAL CONTRACEPTIVE VAGINAL RINGS

A flexible vaginal ring is available, which releases 120 μg of etonogestrel (a progestin) and 15 μg of ethinyl estradiol (an estrogen) each day of use. The ring is inserted into the vagina for a three-week period, then removed for one week, during which the woman has a menstrual period.

## TRANSDERMAL CONTRACEPTIVE PATCH

It delivers 150 μg of the progestogen norelgestromin and 20 μg of ethinyl estradiol per day over 7 days. The levels needed for medication are maintained for 2 days beyond the recommended duration. Failure rate is 0.7 per 100 women years.

# PERMANENT CONTRACEPTIVE METHODS

## 1. FEMALE STERILISATION

For women who have decided not to have any more children, tubal sterilisation is one of the best and effective methods. Sterilisation of the woman can be carried out at any time and also as a postpartum procedure.

## A. Postpartum Sterilisation

Postpartum sterilisation has now become a fairly common procedure, especially in cases where further childbearing is considered inadvisable for various medical reasons and also where the couple is not anxious to have any more children. **It is imperative that the surgeon familiarises himself/herself with all the provisions of the Standards of Female (and Male) Sterilisation, published by Government of India, Ministry of Health and Family Welfare to avoid any technical and/or legal complications.**

Before the patient is submitted to an operation, it is essential to get the consent in writing of both partners to avoid legal complications and as a safeguard to the surgeon who carries out the operation (as per the provisions of sterilisation rules, the consent of the male partner is not necessary so long as the female partner is over the age of 18 and is mentally normal).

### Timing of operation

**It is customary to perform the operation within the first 72 hours of delivery.** There are many centres in the world where this operation is performed soon after delivery, within the first 12 hours. The uterus during this period is well above the symphysis. In an uncomplicated delivery, usually the uterine cavity is free from pathogenic organisms for the first 48–72 hours. Hence, it has been suggested that if the operation is performed within this period, the chances of infection are minimised. Another advantage of postpartum sterilisation is that, if performed within the first 72 hours of delivery, it does not prolong hospital stay.

**Caesarean ligation** The two procedures are combined or after a menstrual period in non-pregnant women.

**Interval ligation** This is done six weeks after delivery.

**Postabortal ligation** Immediately following evacuation of the uterus, after induced or incomplete abortion.

**Gynecological ligation** Combined with gynecological surgeries (benign conditions) like myomectomy or cystectomy.

**Vaginal tubal ligation** Though once popular, at present this method is restricted as an additional procedure during surgeries like Manchester operation for uterine prolapse.

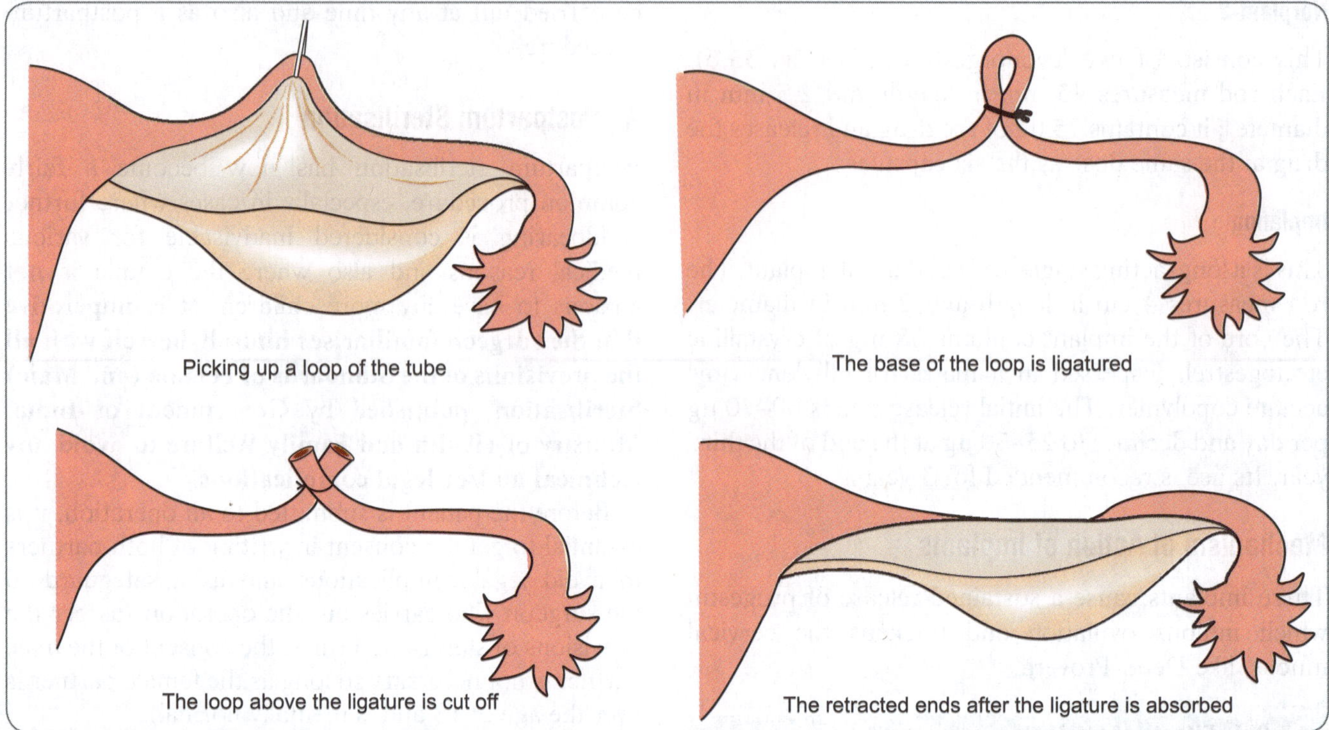


**Fig. 33.7** Tubal sterilisation

## B. Laparoscopic Sterilisation

Tubal sterilisation through a laparoscope is popular all over the world. In India, it is widely used as a routine procedure and also in mass programmes. A ring or band is applied over a knuckle of the tube by an applicator through a laparoscope under vision (Figs. 33.7 and 33.8). In many cases, this can be done in a short time. There is only one stitch over the wound and the patient can go home the same day or the next. The anaesthesia is usually local with supplementation of sedation. A comparison of the

**Table 33.1** Comparison of minilap and laparoscopic sterilisation

| Minilap | Laparoscopic sterilisation |
|---|---|
| Usual surgical equipment available in any operation theatre | Special costly equipment necessary |
| Training is easy | Experience and skill necessary |
| Can be completed even during power failure | Electricity is absolutely necessary throughout the procedure |
| Done under direct vision | Done through an endoscope |
| Risks are minimal | Risks, even though rare, may be serious |
| Time taken may be 6–10 minutes | A few minutes |
| Postoperative: more pain | Postoperative: less pain |
| Failure rate is minimal | Failure rate is higher |

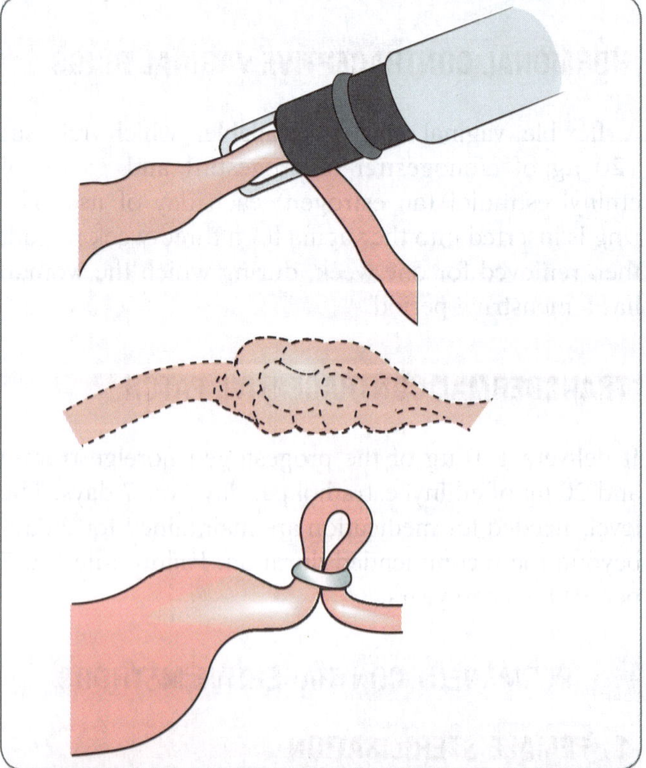

**Fig. 33.8** Laparoscopic sterilisation by silastic band (Falope ring). (a) The tube is picked up by operating laparoscope, so as to push the silastic band into the loop of the tube; (b) Silastic band is placed on the tube.

two methods (laparoscopic sterilisation and minilap) is given in Table 33.1. Other laparoscopic methods of tubal occlusion include bipolar electrocautery and clips. However, use of cautery for sterilisation is not approved by Govt. of India.

### C. Minilap Sterilisation

In interval cases and in patients undergoing MTP, **Pomeroy's technique of tubal ligation** can be employed. Even though the uterus is not palpable, as in the puerperal cases, the operation can be done easily with some training. A pre-op packing of the vagina or elevation of the uterus using a uterine elevator can help in pushing the uterus out of the pelvis and then the tubes could be easily identified. The only difference is that the small incision is made just above the pubic hair line. Precautions, like emptying the bladder, are important. As in puerperal sterilisation, this can be performed under intravenous anaesthesia, or general anaesthesia. A suprapubic incision is made over the skin which is extended downwards and the peritoneum is carefully opened avoiding injury to the bladder. Once the peritoneum is opened, by using a retractor, the tubes are identified under vision and picked up by a Babcock's forceps. The entire length of the tube is examined and the fimbria identified, which ensures that what is picked up is the Fallopian tube. The isthmial portion of the tube is caught and the tube cut. The cut ends of the tubes are ligated with a single round suture using 1-0 chromic catgut. Generally there is a tendency to crush the tubes before cutting which should be avoided. Hemostasis is confirmed and the same procedure is repeated on the opposite side also. After ensuring perfect hemostasis, the peritoneum, rectus sheath and the skin incision are closed in that order. If a vaginal pack is kept prior to surgery for elevating the uterus, it should be removed without fail.

### Failure Following Female Sterilisation

The failure rate varies from 0.1 to 0.5 per cent depending on the method. It is higher in Madlener's than in Pomeroy's method of sterilisation, more in vaginal than in abdominal methods, and more in laparoscopic sterilisation than in a minilaparotomy. The failure rate is slightly higher when associated with other procedures such as hysterotomy or cesarean section. In a large collaborative study of risk of pregnancy after tubal sterilisation involving over 10,000 women and follow-up of ten years, the failure rate varied from 3.6 per cent (after clip sterilisation) to 0.75 per cent (for puerperal and unipolar sterilisation). The failure rate (Table 33.2) also depends on the age of the patient (higher in the younger age group) and the method of sterilisation. Of the pregnancies, a third was in the tube and the others were intrauterine.

### Reversibility Following Sterilisation

This may be requested when a woman loses a child or when she remarries. The success following recanalisation has increased with microsurgical techniques to about 80–85 per cent provided that at the primary operation only a small bit of the tube was removed or clamped with a clip or ring. Isthmial anastomosis has the best results. In a 7 year study from Chennai involving over 400 microsurgical tubal recanalisations, the follow-up showed a 65 per cent pregnancy rate (ectopic rate of 8 per cent) and a live birth rate of 50 per cent.

## 2. MALE STERILISATION

Vasectomy is the procedure employed for sterilisation in men (Fig. 33.9). It is easier than tubal sterilisation and equally effective. Untoward complications are rare. Vasectomy is easier, less expensive and has a lower failure rate than female sterilisation.

### A. Non-scalpel Vasectomy

Non-scalpel vasectomy is a simple method of performing vasectomy; it is now being advocated by the Government of India to promote male sterilisation.

**Table 33.2** Contraceptive failure rate (Rounded-off figures)

| Method | Failure rate* |
|---|---|
| Female sterilisation | 0.4 |
| Vasectomy | 0.2 |
| **Implants** | |
| Norplant | 0.4 |
| Implanon | none reported |
| **Injectables** | |
| Progesterone only | 0.4 |
| Estrogen and progesterone | 0.2 |
| **Oral contraceptives** | |
| Mini-pill (progesterone only) | 3–10 |
| Combined (estrogen and progesterone) | 0.1 |
| Intrauterine contraceptive devices | 3.0 |
| Condoms | 12 |
| Vaginal spermicides | 21 |
| Other vaginal barrier methods | 18–28 |

*Pregnancies per 100 women years of exposure.

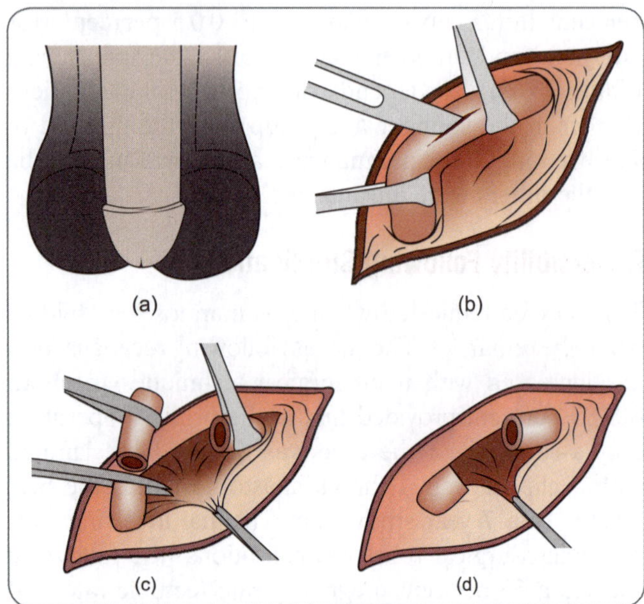


**Fig. 33.9** Steps of vasectomy: (a) Incisions on the skin; (b) The sheath of the vas is being cut open; (c) A portion of the vas is being removed; (d) The vas is ligated at the cut ends.

In this procedure, after local anaesthesia, instead of making an incision, the skin of the scrotum is pierced with a specially designed dissection forceps, at the level of the junction of the middle and upper thirds of the median raphe. The puncture is enlarged with dissecting forceps; the vas deferens is held in position and lifted out of the skin opening with a 'fixing clamp'. Each vas can be occluded through the same skin opening by ligation, heat or by using a clamp.

## 3. EMERGENCY CONTRACEPTION

Emergency contraception, or postcoital contraception, refers to methods of contraception that can be used to prevent pregnancy in the first few days after intercourse. It is intended for emergency use following unprotected intercourse, contraceptive failure (such as forgotten pills or torn condoms), rape or coerced sex. It is no substitute for contraception and should not be used for that purpose.

### Methods of Emergency Contraception

There are two methods of emergency contraception:
1. Emergency contraception pills (ECPs)
2. Copper-bearing intrauterine devices (IUDs).

#### Emergency contraceptive pills (ECPs)

Though many formulations are available, WHO recommends levonorgestrel for emergency contraceptive pill use. Ideally, this should be taken as a single dose of 1.5 mg within five days of unprotected coitus. Alternatively, two doses of 0.75 mg can be taken on the same day 12 hours apart.

##### *Mode of Action*

It acts by preventing or delaying ovulation. It can also act by making the cervical mucus hostile for transportation of sperms and also by affecting the ability of the sperm to bind with the egg.

#### Copper-bearing intrauterine devices (IUDs)

Ideally, a copper IUD can be inserted within five days of unprotected coitus. Fertilisation is prevented by causing a chemical change that damages sperm and egg before they can meet.

## CONTRACEPTION AND CANCER

Hormonal contraception is definitely protective against endometrial and ovarian carcinoma, the protection lasting for several years after discontinuing its use. With oral contraception there is conflicting evidence about predisposition to breast cancer. It showed a 15 per cent greater chance of breast malignancy in the younger age groups and in those with positive family history. Women currently using combined OC or who have used them in the past 10 years are at a slightly increased risk of having breast cancer diagnosed, though the cancers diagnosed tend to be localised to the breast. There is no evidence of an increase in the risk of having breast cancer diagnosed 10 or more years after cessation of use. The hormonal injectables like DMPA do not lead to breast cancer. Long-term use of oral contraceptive appears to slightly increase chances of cervical cancer. However, there are confounding factors like age, sexual behaviour and smoking. The condom is more protective against cervical cancer as it eliminates causative HPV (human papilloma virus) infections. There is no evidence on long-term follow-up of these men that vasectomy leads to prostatic cancer.

There are thus several methods of fertility control, and research is being carried out all over the world to discover safer and more effective methods of contraception. But there is no doubt that there is a need for adoption of contraception to prevent 'population explosion' and to promote family health. The choice of the contraceptive method depends on age, parity, the age of the last child, whether or not the child is breast-fed, religious and cultural beliefs, and socioeconomic conditions.

## RECAP

- Overpopulation is a global problem but mainly concerns the developing world.
- In India only 10 per cent of the population used contraception in 1960 compared to 45 per cent in 1990. The use of contraceptives rose to 59.8 percent by 2015.
- Methods of fertility control—fertility awareness methods (natural family planning methods), barrier methods of contraception, intrauterine contraceptive devices, permanent contraceptive methods, female sterilisation, male sterilisation, emergency contraception.
- Medical eligibility criteria are a set of guidelines published by WHO which helps in decision making as to the suitability of a particular method to the client.
- Lactational amenorrhea method (LAM): It is based on the fact the lactation protects against ovulation. For this method to be effective, three conditions have to be fulfilled.
- Barrier method of contraception: Female: The traditional methods of contraception used by men or women were designed to prevent the entry of live sperm into the cervical canal and include the diaphragm, cervical cap, female condom and spermicides.
- Male condom: The condom is an effective contraceptive method as well as a protector against STDs. It is the only barrier method that can be used by men. The male condom is the only one proven to be effective against HIV infection.
- Intrauterine Contraceptive Devices (IUCD): The copper-bearing intrauterine device (IUD) is a small, flexible plastic frame with copper sleeves or wire around it. It works primarily by causing a chemical change that damages the sperm and egg before they can meet.
- Hormone-releasing IUDs: The LNG-20 contains 52 mg levonorgestrel, which is released at the rate of 20 µg per day. Lifespan of LNG 20 is 5 years and it is being used successfully in dysfunctional uterine bleeding, simple hyperplasia, adenomyosis and fibroids.
- Three types of oral contraceptive pills are now used in contraception.
- Combination pills containing both estrogen and progestogen.
- The sequential regimen: estrogens 14–16 days and progestogen added in the last 5–6 days.
- Progestogens only: this is known as the 'mini pill' or progestogen-only pill (POP).
- Non-contraceptive benefits of oral contraceptives: Less risk of endometrial and ovarian cancer.
- Regular menstrual cycles.
- Probably less endometriosis, benign breast disease, rheumatoid arthritis and increased bone density.
- Pills that contain very low doses of a progestin do not contain estrogen, and so can be used throughout the period of breastfeeding and by women who cannot use preparations with estrogen. These pills work primarily by thickening cervical mucus, disrupting the menstrual cycle, and preventing ovulation.
- Injectible contraceptive: These are depot medroxyprogesterone acetate (DMPA) and norethindrone enanthate (NET-EN).
- Implants: Norplant containing six capsules or rods, Jadelle and Norplant-2 containing two rods, Implanon containing one rod.
- Female sterilisation: This includes postpartum sterilisation, caesarean ligation, interval ligation, postabortal ligation, gynecological ligation, laparoscopic sterilisation and minilap sterilisation.
- The failure rate varies from 0.1 to 0.5 per cent depending on the method.
- Vasectomy is the procedure employed for sterilisation in men.
- Emergency contraception, or postcoital contraception, refers to methods of contraception that can be used to prevent pregnancy in the first few days after intercourse and includes emergency contraception pills (ECPs) and copper-bearing intrauterine devices (IUDs).

## REVIEW QUESTIONS

### I. Long-Answer Question

Discuss the various barrier methods of contraception for female

### II. Short-Answer Questions

1. Types of intrauterine contraceptive devices
2. Male condom

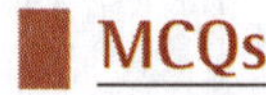

### MCQs

**1. Rhythm or calendar method is not suitable for**
   a) Women with regular cycles
   b) Partners who both understand the method
   c) Women with irregular cycles
   d) None of the above

**2. Which of these is not a medicated IUD?**
   a) Saf-T-coil
   b) Copper 7
   c) Nova T
   d) LNG 20

**3. Implanon consists of**
   a) 6 rods
   b) 2 rods
   c) 8 rods
   d) Single rod

**Further Reading**

Collaborative group on hormonal factors in breast cancer. Breast cancer and hormonal contraception. Lancet. 1996;347:1713–27.
Grimes DA, Economy KE. Primary prevention of gynaecological cancer. Am J Obstet Gynecol. 1995;172:227–35.
Family Planning: A Global Handbook for Providers; WHO, 2007.
Gopalan S, Rathnakumar S, Jain V. editors. Mudaliar and Menon's clinical obstetrics. 12th ed. Chennai: Orient Blackswan; 2014.
Mascarenhas L. Long acting methods of contraception. B M J. 1994;308:90–2.
Peterson HB et al. The risk of pregnancy after tubal sterilisations. Am J Obstet Gynecol. 1996;174:1161–70.
World Health Forum. Contraception and Cancer. 1994;15:1–8.
WHO. Intra-uterine devices. Tech Report Series 753, Geneva, 1987.
WHO. Challenges in reproductive health research. Biennial Report 1992–1993. Geneva, 1994;35–9.

# Appendix

## 1. SALIENT FEATURES OF NATIONAL GUIDELINES FOR ASSISTED REPRODUCTIVE CENTRES

The national guidelines for assisted reproductive centres have been drafted by the Ministry of Health & Family Welfare of the Govt. of India, New Delhi, and the Indian Council of Medical Research, New Delhi.

It is estimated that 15 percent of couples around the world are infertile. The magnitude of the infertility problem also has enormous social implications. Besides the fact that every couple has the right to have a child, in India infertility widely carries with it a social stigma. The various technologies used in ART not only require expertise but also open up many avenues for unethical practices which can adversely affect the recipient of the treatment, medically, socially and legally. The ART bill details procedures for accreditation and supervision of infertility clinics (and related organisations such as semen banks) handling spermatozoa or oocytes outside of the body, or dealing with gamete donors and surrogacy, ensuring that the legitimate rights of all concerned are protected, with maximum benefit to the infertile couples/individuals within a recognised framework of ethics and good medical practice.

### Information and Counselling to be given to Patients

The following information must be given to couples seeking treatment, which will help the couple make an informed choice.

- The basis, limitations and possible outcome of the procedure and its effectiveness including the success rates
- The possible side-effects (e.g., of the drug used) and the risks of treatment to the women and the resulting child, including (where relevant) the risks associated with multiple pregnancy
- The advantages and disadvantages of continuing treatment after a certain number of attempts.
- Pamphlets (one-page on each technique in all local languages and English) which give clear, precise and honest information about the procedure recommended to be used.

### Institutional Ethics Committee

Each ART clinic of level 1B (units engaging in IUI), level 2 (secondary level units) and level 3 (tertiary level units) must have its own ethics committee constituted according to ICMR guidelines, comprising reputed ART practitioners, scientists who are knowledgeable in developmental biology or in clinical embryology, a social scientist, a member of the judiciary and a person who is well-versed in comparative theology. Should the local ART clinic have difficulty in establishing such a body, the state accreditation authority should constitute such a body, co-opting a representative of the ART clinic.

A detailed account of the Code of Practice, Ethical Considerations and Legal Issues is available in the original draft.

The various techniques and the drugs used in ART are discussed in detail in Chapter 13 (Infertility).

In the process of curing infertility in the patient, there is a high iatrogenic risk of transmitting an abnormal paternal geno-(pheno-)type to the ART-born child. Establishing an appropriate database for human infertility would allow the quantification of such risks.

**The National Advisory Committee** under the leadership of the Chairman who is the Secretary, Ministry of Health and Family Welfare, comprises the Director General, Indian Council of Medical Research and several other representatives from various departments and facets of related fields to ensure the proper planning and implementation of the guidelines.

The complete draft is too elaborate to be included in this book. (The complete drfaft can be accessed from: https://www.icmr.nic.in/guidelines?field_select_disease_tid=90)

◆

## 2. EXAMINATION OF A RAPE VICTIM

The gynecologist is often called to examine a rape victim. This is more frequent in small hospitals where there may not be any forensic specialist to examine them. Hence it is imperative that a knowledge of how to examine a rape victim is essential for all doctors.

- **Pre-requisites for the examination of victim** The examination of an alleged rape victim should be done on the request of an authorised person. However if the victim reports directly, she should be examined after obtaining necessary consent and police intimation should be given. An authorised person should match the identity of the victim with the person mentioned in the request. This is in addition to the two identification marks mentioned and verified by the examining doctor.

- **Written witnessed consent** This should be obtained if the victim is 12 years of age, or above 12 years of age. If the victim is below 12 years of age, is mentally unsound, or is intoxicated, consent should be obtained from her parents or legal guardians. Further, the consent must be **'informed consent'** informing her that any evidence obtained may be used in the court and may go for, or against her. **The court or the police have no power to compel a woman.**
- **Presence of an adult female attendant/ nurse** Though the victims are preferably examined by a lady doctor, it may not be possible at all times in peripheral facilities. Where no female doctor is available, the victim can be examined by any registered medical practitioner preferably working in a government facility. The victim can demand the presence of a female attendant and also a female nurse during the entire examination and should be arranged. If the examination is being conducted by a medical board, at least one member of the board should be a female doctor.
- **Vaginal examination** This is not mandatory for establishing sexual violence. Similarly no mention on the size and elasticity of vaginal introitus, elasticity of hymen or about the woman's past sexual habits should be made unless it has any bearing on the present case of sexual violence.
- **Carrying out examination without delay** The examination should be done as early as possible since minor degree of injuries may rapidly fade and the swelling and tenderness of vulva may disappear within a few hours. Chances of detecting sperm from female genital tract also diminish with the passage of time.

## Duties of a Doctor towards an Alleged Victim of Rape

A female of any age, claiming to be a victim of rape, should always be treated as a possible rape victim and must be treated as a **priority patient,** with dignity and respect by the hospital staff and doctors.

**Guardians can request medical treatment** on behalf of a rape victim, if she is below 18 years of age, is mentally retarded or unconscious, or under the influence of alcohol.

The doctor should prepare a **detailed report** mentioning the reasons for each conclusion arrived at, and the description of material collected as sample for DNA profiling.

Even if the rape occurred **outside the jurisdiction of the hospital**, the victim must be examined and treated first, before referring her to the hospital in the appropriate area.

**Forensic evidence** should be collected as soon as possible during the process of examination. However, serious injuries of the victim must be treated first before collecting forensic evidences.

A brief description of the general and specific examination to be conducted is outlined here. Detailed description can be obtained from forensic textbooks.

### General Examination

It should include the patient's height, weight and general build and a routine examination of all the systems. Examination of teeth and secondary sex characters is of particular importance in the assessment of the age of the victim. Where the age is uncertain, radiological examination can help in determining the age. This is more important when the victim is a minor.

The other areas to be examined are:

1. Skin
2. Fingernails
3. Injuries—abrasions, bruises, laceration and incised wounds, bite marks
4. Eyes

### Specific Examination

Examination of the genital area should be carried out under good light with the patient in a lithotomy position so as to allow full exposure of the genital area. At the outset, it needs be remembered that there is a great variation in the appearance of the external female genitalia, with age, sexual maturation, body size/ shape, and other attending factors depending upon the circumstances of each case. The following need to be systematically examined:

1. Pubic hair
2. Thighs, vulva and perineum
3. Injuries
4. Hymen—recent rupture is of maximum corroborative value. Note the site and degree of tears. Signs of recent rupture of hymen are ragged

tears with lack of epithelial healing, but with edema and haemorrhage.

5. Semen—in the vagina (in fornices) or vulva, or garments worn. The presence of semen may be confirmed by vaginal smear.
6. Evidence of struggle

### Opinion

Occurrence of rape or sexual violence is a legal issue. Hence the examining doctor, based on medical examination, should not comment whether rape has been committed or not. Only findings in accordance with medical examination findings should be recorded.

——◆——

## 3. NATIONAL CANCER REGISTRY

Cancer registration is a mechanism to collect and collate all the information about cancer patients so that there is a data as to the number of cases, type of disease and also the prevalence of any particular type of cancer in a selected population. There are two types of cancer registry, viz. **Population-Based Cancer Registry** and **Hospital-Based Cancer Registry.** The former deals with cancer cases in a geographical area whereas the latter deals with individual hospital-based data.

A major activity of the cancer registries is to calculate the incidence of cancer. **Incidence rate** is defined as the number of new cases of disease, which occur in a defined population of disease-free individuals, over a specified period of time. The incidence rate of cancer is generally expressed for 100,000 population over a period of time. Usually the cancer registries calculate incidence rates for every 5 years.

Though cancer registries were in existence in India from as early as 1964, it was in 1982 that ICMR initiated the **National Cancer Registry programme (NCRP).** To begin with, there were three population-based cancer registries at Mumbai, Bengaluru and Chennai. ICMR also started with three hospital-based registries at Chandigarh, Dibrugarh and Thiruvanathapuram. Subsequently more such population and hospital-based registries were included and this helped in planning the National Cancer Control Programme.

Cancer registries provide high-quality reliable data. This is useful in estimating the load of the disease and also to plan expansion of screening, diagnosis and treatment of cancer in the country. These registries also provide information on age and stage-specific survival and mortality rates, which helps in further planning of the various strategies.

——◆——

## 4. COUNSELLING IN MALIGNANCY

In spite of much publicity in lay and technical press about the improvement in the management of malignancy and also improved life expectancy, there is a general feeling amongst most of the patients, that it is the end of the road. This leads to depression and very often to the extent of rejecting further treatment. Hence there is a need to counsel these patients, preferably by a trained counselor.

The counseling should begin with the type and nature of the malignancy and the extent of its involvement (staging). This should be followed by a discussion on life expectancy (5 year survival period) ensuring that no false hope is given to the patient. The counselling should include:

i. Types of therapy available for the particular malignancy the patient is suffering from
ii. Why this particular type of therapy is chosen for the patient
iii. Side effects to be expected after the first therapy and subsequently
iv. Success rate of various forms of therapy including the one the patient would be getting
v. Information about pain and palliative care and the facilities available in the area, for patients with very late-stage malignancies.

In addition, all the doubts the patient may have should be answered clearly and in simple lay terms. The counsellor should realise that the patient is in extreme stress and should have a patient approach towards the affected person.

——◆——

## 5. SYNDROMIC APPROACH IN THE MANAGEMENT OF STI/RTI

In many low-resource settings or in some areas even in the same country, diagnostic facilities may not be available or may be inadequate to arrive at an etiological diagnosis. In addition, even in places where diagnostic facilities are available, the sensitivity and specificity of available tests may vary giving inconsistent results. The other problem is the availability of trained human

## STI/RTI SYNDROMI

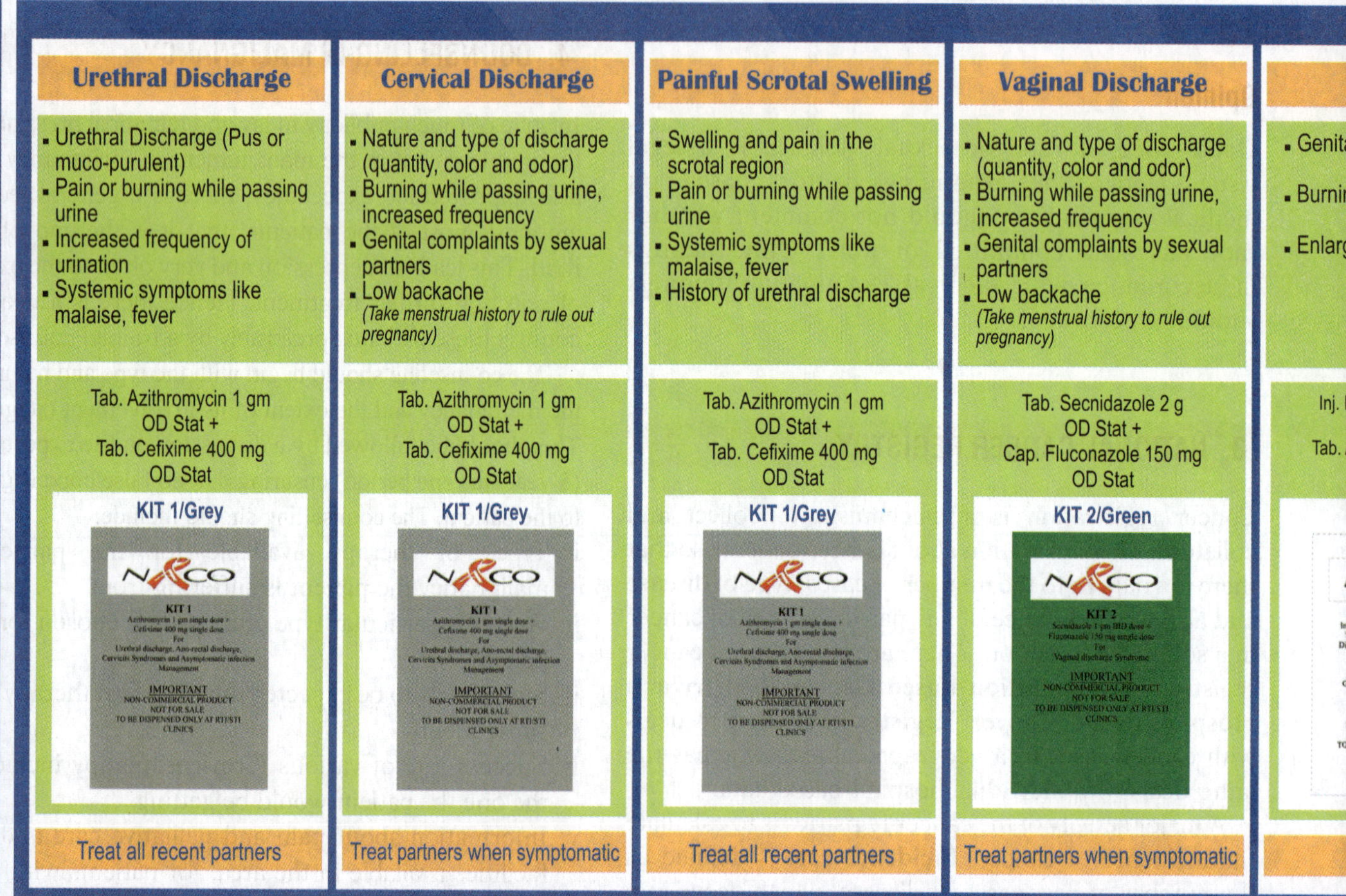


### IMPORTANT CONSIDERATIONS FOR MANAGEMENT OF ALL STI/RT

- Educate and counsel client and sexual partner/s regarding STI/RTI, safer se
- Treat partner/s
- Advise sexual abstinence or condom use during the course of treatment
- Provide condoms, educate about correct and consistent use
- Refer all patients to ICTC
- Follow up after 7 days for all STI, 3rd, 7th, and 14th day for LAP and 7th, 14th,
- If symptoms persist, assess whether it is due to re-infection and advise
- Consider immunization against Hepatitis B

**Fig. A1** A sample STI/RTI syndromic management poster

# ...ASE MANAGEMENT

| ...al Ulcer-Non Herpetic | Genital Ulcer - Herpetic | Lower Abdominal Pain (LAP) | Inguinal Bubo (IB) |
|---|---|---|---|
| ...le or multiple, painful or painless<br>...in the genital area<br>...odes | ▪ Genital ulcer or vesicles, single or multiple, painful, recurrent<br>▪ Burning sensation in the genital area | ▪ Lower Abdominal Pain<br>▪ Fever<br>▪ Vaginal Discharge<br>▪ Menstrual irregularities like heavy, irregular vaginal bleeding<br>▪ Dysmenorrhoea, dysparenunia, dysuria, tenesmus<br>▪ Lower backache<br>▪ Cervical motion tenderness | ▪ Swelling in inguinal region which may be painful<br>▪ Preceding history of genital ulcer or discharge<br>▪ Systemic symptoms like malaise, fever etc |
| ...nicillin ...al ...1 gm) -<br>**If allergic to Inj. Penicillin:** Doxycycline 100 MG (Bid for 15 days) Azithromycin 1GM (Single dose) | Tab. Acyclovir 400 mg<br>TDS for 7 days | Tab. Cefixime 400 mg OD stat +<br>Tab. Metronidazole 400 mg BD X 14 days +<br>Doxycycline 100 mg BD X 14 days | Tab. Azithromycin 1 gm OD Stat +<br>Tab. Doxycycline 100 mg BD for 21 days |
| **KIT 4/Blue**<br>KIT 4<br>Doxycycline 100 mg BID for 15 days + Azithromycin 1 gm single dose<br>For<br>GENITAL ULCER DISEASE - Non-HERPETIC SYNDROME<br>IMPORTANT<br>NON-COMMERCIAL PRODUCT<br>NOT FOR SALE<br>TO BE DISPENSED ONLY AT RTI/STI CLINICS | **KIT 5/Red**<br>KIT 5<br>ACYCLOVIR 400 MG ORALLY TID FOR 7 DAYS<br>For<br>GENITAL ULCER DISEASE - HERPETIC (GUD-HERPETIC) SYNDROME<br>IMPORTANT<br>NON-COMMERCIAL PRODUCT<br>NOT FOR SALE<br>TO BE DISPENSED ONLY AT RTI/STI CLINICS | **Kit 6/Yellow**<br>KIT 6<br>Cefixime 400 mg single dose +<br>Metronidazole 400 mg BID for 14 days +<br>Doxycycline 100 mg BID for 14 days<br>For<br>Lowr abdominal pain Syndrome<br>IMPORTANT<br>NON-COMMERCIAL PRODUCT<br>NOT FOR SALE<br>TO BE DISPENSED ONLY AT RTI/STI CLINICS | **Kit 7/Black**<br>KIT 6<br>Doxycycline 100 mg BID for 21 days + Azithromycin 1 gm single dose<br>For<br>Inguinal Bubo Syndrome<br>IMPORTANT<br>NON-COMMERCIAL PRODUCT<br>NOT FOR SALE<br>TO BE DISPENSED ONLY AT RTI/STI CLINICS |
| ...exual partners for past 3 months | No partner treatment | Treat male partners with Kit 1 | Treat all sexual partners for past 3 weeks |

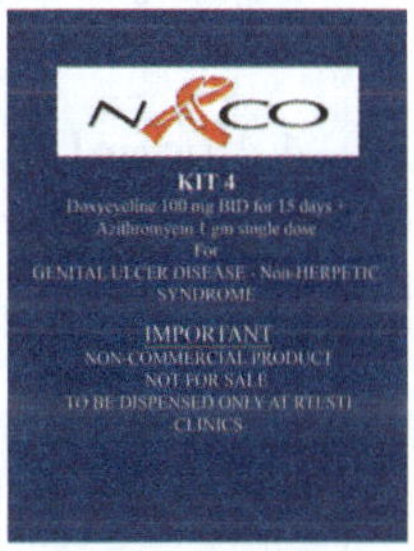

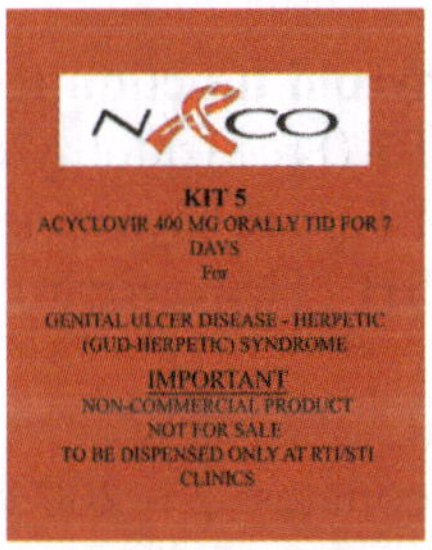

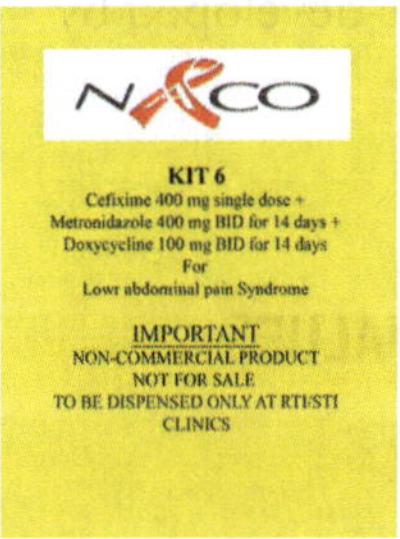

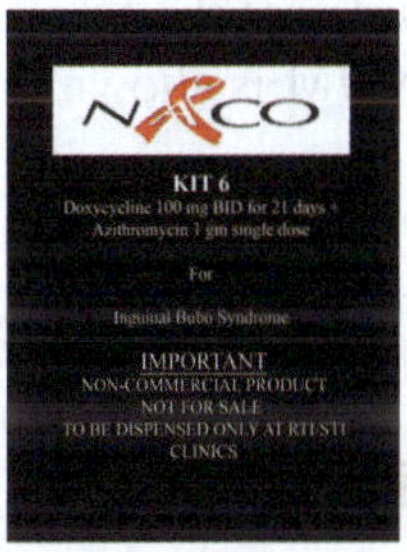

...ctices and importance of taking complete treatment

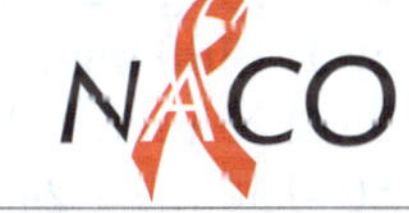

National AIDS Control Organisation

India's voice against AIDS

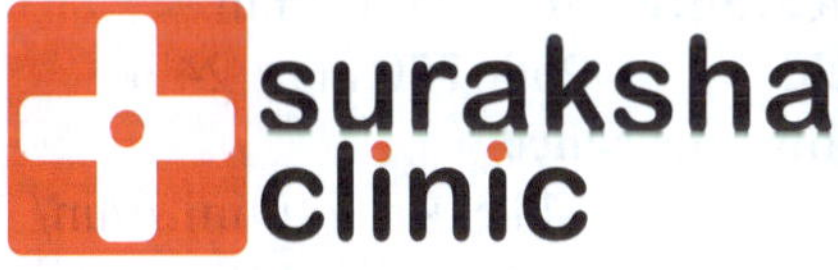


...d 21st day for IB

...mpt referral

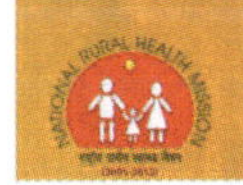

resources at all times and also periodical external quality control.

To overcome all these hurdles, a syndrome-based approach for the management of STI / RTI was developed and promoted in developing countries. Syndromic management is based on the identification of consistent groups of symptoms and easily recognised signs (syndromes), and the provision of treatment that will deal with the majority or most serious organisms responsible for producing a syndrome. WHO developed an algorithm for the benefit of health care providers. However, this is not an all-encompassing method, particularly in women with vaginal discharge, where the chances of cervical cancer are equally high.

Thus syndromic approach is a useful tool in low-resource settings with its own limitations. National Aids Control Organisation (NACO) has developed detailed National Guidelines on the management of STI/RTI. A sample syndromic management poster meant for display at the Suraksha Clinic developed by NACO and NHM is shown in Fig. A1.

## 6. NORMAL INDICES—REFERENCE VALUES

### 24 Hours Urine

| | |
|---|---|
| **Calcium** | 100–300 mg / 24 h |
| **Chloride** | 110–250 mEq / 24 h |
| **Creatinine** | 800–1800 mg / 24 h |
| **Magnesium** | 73–122 mg / 24 h |
| **Oxalate** | 20–53 mg / 24 h |
| **Phosphorus** | 400–1300 mg / 24 h |
| **Potassium** | 25–125 mEq / 24 h |
| **Protein** | 50–150 mg / 24 h |
| **Sodium** | 40–220 mEq / 24 h |
| **Urea** | 10–20 g / 24 h |
| **Urea clearance** | 40–70 mL /min. |
| **Uric acid** | 250–750 mg / 24 h |

**Creatinine clearance**

Male: 95–140 mL/min/ 1.73 m
Female: 70–110 mL/min/ 1.73 m

### Serum Electrolytes

**Sodium**

Neonates: 133–146 mEq/L
Children: 138–145 mEq/L
Adult: 136–145 mEq/L

**Potassium**

Neonates: 3.7–5.9 mEq/L
Children: 3.4–4.7 mEq/L
Adult: 3.5–5 mEq/L

**Chloride**

Neonates: 98–113 mEq/L
Children: 98–107 mEq/L
Adult: 98–107 mEq/L

**Bicarbonate**

Neonates: 20–27 mEq/L
Children: 20–27 mEq/L
Adult: 20–27 mEq/L

**FSH (follicle stimulating hormone)**

Men: 1.5–12.4 mIU/mL
Women:

| | |
|---|---|
| Follicular phase | 3.5–12.5 mIU/mL |
| Ovulation phase | 4.7–21.5 mIU/mL |
| Luteal phase | 1.7–7.7 mIU/mL |
| Postmenopause | 25.8–134.8 mIU/mL |

**TFT (thyroid function test)**

| | |
|---|---|
| FT3 (Free tridothyronine) | 2.0–4.4 pg/mL |
| FT4 (Free thyroxine) | 0.93–1.7 ng/dL |
| TSH (Thyrotropin) | 0.27–4.2 μIU/mL |

**Ferritin**

Neonates: 25–200 ng/mL
Children: 7–140 ng/mL
Male: 20–250 ng/mL
Female: 10–120 ng/mL

**Insulin** 2.6–24.9 μU/mL

**Immunoglobulin "E" (IgE)**

| | |
|---|---|
| Neonates: | Up to 1.5 IU/mL |
| Infants 1st year: | Up to 15 IU/mL |
| 1–5 years: | Up to 60 IU/mL |
| 6–9 years: | Up to 90 IU/mL |
| 10–15 years: | Up to 200 IU/mL |
| Adults: | Up to 100 IU/mL |

**LH (luteinising hormone)**

Men: 1.7–8.6 mIU/mL
Women:

| | |
|---|---|
| Follicular phase | 2.4–12.6 mIU/mL |
| Ovulation phase | 14.0–95.6 mIU/mL |
| Luteal phase | 1.0–11.4 mIU/mL |
| Postmenophase | 7.7–58.5 mIU/mL |

## Liver Function Test

**Bilirubin total**

Newborn 24 h: Less than 8.0 mg/dL
Newborn 48 h: Less than 13.0 mg/dL
Children: Up to 1.0 mg/dL
Adult: Up to 1.2 mg/dL

**Bilirubin direct**

Children: 0.2–0.8 mg/dL
Adult: 0.3–0.9 mg/dL

**SGOT**

Male: Up to 35 U/L
Female: Up to 31 U/L

**SGPT** 10–40 U/L

**Alkaline phosphatase**

| | |
|---|---|
| Neonates D1–D5: | Less than 250 U/L |
| Neonates D6 – 1 year: | Less than 462 U/L |
| Children: | 281–300 U/L |
| Adult male: | 40–130 U/L |
| Adult female: | 35–105 U/L |

**Total protein**

| | |
|---|---|
| Neonates: | 4.6–7.6 g/dL |
| Children: | 5.1–8.0 g/dL |
| Adult: | 6.6–8.7 g/dL |
| Albumin | |
| Neonates: | 2.8–4.4 g/dL |
| Children: | 3.8–5.4 g/dL |
| Adult: | 3.5–5.2 g/dL |

**Globulin** 1.8–3.3 g/dL

**Amylase**

Adult: 28–100 U/L

## Serology

| | |
|---|---|
| **CRP** | Up to 6 mg/L |
| **ASO** | Up to 20 0 IU/mL |
| **RA factor** | Up to 20 IU/mL |

## Infectious Elisa

**Anti-HAV IgM**

Less than cut-off: Negative
More than or equal to cut-off: Positive

**Anti-HEV IgM (ELISA)**

Negative: Less than 1.0
Equivocal: 1.0–1.2
Positive: Greater than 1.2

## Biochemistry Normal Ranges

**Blood sugar**

| | |
|---|---|
| Fasting | 60–100 mg/dL |
| Postprandial | 110–140 mg/dL |
| Random | 80–120 mg/dL |
| HBA1c | Up to 4.2–6.2% |

**Urea**

| | |
|---|---|
| Neonates: | 8.56–25.7 mg/dL |
| Children: | 10.7–38.5 mg/dL |
| Adult: | 16.6–25.7 mg/dL |

**Creatinine**

| | |
|---|---|
| Neonates: | 0.29–1.0 mg/dL |
| Children: | 0.17–0.79 mg/dL |
| Adult Male: | 0.70–1.2 mg/dL |
| Adult Female: | 0.50–0.9 mg/dL |

**Uric acid**

| | |
|---|---|
| Children: | 2.0–5.0 mg/dL |
| Adult Male: | 3.4–7.0 mg/dL |
| Adult Female: | 2.6–6.0 mg/dL |

**Calcium**

| | |
|---|---|
| Neonates: | 7.6–11.0 mg/dL |
| Children: | 8.8–10.8 mg/dL |
| Adults: | 8.6–10.2 mg/dL |

**Phosphorus**

| | |
|---|---|
| Children: | 4.0–7.0 mg/dL |
| Adults: | 2.7–4.5 mg/dL |

| | |
|---|---|
| **G6PD** | 6.4–18.7 $\mu$/g |
| **Serum osmolality** | 275–295 mOsm/kg |
| **Lactate** | 4.5–20 mg/dL |

**Prolactin**

Men: 4.04–15.2 ng/mL
Women (non-pregnant): 4.79–23.3 ng/mL

**Progesterone**

Men: 0.2–1.4 ng/mL
Women:
Follicular phase 0.2–1.5 ng/mL
Ovulation phase 0.8–3.0 ng/mL

Luteal phase 1.7–27 ng/mL
Postmenopause 0.1–0.8 ng/mL

**Total PSA (prostate-specific antigen)**
Up to 4.4 ng/mL

**PTH (parathyroid hormone) INTACT**
15–65 pg/mL

**Vitamin D total**
Severe deficiency: Less than10 ng/mL
Insufficiency: 10–30 ng/mL
No deficiency: More than 30 ng/mL

**Alpha-fetoprotein (AFP)** ≤ 7.0 ng/mL
**Microalbumin** Up to 25 mg/L
**Complement C3** 0.9–1.8 g/L
**Complement C4** 0.1–0.4 g/L

## Haematology Normal Ranges

**Haemoglobin**
Male: 14–18 g/dL
Female: 12–16 g/dL

**Haematocrit (HCT)/PCV**
Male: 40–54%
Female: 37–47%

**Red blood cell (RBC) count**
Male: 4.6–6.2 million/mm³
Female: 4.2–6.2 million/mm³
Mean Corpuscular Volume (MCV): 76–96 fL
Mean Corpuscular Haemoglobin (MCH): 27–31 pg
Mean Corpuscular Haemoglobin Concentration (MCHC): 32–36 g%

**Total white blood cell (WBC) count**
4000–11000 cells/mm³

**Differential Count**
**Polymorphs** 40–65%
**Eosinophils** 1–3%
**Basophils** 0–1%
**Monocytes** 3–7%
**Lymphocytes** 20–40%
**Absolute neutrophil count** 3000–5800 cells/mm³
**Absolute lymphocyte count** 1500–3000 cells/mm³
**Absolute eosinophil count** 40–440 cells/mm³

**Reticulocyte count**
Adult: 0.2–2.0%
Children: 2.0–6.0%

**Platelets** 1.5–4.0 lakhs/mm³

**ESR**
Male:
Newborn: 0–2 mm
1 month–17 years: 0–10 mm
17–70 years: 0–15 mm
More than 70 years: 0–30 mm

Female:
Newborn: 0–2 mm
1 month–17 years: 0–12 mm

**Immunoglobin M (IgM)**
1–4 months: 0.17–1.05 g/L
5–9 months: 0.33–1.26 g/L
10 months–1 year: 0.41–1.73 g/L
2–8 years: 0.43–2.07 g/L
9–10 years: 0.52–2.42 g/L
Adult: 0.56–3.52 g/L

**Immunoglobin A (IgA)**
1–3 months: 0.013–1.53 g/L
46 months: 0.044–0.84 g/L
7 months – 1 year: 0.11–1.06 g/L
2–5 years: 0.14–1.59 g/L
6–10 years: 0.33–2.36 g/L
Adult: 0.7–3.12 g/L

**Immunoglobin G (IgG)**
1 month: 2.51–9.06 g/L
2–4 months: 1.76–6.01 g/L
5–12 months: 1.72–10.69 g/L
1–5 years: 3.45–12.36 g/L
6–10 years: 6.08–15.72 g/L
Adult: 6.39–13.49g/L

**Ammonia** 10–47 umol/L

**CK**
Male: Less than 190 u/L
Female: Less than 170 u/L

**CK-MB** Up to 25 u/L

**LDH**
Neonates: 225–600 u/L

Children: 12–300 u/L
Adult male: 136–225 u/L
Adult female: 135–214 u/L

**Gamma GT** Up to 65 u/L

**TROP–I** 0.010–0.023 ng/mL

**NT Pro BNP** 70–300 ng/L

**Magnesium**
Neonates: 1.5–2.2 mg/dL
Children: 1.7–2.1 mg/dL
Adult: 1.6–2.4 mg/dL

**Iron**
Adult: 33–193 ug/dL

**TIBC**
Adult: 250–450 ug/dL

## Hormones and Tumour Markers

**β-hCG (Intact human chorionic gonadotropin)**
Men: Less than 2 mIU/mL
Female: Less than 1 mIU/mL
Non-pregnant Negative
Pregnant
3rd week: 5.8–71.2 mIU/mL
4th week: 9.5–750 mIU/mL
5th week: 217–7138 mIU/mL
6th week: 158–31795 mIU/mL
7th week: 3697–163563 mIU/mL
8th week: 32065–149571 mIU/mL
9th week: 63803–151410 mIU/mL
10th week: 46509–186977 mIU/mL

**CEA (carcinoembryonic antigen)**
Non-smokers: Up to 5 ng/mL
Smokers: Up to 6.5 ng/mL

**CA 125 (cancer antigen 125)** 35 U/mL

**Cortisol**
Morning (7–10 AM): 6.2–19.4 mg/dL
Afternoon (4–8 PM): 2.3–11.9 mg/dL

**Estradiol (E2)**
Men: 7.63–42.6 pg/mL
Women:
Follicular phase: 1.5–166 pg/mL
Ovulation phase: 85.8–498 pg/mL
Luteal phase: 43.8–211 pg/mL
Postmenopause: Less than 5–54.7 pg/mL

## Lipid Profile

**Total cholesterol** Less than 200 mg/dL

**Triglycerides** Less than 200 mg/dL

**HDL cholesterol**
Male: More than 35 mg/dL
Female: More than 45 mg/dL

**LDL cholesterol**
Optimal: Less than 100 mg/dL
Border line high: 139–159 mg/dL
High: 160–180 mg/dL
Very high: More than 190 mg/dL

**VLDL cholesterol** Less than 35 mg/dL

## 7. INSTRUMENTS USED IN GYNECOLOGICAL EXAMINATION

### 1. Sim's Speculum

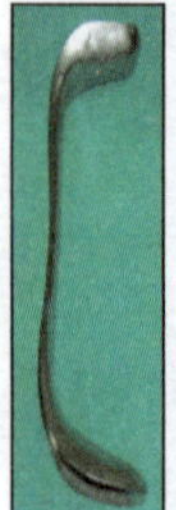
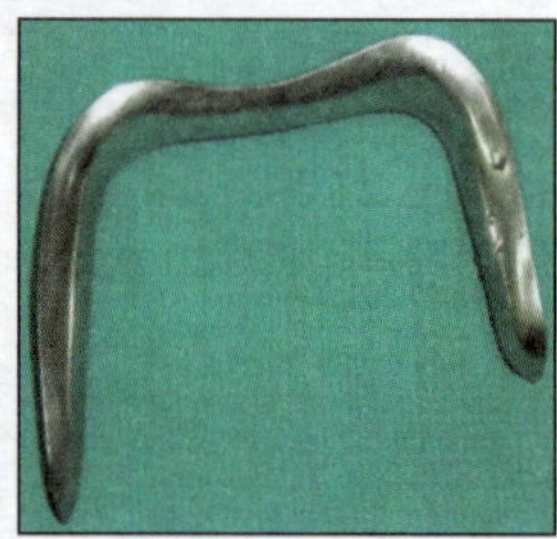

- This is the most commonly used speculum in obstetrics and gynecology.
- It is also known as duck-bill speculum.
- It is used for evacuation of the uterus in missed abortion or inevitable abortion and also in medical termination of pregnancy.
- It is used in dilatation and curettage.

### 2. Cusco's Speculum

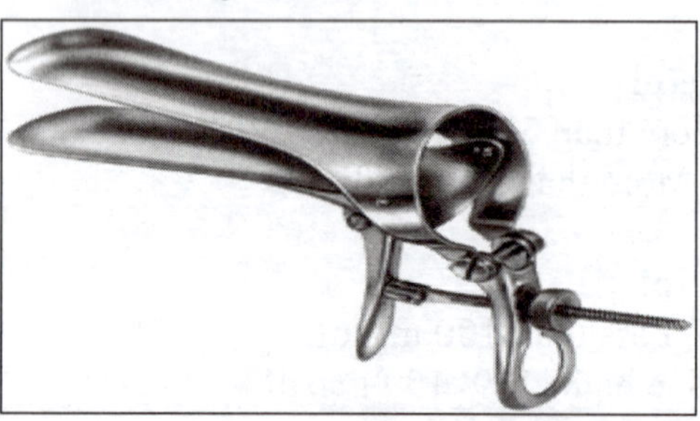

- This is a self-retaining speculum and hence there is no need for an assistant to hold the speculum.
- It can be used in the evacuation of products of conception as in abortion.
- Where a Pap smear is being done routinely, this speculum is useful.

### 3. Hegar's Dilator

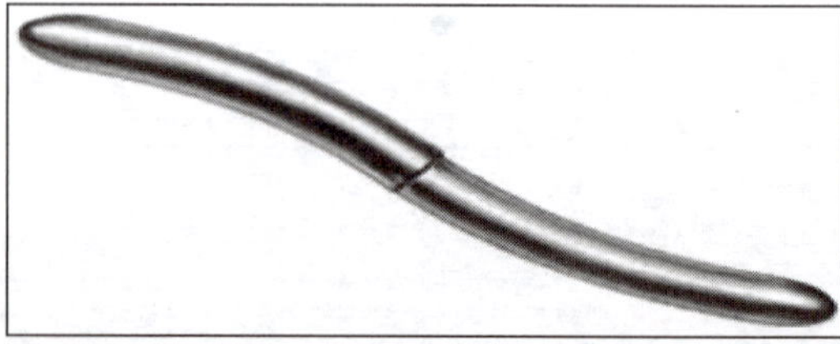

- This dilator is used more commonly in obstetric practice since it is less traumatic.
- It has a round body with tapering ends.
- Both ends are of different size.
- In between pregnancy it can be used as a method to diagnose incompetent cevical os.

### 4. Dilator (Mathew Duncan)

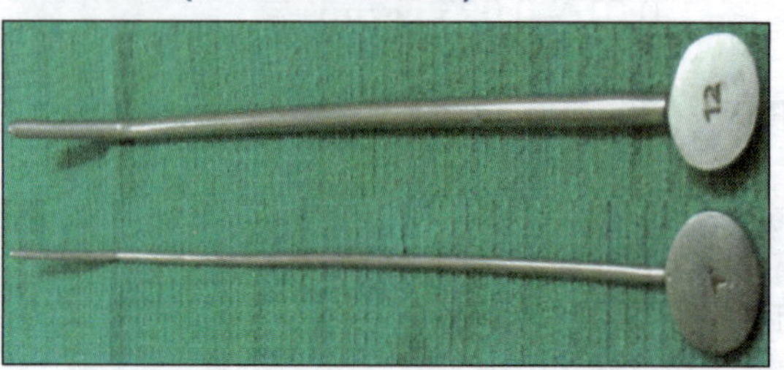

- This dilator is used more commonly in gynecological procedures.
- Each dilator is long and unlike the Hegar's dilator, is only of one size.

### 5. Alli's Tissue Forceps

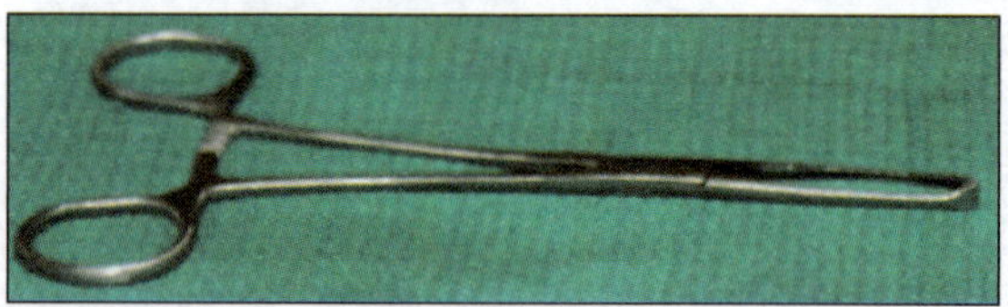

- This instrument is available in two sizes.
- The end of the blade is with 3–4 teeth-like projections.
- A lock is also provided in the handle.
- It is used for holding the rectus sheath both during cutting and also during its suturing.
- Since the teeth could be traumatic, it should be used with caution in obstetric practice.

### 6. Babcock's Forceps

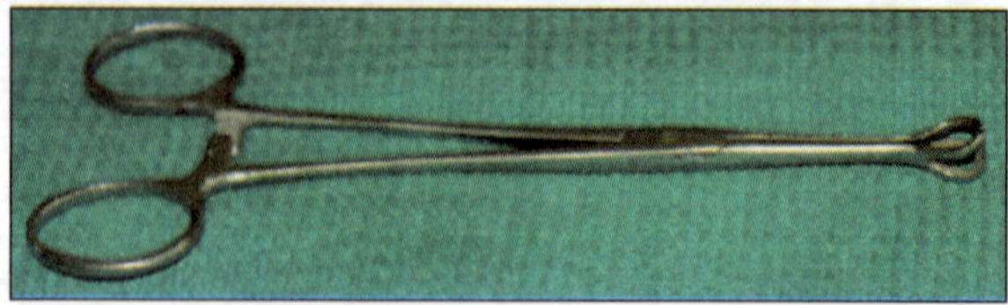

- It is used extensively in female sterilisation to hold the Fallopian tube.
- It can also be used for holding the vas in vasectomy.
- It can be used to hold the appendix.
- It is useful in holding any tissue with minimal trauma.

## 7. Volsellum Forceps

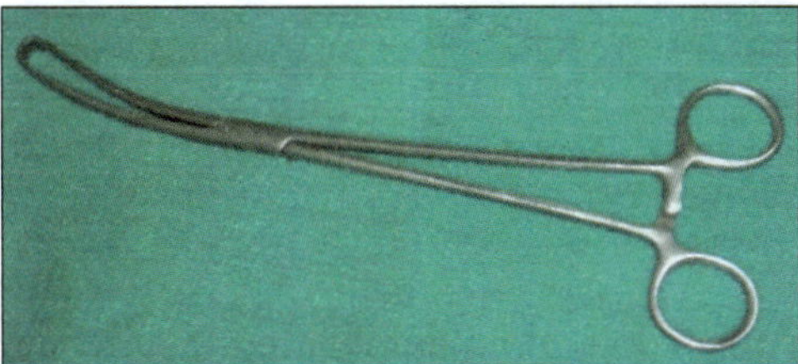

- This is a long instrument with minimal curvature of the blades.
- The tip of the blade has 3 teeth-like projections which fit into the hollow in between two teeth-like projections on the other blade.
- This gives a good grip on the structure held by this forceps.
- It is used for holding the lip of the cervix as in dilatation and curettage.
- Used in dilatation and curettage.

## 8. Uterine Sound

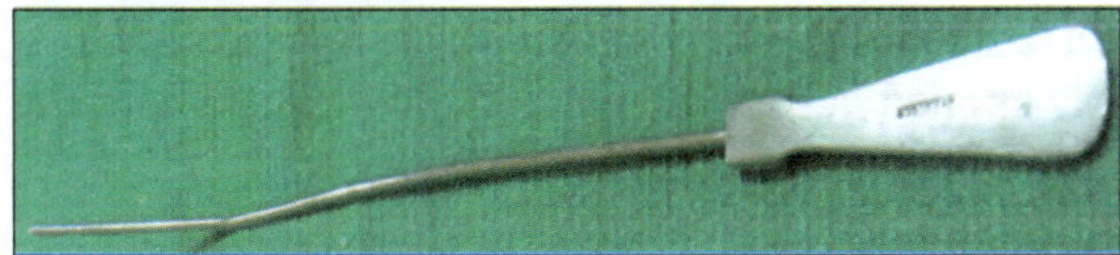

- This instrument is used for measuring the utero cervical length.
- It has a handle with a long portion which is graduated in inches or centimetres to measure the length of the cervix.
- It not only measures the uterine length but also the direction of the uterus, viz., anteversion or retroversion.

## 9. Curette

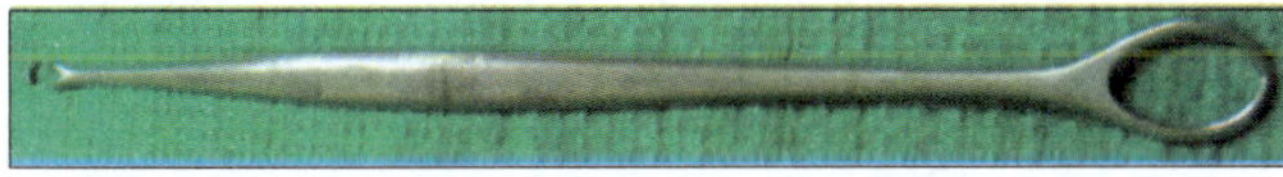

- This instrument has a central shaft with a loop at each end.
- The loop could be either blunt or sharp.
- It is useful in checking curettage following evacuation of uterus or after evacuation of vesicular mole.
- It is used to remove any retained placental bits in postpartum hemorrhage.
- It is used to check and to confirm the completeness of the procedure of termination of pregnancy.
- It is used in dilatation and curettage.

## 10. Curved and Straight Clamp

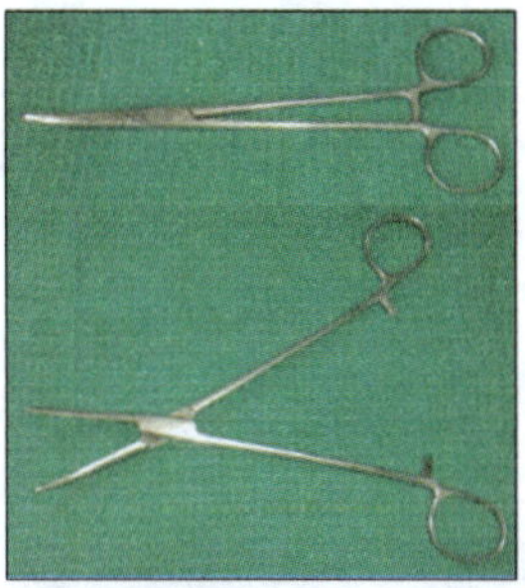

- These are used for clamping tissues and ligaments during abdominal or vaginal hysterectomy.
- They also act as hemostatic clamps.
- Curved clamp is used more often than straight clamp.

## 11. Kocher's Clamp

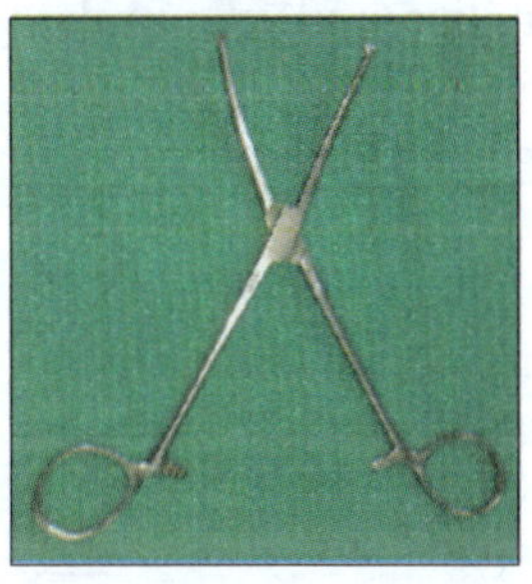

- This is a straight heavy hemostatic clamp with interlocking teeth at its tip.
- This is also used during abdominal or vaginal hysterectomy.

## 12. Cervical Punch Biopsy Forceps

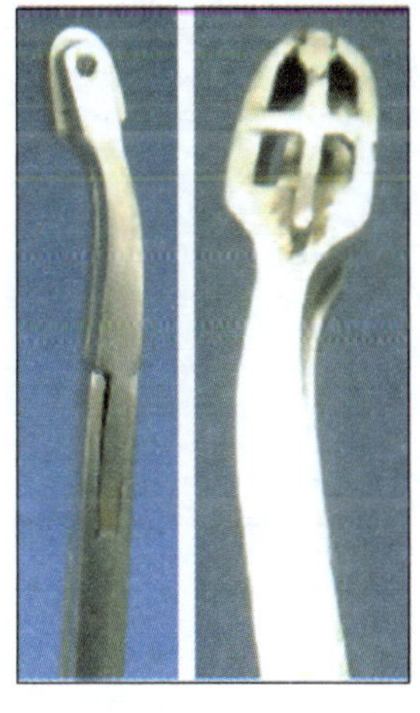

- Cervical punch biopsy forceps is used for taking biopsy from suspected areas in the cervix.

- The instrument has a somewhat sharp upper blade and a concave lower blade.
- Once the area to be biopsied is identified, the sharp end is placed over the area from which biopsy is to be taken and it is locked.
- By twisting the forceps the tissue is obtained.

## 13. Laparoscopic Instruments

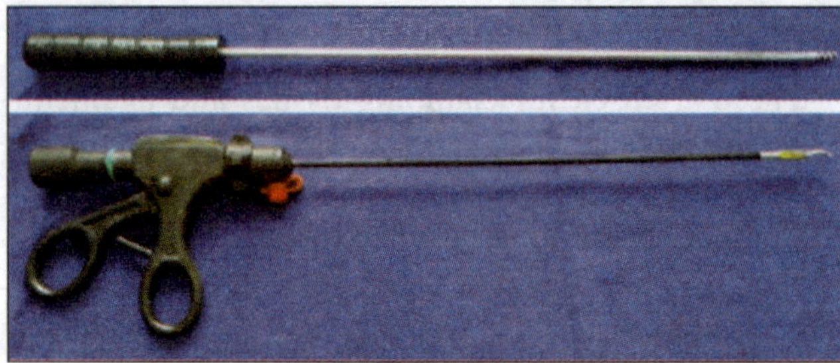

- Myoma screw is used to stabilise and manipulate myoma during laparocsopic procedure.
- Scissors are used for cutting during laparoscopic procedures.
- The scissors usually come with either monopolar or bipolar attachment to facilitate connecting it to a cautery source to minimise bleeding.

## 14. Myoma Screw

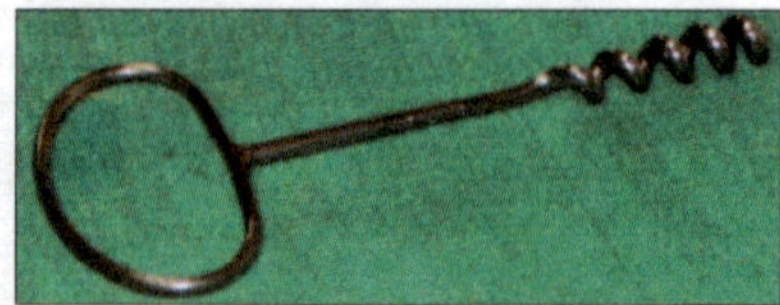

- This is used for fixing and manipulating the myoma during myomectomy and also during hysterectomy.
- There is a tendency to use it to hold the uterus even when there is no myoma.
- This should be avoided since it can cause bleeding.

## 15. Bonney's Myomectomy Clamp

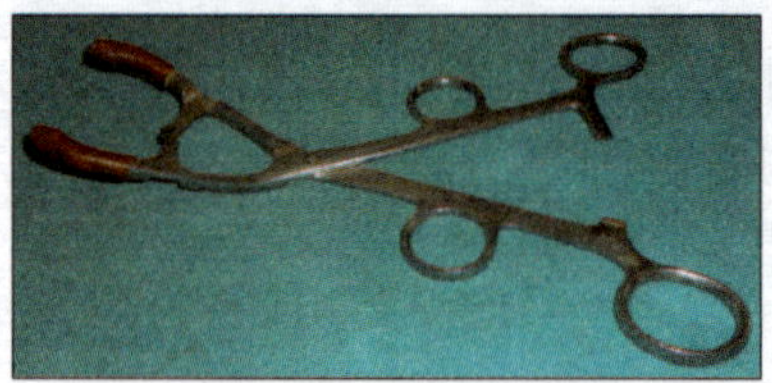

- This is applied during myomectomy to reduce blood loss.
- It is applied across the base of the uterus where the body of the uterus and the cervix meet.
- It helps to occlude the uterine arteries.

# Key to MCQs

*Chapter* 3: **Anatomy of the Female Reproductive System**
1. (b) 2. (a) 3. (b) 4. (a)

*Chapter* 4: **Physiology of Menstruation and Ovulation**
1. (b) 2. (c) 3. (d) 4. (a)

*Chapter* 5: **Congenital Anomalies of the Genital Tract**
1. (b) 2. (c) 3. (c) 4. (a)

*Chapter* 6: **Adolescent Gynecological Problems**
1. (b) 2. (b) 3. (a)

*Chapter* 7: **Abnormal Uterine Bleeding**
1. (a) 2. (b) 3. (a) 4. (a)

*Chapter* 8: **Benign Diseases of the Vulva and Vagina**
1. (c) 2. (b) 3. (a) 4. (a)

*Chapter* 9: **Benign and Premalignant Lesions of the Cervix**
1. (c) 2. (a) 3. (b) 4. (d)

*Chapter* 10: **Benign Diseases of Uterus**
1. (a) 2. (c) 3. (d) 4. (a)

*Chapter* 11: **Benign Tumors of the Ovary and Fallopian Tube**
1. (b) 2. (a) 3. (d) 4. (b)

*Chapter* 12: **Pelvic Inflammatory Disease**
1. (c) 2. (d) 3. (b)

*Chapter* 13: **Infertility**
1. (b) 2. (a) 3. (d) 4. (b)

*Chapter* 14: **Polycystic Ovarian Syndrome**
1. (a) 2. (c) 3. (d) 4. (d)

*Chapter* 15: **Endometriosis**
1. (d) 2. (a) 3. (c) and (d) 4. (b)

*Chapter* 16: **Amenorrhea**
1. (d) 2. (a) 3. (b) 4. (d)

*Chapter* 17: **Menopause**
1. (a) 2. (d) 3. (c) 4. (c)

*Chapter* 18: **Hormones in Gynecology**
1. (d) 2. (a) 3. (b) 4. (c)

*Chapter* 19: **Malignant Diseases of the Vulva, Vagina and Fallopian Tube**
1. (a) 2. (b) 3. (d) 4. (c)

*Chapter* 20: **Malignant Lesions of the Cervix**
1. (c) 2. (b) 3. (a) 4. (d)

*Chapter* 21: **Malignant Neoplasm of the Uterus**
1. (a) 2. (d) 3. (b) 4. (d)

*Chapter* 22: **Malignant Ovarian Tumours**
1. (d) 2. (a) 3. (b)

*Chapter* 23: **Gestational Trophoblastic Disease**
1. (c) 2. (d) 3. (a) 4. (d)

*Chapter* 24: **Chemotherapy in Gynecology**
1. (c) 2. (d)

*Chapter* 25: **Radiotherapy in Gynecological Cancer**
1. (a) 2. (c) 3. (d) 4. (b)

*Chapter* 26: **Uterovaginal Prolapse**
1. (d) 2. (b) 3. (c) 4. (d)

*Chapter* 27: **Disorders of the Urinary System**
1. (b) 2. (a) 3. (b) 4. (c)

*Chapter* 28: **Genitourinary Fistula**
1. (d) 2. (d) 3. (c) 4. (a)

*Chapter* 29: **Radiological Investigations in Gynecology**
1. (d) 2. (a) 3. (b) 4. (a)

*Chapter* 30: **Endoscopy in Gynecology**
1. (b) 2. (c) 3. (a) 4. (c)

*Chapter* 31: **Operative Gynecology**
1. (c) 2. (a) 3. (d) 4. (b)

*Chapter* 33: **Contraception**
1. (c) 2. (a) 3. (d)

# Index


**A**

Abarelix 202
Abdominal tenderness 134
Ablations 109
  endometrial 73
Abnormal uterine bleeding (AUB) 64, 113
Abnormal vaginal bleeding 133
Abscess 133
  pelvic 132, 137
Acanthosis nigricans 141, 159
Acne 141, 142
Actinomycosis 132
Activin 41
Add-back therapy 202
Adenocarcinoma
  clear cell 220
  endometrioid 235
Adenomyoma 108
Adenomyosis 8, 108, 114
  diffuse 108
  focal 108
  resection of 109
Adhesion score 362
Adnexal mass 133
Adrenal hyperplasia 158, 183
  congenital 183
Adrenarche 54, 159
  premature 56
Adult-Onset Congenital Adrenal Hyperplasia (AOCAH) 187
Aerosols 369
Agonists 202
Aldridge's operation 310
Alli's tissue forceps 388
Alopecia 141, 266
  androgenic 160
α-fetoprotein 126
Amenorrhea 58, 142
  exercise-induced 185
  functional hypothalamic 185
  hypothalamic 180
  primary 12, 176
  secondary 184
American Society of Anesthesiologists' Classification 344
Amoebic ulceration 89
Amsel's criteria 88
Anal canal 26
Anal wink sign 290
Androgen receptor antagonist 163
Anechoic 327
Anorexia nervosa 181
Anovulation 142
Anoxic cells 275
Antiandrogens 212
Antibiotic prophylaxis 344
Anti-Müllerian hormone (AMH) 41, 147
Antiovarian antibodies 142
Antiprogesterone 115
Antral follicle count (AFC) 147
Aplasia 46
Aromatase inhibitors (AI) 207
Arrhenoblastoma 182
Artificial insemination 154
ART techniques 138
Ascending carcinogens 246
Asherman syndrome 143, 186, 340
Aspiration 152
  endometrial 347
Assisted reproductive techniques (ART) 154
Asthenospermia 152
Atresia 46
Ayre's spatula 98
Azoospermia 152

**B**

Babcock's forceps 388
Backache 362
Bacterial vaginosis (BV) 87, 134
Baden-Walker system 286
Bartholin's cyst 82, 347
Bartholin's (vulvovaginal) glands 17
  abscess of 80
Basal body temperature (BBT) 40, 144
  method 367
Behcet's syndrome 81
Benzoyl peroxide 163
Billings's method 367
Bio-feedback therapy 309
Biological radiotherapy planning 281
Biopsy 94
  cervical punch 347
  endometrial 117, 145
Bisphosphonates 197
Boari's operation 324
Body mass index 67
Bone marrow toxicity 266
Bonney's myomectomy clamp 390
Bonney's vesical neck elevation test 307
Brachytherapy 276
  interstitial 277
  intracavitary 277
  vaginal (VBT) 240
BRCA1 246
Brenner tumour 121
Bromocriptine 203
Brunschwig operation 230
Burnt match head spots 168
Buserelin 202

**C**

CA 125 126, 127, 171, 238, 241, 252
Cabergoline 203
Calcareous degeneration 112
Calendar method 367
Candida 92
*Candida albicans* 81, 87
Capsular hemorrhage 113
Carboplatin 254
Carcinoma
  embryonal 248
  endometrial 114, 238
  of the cervical stump 277
  of the vagina 218
  of the vulva 215
Carcinosarcoma 272
Cardinal ligaments 29, 284
Care HPV test 99
Carneous degeneration 112
Carnitidine 153
Carunculae myrtiformis 17
Cefotaxime 135
Cefotetan 136
Cefoxitin 135, 136
Ceftriaxone 135
Cell adhesion molecules 147
Cell cycle non-specific agents (CCNSA) 265
Cell cycle specific agents (CCSA) 265
Cervical cancer 223
  during pregnancy 231
Cervical cap 369
Cervical ectopy 227

Cervical intraepithelial neoplasia 61
Cervical motion tenderness 134
Cervical mucus method 367
Cervical punch biopsy forceps 389
Cervical stenosis, acquired 186
Cervical tuberculosis 227
Cervicitis 92, 133
  chronic 93
Cervix 131
  adenocarcinoma of the 278
  amputation of the 349
  carcinoma 61, 231
  uteri 19
Cetrorelix 202
Chemotherapy 254, 269
  adjuvant 240, 265
  adjuvant systemic 265
  combination 264
  dose-dense 254
  in cancer cervix 269
  in cancer endometrium 271
  in ovarian cancer 268
  intra-peritoneal 254
  neoadjuvant 254, 265, 268
  palliative 240, 265
  principles of 263
  toxicity of 266
  treatment for various types of gynecological malignancies 268
Cherney incision 353
*Chlamydia trachomatis* 86, 93, 132, 133, 303
Chocolate cysts 123
Choriocarcinoma 248
Chromosomal inversion 152
CIN 1 101
CIN 2/moderate dysplasia 102
Clindamycin 136
Clinical Breast Examination (CBE) 4
Clinical target volume 276
Clitoris 142
Clomiphene citrate 147, 206
Coccygeus 27
Coelomic cell metaplasia theory 165
Coffee beans 124
Coffey technique, modified 321
Coitus interruptus 367
Cold coagulation 102
Cold knife conisation 102
Colonoscopy 171
Colpocleisis 298, 319
Colpoperineorrhaphy 298, 348
Colporrhaphy 293–295, 297, 298, 343, 348–351
Colposcopy 94, 226
Colposuspension, laparoscopic 311
Combined oral contraceptive (COC) 162, 371
Combined oral pills 72
Complete androgen insensitivity syndrome 180
Compressor urethrae 301
Computed tomography 331
Conception
  mode of action of 365
  products of 227
Condom
  female 369
  male 369
Contraceptives
  barrier 132
Condylomata acuminata 80, 94
Cone beam CT 280
Contact dermatitis 79
Contraception 365
  barrier method of 368
  emergency 378
Contraceptive failure rate 377
Copper T-380 A 370
Copper-T device 370
Corpus cancer syndrome 233
Corpus luteum cysts 122
Cortical dysgenesis 43
Craniopharyngioma 181
C-reactive protein 134
Crohn's disease 80
Cryocautery 102
Cryptomenorrhea 179
*CTNNB1* 235
CT scan 170
Cumulus oophorus 35
Curette 389
Curved and straight clamp 389
Cusco's speculum 388
Cushing's syndrome 158, 182, 183, 184
Cyclofem 374
Cyclo-Provera 374
Cystadenoma
  mucinous 60, 121, 123
  serous 121, 123
Cystic fibrosis 152
Cystitis 303, 304
Cystocele, 288
  central 294
  grades of 294
  lateral 294
Cystometrogram 307
Cystoscopy 171, 307
Cysto-urethrography, lateral 307
Cystourethroscopy 317
Cytokines 147

**D**

Danazol 72, 210
Danocrine 174
Darifenacin 311
Degarelix 202
Dehydroepiandrosterone (DHEA) 158
Depilation 163
Depot medroxyprogesterone acetate (DMPA) 72, 373
Dermatomes, lumbosacral 290
Dermoid cysts 125
Deslorelin 202
Desmopressin 71
Detrusor dyssynergia 305
DEXA scan 195
Diaphragm 167, 368
Diethyl stilboestrol (DBS) 220
Dihydrotestosterone 180
Dilatation and curettage 346
Dilator (Mathew Duncan) 388
Directly Observed Treatment Short course (DOTS) 118
Direct transplantation theory 166
Disruption of the early zygote 366
Disseminated lupus erythematosus 79
Dissemination theory 166
Distension media 339
Doppler study 329
Dose volume histograms 276
Dosimetry 276
Dowager's hump 193
Downregulation 201
Doxycycline 135, 136, 153, 163
DUB (dysfunctional uterine bleeding)
  anovulatory 67
  ovulatory 68
Duloxetine 309
Dutch cap 368
Dydrogesterone 209
Dynamic magnetic resonance imaging 290
Dysfunctional uterine bleeding (DUB) 65
Dysgerminoma 60, 248, 255
Dyslipidemia 160
Dysmenorrhea 57, 108, 113, 141, 169

congestive or secondary 12
primary 57
spasmodic or primary 12
Dysontogenetic cysts 82
Dyspareunia 141, 169

**E**

Echogenic 327
Ectocervix 91
Ectopia vesicae 303
Ectopic pregnancy 114, 137
Ectopy 94
Ectropion 94, 133
Eflorithine hydrochloride 162
Ejaculation 153
Electrical stimulation 309
Electron therapy 275
Elephantiasis, of the vulva 83
ELISA techniques 134
Embryonal rhabdomyosarcoma 220
Empty sella syndrome 181
Endocervical brush 98
Endocervical canal 91
Endocervical crypts 91
Endocervical glands 91
Endocervicitis 93
Endodermal sinus tumour 60, 248
Endometrial cancer 233, 271, 278
TNM classification for 234
Endometrial sampling 68
Endometrioma 121
Endometriosis 59, 114, 123, 165
cervical 95
cutaneous 170
ovarian 168
pelvic 9
Endometriotic cysts 82
Endometritis 132
Endometrium 20
Endosalpingitis 132
Endoscopy, gynecological 335
Enterobiasis 82
Enterocele 288, 297
Epidermal growth factor receptor (EGFR) 267
Epilation 163
Epoophoron 23
ERID1A gene 235
Erosion 94
Erysipelas 80
Erythromycin 163
ESR 134
ESSURE 340
Estradiol (E2) 204
Estriol (E3). 204
Estrogen 40, 72, 115, 142
conjugated equine 69
cream 309
natural 204
Estrone (E1) 204
Ethambutol 118
Ethinyl estradiol 204
Excision 347
External beam radiotherapy (EBRT) 240
External iliac group 31
External os 19

**F**

Factor VIII 71
Fallopian tubes 21, 43, 143, 167
primary carcinoma of the 220
Falloposcopy 146, 341
Fathalla's incessant ovulation theory 246
Fecundablity 140
Fertility control 365, 366
methods of 366
Fibroid
broad ligament 111
cervical 111
intramural 111
polyp 227
submucosal 111
subserous 110
uterus 109
Fibromas 125
FIGO staging
endometrial carcinoma 238
ovarian cancer 253
of carcinoma of the Fallopian tube 221
of GTN 260
Fistula 314, 321
Fitz-Hugh–Curtis syndrome 133, 136
Flap-splitting method 319
Fludeoxyglucose 281
Foam tablets 369
Follicle-stimulating hormone (FSH) 38
Follicular cysts 122
Follistatin 41
Fothergill's operation 297, 349
Frank's method 48
FSH 142
Functional cysts 121
Functional ovarian cyst 59

**G**

$G_0$ phase 263
$G_1$ phase 263
$G_2$ phase 264
Galactorrhea 141, 182
Galactosemia 186
Galen's plethora theory 34
Gametocyte intra-Fallopian transfer (GIFT) 154
Ganirelix 202
Gartner's duct 23, 44, 89
cysts of 89
Genital prolapse 61
Genital tract anomalies 46
Genitofemoral nerve 361
Genitourinary fistula 314
Gentamicin 136
Germ cell tumours 121, 248, 269, 275
extragonadal 249
Gestational surrogates 155
Gestational trophoblastic diseases 257
Gestational trophoblastic neoplasia (GTN) 257
metastatic 260
Gestrinone 174
Gland of Cloquet 31
Gland of the parametrium 30
GLOBOCAN 223, 263
GnRH
analogues 72, 115, 174, 201
antagonists 162
stimulation 202
Godel's operation 298
Gonadal dysgenesis 186
Gonadarche 54
Gonadotropin releasing hormone analogues 212
Gonadotropin-releasing hormone (GnRH) 37
Gonadotropins 202
Gonanes 209
Gonodatropin releasing hormone 142
Gonorrhea 93
Goserelin 72, 202
Graafian follicles 34
Gram-negative diplococci 134
Gram stain 93, 134
*Granuloma pyogenicum* 79
Granulosa cell tumour 249, 255
Grid iron incision 353
Gross tumour volume 276

Growth factors 41
Growth hormone 159
GTD
  high-risk 270
  low-risk 270

**H**
Hairan syndrome 159
Halban's theory 166
Hanging drop method 335
hCG 126, 259
  phantom 260
Heavy menstrual bleeding (HMB) 133
Hegar's dilator 388
Hemangiomas,
  in children 79
  senile 79
Hematocolpos 47, 178, 305
Hematoma 79
Hematometra 47, 114, 178
Hematosalpinx 47
Hemi-zonal assay 153
*Her2/neu* oncogene 235
Herpes simplex 81
Herpes simplex virus 215
Herpes zoster 81
Heymann's packing technique 278
High Dose Rate (HDR) 277
Hilus cell tumour 182
Hirsutism 142, 160
Histrelin 202
HIV 134
HIV infection 59
Hormone replacement therapy (HRT) 197
Hot flashes 141
HPV 94
  testing 99
HPV E6/E7 mRNA testing 99
HSG 145
Human chorionic gonadotropin 134
Human papilloma virus (HPV) 80, 96, 215, 223
Hyaline degeneration 112
Hybrid capture II test 99
Hydrosalpinx 128
Hydrosonography 146
Hydroxyprogesterone 142, 209
Hydroxyprogesterone caproate 240
Hymen 17
  imperforate 78, 179
Hymenectomy 47
Hyperandrogenism 142, 158
Hyperbaric oxygen therapy 275
Hyperprolactinemia 141, 186
Hypoechoic 328
Hypogastric group 30
Hypogonadohypogonadism 141
Hypomenorrhea 64
Hypo-osmotic swelling test 153
Hypopituitarism 181
Hypoplasia 46, 77
Hypotension, prolonged 142
Hypothalamic-pituitary-ovarian axis 37, 177
Hypothalamo-pituitary dysfunction 141
Hypothalamo-pituitary failure 141
Hypothalamus 141, 201
Hypothyroidism 183
Hysterectomy 73, 102, 109, 353
  modified radical 230
  nerve-sparing radical 230
  radical abdominal 356
  total 322
  total abdominal 354
  type 2 radical 230
  type 3 radical 230
  vaginal 298, 322
Hysterosalpingogram 114
Hysterosalpingography 118
Hysteroscope 338
  flexible 339
  rigid 338
Hysteroscopic tubal sterilisation 340
Hysteroscopy 107, 116, 146, 335

**I**
IgA, 143
IgG 143
IgM 143
Iliococcygeus 284
  suspension 296
Ilio-inguinal nerve 361
Imipramine 309, 311
Immune system dysfunction theory 166
Immunisation, active 268
Immunotherapy 267
Implanon 375
Implantation 165
Incisions, types of 351
Incontinence
  false 305
  functional 305
  mixed 311
  true 305
  urge 305
Inferior vena cava 30
Infertility 113, 137, 140
Informed consent 345
Inguinal group 30
Inhibin 41
Inhibitors 267
  5-α-reductase 212
  aromatase 207
  multikinase 267
In-situ hybridisation 99
Insulin-like growth factor-1 (IGF-1) 159
Insulin resistance 159
Insulin sensitivity agents 162
Intensity-modulated radiation therapy 276, 280
Intermenstrual bleeding 13
International Association of Cancer Registries (IARC) 263
Intertrigo 79
Intra-abdominal pressure 335
Intra-cytoplasmic sperm injection (ICSI) 154
Intrauterine adhesions 186
Intrauterine device 369
Intrauterine insemination (IUI) 154
Intrinsic sphincter 305
IOTA group 127
Iron therapy 115
Irregular bleeding 133
Irregular ripening 68
Irregular shedding 68
Irritable bowel syndrome 15
Ischiococcygeus 284
Isoniazid 118
IUD
  hormone-releasing 371
  levonorgestrel 370
  unmedicated 370
IUI 172
IVF 173

**J**
Jeffcoate's system 286

**K**
Kelly's operation 310
Kidney
  absence of one 303
  pelvic 114, 303
Kinase inhibitors 266
Klinefelter's syndrome 43, 61, 152

Kocher's clamp 389
Koilocytes 101
Koplick's jar 99
*KRAS* activation 246
Kraurosis 84
Kruckenberg tumours 249

**L**

Labial adhesions 77
Labia minora 17
Lactate dehydrogenase (LDH) 126
Lactational amenorrhea method (LAM) 367
"Lantern on St.Paul's cathedral" appearance 114
Laparoscopic instruments 390
Laparoscopic ovarian drilling (LOD) 163
Laparoscopy 115, 145, 335
  advantages and disadvantages of 337
  single port access 336
Large loop excision of the transformation zone (LLETZ) 102
Laser vapourisation 102
Latzko's triad of symptoms 221
Latzko technique 319
Le Fort's operation 298
Leiomyoma, tubal 128
Leiomyosarcoma 272
Letrozole 240
Leucorrhea 85
Leukoplakia vulva 84
Leuprolide 72, 202
Levator ani 27, 284
Levonorgestrel-releasing intrauterine system (LNG-IUS) 72, 109
LH 142
  mid-cycle surge 40
Lichen sclerosus (LS) 83
Ligation
  Caesarean 375
  gynecological 375
  interval 375
  postabortal 375
  vaginal tubal 375
Lipid hormones 201
Lippe's loop 370
Liquid-based cytology 96, 97, 99
Low Dose Rate (LDR) 277
Low-grade lesion 101
L-selectin ligand 147
LUNA (Laparoscopic uterosacral nerve ablation) 337
Luteal phase defect 68, 145
Luteinising hormone (LH) 39
Luteolysis 366
Lymphangioma 79

**M**

Mackenrodt's ligament 29, 284
Magnetic Resonance Guided Focused Ultrasound Surgery (MRgFUS) 73, 115
Magnetic resonance imaging (MRI) 108, 332
Manchester operation 297, 349
Manchester technique 279
Mannose fluorescent assay 153
Marshall–Marchetti–Krantz operation 310
Marsupialisation 348
Mayer–Rokitansky–Küster–Hauser (MRKH) syndrome 47, 178
Maylard incision 353
McBurney's incision 353
McCall culdoplasty 297
McIndoe's operation 48
Medical eligibility criteria 366
Medroxyprogesterone 209, 240
Medroxyprogesterone acetate 70
Medullary dysgenesis 43
Megestrol acetate 70, 240
Meig's syndrome 125
Meigs' operation 230
Menarche 54, 141
  delayed 176
  premature 56
Menometrorrhagia, episodic 160
Menopausal transition 197
Menopause 191
  induced 191
  management of 195
  premature 191
Menorrhagia 3, 64, 108, 141
  idiopathic 68
Menstrual calendar 71
Menstrual cycle, phases of 36
Menstruation, theories of 34
Mesenteric cyst 127
Mesonephric duct 44
Mesothelial inclusion cysts 128
Mesotheliomas 128
Metformin 148, 162
Methylene blue test 316
Metronidazole 135
Metropathia hemorrhagica 67
Metrorrhagia 3, 64
Meyer's theory 165
Microassisted Fertilisation Technique (MAF) 154
Microdeletions 152
Microsurgical epididymal sperm aspiration 152
Micturition
  difficulty in 304
  frequency of 304
  painful 304
Millin's operation 310
Minilap sterilisation 377
Minimal clearance 275
Minimally invasive laparoscopic and robotic POP repair 297
Mittelschmerz 12, 141
Mixed germ cell tumours 249
Modern theory 246
Molar evacuation 259
  follow-up after 259
Molecular targets 266
Moles, partial and complete 258
Molluscum contagiosum 81
Monoclonal antibodies 266, 267
Moschcowitz procedure 296
M phase 264
MRI 115
  functional 281
MR-Linac 280
Müllerian duct 22, 43
Müllerian inhibitory factor (MIF) 44, 180
*Mycoplasma fermentas* 144
*Mycoplasma hominis* 144
Myolysis, laparoscopic 116
Myomas 13
Myoma screw 390
Myomatous polyp 114
Myomectomy 73, 116
  laparoscopic 116
Myxomatous degeneration 112

**N**

Nabothian cyst 91
Nabothian follicles 95
Nafarelin 202
*Neisseria gonorrhoeae* 88, 132, 133
Nona vaccine 104
Non-receptor tyrosine kinases 267
Non-steroidal anti-inflammatory drugs (NSAIDs) 363
Norethindrone enanthate 374

Norethisterone 70
Norplant 374, 375
19-nortestosterone 209
NSAID 108, 141

O
Obesity 160
Oblique incisions 353
OC pills, contraindications of 372
Olfactogenital syndrome 181
Oligomenorrhea 64, 142
Oligo-ovulation 142, 158
Oligospermia 152
On-board KV imaging 280
Oocyte donation programme 183
Opioid analgesics 363
Oral contraceptives 371
first-generation 372
low-dose 372
second-generation 372
third-generation 372
Osteopontin 147
Ovarian artery 29
Ovarian cancer 279
early-stage 268
screening for 252
Ovarian failure 142
premature 142
Ovarian fossa 167
Ovarian hyperstimulation syndrome (OHSS) 148
Ovarian hyperthecosis 159
Ovarian insensitivity syndrome 182
Ovarian ligaments 21
Ovarian neoplasms 123
Ovarian tumours 60, 114
Ovaries 22, 34, 167
agenesis of 142
benign epithelial tumours of the 14
Overactive bladder 311
Overweight 142
Ovulation 39, 140
hormones in 40
method 367
methods of detecting 40
pain 169
suppression of 365
Ovulation predictor kits 144
Ovulatory dysfunction 141

P
*p27* 235
*p53* 235
*p53* suppression 246
Paclitaxel 254
Paget's disease 84
Pain 361
chronic 15
chronic pelvic 361
gynecological causes of 361
non-gynecological causes of 362
pelvic 113, 169
PALM-COEIN classification 65
Papanicolaou (Pap) test 223
Papillary cysts 82
Pap smear 67
Parallel organs 275
Paramesonephric ducts 43, 128
Paraovarian cysts 128
Paravaginal defects 290
Paroophoron 23
Partial androgen insensitivity syndrome 180
Particle therapy 275
Passive or adoptive cell therapy 268
PCOS 110, 182
PCR testing 134
PEB regimen 269
*Pediculosis pubis* 81
Pegylated liposomal doxorubicin 268
Pelvic congestion syndrome 12
Pelvic diaphragm 27
Pelvic exenteration 230
Pelvic floor
exercises 309
muscle testing 290
Pelvic inflammatory disease (PID) 59, 131, 370
recurrent 137
Pelvic lymphatics 30
Pelvic muscle exercises 291
Pelvic veins 30
Pemphigus vulgaris 79
Penile implant 154
Pentoxifylline 153
Peptide hormones 201
Peri-hepatic inflammation 132
Perimenopause 191
Perineal body 284
Perineal muscle 27
Peritonitis 133
general 132
pelvic 132
Peritubal adhesions 132
Pernicious anaemia 142
Pessaries, types of 292
PET-CT 229, 281
PET/MRI 281
Pfannenstiel incision 353
Pictorial blood assessment chart (PBAC) 1, 69
Piezoelectric effect 327
Pituitary 202
adenoma 182
infarction 142
tumours 185
Planning CT scan 280
Planning target volume 276
Platelet-derived growth factor receptors (PDGFR a and b) 267
Pneumoperitoneum 335
Polycystic ovarian syndrome 61, 158, 182, 185
Polycystic ovaries 142
sonographic criteria for 161
Polyembryoma 248
Polymenorrhagia 64
Polymenorrhea 3, 64
Polymerase chain reaction 99, 118
Polyp 114
cervical 95, 347
endometrial 106
myomatous 114
Pomeroy's technique 377
POPQ
classification 286
measurements 289
simplified 286
Population of India 365
Positron Emission Tomography (PET) imaging 332
Postcoital bleeding 13, 133
Postcoital test (PCT) 147
Postmenopausal bleeding (PMB) 13, 197
Postoperative care 358
Postpartum hemorrhage 142
Post-traumatic cysts 82
Pouch of Douglas (POD) 7, 9, 21, 167
Powder burn appearance 168
Precocious puberty 55
central 55
heterosexual 56
peripheral 56
true 55
Pregnancy 114
and carcinoma of the cervix 278
Premature ovarian insufficiency (POI) 186
Premenstrual syndrome (PMS) 58
Pre-operative investigations 343

Pre-operative preparation 343
Presacral neurectomy 322
Primary ovarian failure (POF) 186
Probenecid 135
Proctitis 133
Progestasert 371
Progesterone 40, 142
 micronised 208
Progesterone-only pill (POP) 373
Progesterone withdrawal test 187
Progestogens 71
 cyclic 162
Prolactin 142, 203
Prolactinoma 182
Prolapse
 apical 288
 nulliparous 298, 351
 of the apical segment 295
 pelvic organ 283
 uterovaginal 283
Prostaglandin (PG) 68
Protozoa 82
Pseudohermaphroditism 61
Pseudomyxoma peritonei 124
Psoriasis 79
*PTEN* 235
Pubarche 54
Puberty menorrhagia 58
Puberty, variations in normal 56
Pubococcygeus 284
Puborectalis 284
Pubo-vesico-cervical ligament 29, 284
Pudendal artery 30
Pudendal nerve 361
Pulmonary embolism 345
Purandare's cervicopexy 298, 351
Push out technique 370
Pyelonephritis 304
Pyometra 114
Pyosalpinx 132
Pyrazinamide 118
Pyrexial 133

**Q**

QHPV 104
Q-Tip test 307

**R**

Radiation 89
 ionising 274
 megavoltage 274
Radiation oncology
 dose 275
 translational research in 281
 treatment planning 276
Radiation therapy
 3D conformal 280
 image-guided 280
Radiotherapy
 adjuvant 240
 in gynecological cancer 274
Raisinoid 101
Raloxifene 197, 207
Rathke's pouch tumour 181
RCOG Green top guidelines 126
Receptor tyrosine kinases 266
Rectal examination 9
Rectal hiatus 284
Rectocele 288, 295
 high 295
 low 295
 midvaginal 295
Rectovaginal examination 9, 290
Rectovaginal septum 167
Recurrent ovarian cancer
 platinum-resistant 269
 platinum-sensitive 268
Red degeneration 112
Reflex
 anocutaneous 290
 bulbocavernosus reflex 290
 sacral 290
Remnant ovarian syndrome 15, 362
Reproductive aging, stages of 192
Residual ovary syndrome 15, 362
Retinoids 163
Retrograde menstruation theory 165
Re-uptake inhibitors 153
Revised American Fertility Society (AFS) Score 166
Revised National Tuberculosis Control Programme (RNTCP) 118
Rhythm method 367
Rifampicin 118
Robotic assisted laparoscopic surgery 338
Round ligament 21
Rutherford–Morrison incision 353

**S**

Sacral group 30
Sacrocolpopexy, abdominal 296
Sacrospinous ligament fixation 295
Saline infusion sonography 145, 328
Salpingectomy 357
Salpingo-oophoritis 132
Salpingoscope 341
Sampson's theory 165
Sarcoma 114
 endometrial stromal 272
 of the vagina 220
Sarcoma botryoides 220
Sarcomatous changes 112
Savage syndrome 182
Scabies 81
Schistosomiasis 82
Schuchardt's paravaginal incision 319
Scrotal thermography 153
Sebaceous cysts 82
Second look laparotomy 255
Selective estrogen receptor modulator (SERM) 197
Selective progesterone receptor modulator (SPRM) 115, 211
Selective serotonin reuptake inhibitor 309
Semen analysis 144, 151
Sentinel node biopsy 226
Serial organs 275
Serotonin 153
Serous tumours 123
Sertoli–Leydig cell tumour 182, 249
Serum CA 125 171
Sex cord – stromal tumours 249, 269
Sex hormone binding globulin (SHBG) 110, 160
Sexually transmitted diseases 59, 83
Shaw's system 286
Sheehan's syndrome 142, 185
Shirodkar's method 298, 351
Sigmoidoscopy 171
Sildenafil 153
Sim's speculum 388
Simulated apical support 290
Simulator unit 276
Small molecules 266
Solifenacin 311
Selective muscarinic-receptor antagonists 311
Sonography 146
 transabdominal 328
 transrectal and transperineal 328
 transvaginal 107, 146, 328
Sonohysterography 328
Sonosalpingography (SIS) 107, 114
Spermatogenesis, suppression of 365, 152
Sperm cervical mucus contact test 153
Spermicides 369
Sperm penetration assay 153

S phase 264
Squamo-columnar junction 91
Squamous papilloma 95
Staging, of carcinoma of the cervix uteri 229
Staging laparotomy 253
Stamey–Pereyra procedure 310
Stereotactic ablative radiation 279
Sterilisation
failure following female 377
laparoscopic 376
minilap 377
postpartum 375
reversibility following 377
tubal 375
Storage phase 302
Stress urinary incontinence 306
Stromal tumours 121
Stump carcinoma 231
Subdermal implant system 374
Superior hemorrhoidal artery 30
Super-ovulation 172
Surgical anatomy 351
Surgical wound, classification of 344
Surrogacy 155
Suture material 345
Swiss-cheese appearance 68
Sympathetic nerve 361
Symptothermal methods 367
Syphilitic ulcer 227
Syringe barrel test 335

T
Tamoxifen 110, 153, 206, 240
Tanner staging 55
Targeted therapy 266
Teletherapy 276
Tension-free vaginal kits 297
Tension-free vaginal tape procedure 310
Teratomas 61, 125, 248
mature cystic 125
Teratospermia 152
Testicular biposy 152
Testicular determining factor (TDF) 43
Testosterone 158
Thayer-Martin medium 134
Theca cell tumours 60, 124
Theca lutein cysts 123
Thelarche 54
premature 56
Threshold bleeding 68
Thyroid disease 141
Thyrotropin releasing hormone 183
Tibolone 197
Time-dose fraction system 275
Tinea cruris 81
Tinea versicolor 81
Tissue tolerance 275
TNM classification 234
Torsion 111, 113, 127
Total fertility rate (TFR) 365
Toxic shock syndrome 62
Trachelectomy 230
Traditional Risk Classification for Gynecologic Surgery 345
Tranexamic acid 70, 115
Transdermal contraceptive patch 375
Transformation zone 91
Translocations 152
Transobturator tape sling 311
Transperitoneal operation 320
Transvaginal transducer 327
Transverse incisions 353
Transvesical suprapubic approach 320
Trendelenburg position 335
Tretinoin 163
Trichomonal infection 92
*Trichomonas vaginalis* 3, 59, 86
Trichomoniasis 134
Trigone of the bladder 23
Triptorelin 202
Trocar and cannula 335
Trophoblastic tumour
epithelioid 261
placental site 261
Trospium chloride 311
True hermaphrodite 43
Tuberculosis 83
endometrial 117
Tuberculous ulceration 89
Tubo-ovarian abscess 132, 137
Tubo-ovarian masses 14
Tubo-ovarian torsion 59
Tumours
androgen-secreting 158
Turner mosaic 142
Turner's stigmata 180
Turner's syndrome 43, 61, 179
*T. vaginalis* 88
Two cell – two gonadotropin hypothesis 37
Type II endometrial carcinomas 235

U
Ultra-radical surgery 230
Ultrasonography 114, 117
Umbilicus 167
*Ureaplasma urealyticum* 144
Ureter 24
accessory and aberrant 303
bifid 303
double 303
ectopic 303
Ureteric injury 321, 322
Ureterocele 303
Ureterosigmoidostomy 319
Ureterovaginal fistula 321
Urethra 301
female 23
Urethral hypermobility 305
Urethral sphincter 301
Urethroscopy 307
Urethritis, non-gonococcal 303
Urethrovaginal sphincter 301
Urinary fistulae 314
Urine
culture 134
residual 307
retention of 305
Urogenital diaphragm 27
Urogenital hiatus 284
Urography, intravenous 318
Uterine artery 29
Uterine artery embolisation (UAE) 73, 109, 115
Uterine fibroid embolisation (UFE) 115
Uterine sound 389
Uterosacral ligaments 29, 167, 284
Uterosacral vaginal vault suspension 296
Uterus 19, 114, 143
arcuate 48
bicornuate 48, 114
chronic inversion of 114
didelphys 48
inversion of the 113
perforation of the 347
sarcoma of the 242

V
Vaccine 104
quadrivalent 104
Vaccine BHPV 104
Vagina 18
absence of 48, 178
agenesis of the upper third of the 178
carcinoma of the 218
FIGO staging of 219

pre-malignant epithelial changes of 218
primary adenocarcinoma of the 220
sarcoma of the 220
Vaginal acidity 131
Vaginal adenosis 220
Vaginal arteries 30
Vaginal cancer 279
Vaginal cones/pessaries 309
Vaginal discharge 11, 133
Vaginal ring 375
Vaginal support devices 291
Vaginal ulcers 88, 89
Vaginal wall points 289
Vaginitis, senile 88
Valsalva maneuver 288
VaIN 218
high-grade 218
low-grade 218
Varicocele 153
Vascular endothelial growth factor receptor (VEGFR) 267
Vascular endothelial growth factor (VEGF) 149
Vasectomy 377
non-scalpel 377
Vasogram 153
Vault cap 368
Venereal ulcers 88
Venous thromboembolism 345
Veress needle 335
Verrucous carcinoma 220
Vertical incisions 351
Vestibule 17
Video cysto-urethrography 307
VIN
classification of 215
VIN1 215
VIN 2 and 3 215
Violin string adhesions 137
Virilisation 159
Visual inspection with acetic acid (VIA) 96
Visual inspection with Lugol's iodine (VILI) 96
Vitiligo 80
Voiding diary 307
Voiding phase 302
Volsellum forceps 389
von Willebrand factor 71
Vulva 16
benign diseases of the 77
carcinoma of the 215
Crohn's disease of the 80
elephantiasis of the 83
injuries to the 78
lymphatics of the 217
ulcerations of the 82
varicosities of the 79
Vulvar cancer 279
Vulvar intraepithelial neoplasia (VIN) 215
Vulvar synechia 77
Vulvitis 80
Vulvo-vaginitis
gonococcal 85
gonorrheal 80

W

Walthard cell 124
Ward–Mayo's operation 298, 350
WBC 134, 135, 152, 265
Wertheim's operation 32, 230
WHO classification of GTD 257
Wide clearance 275
William's operation 48
Withdrawal method 367, 370
Wolffian duct 23
Wolffian system 44

Y

Yolk sac tumours 248

Z

Zygote intra-Fallopian transfer (ZIFT) 154